TEXTBOOK OF

ANTISOCIAL
PERSONALITY DISORDER

TEXTBOOK OF
ANTISOCIAL
PERSONALITY DISORDER

EDITED BY

Donald W. Black, M.D.
Nathan J. Kolla, M.D., Ph.D., FRCPC

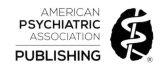

If you wish to buy 50 or more copies of the same title, please go to www.appi.org/specialdiscounts for more information.

Copyright © 2022 American Psychiatric Association Publishing

ALL RIGHTS RESERVED

First Edition

Manufactured in the United States of America on acid-free paper
26 25 24 23 22   5 4 3 2 1

American Psychiatric Association Publishing
800 Maine Avenue SW, Suite 900
Washington, DC 20024-2812
www.appi.org

Library of Congress Cataloging-in-Publication Data
Names: Black, Donald W., 1956- editor. | Kolla, Nathan J., editor.

Title: Textbook of antisocial personality disorder / edited by Donald W. Black, Nathan J. Kolla.

Description: First edition. | Washington, DC : American Psychiatric Association Publishing, [2022] | Includes bibliographical references and index.

Identifiers: LCCN 2021061086 (print) | LCCN 2021061087 (ebook) | ISBN 9781615373239 (hardcover) | ISBN 9781615373222 (ebook)

Subjects: MESH: Antisocial Personality Disorder

Classification: LCC RC555 (print) | LCC RC555 (ebook) | NLM WM 190.5.A2 | DDC 616.85/82—dc23/eng/20220113

LC record available at https://lccn.loc.gov/2021061086

LC ebook record available at https://lccn.loc.gov/2021061087

British Library Cataloguing in Publication Data
A CIP record is available from the British Library.

Contents

Donald W. Black, M.D.
Nathan J. Kolla, M.D., Ph.D., FRCPC

PART I
Definition and History

Peter Tyrer, M.D.
Alireza Farnam, M.D.
Alireza Zahmatkesh, M.D.
Rahil Sanatinia, M.D., Ph.D.

Erik Simonsen, M.D.

PART II
Clinical Concepts

Risë B. Goldstein, Ph.D., M.P.H.

Patrick T. McGonigal, M.A.
Mark Zimmerman, M.D.
Mario J. Scalora, Ph.D.

PART III
Etiology and Pathophysiology

PART IV
Clinical Management

PART V
Special Problems,
Populations, and Settings

Contributors

Christopher Adanty, B.Sc.
Graduate Student, Department of Psychiatry, University of Toronto, Toronto, Ontario, Canada; Centre for Addiction and Mental Health, Toronto, Ontario, Canada

Allan M. Andersen, M.D.
Assistant Professor, Department of Psychiatry, University of Iowa Carver College of Medicine, Iowa City, Iowa

Nayan Bhatia, M.D.
Resident Physician, Virginia Tech Carilion School of Medicine and Carilion Clinic, Roanoke, Virginia

Brittany Bishop, M.Sc.F.S.
Master of Science in Forensic Science, Trent University, Peterborough, Ontario, Canada

Donald W. Black, M.D.
Professor Emeritus, Department of Psychiatry, University of Iowa Roy J. and Lucille A. Carver College of Medicine, Iowa City, Iowa; and Associate Chief of Staff for Mental Health, Iowa City Veterans Administration Health Care, Iowa City, Iowa

R. James Blair, Ph.D.
Director, Center for Neurobehavioral Research in Children, Boys Town National Research Hospital, Boys Town, Nebraska

Nancee Blum, M.S.W.
Retired Adjunct Instructor, University of Iowa Roy J. and Lucille A. Carver College of Medicine, Iowa City, Iowa

Olivia Choy, Ph.D.
Assistant Professor, Department of Psychology, Nanyang Technological University, Singapore

Nasia Dai, B.Sc.
Graduate Student, Department of Psychiatry, University of Toronto, Toronto, Ontario, Canada; Centre for Addiction and Mental Health, Toronto, Ontario, Canada

Christal N. Davis, M.A.
Doctoral Candidate, Department of Psychological Sciences, University of Missouri, Columbia, Missouri

Vincenzo De Luca, M.D., Ph.D.
Professor, Department of Psychiatry, University of Toronto, Toronto, Ontario, Canada; Centre for Addiction and Mental Health, Toronto, Ontario, Canada

Laura Dellazizzo, M.Sc.
M.D.-Ph.D. student, Research Center of the Institut Universitaire en Santé Mentale de Montréal; and Department of Psychiatry and Addictology, Faculty of Medicine, University of Montreal, Montreal, Quebec, Canada

Alexandre Dumais, M.D., Ph.D., FRCPC
Clinician-Researcher, Research Center of the Institut Universitaire en Santé Mentale de Montréal; Department of Psychiatry and Addictology, Faculty of Medicine, University of Montreal; Institut National de Psychiatrie Légale Philippe-Pinel, Montreal, Quebec, Canada

Dylan A. Fall, M.D.
MS4 Medical Student, Mental Health Line, Michael E. DeBakey VA Medical Center; and MS4 Medical Student, Menninger Department of Psychiatry and Behavioral Sciences, Baylor College of Medicine, Houston, Texas

Alireza Farnam, M.D.
Professor of Psychiatry, Medical Faculty, Tabriz University of Medical Sciences, Tabriz, Iran

Georgette E. Fleming, Ph.D.
Lecturer, School of Psychology, The University of New South Wales, Sydney, Australia

Risë B. Goldstein, Ph.D., M.P.H.
Staff Scientist, Social and Behavioral Sciences Branch, Division of Intramural Population Health Research, *Eunice Kennedy Shriver* National Institute of Child Health and Human Development, Bethesda, Maryland

Sheilagh Hodgins, Ph.D., FRSC
Professeur, Département de Psychiatrie et Addictologie, Université de Montréal, and Centre de Recherche de l'Institut Universitaire en Santé Mentale de Montréal, Montreal, Quebec, Canada

Sylvain Houle, M.D., Ph.D., FRCPC
Brain Health Imaging Centre, Centre for Addiction and Mental Health, Toronto, Ontario, Canada

Roland M. Jones, M.B.Ch.B., B.Sc., M.Sc., Ph.D., FRCPsych
Forensic Psychiatrist and Clinician Scientist, Department of Forensic Psychiatry, Centre for Addiction and Mental Health; and Assistant Professor, University of Toronto, Toronto, Ontario, Canada

Najat Khalifa, M.D.
Associate Professor in Forensic Psychiatry, Department of Psychiatry, Queen's University; and Regional Psychiatry Lead, Correctional Service Canada, Ontario, Canada

Eva R. Kimonis, Ph.D.
Professor, School of Psychology; and Director, Parent-Child Research Clinic, The University of New South Wales, Sydney, Australia

Nathan J. Kolla, M.D., Ph.D., FRCPC
Clinician Scientist, Brain Health Imaging Centre, Centre for Addiction and Mental Health, Toronto, Ontario, Canada; Head, Violence Prevention Neurobiological Research Unit, Centre for Addiction and Mental Health; Associate Professor of Psychi-

atry, Criminology and Sociolegal Studies, Pharmacology and Toxicology, University of Toronto, Toronto, Ontario, Canada; and Waypoint/University of Toronto Research Chair in Forensic Mental Health Science, Penetanguishene, Ontario, Canada

Samuel Kuperman, M.D.
Professor, Departments of Psychiatry and Pediatrics, University of Iowa Carver College of Medicine, Iowa City, Iowa

Jaeger Lam, M.A.
Doctoral Candidate, York University, Toronto, Ontario, Canada

Marijn Lijffijt, Ph.D.
Principal Investigator, Research Service Line, Michael E. DeBakey VA Medical Center; and Assistant Professor, Menninger Department of Psychiatry and Behavioral Sciences, Baylor College of Medicine, Houston, Texas

Zhuoran Ma, B.S.
Graduate Student, Department of Psychiatry, University of Toronto, Toronto, Ontario, Canada; Centre for Addiction and Mental Health, Toronto, Ontario, Canada

Liam E. Marshall, Ph.D.
Research Clinician, Waypoint Centre for Mental Health Care and Rockwood Psychotherapy and Consulting, Penetanguishene, Ontario, Canada; and Assistant Professor, Department of Psychiatry, University of Toronto, Toronto, Ontario, Canada

Patrick T. McGonigal, M.A.
Doctoral Student, Department of Psychology, University of Nebraska-Lincoln, Lincoln, Nebraska

James McGuire, Ph.D.
Emeritus Professor, Institute of Population Health, University of Liverpool, Liverpool, United Kingdom

Mario Moscovici, M.D.
Psychiatry Resident, Department of Forensic Psychiatry, Centre for Addiction and Mental Health, Toronto, Ontario, Canada

Nicholas Murphy, Ph.D.
Investigator, Research Service Line, Michael E. DeBakey VA Medical Center; and Assistant Professor, Menninger Department of Psychiatry and Behavioral Sciences, Baylor College of Medicine, Houston, Texas

Joel Paris, M.D.
Emeritus Professor of Psychiatry, Department of Psychiatry, McGill University, Montreal, Quebec, Canada; and Research Associate, Jewish General Hospital, Montreal, Quebec, Canada

Elham Rahmani, M.D., M.P.H.
Resident Physician, Virginia Tech Carilion School of Medicine and Carilion Clinic, Roanoke, Virginia

Nithya Ramakrishnan, B.E., M.S.
Investigator, Research Service Line, Michael E. DeBakey VA Medical Center; and Senior Scientific Programmer, Menninger Department of Psychiatry and Behavioral Sciences, Baylor College of Medicine, Houston, Texas

Anvesh Roy, M.D.
Lecturer, Department of Psychiatry, University of Toronto, Toronto, Ontario, Canada; Centre for Addiction and Mental Health, Toronto, Ontario, Canada

Anthony C. Ruocco, Ph.D.
Professor of Psychology and Psychological Clinical Science, University of Toronto, Toronto, Ontario, Canada

Rahil Sanatinia, M.D., Ph.D.
Research Associate, Division of Psychiatry, Imperial College, London, United Kingdom

Mario J. Scalora, Ph.D.
Associate Professor, Department of Psychology, University of Nebraska-Lincoln, Lincoln, Nebraska

Erik Simonsen, M.D.
Professor of Psychiatry, University of Copenhagen, Copenhagen, Denmark; and Director, Psychiatric Research Unit, Slagelse, Denmark

Wendy S. Slutske, Ph.D.
Curators' Distinguished Professor, Department of Psychological Sciences, University of Missouri, Columbia, Missouri

Anil Srivastava, M.D.
Staff Physician, Department of Psychiatry, Humber River Hospital, Toronto, Ontario, Canada

Alan C. Swann, M.D.
Staff Psychiatrist, Mental Health Line, Michael E. DeBakey VA Medical Center; and Professor, Menninger Department of Psychiatry and Behavioral Sciences, Baylor College of Medicine, Houston, Texas

Robert L. Trestman, M.D., Ph.D.
Professor and Chair, Virginia Tech Carilion School of Medicine and Carilion Clinic, Roanoke, Virginia

Peter Tyrer, M.D.
Consultant in Transformation Psychiatry, Lincolnshire Partnership NHS Trust; and Emeritus Professor of Community Psychiatry, Imperial College, London, United Kingdom

Birgit Völlm, M.D., Ph.D.
Professor of Forensic Psychiatry, Department of Forensic Psychiatry, University Medicine, Rostock, Germany

Alireza Zahmatkesh, M.D.
Faculty of Psychology, Department of Clinical Psychology, Semnan University, Semnan, Iran

Mark Zimmerman, M.D.
Director of Partial Hospital Program and Adult Outpatient Psychiatry, Department of Psychiatry, Rhode Island Hospital, Providence, Rhode Island

Foreword

It has long been recognized that antisocial personality disorder (ASPD) accounts for greater cost and burden to society than any other major mental illness (National Institute for Clinical Excellence 2009). Yet investment to support scientific exploration of this disabling and socially and interpersonally disruptive condition has been woefully inadequate. National Institute of Mental Health funding to study ASPD—from etiology to prevention to treatment—has been negligble. In fairness, this imbalance may in part reflect the nature of the illness itself, because individuals with ASPD deny that they are ill or that they need treatment. Furthermore, the first diagnostic criterion for ASPD in DSM-5 is "Failure to conform to social norms with respect to lawful behaviors, as indicated by repeatedly performing acts that are grounds for arrest" (American Psychiatric Association 2013, p. 659). Although many prisoners meet the full diagnostic criteria for ASPD, prisoners are designated as a "protected class," making it difficult, but not impossible, to carry out research with these large populations. In 1993, an interesting book was published entitled *The Psychopathology of Crime: Criminal Behavior as a Clinical Disorder*, by Adrian Raine (1993). Raine made the argument that if you get the best consensus you can on a definition of psychopathology, then criminal behavior, for the most part, fits the definition. Does that mean that all prisoners should be classified as mentally ill? Certainly not, even though we know that many incarcerated individuals have diagnosable psychiatric disorders, including ASPD, and that criminal behavior is often illness-driven behavior.

Early in my career, I was on the faculty at Columbia University in New York City along with Robert Spitzer, M.D., chair of the DSM-III Task Force, during the development of that new and groundbreaking diagnostic system (American Psychiatric Association 1980). Regarding ASPD, I recall Bob's often-repeated caveat that "antisocial personality disorder is not the same thing as social deviance." I thought I understood that because certainly "social deviance" covers a lot of behavioral territory, such as white-collar crime, illegal drug use, and shoplifting, which would not necessarily reflect the presence of ASPD. But where to draw the line between ASPD and social deviance is not so straightforward because to do so would require defining social norms, which vary widely across cultures and subcultures.

Other debates about definitional terms and boundaries are frequently encountered because antisocial behavior comes in many stripes and covers a wide swath. What do we mean, for example, by "psychopathy" and "sociopathy," and how do they differ from ASPD? Discussions of these behavioral boundaries can become thorny and often contentious, but they are explored elegantly and extensively in this welcome new volume edited by Drs. Black and Kolla. This compendium brings together international experts on ASPD to provide, in a single source, the best knowledge we have about this challenging condition. It is important to add that we now know quite a lot, despite the historical insufficiency of research support. Look inside these pages and you will learn about not only the phenomenology and natural course of ASPD but also its neuropathology, neurophysiology, genetic risk factors, epigenetics, and social determinants. Even some promising directions regarding prevention and treatment are included. All in all, the *Textbook of Antisocial Personality Disorder* is an urgently needed, scholarly, and comprehensive review of one of the most daunting areas of psychopathology in our field.

John M. Oldham, M.D.
Distinguished Emeritus Professor
Baylor College of Medicine, Houston, Texas

References

American Psychiatric Association: Diagnostic and Statistical Manual of Mental Disorders, 3rd Edition. Washington, DC, American Psychiatric Association, 1980

American Psychiatric Association: Diagnostic and Statistical Manual of Mental Disorders, 5th Edition. Arlington, VA, American Psychiatric Association, 2013

National Institute for Clinical Excellence: Antisocial Personality Disorder: Treatment, Management and Prevention. Clinical Guideline 77. London, National Institute for Clinical Excellence, 2009, pp 25–77

Raine A: The Psychopathology of Crime: Criminal Behavior as a Clinical Disorder. New York, Academic Press, 1993

Introduction

Donald W. Black, M.D.
Nathan J. Kolla, M.D., Ph.D., FRCPC

Antisocial personality disorder (ASPD) is psychiatry's forgotten disorder. Despite its enormous cost to individuals, families, and society, few clinicians diagnose ASPD let alone offer treatment, and few researchers investigate it. Despite high public health significance, clinicians and researchers have largely distanced themselves from ASPD, perhaps in sympathy with family members and friends who react similarly. A stark reminder of the disappointing lack of interest by funding agencies is the fact that in 2020 not a single grant funded by the National Institutes of Health (2020) targeted this disorder.

Psychiatry has wrestled with the problem of chronic antisocial behavior for more than 200 years (Black 2013). Although the terms and definitions used have evolved and shifted over the years, they are unified in describing a discrete group of people with recurrent—typically lifelong—misbehavior. These individuals rebel against every type of regulation and expectation, resist authority, and push the limits of acceptable behavior. Breaking norms is the dominant force in these individuals' lives, all too often leading to lives of poverty, loneliness, addiction, and despair. ASPD arguably wreaks more havoc on society than most other mental disorders do because it primarily involves actions directed *against* the social environment.

Poorly understood in the general population, and even among some psychiatrists and psychologists, Goodwin and Guze (1989) have provided one of the best brief definitions. They describe ASPD as "a pattern of recurrent, delinquent, or criminal behavior that begins in early childhood or early adolescence and is manifested by disturbances in many areas of life: family relations, schooling, work, military service, and marriage" (p. 240). The spectrum of behaviors manifested range from relatively minor acts at one end (e.g., lying, cheating) to rape and murder at the other. ASPD is common and culturally universal, but its presence is rarely acknowledged, and determining its causes is as elusive as understanding its treatment.

In the early nineteenth century, Philippe Pinel, leader in the French Revolution and founding father of modern psychiatry, used the term *manie sans delire* to describe individuals who were not insane but had irrational outbursts of rage and violence. Scottish physician William Pritchard used the term *moral insanity* to describe otherwise normally functioning people who willfully engaged in antisocial conduct. Pritchard's use of the term *moral* is prescient because many of the people he described appeared to lack a moral compass, which remains perhaps the most disturbing aspect in many individuals who have ASPD. In the twentieth century, American psychiatrist Hervey Cleckley (1976) provided the first coherent description of the disorder, which he termed *psychopathy*. In his book *The Mask of Sanity*, he outlined a set of criteria that have influenced generations of researchers. While sharing some similarities with psychopathy, ASPD is a different entity, and in this textbook, we highlight these important differences.

By the mid-twentieth century, psychiatry was ripe for a more formal and focused approach to describing antisocial behavior. Sociologist Lee Robins, working at Washington University, conducted a remarkable follow-up study of former child guidance clinic patients. Documented in *Deviant Children Grown Up*, Robins (1966) developed the concept of *sociopathy* as a distinct and identifiable disorder for those who always tend to be in trouble, have little sense of responsibility, lack judgment, blame others, and rationalize their behaviors. Her views strongly influenced the ASPD criteria developed in the late 1970s for DSM-III (American Psychiatric Association 1980). The criteria were refined in subsequent DSM editions but essentially remain true to Robins' vision.

Assumed to be a multidetermined disorder, not unlike hypertension or schizophrenia, the cause of ASPD is thought to involve both genetic vulnerability and environmental events. Early family, twin, and adoption studies had suggested a heritable component, yet exactly what is inherited and how the disorder is transmitted are unclear. Many theories have developed to explain the disorder as either the consequence of a neurodevelopmental insult or chronic autonomic underarousal. A role has been suggested for several neurotransmitters, including serotonin, known to modulate impulsivity and aggression. Structural and functional brain imaging studies have suggested that frontal deficits might contribute to impulsivity, poor judgment, and irresponsible behavior, whereas dysfunction in temporal regions might predispose to antisocial features such as inability to follow rules and deficient moral judgment.

The cynical view of most mental health professionals is that ASPD is untreatable. That conclusion is premature because of the lack of relevant treatment research. In the entire world's literature, only one randomized controlled treatment trial has been conducted. In that study, cognitive-behavioral therapy was tested against treatment as usual, and the study had largely negative findings. This leaves clinicians to sift through the literature searching for treatment studies that may be relevant, such as persons with impulsive personalities, prisoners, or youths with conduct disorder. In each case, some of the study participants could be antisocial, but in most of the studies, the presence or absence of ASPD is never specified.

We believe that this is the ideal time for a textbook that pulls together all the known information about ASPD. The contributors describe much of what has been learned about ASPD and other forms of antisocial behavior, including childhood conduct disorder, adult antisocial behavior, and psychopathy. We have brought together a distinguished group of collaborators who approach ASPD from their unique perspectives as researchers and clinicians. Chapters 1 and 2 review the definition and history of ASPD, while Chapters 3 through 6 cover clinical concepts such as epidemiology, comorbidity, symptoms, and course. Chapters 7 through 10 probe suspected causes of the disorder, which appear to involve a complex interplay of genetics and environment, and Chapters 11 through 15 review its neurophysiology, neurotransmitters, and neuroimaging. The relationship of ASPD to psychopathy is reviewed in Chapter 16. Current treatment recommendations for ASPD are explored in Chapters 17 through 19, and other aspects of ASPD are explored in the remaining chapters. We believe that this is the most current and comprehensive textbook on this vexing disorder and will be of great interest to clinicians tasked with caring for these patients and a useful resource for researchers probing its causes and treatments.

We are grateful for the strong interest shown by our distinguished contributors in joining our endeavor. We received invaluable guidance and support from Publisher John McDuffie and Editor-in-Chief Laura Roberts, M.D., M.A., of American Psychiatric Association Publishing. They, and their talented staff, helped make the textbook a reality. Most of all, we are grateful to the many men and women with ASPD, and their families, who opened their lives up to us as we pursued research or provided clinical care. They are the true experts.

References

American Psychiatric Association: Diagnostic and Statistical Manual of Mental Disorders, 3rd Edition. Washington, DC, American Psychiatric Association, 1980

Black DW: Bad Boys, Bad Men: Confronting Antisocial Personality Disorder (Sociopathy), Revised and Updated. New York, Oxford University Press, 2013

Cleckley H: The Mask of Sanity: An Attempt to Clarify Some Issues About the So-Called Psychopathic Personality, 5th Edition. St. Louis, MO, CV Mosby, 1976

Goodwin D, Guze S: Psychiatric Diagnosis, 4th Edition. New York, Oxford University Press, 1989

National Institutes of Health: NIH RePORTER. 2020. Available at: www.projectreporter.nih.gov/reporter.cfm. Accessed March 18, 2020.

Robins L: Deviant Children Grown Up. Baltimore, MD, Williams & Wilkins, 1966

PART I

Definition and History

CHAPTER 1

Classification and Definition of Antisocial Personality Disorder

Peter Tyrer, M.D.

Alireza Farnam, M.D.

Alireza Zahmatkesh, M.D.

Rahil Sanatinia, M.D., Ph.D.

Antisocial personality characteristics are as old as recorded history and consequently not easy to define. They have three different but overlapping features. These can be summarized as the three *I*'s:

1. Insensitivity: lack of awareness and consideration for the needs of others
2. Infringement: violation of the basic rights of another person
3. Injury: deliberately aggressive behavior intended to harm

The first of these is a self-concept, and the other two are components of interpersonal social function that can range from sudden impulsive behavior to planned sadism. The three *I*'s set the stage for more formal considerations of antisocial behavior.

DSM-I and DSM-II

Clinical descriptions of antisocial behavior date to the early nineteenth century, but formal definitions are more recent. The first official definition was included in DSM-I (American Psychiatric Association 1952). The stimulus for the development of DSM was World War II. Existing systems of classification had failed to fully capture the range of mental disorders apparent among war veterans, leading the American Psy-

3

chiatric Association to conclude that a classification acceptable to all its members was needed. The DSM, later known as DSM-I, came in at 132 pages and contained 106 diagnoses (Black and Grant 2014). It was published as a slim paperback with a plastic binder, contributing to its relative rarity today.

Personality disorders were relegated to their own category independent of other disorders and were considered "disorders of psychogenic origin or without clearly defined tangible cause or structural change" (American Psychiatric Association 1952, p. 7). DSM-I descriptions were prose paragraphs that incorporated behavioral and traitlike criteria. These descriptions tended to be short and were intended to serve as a diagnostic guide for clinicians.

Sociopathic personality disturbance, generally abbreviated as *sociopathy*, was a new category used to describe individuals whose maladaptive behavior was directed toward the social environment: "Individuals to be placed in this category are ill primarily in terms of society and of conformity with the prevailing cultural milieu, and not only in terms of personal discomfort and relations with other individuals" (American Psychiatric Association 1952, p. 38). Subtypes included antisocial reaction, dyssocial reaction, sexual deviation, and addiction, which included alcoholism and drug addiction.

Diagnosis in DSM-I and DSM-II (American Psychiatric Association 1968) was influenced greatly by the work of Adolf Meyer, who believed that all mental illnesses should be viewed in the context of the whole person and should be regarded as reactions rather than discrete illnesses. Hence, the term *antisocial reaction* was applied to those who were "always in trouble, profiting neither from experience nor punishment, and maintaining no real loyalties to any person, group, or code" (p. 38). Those with the *dyssocial reaction* "manifest disregard for the usual social codes, and often come into conflict with them, as a result of having lived all their lives in an abnormal moral environment" (p. 38). In other words, such individuals had no manifest psychiatric disorder but followed criminal lifestyles.

Personality disorders were generally regarded as developmental defects along the lines of the nineteenth-century ideas of degeneration and, as such, were not regarded as treatable through any form of clinical intervention. The modern notion of *psychopathy* and, indirectly, the path of antisocial personality developed from the work of American psychiatrist Hervey Cleckley (1976), detailed in his book *The Mask of Sanity: An Attempt to Clarify Some Issues About the So-Called Psychopathic Personality*, a remarkable example of psychiatric progress being made by clinical observation. Cleckley identified 21 characteristics of psychopathy, perhaps the first attempt in psychiatry to list criteria (Table 1–1). Indicating which of these characteristics have been retained in about the same form in later classifications (and referred to later in this chapter) is useful. It is a measure of Cleckley's impact that his original concepts have been widely adopted, most significantly by psychologist Robert Hare, whose work is discussed elsewhere (see Chapter 16, "New Insights Into the Causes of and Potential for Prevention of Psychopathy—A Syndrome Distinct From Antisocial Personality Disorder").

One problem with the word *psychopath* is that it has been used indiscriminately over the years. This was most apparent in the work of German psychiatrist Kurt Schneider (1923) who described 10 different personalities that now form the basis of the categorical classification of personality disorder. All were described as *psychopathic*, contributing to later confusion about the appropriate use of the term. Nonetheless, his ambiguous term encapsulated the core of personality disorder—that is, the

---

TABLE 1–1.   Cleckley's characteristics of psychopathy

---

1. Superficial attractiveness
2. Apparently free from any neurotic or psychotic symptom
3. Little or no sense of personal responsibility[a]
4. Disregard for the truth[a]
5. Does not accept blame for his or her actions[a]
6. Has no sense of shame[a]
7. Is "undependable"; cheats and lies without any compunction[a]
8. "Execrable" judgment
9. Inability to learn or profit from experience[a]
10. Gross egocentricity[a]
11. Poverty of affect with no depth of feeling
12. Lacking insight; cannot see self as others see him or her[a]
13. No appreciation for kindness or consideration shown by others
14. Alcohol indulgences[a]
15. When drinking, places self in disgraceful or ignominious position seeking a state of stupefaction
16. Not suicidal
17. Sex life shows peculiarities with interest in casual sex
18. No evidence of familial inferiority or heredity
19. No evidence of early maladjustment
20. Inability to follow any plan consistently[a]
21. Has a life plan that ends in failure

---

[a]Concepts that have been retained.

Source.   Cleckley 1976.

---

inability to form and sustain interpersonal relationships (Tyrer et al. 2015). Only one, the "affectionless psychopathic," would now be regarded as clinically antisocial.

The recognition that psychopathy was better linked to antisocial characteristics was emphasized by David Henderson in his book *Psychopathic States* (1939). He described three groups of psychopaths: 1) those who were predominantly aggressive toward others or themselves, including individuals with drug addiction and alcoholism; 2) those who were predominantly passive or inadequate, their aggressiveness being confined to mild threats, sulks, minor delinquencies, petty thieving, and swindling; and 3) those who were predominantly creative. His descriptions were widely adopted in the United Kingdom in the subsequent 30 years, with the "inadequate psychopath" making more of an impression than the other two but not being of much value in advancing knowledge.

DSM-III and ICD-9

The term *antisocial personality* was first used in DSM-II (American Psychiatric Association 1968). The disorder was listed as a specific type of personality disorder no longer linked to addictions or deviant sexuality. Antisocial personality combined elements of the antisocial and dyssocial reactions of DSM-I. The diagnosis was used for "individuals who are basically unsocialized and whose behavior pattern brings them repeatedly into conflict with society....They are grossly selfish, callous, irresponsible, impulsive, and unable to feel guilt or to learn from experience and punishment" (p. 43).

DSM-III (American Psychiatric Association 1980) introduced diagnostic criteria that were strongly influenced by the work of sociologist Lee Robins (1966) in her seminal monograph, *Deviant Children Grown Up.* (Her book is further discussed in Chapters 2, "Antisocial Personality Disorder Throughout Time—Evolution of the Concept," and 6, "Natural History and Course of Antisocial Personality Disorder.") Robins' painstaking study involved the follow-up of nearly 80% of a total of 150 subjects and a comparison control group. The study was also helped by having accurate descriptions of the behaviors shown by the children rather than by later groups who were described in less informative psychodynamic language. Robins showed that the outcomes of children and adolescents with antisocial propensities were much worse than those of children with "neurotic" disorders, even though it was the latter who predominated in child guidance clinics. The study also placed sociopathy firmly within antisocial behavior and so reverted to supporting Henderson's view that social deprivation and neglect were at the core of the disorder.

DSM-III also introduced a multiaxial system to fully describe an individual's psychiatric condition. In this scheme, antisocial personality disorder (ASPD) was placed on Axis II along with other personality disorders and the developmental disorders. The multiaxial system was eliminated in DSM-5 (American Psychiatric Association 2013), in part because it was frequently ignored by clinicians. Also, the scheme had been criticized for marginalizing personality disorders and for creating an artificial separation between major mental disorders and personality disorders (Black and Grant 2014).

Robert Spitzer, a psychiatrist at Columbia University interested in nomenclature, led the DSM-III Task Force Committee. A major goal of the committee was to improve diagnostic reliability by introducing diagnostic criteria that were objective and based on existing data rather than expert opinion whenever possible (American Psychiatric Association 1980). The ASPD criteria borrowed from the Washington University criteria (Feighner et al. 1972) and the Research Diagnostic Criteria (Spitzer et al. 1978). These criteria sets emphasized the continuity between adult and childhood behavior problems.

ASPD became the most reliably diagnosed personality disorder almost overnight because so many of its diagnostic criteria were not opinions but rather ones that were clearly documented (Coccaro et al. 1997). Criterion B could be achieved by satisfying 3 or more of 12 symptoms: truancy, expulsion from school, referral to juvenile court, running away from home, persistent lying, repeated casual sex, repeated substance abuse, theft, vandalism, poor school grades below those expected, rule-breaking (at home or at school), and the initiation of fights (American Psychiatric Association 1980, p. 320). The symptoms had to have an onset before age 15 years, and the person must be at least 18 years old (Criterion A). These two requirements were a consequence of Robins' (1966) influence, because she was convinced that ASPD could not develop after age 18 years (even though her research was unable to fully answer this question).

A similar list of events and behaviors had to be present after age 18 years. Four or more of the following nine symptoms were required for the diagnosis (Criterion C):

inability to sustain work behavior, failure of parenting (if children in family), inability to accept lawful social norms (e.g., thefts, selling drugs, multiple arrests), inability to sustain enduring attachments, aggressive behavior with physical assaults, failure to honor financial obligations, impulsivity or failure to plan ahead and lack of fixed address, repeated lying, and reckless behavior (American Psychiatric Association 1980, pp. 320–321).

The changes in DSM-III undercut some of the previous definitions of psychopathy, especially Cleckley's "no evidence of early maladjustment," and this separation has persisted ever since. But Cleckley's work on psychopathy was incorporated in part because the text description of DSM-III included several of Cleckley's core traits: "stealing, fighting, truancy, and resisting authority are typical early childhood signs" (American Psychiatric Association 1980, p. 318). "In adolescence, unusually early or aggressive sexual behavior, excessive drinking, and use of illicit drugs are frequent." In adulthood, these types of maladaptive behaviors continue, "with the addition of inability to sustain consistent work performance or to function as a responsible parent and failure to accept social norms with respect to lawful behavior" (p. 318).

The World Health Organization (1977, p. 1108) developed a similar general definition for ICD-9:

> [D]eeply ingrained maladaptive patterns of behavior generally recognisable by the time of adolescence or earlier and continuing throughout most of adult life, although often becoming less obvious in middle or old age. The personality is abnormal either in the balance of its components, their quality and expression or in its total aspect. Because of this deviation or psychopathy the patient suffers or others have to suffer and there is an adverse effect upon the individual or on society.

DSM-III-R, DSM-IV, and ICD-10

ASPD criteria were simplified for DSM-III-R (American Psychiatric Association 1987) and DSM-IV (American Psychiatric Association 1994), based in part on results of data reanalyses and field trials, but the fundamental concept of the disorder did not change. In response to criticism, the authors of DSM-III-R added the symptom "lacks remorse" to acknowledge one of the most striking aspects of ASPD, a trait identified by Cleckley. Changes were made to the text but not to the ASPD criteria from DSM-IV to DSM-5.

DSM-5 criteria specify that the person be at least age 18 years and have three or more of seven maladaptive traits (e.g., deceitfulness, impulsivity, irritability and aggressiveness, recklessness, irresponsibility; Box 1–1). As specified since DSM-III-R, the individual must have met the criteria for conduct disorder before age 15 years. Schizophrenia and mania must be ruled out as a cause of the disturbance.

Box 1–1.   DSM-5 Criteria for Antisocial Personality Disorder

---

A. A pervasive pattern of disregard for and violation of the rights of others, occurring since age 15 years, as indicated by three (or more) of the following:

  1. Failure to conform to social norms with respect to lawful behaviors, as indicated by repeatedly performing acts that are grounds for arrest.

2. Deceitfulness, as indicated by repeated lying, use of aliases, or conning others for personal profit or pleasure.
3. Impulsivity or failure to plan ahead.
4. Irritability and aggressiveness, as indicated by repeated physical fights or assaults.
5. Reckless disregard for safety of self or others.
6. Consistent irresponsibility, as indicated by repeated failure to sustain consistent work behavior or honor financial obligations.
7. Lack of remorse, as indicated by being indifferent to or rationalizing having hurt, mistreated, or stolen from another.

B. The individual is at least age 18 years.
C. There is evidence of conduct disorder with onset before age 15 years.
D. The occurrence of antisocial behavior is not exclusively during the course of schizophrenia or bipolar disorder.

Source.   Reprinted from American Psychiatric Association: *Diagnostic and Statistical Manual of Mental Disorders*, 5th Edition. Arlington, VA, American Psychiatric Association, 2013. Copyright © 2013 American Psychiatric Association. Used with permission.

Dimensional Approaches

Concern was expressed after the introduction of DSM-III that the separation of those with and without personality disorder of all types was blurred (Widiger et al. 1984; Zimmerman and Coryell 1990). This led some experts to consider a dimensional approach in which personality traits are described along a continuum from no dysfunction to severe dysfunction. There has been growing consensus that a major share of differences among individuals can be described by four or five major traits. In the best known ("five-factor") model (Costa and McCrae 1992), the traits are extraversion, agreeableness, conscientiousness, neuroticism, and openness to experience. The antisocial element of this model is the negative pole of agreeableness. The advantage of a trait model was that it allowed persistent traits such as antagonism to be linked to the category of antisocial personality, giving it greater weight as a concept while retaining the category.

Arguments supporting a dimensional definition have taken root, and one approach has been the development of a broad-ranging model that includes clinical syndromes such as personality disorders (Hierarchical Taxonomy of Psychopathology [HiTOP]; Krueger et al. 2018). HiTOP is a new initiative in diagnosis organized by a multidisciplinary group (mainly psychologists) to improve both the terminology and the measurement of psychopathology driven by empirical data. Its aim is to improve the classification of psychopathology beyond traditional diagnostic systems.

Both major classifications in psychiatry, DSM and ICD, have attempted to apply a dimensional system. The DSM-5 Personality and Personality Disorders Work Group developed a hybrid model for the revision of DSM-IV's personality disorders (Box 1–2). The model includes assessment of impairments in personality functioning, a reduction from 10 to 6 categories, and an assessment of 5 broad areas of pathological personality trait domains. The model was at variance with DSM-IV's categorical system and previous ICD classifications. The American Psychiatric Association Board of Trustees rejected the model, which was thought to be unwieldy and premature (Black and Grant 2014).

Box 1–2.   DSM-5 Section III Alternative Model for Antisocial Personality Disorder

---

A. Moderate or greater impairment in personality functioning, manifested by characteristic difficulties in two or more of the following four areas:

1. ***Identity:*** Egocentrism; self-esteem derived from personal gain, power, or pleasure.
2. ***Self-direction:*** Goal setting based on personal gratification; absence of prosocial internal standards, associated with failure to conform to lawful or culturally normative ethical behavior.
3. ***Empathy:*** Lack of concern for feelings, needs, or suffering of others; lack of remorse after hurting or mistreating another.
4. ***Intimacy:*** Incapacity for mutually intimate relationships, as exploitation is a primary means of relating to others, including by deceit and coercion; use of dominance or intimidation to control others.

B. Six or more of the following seven pathological personality traits:

1. ***Manipulativeness*** (an aspect of **Antagonism**): Frequent use of subterfuge to influence or control others; use of seduction, charm, glibness, or ingratiation to achieve one's ends.
2. ***Callousness*** (an aspect of **Antagonism**): Lack of concern for feelings or problems of others; lack of guilt or remorse about the negative or harmful effects of one's actions on others; aggression; sadism.
3. ***Deceitfulness*** (an aspect of **Antagonism**): Dishonesty and fraudulence; misrepresentation of self; embellishment or fabrication when relating events.
4. ***Hostility*** (an aspect of **Antagonism**): Persistent or frequent angry feelings; anger or irritability in response to minor slights and insults; mean, nasty, or vengeful behavior.
5. ***Risk taking*** (an aspect of **Disinhibition**): Engagement in dangerous, risky, and potentially self-damaging activities, unnecessarily and without regard for consequences; boredom proneness and thoughtless initiation of activities to counter boredom; lack of concern for one's limitations and denial of the reality of personal danger.
6. ***Impulsivity*** (an aspect of **Disinhibition**): Acting on the spur of the moment in response to immediate stimuli; acting on a momentary basis without a plan or consideration of outcomes; difficulty establishing and following plans.
7. ***Irresponsibility*** (an aspect of **Disinhibition**): Disregard for—and failure to honor—financial and other obligations or commitments; lack of respect for—and lack of follow-through on—agreements and promises.

Note. The individual is at least 18 years of age.

Specify if:

   With psychopathic features.

What is now referred to as the "alternative model" appears in Section III, "Emerging Measures and Models" (American Psychiatric Association 2013). With the alternative model, all personality disorders—including ASPD—are defined in terms of typical impairments in self (identity and self-direction) and interpersonal (empathy and intimacy) functioning, as well as pathological personality traits shown to be empirically related to the disorder. Regarding ASPD, the first criterion (A) is concerned with an egotistical identity; self-direction concentrating on personal gratification and failure to conform to normal ethical behavior; lack of empathy; lack of remorse; and incapacity for mutual intimate relationships, leading to a tendency to exploitation and control of others. This criterion could equally apply fully to psychopathy. Added to this are pathological personality traits (the dimensional aspect of the classification) separated into antagonism, including manipulative behavior, deceitfulness, callousness, and hostility toward others, and disinhibition, characterized by irresponsibility, impulsivity, and excessive risk taking.

An important qualifying characteristic is that the person concerned is at least age 18 years. Also, with the alternative model definition, a specifier is available for those "with psychopathic features." These individuals have a lack of anxiety or fear and a "bold interpersonal style that may mask maladaptive behaviors" (American Psychiatric Association 2013, p. 765). This definition corresponds to *psychopathy*, a related construct discussed elsewhere (Chapter 16).

ICD-10 and ICD-11

ICD-10 (World Health Organization 1992) categories are similar to those in DSM-IV, and its equivalent to ASPD is "dissocial personality disorder" (dissocial covering more disturbance than just antisocial characteristics), diagnosed by the presence of at least three of six characteristics (Table 1–2). Furthermore, persistent irritability and the presence of conduct disorder during childhood and adolescence are not required for the diagnosis.

The ICD-11 (World Health Organization 2018) working group expressed concern with two major deficiencies in the current classifications of personality disorder, and this affected all its discussions and influenced the description of antisocial personality characteristics (Tyrer et al. 2011). The first was the almost total absence of the recording of any personality disorders in official statistics, with the exception of emotionally unstable and dissocial personality disorders (and then only rarely), and the frequent use of "mixed personality disorder" when clinicians could not decide on any specific label. The same problem had been noted by those involved in using the DSM-IV category "personality disorder not otherwise specified" (Verheul et al. 2007).

Another concern was the high level of comorbidity among personality disorder diagnoses (Tyrer et al. 2011), likely a result of the overlap between the criteria for individual personality categories. It is more accurate to describe these features as *co-occurrence* than as *comorbidity*. It is not surprising that those with ASPD who have strong attention-seeking attributes could easily be described as narcissistic and that those who could easily make relationships but not maintain them could be described as borderline. Another interesting aspect of comorbidity is that individuals with many different categories of personality disorder were generally considered more disturbed than were those with only one or two. This was encapsulated in the assessment criteria for an unusual category called "dangerous and severe personality disorder," identified in England as requiring special attention with regard to treatment and public protection (Maden and Tyrer 2003). Strict conditions were agreed in advance for such offenders:

TABLE 1–2.   **ICD-10 criteria for dissocial personality disorder**

≥3 of the following required for the diagnosis

1. Callous unconcern for the feelings of others
2. Gross disparity between behavior and expected social norms, with irresponsibility and disregard for rules and obligations
3. Incapacity in maintaining enduring relationships, though having no difficulty in establishing them
4. Having a very low tolerance to frustration and a low threshold for aggressive behavior, including violence
5. Incapacity to experience guilt or to profit from experience, particularly punishment
6. Marked readiness to blame others or to offer plausible rationalizations for the behavior that has brought the person into conflict with society

---

Source.   World Health Organization 1992.

A. Psychopathy Checklist—Revised (PCL-R; Hare and Neumann 2006) score of 30 or more
B. PCL-R score of between 25 and 29 (or Short-Version equivalent) *and at least* one personality disorder diagnosis using the International Personality Disorder Examination (IPDE; Loranger et al. 1994) other than antisocial personality disorder
    OR
C. Two personality disorder diagnoses, one of which is antisocial personality disorder (or equivalent on the IPDE).

In actual practice, many of those so diagnosed did not fully share these requirements (Tyrer et al. 2007).

In determining the requirements for severe personality disorder, the ICD-11 working group considered that risk of harm was the most prominent element of severity, and in the case of antisocial personality features, it was mainly the risk of harm to others rather than harm to self. So, *this* element is the most prominent component (Tyrer et al. 2015, 2019):

> Severe personality disorder meets all diagnostic requirements for personality disorder. There are severe problems in interpersonal functioning affecting all areas of life. The individual's general social dysfunction is profound and the ability and/or willingness to perform expected occupational and social roles is absent or severely compromised. Severe personality disorder usually is associated with severe harm to self or others that has caused long-term damage or has endangered life. (Tyrer et al. 2015, p. 722)

ICD-11 adopts a dimensional approach to the classification of personality disorders that focuses on impairments in self and personal functioning classified as mild, moderate, or severe. Personality disorders are then further described by specifying the presence of characteristic maladaptive personality traits. One or more of five trait domains can be specified: negative affectivity, detachment, dissociality, disinhibition, and anankastia. The five trait domains are like those included in DSM-5's alternative model. Antisocial features are subsumed to the status of the trait domain dissociality:

The core of the dissocial trait domain is disregard for social obligations and conventions and the rights and feelings of others. The traits of callousness, lack of empathy, hostility and aggression, ruthlessness, and inability or unwillingness to maintain prosocial behavior are characteristically present but not always displayed at all times. (Tyrer et al. 2015, p. 723)

A proposed crosswalk from ICD-10 dissocial personality disorder to its ICD-11 personality disorder counterpart can be described by a combination of the trait domains dissociality, disinhibition, and low negative affectivity. Disinhibition involves impulsive, reckless, and irresponsible behavior, whereas low negative affectivity involves absence of vulnerability, shame, and anxiety (Bach and First 2018). Over time, the classifications for the alternative DSM-5 model for personality disorder and ICD-11 have converged.

Psychopathy does not appear in ICD-11, and it is difficult to predict how the separate notions of antisociality and psychopathy can be reconciled or whether they might be merged. The differences between them are relatively small, and they can certainly be placed on the same spectrum. The presence of insensitivity, one of the three I's mentioned at the beginning of this chapter, is perhaps the strongest component of psychopathy. It links to callousness, indifference, and absence of remorse, enabling people with these characteristics to carry out particularly brutal and violent acts. One factor that is seldom discussed in this context is intelligence. The typical person described as psychopathic, as Cleckley had observed, is a persuasive, glib individual who cleverly plays on other people's vulnerabilities and exploits them. People who are intelligent can do this effectively. Others who are conventionally described as antisocial do not have these intellectual skills and therefore behave in a much more crude and primitive manner (Yu et al. 2012).

Conclusion

Formal efforts to define and classify antisocial behavior took root with DSM-I in 1952 and have continued to the present. Simple prose descriptions gave way to operational diagnostic criteria in DSM-III influenced mainly by the work of sociologist Lee Robins, who emphasized the continuity between childhood and adult behavior problems. The criteria were simplified for later DSM editions, and "lack of remorse" was added to the list of possible symptoms to acknowledge perhaps the most disturbing aspect of the syndrome. More recently, dimensional models have been developed for DSM-5 and ICD-11 to describe and define personality disorders. The model developed for DSM-5 was not accepted by the American Psychiatric Association's Board of Trustees, but the model is included in DSM-5 Section III ("Alternative DSM-5 Model for Personality Disorders"). The model introduced in ICD-11 involves describing the severity of an individual's personality disorder and specifying the presence of one (or more) of five characteristic maladaptive personality traits. The trait domain dissociality includes antisocial behaviors; disinhibition involves impulsive, reckless, and irresponsible behavior; and low negative affectivity involves absence of vulnerability, shame, and anxiety. Research continues as experts study the dimensional models, assess their reliability and validity, and investigate their clinical utility.

Key Points

- Insensitivity, infringement, and injury (the three *I*'s) are core components of antisocial behavior.

- Formal classification of antisocial behavior began in 1952 with DSM-I and has continued to the present in DSM-5.

- DSM-I and DSM-II included brief prose descriptions, replaced by diagnostic criteria in DSM-III that were later simplified for DSM-III-R and DSM-IV. The criteria did not change in DSM-5.

- DSM-5 Section III includes a hybrid model ("Alternative DSM-5 Model for Personality Disorders") that combines a categorical approach with dimensionality.

- ICD-9 and ICD-10 included categorical definitions for antisocial behavior, replaced in ICD-11 by a dimensional model of personality disorders based on disorder severity and five trait domains; antisociality can be described by a combination of dissociality, disinhibition, and low negative affectivity.

References

American Psychiatric Association: Diagnostic and Statistical Manual: Mental Disorders. Washington, DC, American Psychiatric Association, 1952

American Psychiatric Association: Diagnostic and Statistical Manual of Mental Disorders, 2nd Edition. Washington, DC, American Psychiatric Association, 1968

American Psychiatric Association: Diagnostic and Statistical Manual of Mental Disorders, 3rd Edition. Washington, DC, American Psychiatric Association, 1980

American Psychiatric Association: Diagnostic and Statistical Manual of Mental Disorders, 3rd Edition, Revised. Washington, DC, American Psychiatric Association, 1987

American Psychiatric Association: Diagnostic and Statistical Manual of Mental Disorders, 4th Edition. Washington, DC, American Psychiatric Association, 1994

American Psychiatric Association: Diagnostic and Statistical Manual of Mental Disorders, 5th Edition. Arlington, VA, American Psychiatric Association, 2013

Bach B, First MB: Application of the ICD-11 classification of personality disorders. BMC Psychiatry 18(1):351, 2018 30373564

Black DW, Grant JE: DSM-5 Guidebook: The Essential Companion to the Diagnostic and Statistical Manual of Mental Disorders, Fifth Edition. Washington, DC, American Psychiatric Publishing, 2014

Cleckley H: The Mask of Sanity: An Attempt to Clarify Some Issues About the So-Called Psychopathic Personality, 5th Edition. St. Louis, MO, CV Mosby, 1976

Coccaro EF, Berman ME, Kavoussi RJ: Assessment of life history of aggression: development and psychometric characteristics. Psychiatry Res 73(3):147–157, 1997 9481806

Costa P, McCrae R: The NEO PI-R Professional Manual. Odessa, FL, Psychological Assessment Resources, 1992

Feighner JP, Robins E, Guze SB, et al: Diagnostic criteria for use in psychiatric research. Arch Gen Psychiatry 26(1):57–63, 1972 5009428

Hare RD, Neumann CS: The PCL-R assessment of psychopathy: development, structural properties, and new developments, in Handbook of Psychopathy. Edited by Patrick CJ. New York, Guilford, 2006, pp 58–90

Henderson DK: Psychopathic States. London, WW Norton, 1939

Krueger RF, Kotov R, Watson D, et al: Progress in achieving quantitative classification of psychopathology. World Psychiatry 17(3):282–293, 2018 30229571

Loranger AW, Sartorius N, Andreoli A, et al: The International Personality Disorder Examination: The World Health Organization/Alcohol, Drug Abuse, and Mental Health Administration international pilot study of personality disorders. Arch Gen Psychiatry 51(3):215–224, 1994 8122958

Maden T, Tyrer P: Dangerous and severe personality disorders: a new personality concept from the United Kingdom. J Pers Disord 17(6):489–496, 2003 14744075

Robins LN: Deviant Children Grown Up. Baltimore, MD, Williams & Wilkins, 1966

Schneider K: Die Psychopathischen Persönlichkeiten. Berlin, Germany, Springer, 1923

Spitzer RL, Endicott J, Robins E: Research Diagnostic Criteria: rationale and reliability. Arch Gen Psychiatry 35(6):773–782, 1978 655775

Tyrer P, Barrett B, Byford S, et al: Evaluation of the Assessment Procedure at Two Pilot Sites in the DSPD Programme (IMPALOX Study). London, Home Office, 2007

Tyrer P, Crawford M, Mulder R, et al: The rationale for the reclassification of personality disorder in the 11th Revision of the International Classification of Diseases. Pers Ment Health 5:246–259, 2011

Tyrer P, Reed GM, Crawford MJ: Classification, assessment, prevalence, and effect of personality disorder. Lancet 385(9969):717–726, 2015 25706217

Tyrer P, Mulder R, Kim YR, et al: The development of the ICD-11 classification of personality disorders: an amalgam of science, pragmatism, and politics. Annu Rev Clin Psychol 15:481–502, 2019 30601688

Verheul R, Bartak A, Widiger T: Prevalence and construct validity of personality disorder not otherwise specified (PDNOS). J Pers Disord 21(4):359–370, 2007 17685833

Widiger TA, Hurt SW, Frances A, et al: Diagnostic efficiency and DSM-III. Arch Gen Psychiatry 41(10):1005–1012, 1984 6477052

World Health Organization: International Classification of Diseases, 9th Revision. Geneva, World Health Organization, 1977

World Health Organization: The ICD-10 Classification of Mental and Behavioural Disorders: Clinical Descriptions and Diagnostic Guidelines. Geneva, World Health Organization, 1992

World Health Organization: ICD-11, the 11th Revision of the International Classification of Diseases. 2018. Available at: https://icd.who.int. Geneva, World Health Organization, 2018. Accessed September 6, 2021.

Yu R, Geddes JR, Fazel S: Personality disorders, violence, and antisocial behavior: a systematic review and meta-regression analysis. J Pers Disord 26(5):775–792, 2012 23013345

Zimmerman M, Coryell WH: DSM-III personality disorder dimensions. J Nerv Ment Dis 178(11):686–692, 1990 2230755

CHAPTER 2

Antisocial Personality Disorder Throughout Time—Evolution of the Concept

Erik Simonsen, M.D.

Antisocial personality disorder (ASPD) as a diagnostic construct has had many different labels throughout time: psychopathy, psychopathic personality, constitutional psychopathic state, and sociopathy. It emerged as a formal clinical construct in the late nineteenth century, but over the past two centuries, the clinical characteristics have been reformulated.

ASPD was the first personality disorder to be formally recognized, and it has been included in all versions of DSM since it appeared in the first edition in 1952 (American Psychiatric Association 1952) as *sociopathic personality disturbance*. In DSM-II (American Psychiatric Association 1968), it was renamed *antisocial personality disorder*, and in DSM-III (American Psychiatric Association 1980), criteria were enumerated. It was 1 of 10 defined personality disorders and is still included in DSM-5 (American Psychiatric Association 2013). Although the concept of the antisocial personality is the product of a long and often confusing evolution, it stands out because ASPD is one of the oldest and most researched of the personality disorders. Throughout history, there has been an often-sturdy debate on the concept.

Historical Vacillation Between Clinical Understanding and Social Labeling

The development of the antisocial concept was influenced by different traditions: 1) social maladaptation and moral insanity in England (Pinel 1745–1826; Prichard 1786–1848); 2) a certain fragility of personality, even organic in nature (Koch 1841–1908); and 3) psychopathy as a means of deviation of different prototypes from the norm (Schneider 1887–1967). The evolving of the concept also has had different roots in various countries. In French psychiatry, psychopathic or antisocial personality disorder was conceptualized as an impairment of emotion and social behavior, with undisturbed intellectual functions, whereas Anglo-American conceptualizations restricted the term to *habitual social deviation and criminality*, *moral insanity*, and *sociopathy*. In North America, the term *psychopathic personality* was not used until Cleckley (1903–1984) introduced his concept of psychopathy as a disorder defined by certain psychological deficits. In German psychiatry, focus was on psychopathic inferiorities caused by minor mental defects (Koch) or deviation from normality (Schneider).

Whether the antisocial form is but only one form of several manifestations of a more complex substrate was actively debated. Were antisocial reactions to be regarded as one of many other kinds of diagnostic signs for different mental disorders or as a syndrome in itself?

In the late nineteenth and early twentieth centuries, the term *psychopathic personality* was often used synonymously with personality disorders. The psychopathic persons were considered on a spectrum of severity from normality to mental illness. Only in the mid–twentieth century was *ASPD* coined and separated as one of several specific personality disorders from the rest of the group.

More recently, the concept of psychopathy has achieved renewed interest, particularly as academic psychologists and researchers have increasingly turned to the work of Cleckley and Hare (1986), who disdained the DSM ASPD concept as ignoring psychology in favor of behavior.

Looking back, several complex philosophical, medical, medicolegal, sociological, and academic considerations have been debated in the history of the concept of psychopathy or ASPD. Table 2–1 gives an overview of the historical origins and views of the concepts of psychopathy.

Early Nineteenth Century

Before the nineteenth century, criminals were considered sinners and were treated by execution, harsh punishment, or deportation. The French alienists were the first to call attention to a form of insanity in which the disorder was limited to the field of feelings and conduct. Philippe Pinel (1745–1826) is regarded as the father of modern psychiatry and was the first to observe and document illustrative cases of antisocial personalities in which one could be insane without confusion of the mind (Pinel 1801/1962). He portrayed cases in which persons behaved overly impulsive and engaged in senseless acts of violence despite the fact that their reasoning abilities and

TABLE 2–1.   **Historical origins and views of concepts of antisocial personality disorder or psychopathy**

Name	Year	Origin	Concept
Early nineteenth century			
Pinel	1801	French	*Manie sans delire*
Rush	1812	American	Moral alienation
Prichard	1835	British	Moral insanity
Maudsley	1874	British	Cerebral deficits
Morel	1857	French/Austrian	*Folie morale*
Lombroso	1876	Italian	Born criminal
Late nineteenth century			
Koch	1891	German	Psychopathic inferiority
Kraepelin	1887	German	Mental deformities, premorbid personalities
First quarter of the twentieth century			
Schneider	1957	German	Extreme normal variants
Aichhorn	1925	Austrian	Defective superego, gratification of impulsivity
Reich	1925	Austrian	Instinct-ridden character
Second quarter of the twentieth century			
Partridge	1930	American	Sociopathic personality
Alexander (and Healy)	1935	Hungarian/ American	Criminals
Henderson	1939	Scottish	Primary psychopathic persons
Cleckley	1941	American	Mask of sanity, semantic dementia
Karpman	1948	American	Idiopathic psychopathic persons
Stürup	1951	Danish	Suffering in the untreatable

intellect were unimpaired. He used the term *manie sans delire* (essentially, mania without delirium) to describe these patients. Interestingly, this was the first time that a psychopathological entity was recognized as something apart from the mind. He raised the question of whether it is possible for a human being to consider if his or her act is morally wrong.

An equally well-esteemed early figure, American psychiatrist Benjamin Rush (1746–1813), also described persons with good intellect but a long history of irresponsibility without capacity for guilt and empathy for the suffering of others having derangement of the moral faculties. He characterized Pinel's group as described in a morally bad light and thereby foreshadowed the writings of Prichard (1835) that by using the concept *moral insanity*, scientific language and objectivity were contaminated with moralizing (Rush 1812). James Cowles Prichard (1786–1848), both a British medical doctor and an ethnologist, is generally credited with the formulation and introduction of the concept of *moral insanity* (Prichard 1835):

> the moral and active principles of the mind are strongly perverted or depraved, the power of self-government is lost or greatly impaired and the individual is found to be

incapable not of talking or reasoning upon any subject proposed to, but of conducting himself with decency and propriety in the business of life. (p. 85)

This concept encompassed all diseases in which there was a perverse state of temperaments, dispositions, feelings, habits, or actions, while at the same time intellectual functions were preserved and presented without any apparent abnormalities. The inclusion of moral insanity in psychiatric classification was encouraged by many psychiatrists but hampered by others' concern that jurists would make a contempt of the claim that some persons accused of crimes were morally insane and hence not responsible for their actions. The moral insanity as a disease ceased to be regarded as a separate disease, in part because of its conceivable demoralizing effect of the doctrine on criminal law, and instead became a subtype of imbecility.

However, the concept of *moral insanity* was very influential throughout the latter part of the nineteenth century and prescient because the term implies the lack of a moral compass. The concept was still in use in 1883 in the *American Journal of Insanity*, later renamed the *American Journal of Psychiatry*. Prichard was convinced by the content of original descriptions of Pinel but enlarged the concept by observations of criminals and defined moral insanity as "morbid perversion of the natural feelings, affections, inclinations, temper, habits, moral dispositions and natural impulses, without any remarkable disorder or defect of the intellect of knowing and reasoning faculties and particularly without any insane illusion or hallucination" (Prichard 1835, p. 6). The concept also received support from another prominent psychiatrist in England, Henry Maudsley (1835–1918). He believed that the emotional balance of a person could be so disordered by illness that he or she lost the capacity to appreciate true moral feeling (Maudsley 1874).

Bénédict Augustin Morel (1809–1873), a French psychiatrist of Austrian origin, was the first to present etiological considerations about possible explanations of mental disorder and deviant behavior. He developed the degeneration theory in general terms as a common hereditary origin to explain all mental disorders of different severity (Morel 1857). The least disordered group, named *folie morale*, were untrustworthy, emotionally unstable, and eccentric with sparse cognition functions. A similar neurobiological explanation of defective moral behavior was developed by the Italian psychiatrist Cesare Lombroso (1835–1909). The doctrine of moral insanity was reiterated. Under the term *delinquent nato* (born criminal), he claimed that a lack of higher nervous centers was related to lack of moral behavior (Lombroso 1876). According to Lombroso, as many as 25% of criminals among the murderers carry marks of the born delinquent. These degeneration theories paved the way for the concept of *psychopathic inferiority*, thus naively ascribing the sole responsibility to genetic factors.

Late Nineteenth Century

Julius Ludwig August Koch (1841–1908), a German philosopher and psychiatrist, first presented the terms *psychopathic inferiority* and *constitutional psychopathic inferiority* in 1888 to describe a group of criminals and others who committed antisocial acts (Koch 1891). Psychopathy (like cardiopathy, myopathy, or nephropathy for sick heart, muscles, or kidney, respectively) literally conveyed the idea of a sick mind—a mental illness—officially regarded as mentally competent and legally responsible in contrast to the psychotic patient. Such persons with psychopathy would not be eligible for social or medical compensation because of genuine disability, and he or she also would be held legally responsible for his or her antisocial conduct. This understanding was stable in the first quarter of the twentieth century.

As Prichard widened the boundaries of insanity to the point that symptoms affecting other mental functions might be enough to make a diagnosis, it later became apparent that more and more dissimilar entities belonged to a single vaguely defined label (psychopathy). There was a need to subdivide to different kinds of psychopathy and refine the differentiation into different types.

In the twentieth century, Koch's term *constitutional inferiority* was replaced by *psychopathic personality* and was included in the official classification nomenclature as a general term until DSM-I in 1952, in which *sociopathic personality disturbance* was described as a specific disorder.

The German psychiatrists took the lead in this effort to differentiate psychopathy into discrete types, first Emil Kraepelin (1856–1926). Kraepelin was a preeminent descriptive psychopathologist, and based on prodigious numbers of well-documented hospital records and directly observing the varied characteristics of patients, he also identified a wide range of types disposed to criminal activities. However, Kraepelin changed the whole concept of personality throughout the editions (First Edition, 1887, to Eighth Edition, 1915) of his textbook, *Psychiatrie: Ein Lehrbuch* (Kraepelin 1915). In the 1905 edition, he described four types, which today we speak of as antisocial personalities: 1) morbid liars and swindlers, 2) criminals by impulse, 3) professional criminals, and 4) morbid vagabonds. In the Eighth Edition, now under one of the forms of mental diseases (psychopathic personalities), he described four different types: 1) born criminals, 2) the unstable, 3) the morbid liar and swindler, and 4) the pseudo-querulants.

The symptoms of the "born criminal" included a decided lack of comprehensive reflection and foresight, "even early in youth there are conspicuous moral defects such as lack of sympathy shown as barbarous cruelty to animals, malicious teasing, ill-treatment of their playmates, and general unresponsiveness to kindness." Later they develop "selfishness," "duplicity, cunning, callousness, stubbornness and a disposition to lie." The morally defective "professional criminals" become "specialists," exceedingly cunning and skillful. Kraepelin described the morbid liar and swindler as "morbid hyperactivity of imagination, inaccuracy of memory, and a certain instability of emotions and volitions." The emotional attitude is usually "high spirited and self-conscious." They show "occasional dramatic outbreaks of despair or of angry irritability." They are impelled to a career of swindlers, and thirst for adventures leads them to undertake "journeys during which they employ their gift for lying to make credulous people to believe their fabulous tales concerning themselves, their past history" (Kraepelin 1915, p. 518).

The morbid vagabond mentioned in earlier editions was characterized by disposition to wander through life, never taking firm root, and lacking self-confidence and ability to undertake adult responsibility. Kraepelin combined social and psychopathological criteria to define psychopathic personalities as part of the German doctrine.

First Quarter of the Twentieth Century

Kurt Schneider (1887–1967), another prominent German psychiatrist, introduced an "unsystematic theory" and classification of psychopathic personalities, first published in 1923 and revised through several editions. His book *Psychopathic Personalities* marked the beginning of modern ideas of personality disorders because he recognized "all those abnormal personalities who suffer from their abnormalities or cause society to suffer" (Schneider 1957, p. 15). His ideas were extensively used in many countries in Europe influenced by German psychiatry until late in the second half of the twentieth century. He favored a value-free psychological and characterological point of view.

Schneider regarded abnormal personalities as extreme variants of normal personalities. He was the first to define the two sides of personality disorder consequences. He did not use explicit criteria, but under the influence of phenomenology his excellent portrayals of personality types, 10 in the latest editions, are still regarded as descriptions of psychopathology at its best. For example, affectionless psychopathic persons, close to the current concept of ASPD, lack compassion, shame, honor, remorse, and conscience and appear indifferent, distant, callous, and cold. Fanatic personalities are expansive, inclined to be uninhibited, aggressive and combative, often querulous, and litigious, close to the current concept of paranoid personality.

Thus, in the twentieth century in both European and North American literature, the term *psychopathic personalities* appeared as a broad category of personality disorders with intermittent efforts to separate the criminals from the broader category by the terms *antisocial* and *sociopathic* (i.e., the term *psychopathy* was used inconsistently to refer to all personality disorders or to a subgroup of aggressive, antisocial personalities).

August Aichhorn (1878–1949) was an Austrian psychoanalyst, teacher, and training analyst for psychiatrists. He studied juvenile delinquent behavior and disadvantaged youths (Aichhorn 1925). He was known for his intuitive talents for dealing with the antisocial nature of troubled adolescents and their aggressive tendencies. He argued that truancy, vagrancy, stealing, and the like as symptoms of delinquency are parallel to fever, inflammation, and pain as symptoms of disease. Aichhorn asserted that either extreme indulgence and overvaluation or excessive harshness and depredation can set the groundwork for a child's rejection of social values. Viewing these defects of the superego, he noted that these children are not disposed to internalize parental norms and will be inclined to seek immediate gratification through impulsive behaviors. These were the first attempts at analytically based understanding of delinquent behavior, and surface control was not enough to withstand the underlying unconscious forces of the patient. Austrian medical doctor and psychoanalyst Wilhelm Reich (1897–1957) earlier termed the impulsive personalities *instinct-ridden characters*, in which the superego fails to gain expression under the ego's unyielding control and cannot adequately restrain the id's seduction, hence resulting in the free expression of impulses (Reich 1925). Reich contrasted impulsive character with what he and others (Alexander) called the neurotic character.

Table 2–2 provides early etiological models on conceptualization of ASPD.

TABLE 2–2. **Early etiological models on conceptualization of antisocial personality disorder**

Model	Conceptualization	Proponent
Trait	Extreme normal variant	Schneider
Moral	Moral insanity	Prichard, Henderson
Neurological degenerative	Degeneration	Morel
Psychodynamic	Defective superego	Aichhorn, Reich
Neurobiological	Frontal lobe damage	Kraepelin
Attachment	Rejection, trauma	Alexander
Sociobiological	Vagabond, nomadic	Partridge
Developmental	Psychopathological	Cleckley

Second Quarter of the Twentieth Century

George Everett Partridge (1870–1953) was an American psychologist who narrowed the concept of psychopathy to persistent social maladjustments. He introduced the term *sociopathic personality disturbances* in 1930 to carefully distinguish the true psychopathic person from other psychopathic personalities (Partridge 1930). He described three different categories, one based on criminal behavior (delinquent) and biologically determined. He described these individuals as liars, swindlers, and vagabonds. The other two, the inadequate and generally incompatible or emotionally unstable, he regarded as linked to negative upbringing.

Partridge questioned whether the focus on antisocial behaviors might reflect that these acts were obvious and objective at the expense of a deeper understanding of the personality structure. He acknowledged that from a pragmatic point of view, the concept of psychopathy is reduced to focus on types of importance from the standpoint of society and the effect of personalities on social life. Because of the persistent social maladjustment with adverse effects on others, he suggested that *sociopathy* might be a more accurate term. Partridge's focus on deviations, pathological social relationships, and the chronic antisocial motivations of sociopathic persons subsequently dominated conceptualizations in American and British psychiatry more than in the German and French tradition.

David K. Henderson (1884–1965), an influential Scottish physician and psychiatrist, allied himself with Partridge's focus (Henderson 1939). Henderson gave several lectures in New York and ended up narrowing the concept of the violent, antisocial psychopathic person, although he differentiated between three groups: one predominantly aggressive, one passive and inadequate, and one predominantly creative. Only the first two were characterized by their antisocial traits, but this conceptualization was important for the inclusion of the concept in the 1959 Mental Health Act in the United Kingdom and assigned a special role in forensic psychiatry. However, an interesting observation was also that these individuals often feel themselves as outcasts, rarely understood by others, and stigmatized and scapegoated unjustly, an understanding that may have paved the way for The Henderson Hospital, a specialist national unit in London founded in 1959 to manage and treat psychopathy.

Hervey Milton Cleckley (1903–1984), an American psychiatrist, provided perhaps the most influential formulation of psychopathy by moving away from the more social, stigmatizing conceptualization held by Partridge and Henderson. In *The Mask of Sanity: An Attempt to Clarify Some Issues About the So-Called Psychopathic Personalities*, Cleckley (1941) presented a series of psychiatric cases in which he emphasized the core psychological traits of guiltlessness, egocentricity and incapacity for love, superficial charm, lack of remorse or shame, lack of insight, and failure to learn from past experiences.

Cleckley believed that the person with psychopathy could appear normal, but his or her "mask" camouflaged a mental disorder. Cleckley's formulation influenced the definition in DSM-I of the antisocial reaction, a subtype of "sociopathic personality disturbance," and later in ICD, dissocial personality disorder, which concerned social maladaptive traits and socially noxious behavior, bringing the definition in line with clinical observation and personality-based descriptions. Cleckley was the first to differentiate the psychopathic personality as a mental disorder and psychiatric diagnosis distinct from criminality. As an indication of his influence, he authored the chapter "Psychopathic Conditions, Deviations, Addictions" in the widely cited *American Handbook of Psychiatry* (Cleckley 1959).

Sociologists William McCord and Joan McCord followed Cleckley with this definition: "The psychopath is a social, aggressive, highly impulsive person, who feels little or no guilt and is unable to form lasting bonds of affection to other human beings" and maintains no real loyalties to any person, group, or code (McCord and McCord 1956, p. 2). They are frequently callous and hedonistic, showing marked emotional moral insanity as a pattern of repeated immoral behaviors for which they are not responsible, immaturity, lack of responsibility, lack of judgment, and an ability to rationalize their behavior so that it appears warranted, reasonable, and justified. The term was previously classified as *constitutional psychopathic state* and *psychopathic personality*. As defined here, the term is more limited, as well as more specific in its application. Canadian psychologist Robert Hare later modified and further developed Cleckley's approach in the forensic context.

Benjamin Karpman (1886–1962), an American psychiatrist, in 1941 described the concept of a primary and secondary form of psychopathy—the idiopathic psychopathic person (the true guiltless criminal) and the symptomatic psychopathic person (Karpman 1941). Karpman was a proponent of psychoanalysis, and the symptomatic psychopathic person was described as the neurotic character depicted earlier by Franz Gabriel Alexander (1891–1964). He was a Hungarian American psychoanalyst and physician who foremost was engaged in psychoanalytic perspective to understand criminology and psychosomatic medicine. In *The Roots of Crime*, Alexander and Healy (1935) reflected on how "emotional conflicts and deprivation in childhood, the resentments of parents and siblings, find a powerful ally in resentment against the social situation, and this combined with emotional tensions seeks a realistic expression in criminal acts" (p. 288). They also claimed that "criminality in some cases is a direct expression of a protest against certain deprivations, a reaction of spite against certain members of the family, the expression of jealousy, envy, hostile competition, all of which are strengthened by early sufferings or lack of love and support on the part of adults" (p. 288). Like Karpman and others, Alexander was among the first psychoanalysts who sought a rationale (unconscious) for development of antisocial behavior with reference to early parent-child relationships and intrapsychic processes.

Georg K. Stürup (1905–1988), a Danish psychiatrist, invented a pioneering treatment effort in Denmark from 1942 and beyond on the perspective of moral and social judgment. He was inspired by both Cleckley and Henderson in their humanistic and psychologically sensitive approach to the person (Stürup 1968).

From Psychopathic Personalities to Sociopathic Disturbance to Antisocial Personality Disorder

The term *psychopathic personality* was discarded for the DSM nomenclature in 1952, and *personality disorders* was used as the umbrella category that included people with this disorder (American Psychiatric Association 1952). Within that category, the authors included *sociopathic personality disturbance* and described three subtypes: antisocial reaction, dyssocial reaction, and sexual deviation. The first two subtypes correspond with the DSM-II diagnosis ASPD (American Psychiatric Association 1968). The *antisocial reaction* was defined as referring to "chronically antisocial individuals who are always in trouble, profiting neither from experience nor punishment" (American Psychiatric Association 1952, p. 38). The *dyssocial reaction* applied to "individuals who manifest disregard for the usual social codes, and often come in conflict with them." (p. 38). A new category was created for sexual deviation in DSM-II.

In later DSM editions, ASPD became restricted to a description of criminal behavior and behavior problems such as "significant unemployment," irresponsibility as parents, failure to sustain monogamous relationships, and traveling from place to place without a prearranged job.

Sociologist Lee Robins' influential follow-up study, described in the 1966 monograph *Deviant Children Grown Up*, which influenced the term *antisocial personality disorder* in DSM-II, and her descriptions of specific behavioral acts modeled the DSM-III diagnostic criteria (Robins 1966). The criteria remained consistent in subsequent editions, except for the additional characterological criteria to underline the absence of guilt and remorse.

Despite the change in nomenclature, many psychiatrists continued to use the terms *psychopathy, psychopaths, constitutional psychopathic inferiority, psychopathic personality*, and *psychopathic states*.

Similarly, the term *psychopathic personalities* disappeared from ICD between ICD-9 and ICD-10, and antisocial tendencies were named *dissocial personality disorder*.

Conclusion

Even as psychiatry has described the use of the diagnosis ASPD for explaining antisocial acts, it has been persistent in recognizing that such persons have significant psychological impairments.

The balance between focus on value-laden criteria of social aberration and psychopathological elaboration has shifted over the last centuries. There has been a tendency in the American-British tradition to focus more on deviance and social issues and in the French, German, and Scandinavian practice to focus on the psychological deficits and typical variations.

ASPD criteria focus on lack of remorse or guilt, callous lack of empathy, and failure to accept responsibility over antisocial acts. This focus on diminishing inferences and judgments in the assessment was in favor of the goal for the researcher rather than for the clinician.

The early history captured the controversy about the concept that this is a mixture of trait terms and items that index examples of social behavior within a moral frame of reference. The personal characteristics should explain the social behavior, including antisocial examples.

Key Points

- The antisocial and psychopathy construct has oscillated between clinical descriptions of personality features and social labeling.

- German, French, and Scandinavian schools of psychiatry have tended to focus on personal deficits, typical variations, and distinctions between personality disorder and neurosis versus psychosis, but British-American psychiatry has tended to focus on socially irresponsible and aggressive behaviors.

- Controversy remains about the classification of antisocial individuals and how different societies should manage them.

References

Aichhorn A: Wayward Youth. New York, Viking Press, 1925

Alexander F, Healy W: The Roots of Crime. New York, Knopf, 1935

American Psychiatric Association: Diagnostic and Statistical Manual: Mental Disorders. Washington, DC, American Psychiatric Association, 1952

American Psychiatric Association: Diagnostic and Statistical Manual of Mental Disorders, 2nd Edition. Washington, DC, American Psychiatric Association, 1968

American Psychiatric Association: Diagnostic and Statistical Manual of Mental Disorders, 3rd Edition. Washington, DC, American Psychiatric Association, 1980

American Psychiatric Association: Diagnostic and Statistical Manual of Mental Disorders, 5th Edition. Arlington, VA, American Psychiatric Association, 2013

Cleckley H: The Mask of Sanity: An Attempt to Clarify Some Issues About the So-Called Psychopathic Personalities. St. Louis, MO, CV Mosby, 1941

Cleckley H: Psychopathic conditions, deviations, addictions, in American Handbook of Psychiatry, Vol 2. Edited by Arieti S. New York, Basic Books, 1959, p 567

Hare RD: The Hare Psychopathy Checklist. Toronto, ON, Canada, Multi-Health Systems, 1986

Henderson DK: Psychopathic States. London, Chapman & Hall, 1939

Karpman B: On the need for separating psychopathy into two distinct clinical types: symptomatic and idiopathic. J Clin Psychopathol 3:112–137, 1941

Karpman B: The myth of the psychopathic personality. Am J Psychiatry 104(9):523–534, 1948 18911629

Koch JL: Die Psychopathischen Minderwertigkeiten. Ravensburg, Germany, Maier, 1891

Kraepelin E: Psychiatrie: Ein Lehrbuch, 2nd Edition. Leipzig, Germany, Abel, 1887

Kraepelin E: Psychiatrie: Ein Lehrbuch, 8th Edition. Leipzig, Germany, Barth, 1915

Lombroso C: L'Uomo delinquente. Milano, Italy, Hoepli, 1876

Maudsley H: Responsibility in Mental Disease. London, King, 1874

McCord W, McCord J: Psychopathy and Delinquency. New York, Grune & Stratton, 1956

Morel M: Traité de Dégénérescences Physiques, Intellectuelles et Morales de l'Espèce Humaine. Paris, Ballière, 1857

Partridge GE: Current conceptions of psychopathic personality. Am J Psychiatry 10:53–99, 1930

Pinel P: A Treatise on Insanity (1801). Translated by Davis D. New York, Hafner, 1962

Prichard JC: A Treatise on Insanity and Other Disorders Affecting the Mind. London, Sherwood, Gilbert, & Piper, 1835

Reich W: Der Triebhafte Charakter: Eine Psychoanalytische Studie zur Pathologie des Ich. Vienna, Austria, Internationaler Psychoanalytischer Verlag, 1925

Robins L: Deviant Children Grown Up. Baltimore, MD, Williams & Wilkins, 1966

Rush B: Medical Inquiries and Observations Upon the Diseases of the Mind. Philadelphia, PA, Kimber & Richardson, 1812

Schneider K: Clinical Psychopathology. New York, Grune & Stratton, 1957

Stürup GK: Krogede skæbner [Crooked Fates]. Copenhagen, Denmark, Munksgaard, 1951

Stürup GK: Treating the Untreatable. Baltimore, MD, Johns Hopkins University Press, 1968

PART II

Clinical Concepts

CHAPTER 3

Epidemiology of Antisocial Personality Disorder

Risë B. Goldstein, Ph.D., M.P.H.

Over the history of modern psychiatry, antisocial personality disorder (ASPD) has carried multiple names, including *psychopathy*, *sociopathy*, and *constitutional psychopathic inferiority* (Cleckley 1988; Robins 1987), reflecting changing hypotheses about its etiology and the psychological traits and processes underlying its clinical presentation. However, both the epidemiological research literature and the clinical diagnostic criteria since the classification system of Feighner et al. (1972) have defined ASPD primarily in terms of behaviors that violate societal norms, rules, laws, and the rights of others (American Psychiatric Association 1980, 1987, 2000, 2013; Pickersgill 2012; Robins 1987; Robins et al. 1991; Spitzer et al. 1978). This focus on specific antisocial behaviors reflects, in part, that reliable and valid measures of these behaviors

The National Epidemiologic Survey on Alcohol and Related Conditions (NESARC) and the National Epidemiologic Survey on Alcohol and Related Conditions-III (NESARC-III) were funded by the National Institute on Alcohol Abuse and Alcoholism (NIAAA) with supplemental support from the National Institute on Drug Abuse, National Institutes of Health (NIH), Bethesda, MD. This work was supported in part by the Intramural Program of the NIH, NIAAA, and *Eunice Kennedy Shriver* National Institute of Child Health and Human Development. The author expresses appreciation to S. Patricia Chou, Ph.D. (Chief), W. June Ruan, M.A., and Boji Huang, M.D., Ph.D., of the Epidemiology and Biometry Branch, Division of Epidemiology and Prevention Research, NIAAA, for analyses of unpublished data from Wave 1 of the NESARC. Data from the NESARC-III were analyzed using a limited access data set obtained from NIAAA. The NIH had no further role in study design; in the collection, analysis, and interpretation of data; in the writing of the chapter; or in the decision to submit the chapter for publication.

The views, opinions, and assertions expressed in this chapter are those of the author and should not be construed to represent the views or the official policy or position of any of the sponsoring organizations or agencies or the U.S. government.

can be obtained more readily than can measures of underlying personality traits such as self-centeredness, impulsivity, callousness, vindictiveness, and lack of remorse (Pickersgill 2012; Robins 1987). Nevertheless, the few epidemiological studies that defined cases based on personality traits have found high rates of inability to sustain consistent work behavior, repeated arrests, and associated features such as problematic substance use among their case groups. As such, case ascertainment by behavioral and personality-based criteria appears to yield broadly similar groups (Robins 1987).

Over the past four decades, published general population–based studies of the epidemiology of ASPD in the United States have been based on five epidemiological surveys. As summarized in Table 3–1, the New Haven, Connecticut, study (Weissman et al. 1978) examined Research Diagnostic Criteria (RDC; Spitzer et al. 1978), the five-site Epidemiologic Catchment Area (ECA; Robins et al. 1984) survey examined DSM-III (American Psychiatric Association 1980), and a follow-up of the Baltimore ECA sample (Samuels et al. 2002) investigated DSM-IV (American Psychiatric Association 1994) and ICD-10 (World Health Organization 1993) diagnoses. The National Comorbidity Survey (NCS; Kessler et al. 1994) investigated diagnoses according to DSM-III-R criteria (American Psychiatric Association 1987), and the National Epidemiologic Survey on Alcohol and Related Conditions (NESARC; Compton et al. 2005; Grant et al. 2004) focused on DSM-IV/DSM-IV-TR criteria (American Psychiatric Association 2000). Most recently, the National Epidemiologic Survey on Alcohol and Related Conditions-III (NESARC-III; Goldstein et al. 2017) examined ASPD defined according to DSM-5 criteria (unchanged from DSM-IV-TR criteria; American Psychiatric Association 2000, 2013). Outside the United States, the epidemiology of ASPD has been studied in general population samples from English-speaking regions, including Edmonton, Alberta, Canada (Swanson et al. 1994), based on DSM-III; and Christchurch, New Zealand, based on DSM-III (Wells et al. 1989) and DSM-IV (Fergusson et al. 2005). Population-based data also have been published from Oslo, Norway, based on DSM-III-R (Torgersen et al. 2001); the Isle of Gotland, Sweden, based on DSM-IV and ICD-10 (Ekselius et al. 2001); and Taiwan (Hwu et al. 1989) and Korea (Lee et al. 1990a, 1990b), based on DSM-III.

In addition to population-based epidemiological surveys, prevalence and correlates of ASPD have been studied in high-risk populations including unselected series of general psychiatric inpatients and outpatients as well as patients selected for specific presenting conditions such as mood, anxiety, and substance use disorders (SUDs) and borderline, schizotypal, avoidant, and obsessive-compulsive personality disorders. Studies of high-risk groups also have been conducted with adopted-away offspring of parents with serious antisocial behavior or SUDs and inmates in correctional settings.

I review findings published in English regarding the prevalence and sociodemographic and clinical correlates of ASPD. Inasmuch as earlier literature is reviewed elsewhere (Robins 1987; Robins et al. 1991), my primary focus is on investigations reported since the publication of DSM-III in 1980 that are based on DSM-III, DSM-III-R, DSM-IV/DSM-IV-TR, DSM-5, and ICD-10 criteria. In this chapter, I focus on studies from general population, clinical, and correctional samples in which respondents were clinically diagnosed, were given fully structured or semistructured diagnostic interviews, or completed self-report diagnostic questionnaires. Previously unpublished data from the NESARC (Grant et al. 2003) and NESARC-III (Grant et al. 2014), the most recent nationally representative U.S. surveys to examine ASPD, are also presented.

TABLE 3-1.   Lifetime population prevalence estimates for antisocial personality disorder

Study	Location	Diagnostic criteria	Assessment instrument	Sample size	Prevalence (%)
Weissman et al. 1978	New Haven, CT	Research Diagnostic Criteria	Schedule for Affective Disorders and Schizophrenia	511	0.2
Robins et al. 1991	United States	DSM-III	NIMH Diagnostic Interview Schedule	19,182	2.6
Wells et al. 1989	Christchurch, New Zealand	DSM-III	NIMH Diagnostic Interview Schedule	1,498	3.1
Hwu et al. 1989	Taiwan	DSM-III	Chinese Modified Diagnostic Interview Schedule	11,004	0.14 (metropolitan Taipei) 0.07 (small towns) 0.03 (rural villages)
Lee et al. 1990a	Seoul, Korea	DSM-III	NIMH Diagnostic Interview Schedule	3,134	2.1
Lee et al. 1990b	Rural Korea	DSM-III	NIMH Diagnostic Interview Schedule	1,966	0.9
Swanson et al. 1994	Edmonton, Alberta, Canada	DSM-III	NIMH Diagnostic Interview Schedule	3,258	3.7
Kessler et al. 1994	United States	DSM-III-R	WHO Composite International Diagnostic Interview	8,098	3.5
Torgersen et al. 2001	Oslo, Norway	DSM-III-R	Structured Interview for DSM-III-R Personality Disorders	2,053	0.7
Ekselius et al. 2001	Isle of Gotland, Sweden	DSM-IV, ICD-10	DSM-IV and ICD-10 Personality Questionnaire	557	1.8 (DSM-IV antisocial) 3.8 (ICD-10 dissocial)
Samuels et al. 2002	Baltimore, MD	DSM-IV	International Personality Disorder Examination	742	4.1
Compton et al. 2005	United States	DSM-IV	Alcohol Use Disorder and Associated Disabilities Interview Schedule-IV	43,093	3.6
Fergusson et al. 2005	Christchurch, New Zealand	DSM-IV	Custom-written survey items	961	3.1
Goldstein et al. 2017	United States	DSM-5	Alcohol Use Disorder and Associated Disabilities Interview Schedule-5	36,309	4.3

Note.   NIMH=National Institute of Mental Health; WHO=World Health Organization.

Lifetime Prevalence

General Population

As a reflection of evolving diagnostic classification and criteria, and as shown in Table 3–1, epidemiological surveys have used widely varying assessment measures. These considerations and differences in sampling design and study procedures preclude definitive comparisons of prevalence estimates and magnitudes of associations with putative correlates across studies. Nonetheless, the literature allows examinations of the consistency of patterns of prevalence rates and associations with sociodemographic and clinical correlates over time and across study designs, diagnostic classification systems, and instrumentation. It is important to note that the population-based prevalence estimates for ASPD reviewed herein are most likely conservative. Only the ECA survey (Robins et al. 1991) included samples of respondents institutionalized in facilities such as nursing homes, psychiatric hospitals, residential SUD treatment programs, and correctional facilities, as well as those residing in communities (households and noninstitutional group quarters). The other studies sampled only community-dwelling respondents. All of these studies, including the ECA, excluded homeless individuals.

Except for the New Haven study (Weissman et al. 1978), the range of prevalence estimates from English-speaking countries across diagnostic systems and assessment methodology was from 2.6% in the ECA survey according to DSM-III criteria (Robins et al. 1991) to 4.3% in the NESARC-III using DSM-5 criteria (Goldstein et al. 2017). The lower estimate in New Haven may reflect the requirements of the RDC and not those of the DSM criteria sets for evidence of 1) independence of symptomatic behaviors from substance misuse and 2) impaired capacity for sustaining close, responsible adult relationships (Carroll et al. 1993; Rutherford et al. 1995).

In addition to the sampling considerations noted previously, the ECA survey likely yielded underestimates of DSM-III prevalence because the U.S. Office of Management and Budget (OMB) refused to approve questions covering several ASPD criteria. Specifically, OMB disallowed items querying illegal occupations (e.g., fencing stolen goods, pimping, prostitution, and selling drugs), infidelity and sexual activity with multiple partners, financial irresponsibility, and age at sexual debut (Robins et al. 1991). In addition, a symptom item querying child beating was omitted at two sites because of concerns that legally mandated reporting of child abuse might imperil the confidentiality promised to respondents (Robins et al. 1991). However, each ECA site was allowed a 30-minute discretionary section under nonfederal sponsorship. The St. Louis, Missouri, site included in its discretionary section the items disallowed by OMB. Lifetime prevalence of ASPD at that site increased by 50% (from 3.4% to 5.1%) with the addition of those questions. Extrapolating this increase to the U.S. population yields an estimate of 4.0% (Robins et al. 1991) and further tightens the range of estimates from English-speaking countries.

Population-based prevalence estimates from Norway, Sweden, Taiwan, and Korea were considerably lower, ranging from 0.3% in rural Taiwan to 2.1% in Seoul, Korea. Apart from the nosological and methodological considerations noted previously, possible explanations for these lower estimates include cultural factors that suppress versus facilitate the expression of antisocial proclivities (Cooke and Michie 1999). One domain of cross-cultural differences that may partly explain cross-national differences in ASPD prevalence estimates involves the constructs of individualism versus collectivism, each of which may be divided into vertical (emphasizing status differentiation and acceptance of inequality) and horizontal subtypes (presuming equality of status; Singelis et al. 1995).

Individualistic cultures emphasize self-confidence and independence from others. Vertically individualistic cultures such as the United States, Canada, and New Zealand further emphasize status hierarchies, look to competition as a means for individuals to better their status and distinguish themselves from others, and view winning as everything (Shavitt et al. 2011; Triandis and Gelfand 1998). Within these cultures, individuals typically place lower priority on the goals of groups with which they affiliate than on their own personal goals and achievements. By contrast, horizontally individualistic cultures such as Norway and Sweden focus on demonstrating personal uniqueness and self-reliance, but with emphasis on modesty and humility rather than competitiveness and boastfulness (Shavitt et al. 2011; Triandis and Gelfand 1998).

Collectivistic cultures value interdependence and subordination of personal goals to the needs of the groups within which individuals are situated. Vertically collectivistic cultures such as those in Taiwan and Korea emphasize acceptance of authority, filial piety, and maintenance of harmonious hierarchical relationships (Caldwell-Harris and Ayçiçegi 2006; Cooke and Michie 1999; Shavitt et al. 2011). Horizontally collectivistic cultures such as kibbutzim in Israel are not represented among the epidemiological studies reviewed herein but presume equality of status and emphasize honesty, directness, and cooperation.

Vertically individualistic values may support and encourage the expression and cultural transmission of traits related to antisociality such as grandiosity, glibness, superficiality, lack of commitment to faithful sexual partnerships, and more generally irresponsible and exploitive behavior toward other people. Conversely, although they differ in kind from one another, the value sets of horizontally individualistic and both subtypes of collectivistic cultures may have important deterrent effects against traits associated with antisociality (Caldwell-Harris and Ayçiçegi 2006; Cooke and Michie 1999; Shavitt et al. 2011).

Other potential contributors to cross-national differences in ASPD prevalence include differential willingness to report symptoms of psychopathology in general and deviant behaviors in particular. In addition, the types of behaviors that would constitute severe deviance in these cultures may be incompletely covered within nosological frameworks informed primarily by cultural norms prevalent in Western, particularly English-speaking, countries.

Clinical Samples

One might expect ASPD prevalence to be increased in clinical samples as compared with general population samples (Robins 1987). In fact, ASPD prevalence rates in clinical settings are highly variable, reflecting the broad range of factors selecting antisocial patients into or out of treatment, including the primary diagnoses that prompt help seeking and the characteristics of the treatment environments (Goldstein and Grant 2011; Robins 1987; Zimmerman et al. 2008). Help seeking specifically for antisociality is uncommon. In the ECA sample, 14.5% of the respondents with ASPD (Robins et al. 1991) and in the NESARC-III, 27.2% of those so affected (Goldstein et al. 2017) reported seeking treatment for antisocial symptomatology.

Many clinical samples from which ASPD prevalence data have been reported were ascertained in tertiary care settings, including clinical trials of treatments for other disorders. These settings may explicitly exclude individuals with "severe" or "significant" antisocial symptomatology. Others exclude or defer patients with current SUDs (e.g., Blanco et al. 2008; Dunn et al. 2004; Golomb et al. 1995; Markowitz et al. 2015; Mulder et al. 2010; Starcevic et al. 2008; Zimmerman et al. 2004). The well-documented association of ASPD with SUDs (e.g., Compton et al. 2005; Goldstein et al. 2017; Robins et al. 1991) means that selecting patients with active SUDs out of clinical settings would tend also to exclude those with ASPD.

As reviewed by Goldstein and Grant (2011) and Zimmerman et al. (2008), ASPD prevalence rates in most samples of patients ascertained for diagnoses other than PTSD, SUDs, and other personality disorders were less than, equal to, or only modestly greater than those in the general population, ranging from 0% to 6%. They are somewhat higher based on self-report questionnaires (e.g., Golomb et al. 1995; Zimmerman et al. 1991), reflecting the latter's greater sensitivity but poorer specificity (Goldstein and Grant 2011; Robins 1987; Zimmerman et al. 2008). Notably higher prevalence rates (10.1%–18.3%) were obtained through interview assessments in several heterogeneous inpatient samples (Dahl 1986; Grilo et al. 1998; Marinangeli et al. 2000; Ottosson et al. 1998), inpatients with major depressive disorder (Zimmerman et al. 1988), and outpatients in treatment for bipolar disorders (Peselow et al. 1995). The reasons for these higher rates are unclear but may include the relatively young ages (18–40 years) of the samples reported by Dahl (1986) and Grilo et al. (1998) and variations in the distributions of clinical syndromes, particularly SUDs, as presenting diagnoses. Symptomatic overlap, mainly involving impulsivity and irritability, between bipolar disorders and ASPD also may be contributory. The two studies of heterogeneous inpatient samples from which presenting Axis I diagnoses were reported, by Marinangeli et al. (2000) and Ottosson et al. (1998), indicated that modal presenting diagnoses were mood disorders. Prevalence rates of SUDs were reported by only Dahl (1986) and Marinangeli et al. (2000): 57.6% and 14.7%, respectively.

Many estimates of comorbid ASPD prevalence among patients with PTSD are based on samples of male veterans attending Veterans Affairs Medical Center treatment programs (Bollinger et al. 2000; Dunn et al. 2004; Miller et al. 2004; Orsillo et al. 1996; Southwick et al. 1993). In these settings, estimates ranged from 7.0% to 15.0%. In mixed-sex samples drawn from outpatient psychiatry practices in academic medical settings, rates are somewhat lower, from 4.3% to 9.8% (e.g., Ray et al. 2009; Zimmerman et al. 2005; Zlotnick et al. 2001).

The high comorbidity of ASPD in patients with SUDs has been extensively documented over several decades, but prevalence estimates range broadly. As reviewed by Goldstein and Grant (2011), estimates from mixed-sex alcohol use disorder treatment samples based on DSM-III and DSM-III-R criteria ranged from 14.2% to 42.1%. The range is even wider among inpatient, residential, and outpatient drug use disorder treatment samples, most of whom were ascertained for cocaine or opioid use disorders. Based on RDC, under which symptomatic behaviors must be independent of substance use, estimates ranged from 7.7% (Rounsaville et al. 1991) to 26.5% (Rounsaville et al. 1982) in mixed-sex samples. Estimates based on DSM-III, DSM-III-R, and DSM-IV criteria ranged from 15.2% (Mariani et al. 2008) according to DSM-IV, with criteria counted positive only if they were independent of substance use, to more than 40% when criteria were counted positive irrespective of substance relatedness (Broome et al. 1999; Brooner et al. 1992; Compton et al. 2000; Easton et al. 2012; Grella et al. 2003; Kidorf et al. 2018; Rounsaville et al. 1998).

Among patients ascertained for other personality disorders, borderline personality disorder is the presenting diagnosis for which the most extensive ASPD comorbidity data are available (Goldstein and Grant 2011). In studies of mixed-sex inpatient samples based on DSM-III-R criteria, ASPD was identified in 22.7% (Zanarini et al. 1998) and 26.0% (Becker et al. 2000); among outpatients, 15.4% had ASPD (McGlashan et al. 2000). In the Collaborative Longitudinal Study of Personality Disorders (McGlashan et al. 2000), prevalence rates of DSM-IV ASPD were 12.8%, 5.2%, and 2.0% among outpatients ascertained for schizotypal, avoidant, and obsessive-compulsive personality disorders, respectively.

Correctional Samples

As with estimates among SUD treatment patients, ASPD prevalence estimates among individuals incarcerated in correctional institutions vary widely. This variation appears most pronounced in the United States. Based on DSM-III criteria, 33% of the mixed-sex ECA prison sample (Regier et al. 1990), 13.8% of female jail detainees awaiting trial (Teplin et al. 1996), and 49% of male jail detainees awaiting trial (Teplin 1994) carried ASPD diagnoses. Based on DSM-III-R criteria, 56% of incarcerated men (Walters and Chlumsky 1993) and 11.9% of incarcerated women (Jordan et al. 1996) were diagnosed with ASPD. Estimates based on DSM-IV criteria ranged from 21% to 58% (Black et al. 2010; Coolidge et al. 2011; Marcus et al. 2006; Trestman et al. 2007; Warren et al. 2002; Zlotnick 1999). Rates in Canada were 41% among an all-female prison sample (Chapman and Cellucci 2007) and 45.3%–56.7% among male prisoners according to DSM-III criteria (Bland et al. 1990; Hare 1983). Estimates from the United Kingdom ranged from 44% according to DSM-III-R criteria in a mixed-sex sample (Coid et al. 1999) to 58% based on DSM-IV criteria in an all-female sample admitted to secure forensic psychiatry services (Logan and Blackburn 2009). In Australia, Ogloff et al. (2015) found that 43% of an all-male sample recruited from a forensic mental health institute met DSM-IV criteria.

Although these prevalence estimates are much higher than those observed in general population samples, they are lower than some reported from earlier studies, including 78% among male and 65% among female prisoners diagnosed according to the criteria of Feighner et al. (1972; Guze 1976). Changes in diagnostic classification, as well as differences in sample ascertainment and assessment methodology, may have contributed to these discrepant findings. In addition, an upsurge in incarceration rates and durations began in the early 1970s and continued into the first decade of the twenty-first century in the United States, reflecting increasingly punitive approaches to crime in general and violent crime and drug offenses in particular. Manifestations of these shifts include mandatory minimum sentences, truth-in-sentencing laws that require offenders to serve the majority of their sentences before becoming eligible for parole, and "three strikes" provisions typically requiring sentences of at least 25 years for even a relatively minor third felony conviction (National Research

Council 2014). These legal trends may have disproportionately added individuals with relatively limited antisocial proclivities to prison populations, thereby lowering ASPD prevalence estimates.

Age at Onset

By definition, DSM-III, DSM-III-R, DSM-IV/DSM-IV-TR, and DSM-5, as well as the RDC and the criteria of Feighner et al. (1972), require evidence of conduct problems with onset before age 15 as a component of an ASPD diagnosis. The ECA (Robins et al. 1991) and the Edmonton survey (Swanson et al. 1994) queried age at first onset of every endorsed childhood symptom and defined age at ASPD onset as the earliest of these ages. In the ECA survey, on average, onset occurred during respondents' ninth year of age (Robins et al. 1991). In Edmonton, mean age at onset was a little more than a year and a half earlier (7.6 years) for men than for women (9.2 years; Swanson et al. 1994).

The NESARC (Alegría et al. 2013; Grant et al. 2003) and NESARC-III (Grant et al. 2011) asked respondents to report the age at which two or more conduct disorder symptoms occurring before age 15 years began to cluster in time: "About how old were you the FIRST time SOME of these experiences BEGAN to happen?" In addition, to assess "childhood" versus "adolescence" onset (Goldstein et al. 2006), the NESARC and NESARC-III asked respondents with at least three symptoms occurring before age 15: "Did ANY of these experiences you mentioned happen BEFORE you were 10 years old?" Mean age at onset in the NESARC was about a year earlier (12.4 years) among men than among women (13.5 years; Alegría et al. 2013). Slightly fewer than one in three affected respondents reported any symptoms before age 10 years. In the NESARC-III, the mean age at onset was 12.0 years overall and among men, and 11.8 years among women, with 27.8% of affected respondents reporting symptoms before age 10 years (R.B. Goldstein, S.P. Chou, unpublished data, June 2019).

Sociodemographic Correlates

Sex

Among the most consistent findings concerning the epidemiology of ASPD is the overrepresentation of men. Robins et al. (1991), among others, noted the potential for the change in diagnostic criteria for conduct disorder from DSM-III to DSM-III-R to increase still further the male excess of ASPD. DSM-III-R eliminated symptoms such as early substance use, casual sexual activity, rule breaking at home and at school, expulsion from school, delinquency, and academic underachievement, whose sex-specific prevalence rates were relatively similar. The revised criteria added aggressive behaviors including weapon use, cruelty to animals, cruelty to people, forcing others into sexual activity, and confrontational stealing; this emphasis on aggressive symptomatology was maintained through DSM-IV/DSM-IV-TR to DSM-5. Among general population–based samples, however, both the lowest and the highest unadjusted lifetime sex (male-to-female) ratios, from 2.2 in Christchurch (Wells et al. 1989) to 8.1 in

Edmonton (Swanson et al. 1994), were based on DSM-III criteria; in the ECA survey (Robins et al. 1991), the ratio was 5.6. Past-year sex ratios in the ECA (Robins et al. 1991) and NESARC-III (R.B. Goldstein, S.P. Chou, unpublished data, June 2019), and 6-month sex ratios in Christchurch (Oakley-Brown et al. 1989), were similar to their respective lifetime estimates.

Surprisingly few clinical studies have reported sex-specific ASPD prevalence rates. As with overall rates, male-to-female ratios appear to vary by setting and presenting diagnoses, ranging from 4.4- to 7.2-fold greater among men than among women in samples ascertained for conditions other than PTSD, SUDs, and other personality disorders (Golomb et al. 1995; Starcevic et al. 2008; also see review by Goldstein and Grant 2011). Zlotnick et al. (2001) showed a male-to-female ratio of 13.4 among one of the few mixed-sex outpatient samples ascertained for PTSD from which such data have been published. Among SUD treatment samples, sex ratios are considerably smaller, generally less than 2.0 among drug use disorder treatment patients and less than 3.0 for alcohol use disorder treatment patients (Goldstein and Grant 2011; Kidorf et al. 2018). In the few mixed-sex correctional samples to report sex-specific prevalence rates, the male-to-female ratios ranged from around unity (Coolidge et al. 2011) to 1.4 (Black et al. 2010). Among patients ascertained for borderline personality disorder, male-to-female ratios of DSM-III-R and DSM-IV ASPD ranged from 1.9 to 3.1, respectively (Johnson et al. 2003; McCormick et al. 2007; Tadić et al. 2009; Zanarini et al. 1998).

In addition to higher prevalence rates, several factors suggest that men are more intrinsically vulnerable than women to ASPD, requiring exposure to fewer risk factors before manifesting the disorder. As noted previously, mean age at onset was somewhat earlier among men than among women in Edmonton (Swanson et al. 1994) and in the NESARC (Alegría et al. 2013), although it was virtually identical in both sexes in the NESARC-III. Women also appear to remit earlier: in Edmonton (Bland et al. 1997), all men with ASPD had achieved 1-year remission by age 65 and all women by age 35; in the NESARC-III, all men had remitted by age 64 and all women by age 59 (R.B. Goldstein, S.P. Chou, unpublished data, June 2019). Mean age at remission (24.7 years in men, 23.5 years in women) did not differ significantly in the NESARC-III nor did duration (12.7 years in men and 11.8 years in women). Conversely, antisocial women report a far broader range of childhood adversities, including family histories of SUDs and antisocial behavior (Alegría et al. 2013; Goldstein et al. 2007a, 2007b; Robins 1966) and childhood maltreatment (Alegría et al. 2013), compared with antisocial men.

Age at Assessment

As shown in Table 3–2, ASPD is a disorder of young and early-middle adulthood. Symptomatic remission that picks up momentum in midlife and beyond is clearly contributory. However, individuals with ASPD from both general population (Badawi et al. 1999; Krasnova et al. 2019) and clinical (Black et al. 1996; Martin et al. 1985a, 1985b) samples are also at significantly elevated risk for premature mortality, both from natural causes such as cancer, respiratory disease, and HIV/AIDS and from unnatural causes including homicide, suicide, and unintentional injuries. Therefore, affected individuals who are available for epidemiological surveys, and in particular those who remain accessible for prospective follow-ups, may disproportionately rep-

TABLE 3–2.   **Lifetime population prevalence estimates (%) of antisocial personality disorder, by sex and age at interview**

	Sex		Age (y) at interview			
Study	Male	Female	18–29	30–44	45–64	≥65
Robins et al. 1991[a]	4.5	0.8	3.8	3.7	1.4	0.3
Wells et al. 1989	4.2	1.9	5.7	3.9	0.0	NA[b]
Hwu et al. 1989						
Metropolitan Taipei	2.4	0.4	NR	NR	NR	NR
Small towns	1.3	0.0	NR	NR	NR	NR
Rural villages	0.6	0.0	NR	NR	NR	NR
Lee et al. 1990a	3.5	0.8	2.0[c]	2.2[c]	1.8[c]	
Lee et al. 1990b	1.6	0.3	1.5[c]	1.0[c]	0.3[c]	
Swanson et al. 1994	6.5	0.8	4.8 (18–24) 5.1 (25–34)	3.1 (35–44)	2.2 (45–54) 2.7 (55–64)	0.3
Kessler et al. 1994	3.5	1.2	NR	NR	NR	NR
Torgersen et al. 2001	1.3	0.0	NR	NR	NR	NR
Grant et al. 2004	5.5	1.9	6.2	4.2	2.8	0.6
Goldstein et al. 2017	6.4	2.4	5.8	5.0	4.2	1.8

Note.   NR=not reported.
[a]Epidemiologic Catchment Area survey (five sites, household plus institutionalized samples).
[b]Not applicable; individuals 65 and older were not included in the sample.
[c]Ages in this study were categorized as 18–24, 25–44, and 45–65 years.

resent survivor populations; characteristics that differentiate such survivors from premature decedents with ASPD have not been identified.

Is There Evidence for a Secular Increase in ASPD?

On the basis of ECA data, Robins (1987) and colleagues (Robins et al. 1991) posited the existence of a cohort effect leading to increasing rates of ASPD in the United States. Their evidence included the peak prevalence of the disorder in the youngest age group (<30 years). In addition, they noted that respondents in this age group who met childhood criteria still had considerable opportunity to manifest additional symptoms that would qualify them for the ASPD diagnosis, whereas those in the next older group, ages 30–44 years, were less likely to do so. To estimate the lifetime prevalence that would plausibly be observed in the youngest cohort if they were observed up to age 44, they extrapolated the conditional probability of progressing to ASPD among the members of the cohort ages 30–44 years who endorsed three or more childhood criteria (0.34) to the same subset of the youngest group, whose observed conditional probability of progression was 0.22. The result was nearly a doubling of lifetime prevalence in the youngest group (6.4% vs. 3.8% in the cohort younger than 30 years and vs. 3.7% in the cohort ages 30–44 years). Additional evidence cited for a possible cohort effect included parallel increases in crime in general and violent crime in particular based on U.S. Federal Bureau of Investigation statistics, as well as increasing mortality due to sexually transmitted diseases such as cervical cancer, motorcycle crashes, and alcohol and drug use disorders, at the same time that mortality from a wide variety of other causes was declining (Robins 1987; Robins et al. 1991).

More recently, data from the NESARC (S.P. Chou, W.J. Ruan, B. Huang, unpublished data, July 2019) and NESARC-III (R.B. Goldstein, S.P. Chou, unpublished data, July 2019) suggest different conclusions. Conditional probability of progression from childhood symptomatology to ASPD in the total NESARC-III sample was much higher, at 0.90, than was observed in the ECA survey and, more recently, in the NESARC (0.77; see Compton et al. 2005). It is important to note that the extent to which childhood ASPD symptomatology is synonymous with diagnoses of conduct disorder was not as great under DSM-III as it has been under subsequent DSM classifications. Beyond these considerations and differences in survey methodology, the dramatically greater likelihood of progression from childhood deviance to ASPD in the NESARC and NESARC-III than in the ECA survey may reflect a more severe form of antisociality defined by DSM-IV/DSM-IV-TR and DSM-5 criteria, with their emphases on aggressive behaviors, than defined by DSM-III. It could also reflect that numerous cases of nonprogressive conduct disorder were probably missed in the NESARC and NESARC-III, perhaps because once respondents had remitted, they were more likely to forget or simply not to report the defining behaviors (Rueter et al. 2000). Age-specific conditional probabilities of progression from conduct disorder to ASPD in the NESARC were 0.79 among both the youngest (<30 years) and the next older (30–44 years) cohorts. In the NESARC-III, conditional probabilities of progression were 0.93 among respondents younger than 30 years and 0.91 among those ages 30–44 years. Accordingly, the estimated lifetime ASPD prevalence among the youngest NESARC respondents would be unchanged at 6.2%. In the NESARC-III, estimated ASPD prevalence would be trivially lower, at 5.7% rather than 5.8% as actually observed.

Attempts to infer secular trends from the available epidemiological data require considerable caution because of the methodological considerations discussed previously. Nevertheless, the relatively narrow ranges of total population and age-specific prevalence estimates, the consistency of the patterns of inverse associations of ASPD with current age, and the identical or very similar conditional probabilities of progression to ASPD among NESARC and NESARC-III respondents ages 30–44 versus those younger than 30 years who met criteria for conduct disorder suggest that if a secular increase is occurring, it is probably quite modest. Any attempt to contextualize findings pertaining to ASPD in the setting of crime statistics must also be made with considerable caution and the recognition that criminality is neither necessary nor sufficient for an ASPD diagnosis. Nevertheless, it is noteworthy that data from both the FBI and the Bureau of Justice Statistics (Pew Research Center 2018) indicate decreases in violent crime of about 50% and in property crime of between 69% and 74% in the United States between 1993 and 2017, whereas ASPD prevalence rates appear to have remained relatively stable since the 1980s.

Race and Ethnicity

General population ASPD prevalence rates have been reported by race and ethnicity only from the United States, perhaps reflecting the much greater racial and ethnic heterogeneity than seen in other countries from which epidemiological data are available. Robins (1987) and colleagues (Robins et al. 1991) noted with some surprise the lack of differences among non-Hispanic white, non-Hispanic Black or African American, and Hispanic or Latinx respondents in ASPD prevalence based on the ECA survey. Because many individuals incarcerated in prisons, among whom these racial and ethnic minority groups are overrepresented, meet criteria for ASPD diagnoses, elevated rates of the disorder might plausibly be expected among them (Robins et al. 1991). As they themselves noted, however, most antisocial individuals are not criminals. Moreover, most studies based on correctional samples that were reviewed earlier in this chapter found that fewer than half of incarcerated individuals met criteria for an ASPD diagnosis. In their examination of ASPD symptom patterns by racial and ethnic group, and consistent with well-documented racial disparities in criminal justice system involvement (Hetey and Eberhardt 2018), Robins et al. (1991) found that non-Hispanic Black male respondents were more likely than white male respondents to have been arrested twice or more for nontraffic arrests and to have had at least one felony conviction. Beyond these two symptoms of DSM-III ASPD, however, they observed elevated Black-to-white prevalence ratios only for weapon use and unemployment for 6 or more months in the preceding 5 years. Robins et al. (1991) interpreted these findings as suggesting that non-Hispanic Black male respondents may have been more likely than non-Hispanic white male respondents to engage in arrestable behaviors but also that Black men were more vulnerable than white men to arrest, felony conviction, and incarceration given engagement in the same behaviors. Of note, Black male ECA survey respondents' increased likelihood of endorsing these symptoms was counterbalanced by their reduced likelihood, relative to white male respondents, of endorsing traveling for a month with no planned itinerary or arrangements for lodging or work, having no fixed address for a month or more, changing jobs three or more times in the preceding 5 years, quitting a job three times or more since the age of 18, and engaging in child abuse.

Since the ECA survey, and as shown in Table 3–3, similarity also has been observed among non-Hispanic white, non-Hispanic Black, and Hispanic or Latinx population subgroups in the NCS (Kessler et al. 1994) and the NESARC (Grant et al. 2004). ASPD rates also did not differ between non-Hispanic white and non-Hispanic Black individuals but were lower among Hispanic or Latinx than among white respondents in the NESARC-III (Goldstein et al. 2017). In addition to methodological differences among the surveys noted previously, the inconsistent findings for Hispanics could result from differences in rates among subethnic groups and differences in subethnic distributions between the two samples. Differences among subethnic groups and over time in willingness to report antisocial behaviors also could be contributory, particularly among respondents who might have perceived themselves to be at risk for adverse outcomes such as deportation.

The NESARC (Grant et al. 2004) and NESARC-III (Goldstein et al. 2017) extended racial and ethnic comparisons of ASPD prevalence estimates by examining them separately in Asian/Native Hawaiian/other Pacific Islander and Native American (American Indian or Alaska Native) respondents. Although these subgroups were relatively small in both samples, they yielded significantly lower rates among the former and significantly higher rates among the latter than among non-Hispanic white persons. As noted previously with regard to the low prevalence estimates of ASPD observed in Taiwan and Korea (Hwu et al. 1989; Lee et al. 1990a, 1990b), the relatively low rates among Asian and Pacific Islander respondents may reflect protective cul-

TABLE 3–3. Lifetime U.S. prevalence estimates and ORs of antisocial personality disorder, by race and ethnicity

Study	Non-Hispanic white	Non-Hispanic Black	Native American	Asian or Pacific Islander	Hispanic
			Prevalence (%)		
Robins et al. 1991	2.6	2.3	NR	NR	3.4
Grant et al. 2004	3.6	3.7	9.7	1.8	3.3
Goldstein et al. 2017	4.3	5.3	11.9	1.9	4.0
			OR (95% CI)		
Kessler et al. 1994[a]	1.00 (referent)	0.9 (0.6–1.4)	NR	NR	1.4 (0.9–2.2)
Compton et al. 2005[b]	1.00 (referent)	0.9 (0.7–1.0)	2.3 (1.7–3.3)	0.4 (0.2–0.6)	0.5 (0.4–0.6)
Goldstein et al. 2017[b]	1.00 (referent)	1.0 (0.8–1.2)	3.0 (2.0–4.5)	0.3 (0.2–0.4)	0.5 (0.4–0.6)

Note. NR=not reported.
[a]Unadjusted.
[b]Adjusted for respondent sex, age, marital status, educational attainment, region and urbanicity of residence, and past-year income.

tural factors, including strong family orientation and the availability of social networks that provide support and deter deviance (Xu et al. 2011; Zhang and Ta 2009), as well as differential willingness to report potentially stigmatizing symptoms (Xu et al. 2011).

No population-based studies have examined ASPD specifically among Alaska Natives, and population-based studies of ASPD among American Indians are scarce. However, both the NESARC and the NESARC-III reported lower prevalence estimates among the combined group of Native Americans (American Indians plus Alaska Natives) than the 17% observed among American Indians by Ehlers et al. (2008) according to DSM-III-R criteria in a sample ascertained through a combination of venue-based and respondent-driven methods from eight geographically contiguous reservations. A comprehensive treatment of the disparities in ASPD between Native Americans and other U.S. racial and ethnic groups is beyond the scope of this chapter. However, possible contributors to the high rates of ASPD observed specifically in American Indians include both problems of cross-cultural validity and differential exposures to both risk and protective factors. In addition to differences in the cultural meanings of behaviors that are labeled symptomatic by DSM criteria, epidemiological surveys typically lack the resources to assess and account appropriately, as dictated by DSM-IV/DSM-IV-TR and DSM-5, for the contexts in which ostensibly symptomatic behaviors occur.

For example, the DSM-defined conduct disorder criterion of truancy might result from social or geographic isolation, long distances from residence to school, and inadequate transportation options, which disproportionately affect American Indians. Similarly, children and adolescents might have run away from boarding schools. In addition to being separated from their families at those schools, they often faced multiple varieties of abuse and forcible separations from their traditional languages and cultures (Beals et al. 1997; Brave Heart et al. 2011; Nutton and Fast 2015).

In adolescence and adulthood, spur-of-the-moment decisions about quitting school, moving residence, changing jobs, traveling around for a month or more without planning where to live or work, living with relatives because one did not have one's own place, and having no fixed address for a month or more are subsumed under the DSM criterion of impulsivity. Similarly, repeated absences from work and repeatedly quitting jobs without others lined up are subsumed under the criterion of consistent irresponsibility. However, for American Indians, these behaviors may reflect conformity with spiritual and cultural norms regarding family obligations. In this context, circumstances such as an urgent need to perform family caregiving or to attend to culturally mandated rituals in the wake of a family member's death, would take precedence over performance of other roles. Similarly, living with relatives rather than on one's own, subsumed under the criterion of impulsivity, may reflect social and cultural norms of attachment and commitment to family members (Brave Heart et al. 2016).

Other symptomatology subsumed under ASPD criteria such as failure to conform to social norms (e.g., stealing that could be motivated by the need to feed oneself or one's family) and irresponsibility (e.g., failing to pay off debts), as well as having no fixed address and living doubled up with relatives or friends, may represent the consequences of, or attempts to survive amidst, extremely adverse social and economic conditions, including high rates of unemployment and poverty (Brave Heart et al. 2016; U.S. Census Bureau 2017). These conditions and others, such as racial and ethnic segregation and oppression and enrollment of multiple generations of children in boarding schools where they were maltreated, have contributed to historical trauma (Brave Heart et al. 2011; Gone and Trimble 2012; Kirmayer et al. 2014). This, along with continuing, severe socioeconomic disadvantage (U.S. Census Bureau 2017), may yield severe family stress with adverse effects on parenting, potentially increasing the risks that parents will administer harsh, coercive, or inconsistent discipline and fail to provide consistent monitoring as well as warmth and nurturance. All these aspects of problematic parenting have been implicated as risk factors for the development of antisocial behavior, particularly in the setting of genetic vulnerabilities to externalizing psychopathology (e.g., Boden et al. 2010; Ehlers et al. 2008; Jaffee et al. 2012; Kim-Cohen et al. 2006). In addition to potentially shared genetic liabilities between alcohol use disorders and antisociality, high rates of alcohol use disorders among women may involve extensive prenatal exposure to alcohol, which can contribute to antisocial behavior in offspring (Khoury et al. 2018; Ruisch et al. 2018; Wetherill et al. 2018).

Nativity

During the eighteenth and nineteenth centuries, British law and policy provided for the deportation of convicts to its colonies, including the United States and Australia (Foxhall 2011). It has therefore been suggested (e.g., Robins 1987) that the relatively high rates of ASPD observed in former colonies that were destinations for such individuals could reflect familial transmission through either genetic traits or deleterious parenting practices. By contrast, recent data show lower rather than higher prevalence rates of ASPD among immigrant than among U.S.-born respondents in both the NESARC (1.5% vs. 4.0% among native-born; Salas-Wright et al. 2014) and the NESARC-III (1.7% vs. 4.8%; R.B. Goldstein, S.P. Chou, unpublished data, May 2019). After adjustment for age, sex, race or ethnicity, household income, education, marital status, region and urbanicity of residence, and lifetime SUDs, the OR (95% CI) for ASPD among first-generation immigrants compared with native-born respondents in the NESARC was 0.39 (0.32–0.48); in the second generation (i.e., offspring of first-generation immigrants), it was 0.81 (0.74–0.89). In the NESARC-III (R.B. Goldstein, S.P. Chou, unpublished data, May 2019), after adjustment for the same covariates, ORs (95% CIs) for first- and second-generation immigrants were 0.35 (0.25–0.48) and 1.08 (0.88–1.33), respectively.

Reasons for the inconsistent findings regarding second-generation immigrants are not clear. However, the lower odds in both surveys for first-generation immigrants could reflect U.S. immigration policies that tend to exclude antisocial individuals. First-generation immigrants also may have hesitated to report antisocial symptomatology, perhaps for fear of consequences such as deportation despite rigorous guarantees of confidentiality. Whether ASPD rates in immigrants vary by characteristics such as country of origin, age at or time since arrival in the United States, or the circumstances of their migration has not been examined.

Urbanicity

Urban residence might be associated with ASPD for reasons such as increased opportunity to engage in deviant behavior, overcrowding and perceived scarcity of resources that might break down respect for social norms and rules, and reduced interaction with external sources of social controls such as consistently administered family or community sanctions (Robins 1987; Robins et al. 1991). Evidence for associations of ASPD with urban versus suburban or rural residence at the time of assessment, however, is inconsistent. In the United States, the ECA survey (Robins et al. 1984) and the NESARC (Compton et al. 2005) found ASPD to be more prevalent in urban than in rural residents. Similar patterns were observed in Taiwan (Hwu et al. 1989) and Korea (Lee et al. 1990a, 1990b). By contrast, urbanicity at interview was not associated with ASPD in the NCS (Kessler et al. 1994) or the NESARC-III (Goldstein et al. 2017). Urban versus rural residence earlier in the life course might be associated with the development of ASPD, but this question has not been examined. Some studies have found urbanicity to be a risk factor for antisocial behaviors in childhood or adolescence (e.g., Rutter et al. 1975; Wichstrøm et al. 1996), whereas others have not (e.g., Costello et al. 1996; Harden et al. 2009; Offord et al. 1987); none to date have investigated whether it is associated with progression to ASPD from conduct disorder in childhood or adolescence.

Socioeconomic Status: Educational Attainment, Income, and Receipt of Public Assistance

Current

Associations of antisociality with socioeconomic status (SES) in adulthood have been defined in terms of educational attainment, current income, and receipt of public assistance. Robins et al. (1991) showed in the ECA survey that the number of years of education completed was less important than failure to complete the last unit of education begun, whether elementary, junior high, or high school. However, the interpretation of this finding is complicated by the fact that under DSM-III, not only truancy but also academic underperformance, school discipline problems, and expulsion for misbehavior are criterion symptoms, as well as associated with premature termination of affected individuals' educational careers. In addition, norms shifted drastically during the twentieth century regarding the appropriate point at which to leave school for the workforce, particularly as postsecondary education became increasingly necessary to secure many well-paying jobs. As shown in Table 3–4, more recent U.S. surveys, based on criteria that include fewer manifestations of educational problems and fielded in the late twentieth and twenty-first centuries, showed a consistently inverse association between educational attainment and ASPD (Compton et al. 2005; Goldstein et al. 2017; Kessler et al. 1994).

As might be expected given the prominence of job troubles and financial irresponsibility as symptoms of ASPD, and of low educational attainment as an associated feature, ASPD also bears a consistently inverse association with past-year income at assessment (Table 3–5). Moreover, ASPD is more than twice as prevalent among individuals reporting past-year receipt of public assistance (any of the following: Supplemental Security Income, welfare, food stamps, or Special Supplemental Nutrition Program for Women, Infants, and Children) as among those not receiving assistance (8.3% vs. 3.5%; R.B. Goldstein, S.P. Chou, unpublished data, July 2019). Increased rates of ASPD among recipients of public assistance were observed in both sexes and among non-Hispanic white, non-Hispanic Black, and Hispanic respondents but not among Native American or Asian or Pacific Islander respondents. In the only longi-

TABLE 3–4. Lifetime U.S. prevalence estimates and ORs of antisocial personality disorder, by educational attainment

Study	Prevalence (%)			
	Less than high school	High school graduation	Postsecondary education	
Grant et al. 2004	5.4	3.9	3.7[a]	2.1[b]
Goldstein et al. 2017	6.2	5.1	3.6	
	OR (95% CI)			
Kessler et al. 1994[c]	4.1 (6.1–33.0)	4.3 (2.1–8.9)	3.3 (1.4–7.7)[a]	1.0 (referent)[b]
Compton et al. 2005[d]	2.2 (1.7–2.7)	1.3 (1.1–1.6)	1.0 (referent)	
Goldstein et al. 2017[d]	1.7 (1.4–2.1)	1.3 (1.1–1.6)	1.0 (referent)	

[a]Some college or 2-year degree.
[b]Bachelor's degree or higher.
[c]Unadjusted.
[d]Adjusted for respondent sex, age, race or ethnicity, marital status, region and urbanicity of residence, and past-year income.

TABLE 3–5. Lifetime U.S. prevalence estimates and ORs of antisocial personality disorder, by past-year income

Study	Prevalence (%)			
	<$20,000	$20,000–$34,999	$35,000–$69,999	≥$70,000
Grant et al. 2004	3.8	4.0	3.1	2.8
Goldstein et al. 2017	6.3	4.7	4.1	2.8
	OR (95% CI)			
Kessler et al. 1994[a]	3.0 (1.7–5.2)	2.2 (1.2–4.1)	1.6 (0.8–3.1)	1.0 (referent)
Compton et al. 2005[b]	1.6 (1.2–2.3)	1.5 (1.1–2.0)	1.1 (0.8–1.6)	1.0 (referent)
Goldstein et al. 2017[b]	2.5 (2.0–3.1)	1.9 (1.5–2.4)	1.5 (1.3–1.9)	1.0 (referent)

[a]Unadjusted.
[b]Adjusted for respondent sex, age, race or ethnicity, marital status, educational attainment, and region and urbanicity of residence.

tudinal follow-up of individuals with ASPD in a nationally representative sample, Goldstein et al. (2012) found that the excesses of recent financial dependency persist even among symptomatically remitted respondents, suggesting that the enduring consequences to their prospects for employability and self-sufficiency of their earlier misdeeds are difficult to overcome.

Childhood

Although current financial woes may be both symptoms and consequences of antisociality, family socioeconomic disadvantage in childhood has been postulated as a risk factor for its development. Findings to date, however, have been inconsistent.

Robins (1966) noted that former child guidance clinic patients who went on to become antisocial came from families who had lower SES and were more likely to have received public assistance than those receiving other or no diagnoses. Moreover, in adulthood, their SES was lower than the SES of their parents. However, associations with childhood disadvantage became nonsignificant once paternal antisociality and number of childhood antisocial symptoms were accounted for. This finding was interpreted to suggest that childhood disadvantage could reflect downward mobility of families caused by paternal antisociality, which could be transmitted through a combination of genetic and environmental influences to their offspring.

In the NESARC-III, the prevalence of ASPD was substantially higher (10.1% vs. 3.2%) among adults who retrospectively reported that their families had received public assistance before respondents were 18 years old. Regardless of whether the differences were statistically significant, respondents with ASPD who had at least one antisocial parent were more likely to report that their families had received public assistance at every level of their own retrospectively endorsed conduct disorder criteria (3, 4–5, or >5) than were those with no antisocial parents (R. B. Goldstein, S. P. Chou, unpublished data, July 2019). Although these findings also suggest the possibility of downward mobility as a contributing factor, the cross-sectional design of the NESARC-III precludes definitive conclusions.

Results of prospective studies of children and adolescents in nonclinical samples suggest a causal mechanism involving childhood poverty. Offspring in poor households have more conduct problems, even when compared with siblings and cousins exposed to varying household incomes (D'Onofrio et al. 2009). Levels of antisocial behavior increase more rapidly among offspring with higher cumulative exposure to household poverty but decrease if household income improves (Akee et al. 2010; Costello et al. 2003; Dearing et al. 2006; Mcleod and Shanahan 1996; Strohschein 2005). The observed relationships may reflect the broad range of adversities associated with childhood poverty. These include dangerous, often violent neighborhoods, as well as exposures to toxicants such as pesticides and lead and poor-quality housing stock. As noted previously, in consideration of elevated rates of ASPD among American Indians, adversities also include family stress that may increase risks for maltreatment, deleterious disciplinary practices, and lack of parental warmth and monitoring (Akee et al. 2010; Boyle et al. 2019; Costello et al. 2003; Dearing et al. 2006; D'Onofrio et al. 2009; Strohschein 2005).

Does the Requirement of Conduct Disorder Onset Before Age 15 for the ASPD Diagnosis Matter?

Since the publication of the criteria of Feighner et al. (1972), evidence of at least some manifestations of serious antisocial symptomatology before age 15 has been required for the ASPD diagnosis. However, increasing evidence from both clinical (e.g., Black and Braun 1998; Brooner et al. 1992; Cottler et al. 1995; Goldstein et al. 1999) and general population (Compton et al. 2005; Goldstein et al. 2017; Marmorstein 2006; Tweed et al. 1994) samples indicates that syndromal antisocial behavior in adulthood without conduct disorder before age 15 (adulthood antisocial behavioral syndrome, or AABS, not a codable DSM diagnosis; Goldstein et al. 1999) is at least as common as fully diagnosable ASPD. If fully diagnosable ASPD and AABS are essentially similar, AABS may simply reflect underreporting of childhood conduct problems, and eliminating or reducing (e.g., to a single symptom criterion; Cottler et al. 1995) the requirement of conduct disorder before age 15 for the ASPD diagnosis can be considered. Alternatively, if the two groups differ in clinically or epidemiologically relevant ways, consideration might be given to adding a new diagnostic category to capture AABS.

Evidence from both clinical and general population samples suggests that underreporting does not fully explain the existence of AABS. Individuals with AABS show significantly fewer antisocial symptoms in adulthood (Cottler et al. 1995; Goldstein et al. 1999, 2007a), especially violent symptoms, than do those with ASPD (Goldstein et al. 1999, 2007a). Individuals with AABS are also more likely to be female, consistent with findings reviewed earlier in this chapter concerning sex differences in age at onset. In addition, individuals who have AABS tend to be better educated than those with ASPD. This may reflect the later age at onset in the former of the seriously deviant behavior that would be incompatible with academic achievement. Those with AABS are also generally older at assessment and with higher recent incomes than are those with ASPD; findings concerning marital status, race or ethnicity, region of residence, and prevalence of family histories of antisocial behavior are inconsistent (Black and Braun 1998; Compton et al. 2005; Cottler et al. 1995; Goldstein et al. 1999, 2007a, 2017; Marmorstein 2006; Tweed et al. 1994). Although somewhat better off than those with ASPD, individuals with AABS manifest significantly more disadvantage and maladjustment than those who were never syndromally antisocial (Compton et al. 2005; Goldstein et al. 2007b, 2017).

A comprehensive treatment of clinical correlates, course, and outcome of ASPD versus AABS is beyond the scope of this chapter. Nevertheless, it should be noted that the differences in these characteristics, even when statistically significant, are generally of degree rather than kind (Black and Braun 1998; Compton et al. 2005; Goldstein and Grant 2009; Goldstein et al. 2008, 2012, 2017). These findings suggest that AABS has clinical and public health relevance. Nevertheless, the fact that differences do exist between the groups and the stigmatizing nature of the ASPD diagnosis also argue for caution in eliminating or modifying the requirement of conduct disorder manifestations before age 15 within the ASPD criteria set.

Conclusion

Over the past four decades, multiple diagnostic classification systems, and multiple assessment instruments, the lifetime general population prevalence of ASPD has been estimated at 3%–5% in English-speaking countries. Although some earlier findings suggested secular increases consistent with cohort effects, more recent ones suggest that ASPD prevalence has remained relatively stable. In clinical samples, prevalence estimates are highest among patients in SUD treatment settings and less than or equal to general population estimates among those ascertained for conditions other than SUDs, PTSD, or other personality disorders. In correctional settings, prevalence estimates vary widely but for unclear reasons. By definition, onset occurs in childhood or early adolescence.

ASPD disproportionately affects men and begins in childhood or early adolescence; by definition, it cannot be diagnosed until age 18 years. In addition to male sex and age at assessment in early to middle adulthood, ASPD is associated with low SES in adulthood. Findings pertaining to the role of childhood poverty as a risk factor, however, are inconsistent, with some studies suggesting selection effects of downward mobility related to parental antisociality and others suggesting causal roles of disadvantage. Findings of studies examining urbanicity as a risk factor are also inconsistent. Rates do not differ between non-Hispanic white and non-Hispanic Black population subgroups but are significantly lower in Asian or Pacific Islander and higher among Native American individuals. Although not a codable DSM diagnosis, AABS is at least as common as ASPD. In addition to a higher representation of women, individuals with AABS have somewhat less severe but still substantial antisocial symptomatology, particularly violent behavior, and social maladjustment in adulthood.

Key Points

- Antisocial personality disorder (ASPD) prevalence estimates range from 3% to 5% in English-speaking countries, with lower estimates from Norway, Sweden, Taiwan, and Korea.

- Prevalence estimates from clinical samples ascertained for most diagnoses are generally less than or similar to those from general population samples. Estimates from substance use disorder treatment and correctional samples are higher and more variable.

- Sociodemographic correlates include male sex, age in young or early middle adulthood, and low educational attainment and current income. Rates are lower among first-generation immigrants than among individuals who were born and whose parents were born in the United States.

- Data indicate relatively stable ASPD prevalence over time.

- Individuals with syndromal antisocial behavior in adulthood but without evidence of conduct disorder before age 15 have less severe but still substantial antisocial symptomatology and maladjustment in adulthood.

References

Akee RK, Copeland WE, Keeler G, et al: Parents' incomes and children's outcomes: a quasi-experiment. Am Econ J Appl Econ 2(1):86–115, 2010 20582231

Alegría AA, Blanco C, Petry NM, et al: Sex differences in antisocial personality disorder: results from the National Epidemiological Survey on Alcohol and Related Conditions. Pers Disord 4(3):214–222, 2013 23544428

American Psychiatric Association: Diagnostic and Statistical Manual of Mental Disorders, 3rd Edition. Washington, DC, American Psychiatric Association, 1980

American Psychiatric Association: Diagnostic and Statistical Manual of Mental Disorders, 3rd Edition, Revised. Washington, DC, American Psychiatric Association, 1987

American Psychiatric Association: Diagnostic and Statistical Manual of Mental Disorders, 4th Edition. Washington, DC, American Psychiatric Association, 1994

American Psychiatric Association: Diagnostic and Statistical Manual of Mental Disorders, 4th Edition, Text Revision. Washington, DC, American Psychiatric Association, 2000

American Psychiatric Association: Diagnostic and Statistical Manual of Mental Disorders, 5th Edition. Arlington, VA, American Psychiatric Association, 2013

Badawi MA, Eaton WW, Myllyluoma J, et al: Psychopathology and attrition in the Baltimore ECA 15-year follow-up 1981–1996. Soc Psychiatry Psychiatr Epidemiol 34(2):91–98, 1999 10189815

Beals J, Piasecki J, Nelson S, et al: Psychiatric disorder among American Indian adolescents: prevalence in Northern Plains youth. J Am Acad Child Adolesc Psychiatry 36(9):1252–1259, 1997 9291727

Becker DF, Grilo CM, Edell WS, et al: Comorbidity of borderline personality disorder with other personality disorders in hospitalized adolescents and adults. Am J Psychiatry 157(12):2011–2016, 2000 11097968

Black DW, Braun D. Antisocial patients: a comparison of those with and those without childhood conduct disorder. Ann Clin Psychiatry 10(2):53–57, 1998 9669536

Black DW, Baumgard CH, Bell SE, et al: Death rates in 71 men with antisocial personality disorder: a comparison with general population mortality. Psychosomatics 37(2):131–136, 1996 8742541

Black DW, Gunter T, Loveless P, et al: Antisocial personality disorder in incarcerated offenders: psychiatric comorbidity and quality of life. Ann Clin Psychiatry 22(2):113–120, 2010 20445838

Blanco C, Olfson M, Goodwin RD, et al: Generalizability of clinical trial results for major depression to community samples: results from the National Epidemiologic Survey on Alcohol and Related Conditions. J Clin Psychiatry 69(8):1276–1280, 2008 18557666

Bland RC, Newman SC, Dyck RJ, et al: Prevalence of psychiatric disorders and suicide attempts in a prison population. Can J Psychiatry 35(5):407–413, 1990 2372751

Bland RC, Newman SC, Orn H: Age and remission of psychiatric disorders. Can J Psychiatry 42(7):722–729, 1997 9307832

Boden JM, Fergusson DM, Horwood LJ: Risk factors for conduct disorder and oppositional/defiant disorder: evidence from a New Zealand birth cohort. J Am Acad Child Adolesc Psychiatry 49(11):1125–1133, 2010 20970700

Bollinger AR, Riggs DS, Blake DD, et al: Prevalence of personality disorders among combat veterans with posttraumatic stress disorder. J Trauma Stress 13(2):255–270, 2000 10838674

Boyle MH, Georgiades K, Duncan L, et al: Poverty, neighbourhood antisocial behaviour, and children's mental health problems: findings from the 2014 Ontario Child Health Study. Can J Psychiatry 64(4):285–293, 2019 30978142

Brave Heart MY, Chase J, Elkins J, et al: Historical trauma among Indigenous Peoples of the Americas: concepts, research, and clinical considerations. J Psychoactive Drugs 43(4):282–290, 2011 22400458

Brave Heart MY, Lewis-Fernández R, Beals J, et al: Psychiatric disorders and mental health treatment in American Indians and Alaska Natives: results of the National Epidemiologic Survey on Alcohol and Related Conditions. Soc Psychiatry Psychiatr Epidemiol 51(7):1033–1046, 2016 27138948

Broome KM, Flynn PM, Simpson DD: Psychiatric comorbidity measures as predictors of retention in drug abuse treatment programs. Health Serv Res 34(3):791–806, 1999 10445903

Brooner RK, Schmidt CW, Felch LJ, et al: Antisocial behavior of intravenous drug abusers: implications for diagnosis of antisocial personality disorder. Am J Psychiatry 149(4):482–487, 1992 1554033

Caldwell-Harris CL, Ayçiçegi A: When personality and culture clash: the psychological distress of allocentrics in an individualist culture and idiocentrics in a collectivist culture. Transcult Psychiatry 43(3):331–361, 2006 17090622

Carroll KM, Ball SA, Rounsaville BJ: A comparison of alternate systems for diagnosing antisocial personality disorder in cocaine abusers. J Nerv Ment Dis 181(7):436–443, 1993 8320546

Chapman AL, Cellucci T: The role of antisocial and borderline personality features in substance dependence among incarcerated females. Addict Behav 32(6):1131–1145, 2007 16962249

Cleckley H: The Mask of Sanity, 5th Edition. Augusta, GA, Private Printing by Emily S. Cleckley, 1988

Coid J, Kahtan N, Gault S, et al: Patients with personality disorder admitted to secure forensic psychiatry services. Br J Psychiatry 175(12):528–536, 1999 10789349

Compton WM 3rd, Cottler LB, Ben Abdallah A, et al: Substance dependence and other psychiatric disorders among drug dependent subjects: race and gender correlates. Am J Addict 9(2):113–125, 2000 10934573

Compton WM, Conway KP, Stinson FS, et al: Prevalence, correlates, and comorbidity of DSM-IV antisocial personality syndromes and alcohol and specific drug use disorders in the United States: results from the National Epidemiologic Survey on Alcohol and Related Conditions. J Clin Psychiatry 66(6):677–685, 2005 15960559

Cooke DJ, Michie C: Psychopathy across cultures: North America and Scotland compared. J Abnorm Psychol 108(1):58–68, 1999 10066993

Coolidge FL, Marle PD, Van Horn SA, et al: Clinical syndromes, personality disorders, and neurocognitive differences in male and female inmates. Behav Sci Law 29(5):741–751, 2011 21815201

Costello EJ, Angold A, Burns BJ, et al: The Great Smoky Mountains Study of Youth: goals, design, methods, and the prevalence of DSM-III-R disorders. Arch Gen Psychiatry 53(12):1129–1136, 1996 8956679

Costello EJ, Compton SN, Keeler G, et al: Relationships between poverty and psychopathology: a natural experiment. JAMA 290(15):2023–2029, 2003 14559956

Cottler LB, Price RK, Compton WM, et al: Subtypes of adult antisocial behavior among drug abusers. J Nerv Ment Dis 183(3):154–161, 1995 7891061

Dahl AA: Some aspects of the DSM-III personality disorders illustrated by a consecutive sample of hospitalized patients. Acta Psychiatr Scand Suppl 328:61–67, 1986 3463140

Dearing E, McCartney K, Taylor BA: Within-child associations between family income and externalizing and internalizing problems. Dev Psychol 42(2):237–252, 2006 16569163

D'Onofrio BM, Goodnight JA, Van Hulle CA, et al: A quasi-experimental analysis of the association between family income and offspring conduct problems. J Abnorm Child Psychol 37(3):415–429, 2009 19023655

Dunn NJ, Yanasak E, Schillaci J, et al: Personality disorders in veterans with posttraumatic stress disorder and depression. J Trauma Stress 17(1):75–82, 2004 15027797

Easton CJ, Oberleitner LM, Scott MC, et al: Differences in treatment outcome among marijuana-dependent young adults with and without antisocial personality disorder. Am J Drug Alcohol Abuse 38(4):305–313, 2012 22242558

Ehlers CL, Gilder DA, Slutske WS, et al: Externalizing disorders in American Indians: comorbidity and a genome wide linkage analysis. Am J Med Genet B Neuropsychiatr Genet 147B(6):690–698, 2008 18286631

Ekselius L, Tillfors M, Furmark T, et al: Personality disorders in the general population: DSM-IV and ICD-10 defined prevalence as related to sociodemographic profile. Pers Individ Dif 30(2):311–320, 2001

Feighner JP, Robins E, Guze SB, et al: Diagnostic criteria for use in psychiatric research. Arch Gen Psychiatry 26(1):57–63, 1972 5009428

Fergusson DM, Horwood LJ, Ridder EM: Show me the child at seven: the consequences of conduct problems in childhood for psychosocial functioning in adulthood. J Child Psychol Psychiatry 46(8):837–849, 2005 16033632

Foxhall K: From convicts to colonists: the health of prisoners and the voyage to Australia, 1823–53. J Imp Commonw Hist 39(1):1–19, 2011 21584986

Goldstein RB, Grant BF: Three-year follow-up of syndromal antisocial behavior in adults: results from the Wave 2 National Epidemiologic Survey on Alcohol and Related Conditions. J Clin Psychiatry 70(9):1237–1249, 2009 19538901

Goldstein RB, Grant BF: Burden of syndromal antisocial behavior in adulthood, in Antisocial Behavior: Causes, Correlations, and Treatments. Edited by Clark RM. Hauppauge, NY, Nova Science Publishers, 2011, pp 1–74

Goldstein RB, Powers SI, McCusker J, et al: Antisocial behavioral syndromes among residential drug abuse treatment clients. Drug Alcohol Depend 53(2):171–187, 1999 10080043

Goldstein RB, Grant BF, Ruan WJ, et al: Antisocial personality disorder with childhood- vs. adolescence-onset conduct disorder: results from the National Epidemiologic Survey on Alcohol and Related Conditions. J Nerv Ment Dis 194(9):667–675, 2006 16971818

Goldstein RB, Dawson DA, Saha TD, et al: Antisocial behavioral syndromes and DSM-IV alcohol use disorders: results from the National Epidemiologic Survey on Alcohol and Related Conditions. Alcohol Clin Exp Res 31(5):814–828, 2007a 17391341

Goldstein RB, Compton WM, Pulay AJ, et al: Antisocial behavioral syndromes and DSM-IV drug use disorders in the United States: results from the National Epidemiologic Survey on Alcohol and Related Conditions. Drug Alcohol Depend 90(2–3):145–158, 2007b 17433571

Goldstein RB, Dawson DA, Chou SP, et al: Antisocial behavioral syndromes and past-year physical health among adults in the United States: results from the National Epidemiologic Survey on Alcohol and Related Conditions. J Clin Psychiatry 69(3):368–380, 2008 18348594

Goldstein RB, Dawson DA, Smith SM, et al: Antisocial behavioral syndromes and 3-year quality-of-life outcomes in United States adults. Acta Psychiatr Scand 126(2):137–150, 2012 22375904

Goldstein RB, Chou SP, Saha TD, et al: The epidemiology of antisocial behavioral syndromes in adulthood: results from the National Epidemiologic Survey on Alcohol and Related Conditions-III. J Clin Psychiatry 78(1):90–98, 2017 27035627

Golomb M, Fava M, Abraham M, et al: Gender differences in personality disorders. Am J Psychiatry 152(4):579–582, 1995 7694907

Gone JP, Trimble JE: American Indian and Alaska Native mental health: diverse perspectives on enduring disparities. Annu Rev Clin Psychol 8:131–160, 2012 22149479

Grant BF, Dawson DA, Stinson FS, et al: The Alcohol Use Disorder and Associated Disabilities Interview Schedule-IV (AUDADIS-IV): reliability of alcohol consumption, tobacco use, family history of depression and psychiatric diagnostic modules in a general population sample. Drug Alcohol Depend 71(1):7–16, 2003 12821201

Grant BF, Hasin DS, Stinson FS, et al: Prevalence, correlates, and disability of personality disorders in the United States: results from the National Epidemiologic Survey on Alcohol and Related Conditions. J Clin Psychiatry 65(7):948–958, 2004 15291684

Grant BF, Goldstein RB, Chou SP, et al: The Alcohol Use Disorder and Associated Disabilities Interview Schedule—Diagnostic and Statistical Manual of Mental Disorders, 5th Edition Version (AUDADIS-5). Rockville, MD, National Institute on Alcohol Abuse and Alcoholism, 2011

Grant BF, Chu A, Sigman R, et al: Source and accuracy statement: National Epidemiologic Survey on Alcohol and Related Conditions-III (NESARC-III). Rockville, MD, National Institute on Alcohol Abuse and Alcoholism, 2014

Grella CE, Joshi V, Hser Y-I: Followup of cocaine-dependent men and women with antisocial personality disorder. J Subst Abuse Treat 25(3):155–164, 2003 14670521

Grilo CM, McGlashan TH, Quinlan DM, et al: Frequency of personality disorders in two age cohorts of psychiatric inpatients. Am J Psychiatry 155(1):140–142, 1998 9433356

Guze SB: Criminality and Psychiatric Disorders. New York, Oxford University Press, 1976

Harden KP, D'Onofrio BM, Van Hulle C, et al: Population density and youth antisocial behavior. J Child Psychol Psychiatry 50(8):999–1008, 2009 19490315

Hare RD: Diagnosis of antisocial personality disorder in two prison populations. Am J Psychiatry 140(7):887–890, 1983 6859306

Hetey RC, Eberhardt JL: The numbers don't speak for themselves: racial disparities and the persistence of inequality in the criminal justice system. Curr Dir Psychol Sci 27(3):183–187, 2018

Hwu H-G, Yeh E-K, Chang L-Y: Prevalence of psychiatric disorders in Taiwan defined by the Chinese Diagnostic Interview Schedule. Acta Psychiatr Scand 79(2):136–147, 1989 2923007

Jaffee SR, Strait LB, Odgers CL: From correlates to causes: can quasi-experimental studies and statistical innovations bring us closer to identifying the causes of antisocial behavior? Psychol Bull 138(2):272–295, 2012 22023141

Johnson DM, Shea MT, Yen S, et al: Gender differences in borderline personality disorder: findings from the Collaborative Longitudinal Personality Disorders Study. Compr Psychiatry 44(4):284–292, 2003 12923706

Jordan BK, Schlenger WE, Fairbank JA, et al: Prevalence of psychiatric disorders among incarcerated women, II: convicted felons entering prison. Arch Gen Psychiatry 53(6):513–519, 1996 8639034

Kessler RC, McGonagle KA, Zhao S, et al: Lifetime and 12-month prevalence of DSM-III-R psychiatric disorders in the United States: results from the National Comorbidity Survey. Arch Gen Psychiatry 51(1):8–19, 1994 8279933

Khoury JE, Jamieson B, Milligan K: Risk for childhood internalizing and externalizing behavior problems in the context of prenatal alcohol exposure: a meta-analysis and comprehensive examination of moderators. Alcohol Clin Exp Res 42(8):1358–1377, 2018 29852057

Kidorf M, Solazzo S, Yan H, et al: Psychiatric and substance use comorbidity in treatment-seeking injection opioid users referred from syringe exchange. J Dual Diagn 14(4):193–200, 2018 30332349

Kim-Cohen J, Caspi A, Taylor A, et al: MAOA, maltreatment, and gene-environment interaction predicting children's mental health: new evidence and a meta-analysis. Mol Psychiatry 11(10):903–913, 2006 16801953

Kirmayer LJ, Gone JP, Moses J: Rethinking historical trauma. Transcult Psychiatry 51(3):299–319, 2014 24855142

Krasnova A, Eaton WW, Samuels JF: Antisocial personality and risks of cause-specific mortality: results from the Epidemiologic Catchment Area study with 27 years of follow-up. Soc Psychiatry Psychiatr Epidemiol 54(5):617–625, 2019 30506390

Lee CK, Kwak YS, Yamamoto J, et al: Psychiatric epidemiology in Korea, part I: gender and age differences in Seoul. J Nerv Ment Dis 178(4):242–246, 1990a 2319232

Lee CK, Kwak YS, Yamamoto J, et al: Psychiatric epidemiology in Korea, part II: urban and rural differences. J Nerv Ment Dis 178(4):247–252, 1990b 2181056

Logan C, Blackburn R: Mental disorder in violent women in secure settings: potential relevance to risk for future violence. Int J Law Psychiatry 32(1):31–38, 2009 19081630

Marcus DK, Lilienfeld SO, Edens JF, et al: Is antisocial personality disorder continuous or categorical? A taxometric analysis. Psychol Med 36(11):1571–1581, 2006 16836795

Mariani JJ, Horey J, Bisaga A, et al: Antisocial behavioral syndromes in cocaine and cannabis dependence. Am J Drug Alcohol Abuse 34(4):405–414, 2008 18584570

Marinangeli MG, Butti G, Scinto A, et al: Patterns of comorbidity among DSM-III-R personality disorders. Psychopathology 33(2):69–74, 2000 10705249

Markowitz JC, Petkova E, Biyanova T, et al: Exploring personality diagnosis stability following acute psychotherapy for chronic posttraumatic stress disorder. Depress Anxiety 32(12):919–926, 2015 26439430

Marmorstein NR: Adult antisocial behaviour without conduct disorder: demographic characteristics and risk for cooccurring psychopathology. Can J Psychiatry 51(4):226–233, 2006 16629347

Martin RL, Cloninger CR, Guze SB, et al: Mortality in a follow-up of 500 psychiatric outpatients, I: total mortality. Arch Gen Psychiatry 42(1):47–54, 1985a 3966852

Martin RL, Cloninger CR, Guze SB, et al: Mortality in a follow-up of 500 psychiatric outpatients, II: cause-specific mortality. Arch Gen Psychiatry 42(1):58–66, 1985b 3966853

McCormick B, Blum N, Hansel R, et al: Relationship of sex to symptom severity, psychiatric comorbidity, and health care utilization in 163 subjects with borderline personality disorder. Compr Psychiatry 48(5):406–412, 2007 17707247

McGlashan TH, Grilo CM, Skodol AE, et al: The Collaborative Longitudinal Personality Disorders Study: baseline Axis I/II and II/II diagnostic co-occurrence. Acta Psychiatr Scand 102(4):256–264, 2000 11089725

Mcleod JD, Shanahan MJ: Trajectories of poverty and children's mental health. J Health Soc Behav 37(3):207–220, 1996 8898493

Miller MW, Kaloupek DG, Dillon AL, et al: Externalizing and internalizing subtypes of combat-related PTSD: a replication and extension using the PSY-5 scales. J Abnorm Psychol 113(4):636–645, 2004 15535795

Mulder RT, Joyce PR, Frampton CM: Personality disorders improve in patients treated for major depression. Acta Psychiatr Scand 122(3):219–225, 2010 19895619

National Research Council: The Growth of Incarceration in the United States: Exploring Causes and Consequences. Washington, DC, National Academies Press, 2014

Nutton J, Fast E: Historical trauma, substance use, and indigenous peoples: seven generations of harm from a "big event." Subst Use Misuse 50(7):839–847, 2015 26158749

Oakley-Brown MA, Joyce PR, Wells JE, et al: Christchurch Psychiatric Epidemiology Study, Part II: six-month and other period prevalences of specific psychiatric disorders. Aust N Z J Psychiatry 23(3):315–326, 1989 2803145

Offord DR, Boyle MH, Jones BR: Psychiatric disorder and poor school performance among welfare children in Ontario. Can J Psychiatry 32(7):518–525, 1987 3676981

Ogloff JRP, Talevski D, Lemphers A, et al: Co-occurring mental illness, substance use disorders, and antisocial personality disorder among clients of forensic mental health services. Psychiatr Rehabil J 38(1):16–23, 2015 25799303

Orsillo SM, Weathers FW, Litz BT, et al: Current and lifetime psychiatric disorders among veterans with war zone-related posttraumatic stress disorder. J Nerv Ment Dis 184(5):307–313, 1996 8627277

Ottosson H, Bodlund O, Ekselius L, et al: DSM-IV and ICD-10 personality disorders: a comparison of a self-report questionnaire (DIP-Q) with a structured interview. Eur Psychiatry 13(5):246–253, 1998 19698634

Peselow ED, Sanfilipo MP, Fieve RR: Relationship between hypomania and personality disorders before and after successful treatment. Am J Psychiatry 152(2):232–238, 1995 7840357

Pew Research Center: What the data says (and doesn't say) about crime in the United States. November 20, 2020. Available at: www.pewresearch.org/fact-tank/2020/11/20/facts-about-crime-in-the-u-s. Accessed September 19, 2021.

Pickersgill M: Standardising antisocial personality disorder: the social shaping of a psychiatric technology. Sociol Health Illn 34(4):544–559, 2012 22017609

Ray LA, Capone C, Sheets E, et al: Posttraumatic stress disorder with and without alcohol use disorders: diagnostic and clinical correlates in a psychiatric sample. Psychiatry Res 170(2–3):278–281, 2009 19900714

Regier DA, Farmer ME, Rae DS, et al: Comorbidity of mental disorders with alcohol and other drug abuse: results from the Epidemiologic Catchment Area (ECA) Study. JAMA 264(19):2511–2518, 1990 2232018

Robins LN: Deviant Children Grown Up. Baltimore, MD, Williams & Wilkins, 1966

Robins LN: The epidemiology of antisocial personality disorder, in Psychiatry, Volume 3. Edited by Michels RO, Cavenar JO. Philadelphia, PA, Lippincott, 1987, pp 1–14

Robins LN, Helzer JE, Weissman MM, et al: Lifetime prevalence of specific psychiatric disorders in three sites. Arch Gen Psychiatry 41(10):949–958, 1984 6332590

Robins LN, Tipp J, Przybeck T: Antisocial personality disorder, in Psychiatric Disorders in America: The Epidemiologic Catchment Area Study. Edited by Robins LN, Regier DA. New York, Free Press, 1991, pp 258–290

Rounsaville BJ, Weissman MM, Kleber H, et al: Heterogeneity of psychiatric diagnosis in treated opiate addicts. Arch Gen Psychiatry 39(2):161–168, 1982 7065830

Rounsaville BJ, Anton SF, Carroll K, et al: Psychiatric diagnoses of treatment-seeking cocaine abusers. Arch Gen Psychiatry 48(1):43–51, 1991 1984761

Rounsaville BJ, Kranzler HR, Ball S, et al: Personality disorders in substance abusers: relation to substance use. J Nerv Ment Dis 186(2):87–95, 1998 9484308

Rueter MA, Chao W, Conger RD: The effect of systematic variation in retrospective conduct disorder reports on antisocial personality disorder diagnoses. J Consult Clin Psychol 68(2):307–312, 2000 10780131

Ruisch IH, Dietrich A, Glennon JC, et al: Maternal substance use during pregnancy and off-spring conduct problems: a meta-analysis. Neurosci Biobehav Rev 84:325–336, 2018 28847489

Rutherford MJ, Alterman AI, Cacciola JS, et al: Gender differences in diagnosing antisocial personality disorder in methadone patients. Am J Psychiatry 152(9):1309–1316, 1995 7653686

Rutter M, Cox A, Tupling C, et al: Attainment and adjustment in two geographical areas, I—the prevalence of psychiatric disorder. Br J Psychiatry 126(6):493–509, 1975 1174767

Salas-Wright CP, Kagotho N, Vaughn MG: Mood, anxiety, and personality disorders among first and second-generation immigrants to the United States. Psychiatry Res 220(3):1028–1036, 2014 25223256

Samuels J, Eaton WW, Bienvenu OJ 3rd, et al: Prevalence and correlates of personality disorders in a community sample. Br J Psychiatry 180(6):536–542, 2002 12042233

Shavitt S, Johnson TP, Zhang J: Horizontal and vertical cultural differences in the content of advertising appeals. J Int Consum Mark 23(3–4):297–310, 2011 25554720

Singelis TM, Triandis HC, Bhawuk DBS, et al: Horizontal and vertical dimensions of individualism and collectivism: a theoretical and measurement refinement. Cross Cult Res 29(3):240–275, 1995

Southwick SM, Yehuda R, Giller EL Jr: Personality disorders in treatment-seeking combat veterans with posttraumatic stress disorder. Am J Psychiatry 150(7):1020–1023, 1993 8317570

Spitzer RL, Endicott J, Robins E: Research Diagnostic Criteria: rationale and reliability. Arch Gen Psychiatry 35(6):773–782, 1978 655775

Starcevic V, Latas M, Kolar D, et al: Co-occurrence of Axis I and Axis II disorders in female and male patients with panic disorder with agoraphobia. Compr Psychiatry 49(6):537–543, 2008 18970901

Strohschein L: Household income histories and child mental health trajectories. J Health Soc Behav 46(4):359–375, 2005 16433281

Swanson MC, Bland RC, Newman SC: Epidemiology of psychiatric disorders in Edmonton: antisocial personality disorders. Acta Psychiatr Scand Suppl 376:63–70, 1994 8178687

Tadić A, Wagner S, Hoch J, et al: Gender differences in Axis I and Axis II comorbidity in patients with borderline personality disorder. Psychopathology 42(4):257–263, 2009 19521142

Teplin LA: Psychiatric and substance abuse disorders among male urban jail detainees. Am J Public Health 84(2):290–293, 1994 8296957

Teplin LA, Abram KM, McClelland GM: Prevalence of psychiatric disorders among incarcerated women, I: pretrial jail detainees. Arch Gen Psychiatry 53(6):505–512, 1996 8639033

Torgersen S, Kringlen E, Cramer V: The prevalence of personality disorders in a community sample. Arch Gen Psychiatry 58(6):590–596, 2001 11386989

Trestman RL, Ford J, Zhang W, et al: Current and lifetime psychiatric illness among inmates not identified as acutely mentally ill at intake in Connecticut's jails. J Am Acad Psychiatry Law 35(4):490–500, 2007 18086741

Triandis HC, Gelfand MJ: Converging measurement of horizontal and vertical individualism and collectivism. J Pers Soc Psychol 74(1):118–128, 1998

Tweed JL, George LK, Blazer D, et al: Adult onset of severe and pervasive antisocial behavior: a distinct syndrome? J Pers Disord 8(3):192–202, 1994

U.S. Census Bureau: Selected population profile in the United States: 2017 American Community Survey 1-year estimates. Available at: https://data.census.gov/cedsci/table?q=Selected%20population%20profile%20in%20the%20United%20States%3A%202017%20American%20Community%20Survey%201-year%20estimates&t=006%20%20American%20Indian%20and%20Alaska%20Native%20alone%20%28300,%20A01-Z99%29&hidePreview=true. Accessed July 28, 2019.

Walters GD, Chlumsky ML: The Lifestyle Criminality Screening Form and Antisocial Personality Disorder: predicting release outcome in a state prison sample. Behav Sci Law 11(1):111–115, 1993 10150226

Warren JI, Burnette M, South SC, et al: Personality disorders and violence among female prison inmates. J Am Acad Psychiatry Law 30(4):502–509, 2002 12539904

Weissman MM, Myers JK, Harding PS: Psychiatric disorders in a U.S. urban community: 1975–1976. Am J Psychiatry 135(4):459–462, 1978 637143

Wells JE, Bushnell JA, Hornblow AR, et al: Christchurch Psychiatric Epidemiology Study, part I: methodology and lifetime prevalence for specific psychiatric disorders. Aust N Z J Psychiatry 23(3):315–326, 1989 2803144

Wetherill L, Foroud T, Goodlett C: Meta-analyses of externalizing disorders: genetics or prenatal alcohol exposure? Alcohol Clin Exp Res 42(1):162–172, 2018 29063614

Wichstrøm L, Skogen K, Oia T: Increased rate of conduct problems in urban areas: what is the mechanism? J Am Acad Child Adolesc Psychiatry 35(4):471–479, 1996 8919709

World Health Organization: The ICD-10 Classification of Mental and Behavioural Disorders: Diagnostic Criteria for Research. Geneva, World Health Organization, 1993

Xu Y, Okuda M, Hser YI, et al: Twelve-month prevalence of psychiatric disorders and treatment-seeking among Asian Americans/Pacific Islanders in the United States: results from the National Epidemiological Survey on Alcohol and Related Conditions. J Psychiatr Res 45(7):910–918, 2011 21238989

Zanarini MC, Frankenburg FR, Dubo ED, et al: Axis II comorbidity of borderline personality disorder. Compr Psychiatry 39(5):296–302, 1998 9777282

Zhang W, Ta VM: Social connections, immigration-related factors, and self-rated physical and mental health among Asian Americans. Soc Sci Med 68(12):2104–2112, 2009 19427087

Zimmerman M, Pfohl B, Coryell W, et al: Diagnosing personality disorder in depressed patients: a comparison of patient and informant interviews. Arch Gen Psychiatry 45(8):733–737, 1988 3395201

Zimmerman M, Pfohl B, Coryell WH, et al: Major depression and personality disorder. J Affect Disord 22(4):199–210, 1991 1939929

Zimmerman M, Chelminski I, Posternak MA: Exclusion criteria used in antidepressant efficacy trials: consistency across studies and representativeness of samples included. J Nerv Ment Dis 192(2):87–94, 2004 14770052

Zimmerman M, Rothschild L, Chelminski I: The prevalence of DSM-IV personality disorders in psychiatric outpatients. Am J Psychiatry 162(10):1911–1918, 2005 16199838

Zimmerman M, Chelminski I, Young D: The frequency of personality disorders in psychiatric patients. Psychiatr Clin North Am 31(3):405–420, vi, 2008 18638643

Zlotnick C: Antisocial personality disorder, affect dysregulation and childhood abuse among incarcerated women. J Pers Disord 13(1):90–95, 1999 10228930

Zlotnick C, Zimmerman M, Wolfsdorf BA, et al: Gender differences in patients with posttraumatic stress disorder in a general psychiatric practice. Am J Psychiatry 158(11):1923–1925, 2001 11691704

CHAPTER 4

Psychiatric and Medical Comorbidity of Antisocial Personality Disorder

Patrick T. McGonigal, M.A.

Mark Zimmerman, M.D.

Mario J. Scalora, Ph.D.

Antisocial personality disorder (ASPD) rarely occurs in isolation and is typically comorbid with other psychiatric disorders and medical conditions. Comorbidities complicate the assessment and treatment of patients presenting for services. For example, comorbid disorders in the presence of ASPD are more resistant to treatment. In this chapter, we review the current literature and highlight issues of comorbidity that are commonly encountered when assessing and treating ASPD.

Psychiatric Comorbidity

Patients with ASPD often meet criteria for more than one psychiatric disorder, and their chief complaints are rarely related directly to ASPD itself. Table 4–1 provides a brief overview of selected studies that detail the comorbidity prevalence rates among participants with ASPD and other psychiatric conditions in various settings. Patients with ASPD are likely to seek psychiatric services as a stipulation of probation, as a component of a substance use clinic, or within institutional settings. Research suggests that contrary to stereotypes and widely held assumptions, patients with ASPD can respond positively to treatment interventions (Black 2017; Dixon-Gordon et al. 2011). However, high rates of comorbidity and clinical characteristics associated with ASPD (i.e., treatment noncompliance, irresponsibility) often lead to chronic service use and criminal recidivism among this population, which can have considerable personal and societal costs (DeLisi et al. 2018; Gibson et al. 2010). Recurrent reoffending and antisocial behavior require additional law enforcement personnel (i.e., correctional officers, social workers), legal services (i.e., legal counseling, trials, and prosecution), and criminal justice involvement (i.e., incarceration, postrelease monitoring; Reidy et al. 2015). Higher service use may involve recurrent hospitalizations, more clinical interactions with therapists and psychiatrists, and case management.

One reason for high use of services might be that patients with comorbid conditions are significantly less likely to complete and respond to interventions (Bock et al. 2010; Krawczyk et al. 2017). This could be especially true for patients diagnosed with ASPD and comorbid psychiatric disorders (Bock et al. 2010). In correctional settings where the incidence of ASPD is higher, comorbid psychiatric conditions (i.e., mood and anxiety disorders, psychosis) are common and predict higher rates of reoffending (Ogloff et al. 2015). Personality disorder symptoms tend to contribute to the etiology and maintenance of these forms of psychopathology (e.g., depression, anxiety). Thus, the presence of personality disorder symptoms in patients with these seemingly unrelated psychiatric concerns should not be ignored (Tyrer et al. 2015; Zimmerman et al. 2008).

Demographic Considerations

It is well established that ASPD is diagnosed more frequently in men than in women (Alegria et al. 2013), although clinical presentations among patients with ASPD differ between men and women (Alegria et al. 2013; Cale and Lilienfeld 2002; Goldstein et al. 1996; Sher et al. 2015). Some of these differences are early developing; in childhood, females with ASPD are more likely to have shown socially defiant behaviors, such as running away from home, whereas males are more likely to have engaged in interpersonal aggression (i.e., animal cruelty, fire setting, using weapons; Goldstein et al. 1996).

Differences across gender translate to comorbid concerns as well. Females with ASPD report experiencing emotional and sexual abuse in childhood more frequently than do males with ASPD (Sher et al. 2015), so females with ASPD may be more likely to develop PTSD or other traumatic stress responses. In adulthood, women with ASPD may be more likely to meet criteria for a comorbid Cluster B personality disorder (i.e., histrionic, borderline) and comorbid mood disorders (Sher et al. 2015). By contrast, men with ASPD generally interact more frequently with law enforcement and report engaging in more frequent antisocial behaviors (Sher et al. 2015).

Externalizing Disorder Comorbidity

Given the externalizing features of ASPD, it is not surprising that patients with the disorder are significantly more likely to have comorbid externalizing psychiatric conditions (i.e., substance use disorders, impulse-control disorders, ADHD). Because externalizing behavioral issues (i.e., antisocial behavior, anger outbursts, impulsivity, recklessness) are embedded within ASPD criteria, differential diagnosis may become particularly challenging. Specifically, the clinician must decide whether presenting issues are best accounted for by ASPD, a separate diagnosis, or a comorbid presentation. These diagnostic considerations are important because they pose questions for which clinical issues warrant treatment priority and which interventions to implement. The high rate of comorbid externalizing issues and ASPD may predict more

TABLE 4–1. Percentage of comorbidity among participants with antisocial personality disorder (ASPD) reported by study

Study	N	Method	Sample	MDD	BD	GAD	SAD	PTSD	ADHD	AUD/SUD	PG	BPD	NPD	HPD	Any PD
Alegria et al. 2013[a]	1,226	AUDASIS	Community	24.4	24.3	19.9	—	13.4	12.3	88.7	2.4	21.8	19.1	12.3	57.0
Black et al. 2010	320	MINI	Forensic	33.6	66.5	31.0	20.4	20.4	33.6	98.2	—	44.1	—	—	—
Coid 2003	260	SCID	Forensic	51.0	16.0	—	—	—	—	46.0	—	61.0	67.0	68.0	—
Darke et al. 2004	615	DIS	Substance clinic	—	—	—	—	—	—	—	—	38.0	—	—	—
Dowling et al. 2015	2,370	Meta-analysis	Meta-analysis	—	—	—	—	—	—	—	14.0	—	—	—	—
Evren et al. 2006	132	SCID	Inpatient	45.2	—	—	—	—	—	64.5	—	—	—	—	—
Goodwin and Hamilton 2003	5,877	CIDI	Community	30.6[b]	—	14.6	30.9	20.9	—	62.8[b]	—	—	—	—	—
Hodgins et al. 2010	495	DIS	Forensic	—	—	48.4	10.0	15.0	—	—	—	—	—	—	—
Marmorstein 2006[c]	8,098	CIDI	Community	30.3	—	14.8	30.8	21.0	—	82.6	—	—	—	—	—
McGonigal et al. 2019	2,691	SCID	Outpatient	57.6	22.0	—	—	44.1	13.6	83.1	—	—	—	—	52.5
Mueser et al. 2006	178	SCID	Substance clinic	—	21.1	—	—	—	—	89.5	—	—	—	—	—
Ogloff et al. 2015	130	SCID	Forensic	—	—	—	—	—	—	91.1	—	—	—	—	—
Semiz et al. 2008	105	SCID	Forensic	—	—	—	—	—	65.0	—	—	—	—	—	—

TABLE 4–1. Percentage of comorbidity among participants with antisocial personality disorder (ASPD) reported by study *(continued)*

Study	N	Method	Sample	MDD	BD	GAD	SAD	PTSD	ADHD	AUD/SUD	PG	BPD	NPD	HPD	Any PD
Soloff et al. 2005	119	SCID	Inpatient	—	—	—	—	—	—	—	—	23.9	—	—	—
Swann et al. 2013[c]	55	SCID	Community	—	12.1	—	—	—	—	62.7	—	—	—	—	—
Ullrich and Coid 2009[c]	8,395	SCID	Community	4.9	—	11.0	—	—	—	36.9	—	—	—	—	—

Note.   AUD=alcohol use disorder; AUDASIS=Alcohol Use Disorder and Associated Disabilities Interview Schedule for DSM-IV; BD=bipolar disorder; BPD=borderline personality disorder; CIDI=Composite International Diagnostic Interview; DIS=Diagnostic Interview Schedule; GAD=generalized anxiety disorder; HPD=histrionic personality disorder; MDD=major depressive disorder; MINI=Mini-International Neuropsychiatric Interview; NPD=narcissistic personality disorder; PD=personality disorder; PG=pathological gambling; SAD=social anxiety disorder; SCID=Structured Clinical Interview for DSM-IV; SUD=substance use disorder.
Rates provided reflect lifetime prevalence unless otherwise stated. Em dashes indicate that prevalence data on disorder were not included in the reviewed study.
[a]Prevalence rates generated by averaging percentage rates provided between male and female participants.
[b]Prevalence rates generated by averaging percentage rates provided between ASPD/no anxiety disorder and ASPD/anxiety disorder.
[c]Time frame of prevalence is not noted.

negative outcomes, including a greater propensity toward chronic psychosocial issues (i.e., homelessness, incarceration), violent behaviors, interactions with the law, and issues in interpersonal relationships. Furthermore, externalizing disorder comorbidity may augment the severity of antisocial personality traits (e.g., Black et al. 2010; Moeller and Dougherty 2001), highlighting the importance of assessing for comorbid externalizing disorders throughout the course of treatment.

Substance Use and Alcohol Use Disorders

Patients with ASPD are at an increased risk for developing substance use disorders throughout the course of the life span. In a sample of injection drug users, approximately 23% met criteria for ASPD (Havens et al. 2007). In fact, up to 85% of patients with ASPD present to clinical settings with problems relating to drug or alcohol use (Marmorstein 2006; Robins et al. 1991). Such difficulties with alcohol and drugs tend to begin earlier in life for patients with ASPD, and they often have family members who also have substance use concerns (Pietrzak and Petry 2005; Westermeyer and Thuras 2005). Furthermore, patients with comorbid alcohol use disorder and Cluster B personality disorders, such as ASPD, tend to have marked deficits in decision-making compared with patients with comorbid alcohol use disorder and Cluster A and C personality disorders (Dom et al. 2006). This impaired decision-making, along with the other adverse effects of illicit substance use, may underscore the pervasive pattern of behavioral concerns central to patients with ASPD (i.e., engaging in fights, sensation-seeking behavior).

Substance use may compound the severity of antisocial traits and potentially affect treatment engagement and response. For instance, substance use generally amplifies aggressive tendencies, particularly among antisocial patients (Moeller and Dougherty 2001). Although many researchers and clinicians note the difficulties of engaging patients with ASPD in treatment interventions given treatment-interfering behaviors (e.g., difficulties completing homework assignments, ruptures in therapeutic alliance; Bender 2005; Frances and Ross 2001; Freeman and Rosenfield 2002), some evidence suggests that substance use treatment can have positive effects on patients with ASPD (Cacciola et al. 1995). In a sample of injection drug users with ASPD, a greater amount of time spent with case managers predicted the likelihood of initiating substance use treatment (Havens et al. 2007).

Patients with ASPD and comorbid alcohol use disorder may benefit from pharmacotherapy as well. Ralevski et al. (2007) found that patients with comorbid ASPD and alcohol use disorder responded similarly to patients without comorbid ASPD within a randomized trial of disulfiram and naltrexone. Although patients with ASPD are significantly more likely to undergo multiple modalities of substance use treatment compared with patients without ASPD, evidence suggests that these treatments can have benefits for patients with ASPD (Westermeyer and Thuras 2005).

Impulse-Control Disorders

Impulse-control disorders, which may be used in diagnosis to reflect problematic behaviors such as pathological gambling and compulsive sexual behavior, are comorbid to various extents with ASPD (Dowling et al. 2015; Raymond et al. 2003). Impulse-control disorders represent a class of addictive disorders in which repetitive urges are uncontrollable, and engagement in behaviors persists despite negative reactions or consequences (Brewer and Potenza 2008). Given the propensity toward externalizing behaviors and sensation seeking among individuals with ASPD, it may not be surprising that comorbid impulse-control disorders are prevalent. In fact, behaviors reflected in impulse-control disorders are so central to behaviors observed in those with ASPD (i.e., gambling, fire setting, theft, anger) that exclusion criteria instruct clinicians not to diagnose impulse-control disorders if better accounted for by ASPD (American Psychiatric Association 2013). Nevertheless, impulse-control disorders have clinical features (i.e., genetic risk, reward deficits, neurobiological agents) that can be distinguished from ASPD (Brady et al. 1998; Brewer and Potenza 2008), and patients with ASPD do present with comorbid impulse-control disorders above and beyond presenting personality pathology.

The most widely studied comorbid impulse-control disorder for people with ASPD is pathological gambling disorder. Evidence suggests that pathological gambling may serve similar behavioral functions as substance use disorders (Petry 2001) but may share similar familial predispositions as ASPD (Black et al. 2006; Slutske et al. 2001). A large twin study of 4,497 male pairs from the community found that genetic factors accounted for 66% of the relationship between pathological gambling and ASPD and that patients with pathological gambling were 6.4 times more likely to meet criteria for ASPD (Slutske et al. 2001). Patients with comorbid pathological gambling and ASPD are likely to have more severe gambling issues, gamble more frequently, have stolen from family members to gamble, and report beginning habitual gambling (i.e., once a week) at an earlier age (Pietrzak and Petry 2005). Another study found that patients with comorbid ASPD and pathological gambling had neurological deficits in executive functioning and decision-making (Blum et al. 2017).

Research evidence on other impulse-control disorders (i.e., compulsive sexual behavior, pyromania) is scarce compared with evidence on pathological gambling, perhaps because of a lower base rate of incidence. This lower base rate of comorbidity may be due to the ASPD exclusion criteria for diagnosing impulse-control disorders, including intermittent explosive disorder. Nevertheless, some evidence indicates that antisocial personality may be associated with problematic behaviors reflected in these impulse-control disorders. In a small sample of individuals with compulsive sexual behavior, two individuals (11%) met criteria for ASPD (Raymond et al. 2003). In a study of 313 veterans, sexual addiction was modestly correlated with antisocial personality features as measured by the Millon Clinical Multiaxial Inventory-II (Nelson and Oehlert 2008). Furthermore, antisocial personality features may be 22 times more likely to present in fire setters compared with a control group, even after accounting for comorbid substance use (Dickens and Sugarman 2012). As in patients with substance use disorders, evidence suggests that individuals undergoing treatment for impulse-control disorders can experience benefits in certain domains. In a randomized trial of cognitive-behavioral therapy for pathological gambling, individuals with ASPD responded similarly compared with those without ASPD throughout the course of treatment (Ledgerwood et al. 2007).

ADHD

ADHD is characterized by features of pervasive inattention, impulsivity, or hyperactivity typically beginning in childhood. ADHD is indicated in 33%–65% of adults with ASPD and is highly comorbid with conduct disorder in childhood (Black et al.

2010; Semiz et al. 2008). A large meta-analysis suggests that the presence of ADHD predicts the likelihood of developing antisocial personality features in adulthood, particularly when comorbid with conduct disorder in childhood (Holmes et al. 2001; Storebø and Simonsen 2016). The latter, however, is a more robust independent predictor of developing ASPD in adulthood (Lahey et al. 2005). Several theorized mechanisms may contribute to the development of conduct disorder and later ASPD among children with ADHD. For example, children with ADHD may have difficulties complying with authority and learning from past behavior. They may have poorer academic performance and institutional quality and display disruptive classroom behavior (e.g., truancy), all of which may contribute to the etiology of early antisocial behavior (Holmes et al. 2001).

Both ADHD and ASPD are independently predictive of problematic outcomes in adulthood, including experiencing motor vehicle accidents, recidivism among offenders, and alcohol abuse (Dumais et al. 2005; Knop et al. 2009; Roy et al. 2020; Young and Thome 2011). When ADHD is comorbid with conduct disorder, the risk for these behaviors may be even greater (Knop et al. 2009). In adulthood, comorbid ASPD and ADHD additionally heighten the risk for greater psychosocial impairment, suicide attempts, self-injurious behaviors, and expression of other forms of comorbid psychopathology (Black et al. 2010; Semiz et al. 2008). Evidence suggests that interventions that include anger management can be effective for children who have ADHD and aggressive behavior (Miranda and Presentación 2000). In adults, treatment may be particularly effective when conducted in the context of highly structured settings (Ginsberg and Lindefors 2012; Retz and Retz-Junginger 2014). This may be attributable in part to the likelihood of premature dropout from treatment among patients with comorbid ASPD and ADHD.

Learning Disorders and Intellectual Disability

Evidence suggests that difficulties with learning, reading, and educational attainment in childhood are associated with antisocial behavior. Evidence suggests that among males with antisocial behavior, up to half may struggle with reading comprehension (Maughan et al. 1985). In a large twin study, results indicated that the relation between antisocial behavior and reading achievement was more strongly influenced by environmental factors (e.g., stimulating environment, socioeconomic status) than by genetic factors (Trzesniewski et al. 2006). Difficulties with learning and reading may be exacerbated given the likelihood of discontinuing education, truancy, and behavioral misconduct in school environments among students with antisocial behavior and conduct disorder (French and Conrad 2001; Kessler et al. 1995). These difficulties in childhood may have an indirect effect on developing ASPD in adulthood in the context of other important risk factors (i.e., conduct disorder, early criminality; Simonoff et al. 2004). Furthermore, children with learning difficulties and antisocial behavior tend to have worse outcomes after leaving school (i.e., unemployment; Maughan et al. 1985). Assessing for comorbid learning disorders among at-risk children may assist in preventing the development of ASPD in adulthood and associated negative outcomes by promoting educational completion and academic achievement.

Intellectually disabled individuals sometimes meet criteria for ASPD. Full-blown cases of ASPD have been reported in which the individual has engaged in criminal behavior, impulsive and aggressive acts, deceitfulness, and lack of remorse; he or she might even have had a history of arrests or incarceration (Hurley and Sovner 1995). Other individuals with intellectual disability might have difficult behaviors that directly result from the intellectual disability. In those cases, the individual might not fit within the antisocial syndrome. Assessment of ASPD can be complicated by communication difficulties or behavior problems that appear to result from the intellectual disability itself (Morrissey and Hollin 2010).

Internalizing Disorder Comorbidity

Although the relation between ASPD and externalizing syndromes may be more readily apparent, ASPD also can be comorbid with internalizing syndromes. Some may be quick to dismiss the co-occurrence of internalizing symptoms, such as depression or anxiety, among patients with ASPD, perhaps because of an assumption that these patients generally lack empathy and remorse, negative emotion, or regard for others. These assumptions stem from stereotypes and do not generalize to all patients who meet criteria for ASPD. Empirical evidence suggests that certain internalizing disorders are prevalent in this population (Goodwin and Hamilton 2003; McGonigal et al. 2019; Ullrich and Coid 2009). Internalizing symptoms are evidenced to motivate independent treatment seeking among these patients who otherwise may not seek services (Ullrich and Coid 2009), and this distress may be an important predictor of treatment success for patients with ASPD (Modesto-Lowe and Kranzler 1999). The characteristics of these disorders may create unique challenges for clinicians; thus, understanding their comorbidity is essential.

Major Depressive and Bipolar Disorders

Depressive and manic episodes are common among patients with ASPD. Major depressive disorder and bipolar disorder may present in up to 65% and 22% of patients, respectively (McGonigal et al. 2019; Mueser et al. 2006). Patients with ASPD are likely to encounter a range of life stressors, often self-initiated. The occurrence of life stressors is associated with a higher risk for depression recurrence among patients with ASPD, particularly when stressors involve loss or change in relationship (Perry et al. 1992). The incidence of suicide attempts is particularly high for patients with ASPD, and antisocial personality traits are a significant risk factor for attempted suicide (Douglas et al. 2008; Verona et al. 2001; Zimmerman et al. 2012). This may be due to the impulsive and reckless nature of the disorder (Gvion and Apter 2011). However, some evidence suggests that this relationship is accounted for by traits characteristic of other personality disorders (i.e., negative affectivity; Verona et al. 2001). Nevertheless, depressive symptoms in patients with ASPD heighten the risk for suicidality and suicide attempts, particularly among patients with comorbid substance use issues (Evren et al. 2006).

Depressed patients with a history of antisocial behavior are more likely to engage in problematic substance use and experience irritability within the context of depressive episodes (Rowe et al. 1996). Among a sample of patients with bipolar disorder, antisocial personality traits were related to a higher frequency of mood episodes, substance use, and early onset of mania (Swann et al. 2013). Mood disorders may affect the assessment of personality disorders as well; depressed patients tend to underrate symptoms of personality disorder compared with informants (Zimmerman et al. 1988). Taken together, these findings suggest that patients with comorbid ASPD and mood disorders present with several complex clinical issues, including more problematic substance use, suicidality, and course of mood illness. These clinical issues have significant implications for the assessment and treatment of ASPD.

PTSD

Estimates of PTSD range from 14% to 45% in patients with ASPD (Alegria et al. 2013; McGonigal et al. 2019). Experiences of childhood abuse and neglect are common in this population. In a large epidemiological study, childhood physical abuse was indicated in approximately 42% of individuals with ASPD, and sexual abuse was present in 27% of these individuals (Afifi et al. 2011). In adulthood, offenders with ASPD are significantly more likely to have experienced physical trauma and crime-related trauma (i.e., home burglary, being mugged, held at gunpoint; Gobin et al. 2015). Several theories have emerged that implicate childhood trauma as a clinical mechanism of etiology and maintenance of antisocial personality features (e.g., Martens 2006). Researchers suggest that experiences of trauma throughout the life span may result in difficulties regulating emotions and anger experiences, leading to antisocial behavior in adulthood (Gobin et al. 2015). Empirical evidence suggests that early childhood trauma not only is a significant risk factor for antisocial behavior in later childhood and adulthood (Ardino 2012; Armstrong and Kelley 2008; Bruce and Laporte 2015) but also predicts the severity of such behaviors in adulthood (Bruce and Laporte 2015). ASPD features additionally affect the degree to which individuals with PTSD respond to interventions such as anger management, potentially because of lower treatment engagement (Marshall et al. 2010).

Anxiety Disorders

The lifetime prevalence of anxiety disorders, such as generalized anxiety disorder (GAD) and social anxiety disorder, in patients with ASPD is between 30% and 50% (Goodwin and Hamilton 2003; Hodgins et al. 2010; McGonigal et al. 2019; Ullrich and Coid 2009). It is theorized that antisocial behavior may be used as a form of coping with high rates of anxiety among patients with ASPD (Goodwin and Hamilton 2003). The presence of an anxiety disorder may exacerbate risk for major depression, substance use, and suicidality in patients who have ASPD (Goodwin and Hamilton 2003). Patients with ASPD who experience comorbid internalizing disorder symptoms—particularly acute anxiety disorders—are more likely to seek outpatient services from psychologists, psychiatrists, and social workers (Ullrich and Coid 2009). This may be attributable to the high levels of physiological and psychological distress commonly experienced by patients with anxiety disorders. Offenders with ASPD and comorbid anxiety disorders report a higher number of diagnostic criteria and are more likely to meet criteria for comorbid substance use disorders, alcohol use disorders, and persistent depressive disorder. They are also significantly more likely to experience suicidal ideation and suicide attempts (Hodgins et al. 2010). Patients with ASPD and comorbid anxiety disorders may fare worse in treatment given the additive risk of experiencing co-occurring psychopathology and adverse outcomes (i.e., substance relapse, suicidality).

Malingering

Individuals with ASPD and personality pathology may malinger in clinical settings, which may be expected given deceitfulness as a symptom of ASPD. DSM-5 (American

Psychiatric Association 2013) acknowledges that ASPD and malingering behavior are related. Malingering is listed among "Other Conditions That May Be a Focus of Clinical Attention," which are not attributable to mental illness (i.e., Z-code conditions). The essential feature "is the intentional production of false or grossly exaggerated physical or psychological symptoms, motivated by external incentives such as avoiding military duty, avoiding work, obtaining financial compensation, evading criminal prosecution, or obtaining drugs" (American Psychiatric Association 2013, p. 726). According to DSM-5, "Malingering should be strongly suspected...[in] the presence of antisocial personality disorder" (p. 727). For example, an antisocial man seeks hospitalization for suicidal thoughts or plans during winter to escape the cold temperatures.

Empirical evidence establishing malingering as an inherent component of ASPD is somewhat mixed (Niesten et al. 2015). Some studies suggest an association between antisocial and psychopathic traits and malingering behavior (e.g., Delain et al. 2003; Grillo et al. 1994); other researchers have not established such relationships (Poythress et al. 2001; van Impelen et al. 2018). Scholars note that although patients with ASPD are known to malinger or exaggerate symptoms, clinicians should be cautious and avoid assuming that all patients with ASPD are exaggerating symptoms (Hong et al. 2019). When malingering is suspected, clinicians should consider underlying motivations driving the patient's feigned or exaggerated symptoms while communicating clear boundaries (Hong et al. 2019). Just as clinical presentations vary among patients with ASPD, malingering behavior also may vary in this population, depending on setting, context, and motivation. Thus, we suggest the use of evidence-based assessment tools (e.g., Structured Interview of Reported Symptoms, Structured Inventory of Malingered Symptomatology, validity scales) in conjunction with effort tests (e.g., Test of Memory Malingering, Rey 15 Item Test, Dot Counting Test) when possible to formally evaluate feigned or exaggerated symptoms to inform a cohesive case conceptualization.

Personality Disorders

Modern conceptualizations of personality pathology argue that personality disorders lie along a multidimensional continuum representing dysfunctional and maladaptive traits (Kotov et al. 2017; Widiger et al. 2009). This perspective of personality disorders allows for a more nuanced characterization of presentations that do not neatly conform to established standards of outlined criteria. This continued push for new guidelines is partly the result of high rates of comorbidity among personality disorders (Kotov et al. 2018; Widiger et al. 2009). Approximately half of patients with ASPD may meet criteria for more than one personality disorder (McGonigal et al. 2019), namely within the Cluster B group of personality disorders (i.e., borderline, narcissistic, histrionic; Coid 2003). These are generally characterized by negative affectivity (i.e., dysregulation, hostility), antagonism (i.e., manipulation, grandiosity), and disinhibition (i.e., impulsivity; Anderson et al. 2014; Watson and Sinha 1998).

Comorbid Cluster B personality disorders may present with additional challenges for clinicians, including treatment resistance and clinical severity (Ozkan and Altindag 2005; Shea et al. 1992). Patients with comorbid Cluster B personality disorders report more frequent instances of childhood trauma, suicidality, and depression (Garno et al. 2005; Soloff et al. 2005). Cluster B personality symptoms also affect the course of illness among patients with comorbid bipolar disorder because these personality traits are associated with shorter periods of time in between manic and depressive episodes (Ng et al. 2017). The average life expectancy for patients with comorbid Cluster B personality disorders is reduced by 9–13 years, perhaps because of increased associations with suicide attempts and fatal medical conditions (Cailhol et al. 2017). Comorbid Cluster B personality disorders are therefore imperative to identify and target in interventions as they affect the course of comorbid psychiatric conditions and have potentially fatal consequences. This may be especially valuable given the personality traits (e.g., impulsivity, negative affectivity) that increase risk for adverse outcomes within this cluster of disorders.

Special attention to comorbid borderline personality disorder (BPD) and ASPD is certainly warranted given the high degree of comorbidity. Estimates of comorbidity range from approximately 20% in community and inpatient settings (Alegria et al. 2013; Soloff et al. 2005) to upward of 60% in forensic samples (Black et al. 2010; Coid 2003). ASPD and BPD share several commonalities across diagnostic criteria (i.e., anger, impulsivity), but evidence suggests that these characteristics may be experienced differentially depending on the disorder (McGonigal and Dixon-Gordon 2020). Patients with comorbid ASPD and BPD have a particularly severe clinical presentation. Compared with patients with ASPD or BPD alone, patients with this comorbidity tend to pose significantly higher risk for violent offending and suicidal behavior (Freestone et al. 2013; Howard et al. 2014). In addition to violence risk, these patients are more likely to exhibit childhood misconduct across a range of antisocial behaviors and are at higher risk for meeting criteria for substance use and alcohol use disorders (Freestone et al. 2013). Analyses suggest that comorbid borderline personality pathology may better account for deleterious outcomes among patients with ASPD (i.e., suicidality, self-harm; Darke et al. 2004; Verona et al. 2001); thus, clinicians must attend to this comorbidity when diagnosing ASPD.

Symptom Overlap and Differential Diagnosis

In addition to the high rate of psychiatric comorbidity, the symptoms of ASPD are typically shared with other psychiatric disorders. Table 4–2 highlights the potential shared features of ASPD and other forms of psychopathology. This overlap creates significant difficulty distinguishing ASPD from other psychiatric illnesses. The ASPD diagnosis is particularly stigmatizing, and the diagnosis has significant implications within health care and forensic settings (Cunningham and Reidy 1998; Sheehan et al. 2016). For example, individuals with ASPD are less likely to be seen as mentally ill by court officials; are likely to be seen as dangerous, violent, and responsible for criminal offenses; and may be less likely to receive requisite services in criminal justice settings (Sheehan et al. 2016). These potential consequences highlight the importance of understanding symptom overlap and differential diagnosis, to ensure an accurate diagnosis of ASPD and comorbid conditions.

Anger and Irritability

Aggression and behavioral outbursts are central features of ASPD as well as other psychiatric disorders. Targeting anger in treatment settings where ASPD is more common (i.e., correctional settings) is typically prioritized among health care staff

TABLE 4–2.   Antisocial personality disorder (ASPD) symptom overlap across psychiatric disorders

ASPD symptom criteria	Shared criterion or characteristic
Anger, aggression, or irritability	BPD, PTSD, IED, GAD, SUD, psychosis
Violation of social norms	BPD, ODD
Impulsivity	BPD, BD, PTSD, SUD, IC, ADHD
Irresponsibility	ADHD
Deceitfulness	SUD, IC
Recklessness and sensation seeking	BPD, PTSD, ADHD, BD, SUD, IC
Lack of empathy	Psychopathy, NPD, PD
Evidence of conduct disorder before age 15 years[a]	ADHD, ODD

Note.   BD=bipolar disorder; BPD=borderline personality disorder; GAD=generalized anxiety disorder; IC=impulse-control disorder; IED=intermittent explosive disorder; NPD=narcissistic personality disorder; ODD=oppositional defiant disorder; PD=personality disorder; SUD=substance use disorder.
[a]Although evidence of conduct disorder is not required to diagnose ADHD or ODD, behavioral and conduct issues are common among children diagnosed with ADHD and ODD.

within the institution to reduce the risk of violence or recidivism (Jones and Hollin 2004). However, anger in ASPD may be experienced and expressed differentially depending on comorbid conditions (McGonigal and Dixon-Gordon 2020; Scott et al. 2014). Therefore, determining differential diagnosis and attending to psychiatric comorbidity in which anger is a defining feature are important as clinicians weigh potential treatment options.

The presence of anger, irritability, and aggression are diagnostic characteristics of several psychiatric conditions such as bipolar disorder, PTSD, GAD, intermittent explosive disorder, BPD, and substance use disorder (American Psychiatric Association 2013). In these disorders, anger may be a primary facet to the disorder (e.g., intermittent explosive disorder), a consequence of a clinically significant experience (e.g., rumination in GAD, trauma in PTSD), or related to withdrawal (e.g., substance use and addictive disorders). In fact, anger and irritability may permeate across a wide range of other internalizing and externalizing mental disorders in which anger is not a diagnostic feature (Cassiello-Robbins and Barlow 2016). In particular, empirical evidence suggests that the most elevated anger experiences exist within the context of major depression, panic disorder, agoraphobia, PTSD, intermittent explosive disorder, and Cluster B personality disorders (Genovese et al. 2017). This study also suggested that reported levels of anger were generally equivalent to reported experiences of anxiety and depression, indicating the relevance of anger to patients with a variety of psychiatric disorders (Genovese et al. 2017). When a patient with several psychiatric complaints presents to a clinician, the clinician must assess which condition(s) to attribute the overlapping symptoms to. For the example of anger, the clinician must decide whether the anger the patient is experiencing is related to genuine antisocial personality characteristics, trauma in the case of PTSD, worry and rumination in the case of GAD, mania in the case of bipolar disorder, frustration following a loss in the case of bereavement, or withdrawal in the case of substance abuse or whether the case represents comorbidity among several disorders.

Impulsivity and Recklessness

The criterion of impulsivity is complex because this characteristic has several defini- tions in the field with differential consequences and implications (Evenden 1999). As defined in DSM-5, impulsivity refers to "a failure to plan ahead" (American Psychi- atric Association 2013, p. 659). That is, "decisions are made on the spur of the mo- ment, without forethought and without consideration for the consequences to self or others; this may lead to sudden changes of jobs, residences, or relationships" (Amer- ican Psychiatric Association 2013, p. 660). Here, impulsivity may refer to major life changes that have marked effects on the patient or those around him or her. Relatedly, recklessness refers to an apparent lack of disregard for safety as characterized by dan- gerous behaviors such as reckless driving, risky sexual behavior, and drug use. Ex- tending toward the safety and well-being of others, this criterion also may refer to neglect of a child or child endangerment (American Psychiatric Association 2013, p. 660). Impulsivity is an especially concerning clinical feature because it compro- mises the safety of the patient and others. Indeed, impulsivity is associated with higher rates of risky sexual behavior, suicide attempts and ideation, and violent be- havior (Cunradi et al. 2009; Dudley et al. 2004; Klonsky and May 2010; McCoul and Haslam 2001).

　　Like anger, impulsivity and recklessness are characteristics that may be attribut- able to several common comorbid psychiatric conditions among patients with ASPD. Although these behaviors may have differential pathways of etiology and develop- ment depending on the comorbid condition, they may present very similarly across patients. This can create confusion and frustration when deciding on a diagnosis of ASPD. Impulsivity and reckless behavior in patients with BPD and PTSD are more likely to manifest as binge-eating episodes, risky sexual behavior, reckless spending, and substance use (American Psychiatric Association 2013). These behaviors are po- tentially attributable to shared deficits in emotion regulation processes (Chapman et al. 2008; Weiss et al. 2012). Among patients with ADHD, however, impulsivity may be more attributable to differences in neurodevelopment (Winstanley et al. 2006).

　　Although impulsive behavior may intensify in manic episodes among patients with bipolar disorder, evidence suggests that impulsivity may actually serve as a trait component among patients with the disorder because it is experienced and expressed in mood variations outside of manic episodes (Najt et al. 2007). Patients with higher trait-impulsivity are also more likely to develop substance use and addictive disor- ders, potentially as a result of significant genetic vulnerabilities (Verdejo-García et al. 2008). Thus, a patient presenting with high-risk behavioral issues caused by impul- sivity or recklessness may be a candidate for ASPD, an entirely separate diagnostic category, or both.

Distinguishing Features

As reviewed, ASPD has several shared symptoms and features that are common among other forms of psychopathology (e.g., BPD, PTSD, ADHD). These shared features complicate the diagnostic process, especially when a patient presents with several comorbid psychiatric conditions. However, ASPD has several unique characteristics that may assist in distinguishing the disorder from other similar conditions. These features may help clinicians separate ASPD from other common comorbid conditions.

Lack of Empathy

The criterion of lacking empathy is largely unique to personality disorders and may serve as a distinguishing feature when diagnostic uncertainty occurs. Lack of empathy is shared with DSM-5 narcissistic personality disorder and within the interpersonal deficits criteria of the proposed alternative DSM-5 model for personality disorders. This contemporary form of personality disorder conceptualization indicates that deficits in empathy generalize more broadly across personality disorders but present differently depending on the diagnosis. For example, in ASPD, deficits in empathy are defined as a "lack of concern for feelings, needs, or suffering of others; lack of remorse after hurting or mistreating another" (American Psychiatric Association 2013, p. 764). Yet in the alternative model for schizotypal personality disorder, impairment in empathy refers to a "pronounced difficulty understanding [the] impact of own behaviors on others; frequent misinterpretations of others' motivations and behaviors" (American Psychiatric Association 2013, p. 769). The empathy of narcissistic personality disorder refers to self-absorption and a lack of concern with others unless there is a direct effect on the patient (American Psychiatric Association 2013, p. 767). The characteristic of lack of empathy is embedded within the features of personality disorders but not in other forms of psychopathology. Establishing the presence of this symptom when assessing for ASPD may assist in identifying and diagnosing personality pathology when questions of differential diagnosis are apparent.

Differentiating Personality Disorder From Other Psychopathologies

Differentiating between other conditions and ASPD requires a fundamental understanding of unique aspects of personality disorder that are distinct from other forms of psychopathology. Many factors are thought to contribute to the etiology of personality disorders and ASPD in particular (e.g., genetic risk, neuropsychological factors, traumatic experiences), but a defining feature of personality disorders is the longstanding and consistent presentation across the life span, particularly with origins in childhood (Farrington 1991; Reichborn-Kjennerud et al. 2015). Arguably, the requirement of conduct disorder when diagnosing ASPD illustrates this developmental pathway. Of course, other forms of psychopathology may similarly begin in childhood (e.g., depression, PTSD, GAD, bipolar disorder, substance abuse). However, personality disorders are unique in that they represent chronic, rigid, and pervasive patterns of maladaptive behaviors interfering in a range of interpersonal and intrapersonal contexts (Shea et al. 1992; Skodol et al. 2011).

Case Example

Mr. A, a 22-year-old white man, was referred to a psychiatric day hospital from an emergency department. He was brought to the emergency department by his mother who expressed increasing concern about his behavior since he had returned from a study abroad experience and moved in with her 3 months earlier. She reported that he was engaging in reckless behavior and substance abuse and was recently arrested for attempting to evade the police after being pulled over for speeding. Prior to this visit to the emergency department, Mr. A had visited the hospital on two additional occasions: to address symptoms of premature ejaculation and to seek a psychiatric evaluation after an impulsive suicide attempt while incarcerated. During these visits, he was diagnosed with GAD and an unspecified bipolar disorder. At the most recent visit to the emergency department, he was diagnosed with bipolar I disorder and was given a prescription for quetiapine to address manic symptoms. Physicians made a referral for intensive psychiatric treatment through the day hospital on campus.

As part of routine clinical practice, Mr. A was given a comprehensive psychiatric evaluation, which included the Structured Clinical Interview for DSM-IV and the Structured Interview for DSM-IV Personality. On initiation of the interview, Mr. A expressed concern about the bipolar I diagnosis and sought diagnostic clarity, particularly because he felt that the quetiapine was "not working" ("I want to find out if I'm doing these risky activities because I like it or because I'm manic"). He described a long-standing history of experiencing significant anger and initiating physical fights with others, engaging in reckless behavior (i.e., drag racing, drug dealing, driving under the influence), acting irresponsibly by adding significant debts without enough income ("I bought a $40,000 truck, and I don't have a job"), having inconsistent patterns of work behavior, and being deceitful via lying to his mother and feigning suicidality and aggressive behavior in jail ("I wanted to get into a different cell. I punched a wall to portray myself as mentally unstable"). When asked if he felt sorry for his past actions, Mr. A replied: "I do feel sorry. I feel sorry that I tried to convey my message to people, and they didn't get it."

Mr. A noted that he had recently moved back home with his parents after leaving university but that these symptoms were consistently present throughout his lifetime. This behavior even extended into early childhood as Mr. A described slashing tires, breaking and entering, shoplifting, conning others, and skipping school as an early adolescent. Although Mr. A did describe a history of depressive episodes throughout his life, he denied experiencing discrete periods of elevated mood ("I was always doing these things"). He stated, "Other people were noticing things that have just been normal for me, like partying and drugs. I never felt *too* good or *too* hyper. After I was arrested, it really amplified the situation. My mom got even more concerned, and we started getting into even more arguments."

Mr. A has a classic case of ASPD. His antisocial traits began at a young age and evolved into a full-blown antisocial syndrome. In this case example, emergency department providers incorrectly diagnosed bipolar disorder instead of ASPD. Throughout the interview, he endorsed several symptoms that were easily misinterpreted and misconstrued by other professionals as mania but were more indicative of antisocial traits. Within acute psychiatric settings, the likelihood of incorrectly diagnosing a personality disorder when one is contraindicated is significantly higher (Zimmerman et al. 2008), yet the opposite was true in this example. The severity of antisocial symptoms in this case could have led to a diagnostic bias. A careful examination of Mr. A's childhood symptoms would have suggested the presence of a long-standing history of antisocial traits throughout his life span, which could have conditionally ruled out bipolar disorder. Additionally, inquiring about the presence of antisocial behavior in the absence of elevated mood would have uncovered the inflexibility of behaviors across time and conditions, suggesting a personality-related condition. This case example illustrates the importance of diagnostic clarity and how antisocial symptoms might be misinterpreted depending on the context and degree of information available.

Medical Comorbidity

Patients with psychiatric illnesses are at a significantly higher risk for experiencing medical conditions (e.g., diabetes, chronic bronchitis, liver failure) compared with the general population (Sokal et al. 2004). Among medical inpatients, psychiatric conditions are associated with extended lengths of stays as well as medical readmissions (Fulop et al. 1989; Furlanetto et al. 2003; Saravay et al. 1996). This may be especially relevant for patients with greater hostility and anger (Saravay et al. 1996), perhaps because of noncompliance or chronic stress.

Compared with the evidence base on psychiatric comorbidity, the literature regarding ASPD and comorbid medical conditions is significantly less rich. In fact, scholars have commented on the dearth of literature on comorbid medical concerns and personality disorders, with the exception of BPD (Frankenburg and Zanarini 2006). Nevertheless, evidence suggests that ASPD may heighten the risk for several comorbid medical concerns given the nature of the disorder. Compared with those without ASPD, individuals with ASPD report more frequent medical issues (Pietrzak and Petry 2005) and are more likely to receive physical disability benefits, perhaps because of the severity of reported medical conditions (Byrne et al. 2013).

Individuals with ASPD are at a significantly greater risk for experiencing premature death attributable to both natural (i.e., medical conditions) and unnatural causes (i.e., suicide, homicide, injury) compared with the general population (Repo-Tiihonen et al. 2010). This high mortality rate may be due in part to the higher incidence rate of physical trauma reported by individuals with ASPD, as well as other comorbid medical conditions (Black et al. 1996). In addition, comorbid psychiatric disorders can affect medical comorbidity among these patients. For example, substance use issues are markedly high among patients with ASPD, which exacerbates risk for medical comorbidity common among patients with these diagnoses (i.e., diabetes, respiratory issues, skin infections, heart disease, asthma, gastrointestinal disorders; Dickey et al. 2002). Given the clinical features of ASPD, patients are at a heightened risk for experiencing a wide array of medical concerns.

Physical Injuries and Motor Vehicle Accidents

Patients with ASPD present with features that increase the risk for experiencing physical injury. For example, patients with ASPD likely have a behavioral history of aggression and violence. In research literature, the association between ASPD and violent behavior is well established. A large meta-analysis suggested that ASPD was a stronger predictor of violent behavior than any other psychiatric diagnosis (Bonta et al. 1998), and similar findings have been reported in more recent meta-analyses (Yu et al. 2012). Recurrent aggressive behavior poses significant risks for sustaining physical injuries as a result of physical fighting and violence (e.g., broken bones, cuts, bruising). In addition, patients with ASPD likely have a chronic disregard for safety and engage in high-risk physical activities (e.g., high-speed driving, cliff jumping), which may heighten the risk for such injuries.

Aggressive tendencies, sensation-seeking behavior, and substance use may facilitate the risk for motor vehicle accidents. Aggressive behavior while driving is a significant predictor of being involved in a car accident (El Chliaoutakis et al. 2002). In a small sample of aggressive drivers referred by the court for an anger management program, up to 25% met criteria for ASPD (Galovski et al. 2002). These results have implications for the mortality of patients with ASPD; one study suggested that patients with ASPD are more likely to die as a result of a motor vehicle accident compared with an age-matched control sample (Dumais et al. 2005). Comorbid substance use disorders may exacerbate this risk. Empirical evidence indicates that individuals with ASPD tend to have a greater number of driving under the influence charges (McCutcheon et al. 2009), and patients with comorbid alcohol use disorder and ASPD are at a higher risk for experiencing a motor vehicle accident (Yates et al. 1987).

Traumatic Brain Injuries

Another prevalent form of medical comorbidity among patients with ASPD involves an increased risk for traumatic brain injuries (TBIs; Gerring and Vasa 2014). In a retrospective study of personality features among medical patients with TBI, patients were significantly more likely to meet criteria for ASPD *before* their TBI diagnosis (Hibbard et al. 2000). This suggests that patients with ASPD are more likely to experience TBIs at some point throughout the life span. This same study found that an additional 21% of patients met criteria for ASPD *following* their TBI diagnosis, indicating that head injuries may account for some etiological factors of antisocial personality traits (Hibbard et al. 2000). Indeed, changes in aggression and onset of violent behavior have been noted following head injuries (Bannon et al. 2015). The effects of TBIs are particularly deleterious. Patients with a history of TBIs are significantly more likely to experience cognitive difficulties, including memory, sleep, and affect recognition deficits, as well as a higher propensity toward violent and suicidal behavior (Babbage et al. 2011; Bahraini et al. 2013; Farrer et al. 2012; Grima et al. 2016; McAllister et al. 2006). Both TBIs and ASPD are common among incarcerated samples. TBIs may be indicated in approximately 60% of forensic samples, suggesting a considerable degree of comorbidity among patients with ASPD in similar settings (Shiroma et al. 2010).

Sexually Transmitted Infections and Hepatitis

The association between ASPD and sexually transmitted infections (STIs) is relatively strong. Evidence suggests that externalizing psychopathology (i.e., ASPD, substance use disorder) predicts STI diagnoses above and beyond internalizing psychopathology (i.e., major depressive disorder, panic disorder) over time (Magidson et al. 2014). In a sample of 201 patients in an STI clinic, approximately 18% of the patients met criteria for ASPD (Erbelding et al. 2004). This study found that patients with ASPD were significantly more likely to have a history of gonorrhea, chlamydia, and syphilis compared with patients without ASPD and those with other personality disorders (i.e., BPD; Erbelding et al. 2004). These findings are similar to empirical studies conducted in other settings; in a small sample of forensic psychiatric inpatients with ASPD, approximately 23.5% had a history of at least one STI (Cardasis et al. 2008).

　These comorbidities may be caused by high-risk sexual behaviors that are more common among patients with ASPD (i.e., condomless sex, multiple partners, exchanging sex for money or drugs, sex under the influence). These behaviors place patients with ASPD at a higher risk for STIs, including HIV (Compton et al. 2000; Gill et al. 1992). In addition, patients with ASPD are significantly more likely to use injection drugs, which can exacerbate the risk for HIV (Compton et al. 1995). Among a sample of injection drug users, patients with comorbid ASPD reported engaging in significantly higher rates of HIV risk behaviors (i.e., sharing equipment; Brooner et al. 1990). The high incidence of HIV and ASPD has been shown in a wide range of samples, including patients receiving residential substance abuse services and outpatients receiving HIV care (Compton et al. 2000; Shacham et al. 2016). Comorbid ASPD is especially concerning given poorer treatment effects found among patients with ASPD presenting with HIV risk behaviors and HIV-1 seropositive status (Bauer and Shanley 2006; Compton et al. 2000).

In addition to the STIs, individuals with ASPD are at heightened risk for contracting hepatitis. The prevalence rate of comorbid ASPD among samples of hepatitis C–positive patients ranges from 16% to 40% (Batki et al. 2011; Yovtcheva et al. 2001). The presence of comorbid ASPD has important implications for the course of hepatitis treatment; individuals diagnosed with hepatitis C and comorbid ASPD are significantly more likely to consume alcohol during the course of treatment (Stephens and Havens 2013), exacerbating the risk of liver damage.

Conclusion

Comorbid psychiatric conditions augment the already complex nature of assessing, diagnosing, and treating ASPD. Across diagnoses, externalizing conditions such as substance use disorders, impulse-control disorders, and ADHD can complicate treatment adherence and compliance. Internalizing conditions such as mood disorders and anxiety disorders can add to the acuity of psychiatric issues (e.g., suicidality, mania, panic). Comorbid personality disorders additionally complicate diagnostic clarity and may present with more frequent or more severe treatment-interfering behaviors. Across symptoms, ASPD shares diagnostic features with several disorders. Anger, irritability, impulsivity, and recklessness are all facets of both externalizing and internalizing conditions, as well as other personality disorders. These shared symptoms may lead to confusion as the clinician decides to which comorbid disorder each symptom is attributable. Although ASPD is more common in unique clinical settings (i.e., forensic, inpatient), clinicians in any setting may encounter a patient with ASPD. Clinicians who are tasked with assessing and treating ASPD should attend to issues of comorbidity because they typically predict more severe courses of illness, symptoms, and treatment resistance. Although deciding which clinical issues to target will vary on a case-by-case basis, understanding comorbid psychiatric and medical conditions can inform assessment procedures, potential referrals, and course of treatment.

Key Points

- Psychiatric comorbidity among individuals with antisocial personality disorder (ASPD) is associated with negative outcomes such as high service use, poor treatment response, and reoffending.

- Individuals with ASPD often meet criteria for comorbid internalizing and externalizing conditions, including mood disorders, substance use disorders, and ADHD.

- ASPD shares transdiagnostic features (e.g., anger, impulsivity) with a range of psychiatric disorders, highlighting the need to thoroughly assess for comorbid conditions to best inform clinical care and risk management strategies.

- Comorbid personality disorders present in about one-half of individuals with ASPD. The borderline, narcissistic, and histrionic types are more common than other personality disorders.

- A history of aggressive behavior and recklessness increases the odds of developing comorbid medical conditions (e.g., traumatic brain injury, sexually transmitted diseases).

References

Afifi TO, Mather A, Boman J, et al: Childhood adversity and personality disorders: results from a nationally representative population-based study. J Psychiatr Res 45(6):814–822, 2011 21146190

Alegria AA, Blanco C, Petry NM, et al: Sex differences in antisocial personality disorder: results from the National Epidemiological Survey on Alcohol and Related Conditions. Personal Disord 4(3):214–222, 2013 23544428

American Psychiatric Association: Diagnostic and Statistical Manual of Mental Disorders, 5th Edition. Arlington, VA, American Psychiatric Publishing, 2013

Anderson J, Snider S, Sellbom M, et al: A comparison of the DSM-5 Section II and Section III personality disorder structures. Psychiatry Res 216(3):363–372, 2014 24656519

Ardino V: Offending behaviour: the role of trauma and PTSD. Eur J Psychotraumatol 3:2012, 2012 22893844

Armstrong GJ, Kelley SDM: Early trauma and subsequent antisocial behavior in adults. Brief Treatment and Crisis Intervention 8(4):294–303, 2008

Babbage DR, Yim J, Zupan B, et al: Meta-analysis of facial affect recognition difficulties after traumatic brain injury. Neuropsychology 25(3):277–285, 2011 21463043

Bahraini NH, Simpson GK, Brenner LA, et al: Suicidal ideation and behaviours after traumatic brain injury: a systematic review. Brain Impair 14(1):92–112, 2013

Bannon S, Salis KL, O'Leary D: Structural brain abnormalities in aggression and violent behavior. Aggress Violent Behav 25(2015):323–331, 2015

Batki SL, Canfield KM, Ploutz-Snyder R: Psychiatric and substance use disorders among methadone maintenance patients with chronic hepatitis C infection: effects on eligibility for hepatitis C treatment. Am J Addict 20(4):312–318, 2011 21679262

Bauer LO, Shanley JD: ASPD blunts the effects of HIV and antiretroviral treatment on event-related brain potentials. Neuropsychobiology 53(1):17–25, 2006 16319505

Bender DS: The therapeutic alliance in the treatment of personality disorders. J Psychiatr Pract 11(2):73–87, 2005 15803042

Black DW: The treatment of antisocial personality disorder. Curr Treat Options Psychiatry 4(4):295–302, 2017

Black DW, Baumgard CH, Bell SE, et al: Death rates in 71 men with antisocial personality disorder: a comparison with general population mortality. Psychosomatics 37(2):131–136, 1996 8742541

Black DW, Monahan PO, Temkit M, et al: A family study of pathological gambling. Psychiatry Res 141(3):295–303, 2006 16499975

Black DW, Gunter T, Loveless P, et al: Antisocial personality disorder in incarcerated offenders: psychiatric comorbidity and quality of life. Ann Clin Psychiatry 22(2):113–120, 2010 20445838

Blum AW, Leppink EW, Grant JE: Neurocognitive dysfunction in problem gamblers with co-occurring antisocial personality disorder. Compr Psychiatry 76:153–159, 2017 28528231

Bock C, Bukh JD, Vinberg M, et al: The influence of comorbid personality disorder and neuroticism on treatment outcome in first episode depression. Psychopathology 43(3):197–204, 2010 20375542

Bonta J, Law M, Hanson K: The prediction of criminal and violent recidivism among mentally disordered offenders: a meta-analysis. Psychol Bull 123(2):123–142, 1998 9522681

Brady KT, Myrick H, McElroy S: The relationship between substance use disorders, impulse control disorders, and pathological aggression. Am J Addict 7(3):221–230, 1998 9702290

Brewer JA, Potenza MN: The neurobiology and genetics of impulse control disorders: relationships to drug addictions. Biochem Pharmacol 75(1):63–75, 2008 17719013

Brooner RK, Bigelow GE, Strain E, Schmidt CW: Intravenous drug abusers with antisocial personality disorder: increased HIV risk behavior. Drug Alcohol Depend 26(1):39–44, 1990 2209414

Bruce M, Laporte D: Childhood trauma, antisocial personality typologies and recent violent acts among inpatient males with severe mental illness: exploring an explanatory pathway. Schizophr Res 162(1–3):285–290, 2015 25636995

Byrne SA, Cherniack MG, Petry NM: Antisocial personality disorder is associated with receipt of physical disability benefits in substance abuse treatment patients. Drug Alcohol Depend 132(1–2):373–377, 2013 23394688

Cacciola JS, Alterman AI, Rutherford MJ, et al: Treatment response of antisocial substance abusers. J Nerv Ment Dis 183(3):166–171, 1995 7891063

Cailhol L, Pelletier É, Rochette L, et al: Prevalence, mortality, and health care use among patients with Cluster B personality disorders clinically diagnosed in Quebec: a provincial cohort study, 2001–2012. Can J Psychiatry 62(5):336–342, 2017 28403655

Cale EM, Lilienfeld SO: Sex differences in psychopathy and antisocial personality disorder: a review and integration. Clin Psychol Rev 22(8):1179–1207, 2002 12436810

Cardasis W, Huth-Bocks A, Silk KR: Tattoos and antisocial personality disorder. Personal Mental Health 2(3):171–182, 2008

Cassiello-Robbins C, Barlow DH: Anger: the unrecognized emotion in emotional disorders. Clinical Psychology: Science and Practice 23(1):66–85, 2016

Chapman AL, Leung DW, Lynch TR: Impulsivity and emotion dysregulation in borderline personality disorder. J Pers Disord 22(2):148–164, 2008 18419235

Coid J: The co-morbidity of personality disorder and lifetime clinical syndromes in dangerous offenders. J Forensic Psychiatry Psychol 14:341–366, 2003

Compton WM, Cottler LB, Shillington AM, et al: Is antisocial personality disorder associated with increased HIV risk behaviors in cocaine users? Drug Alcohol Depend 37(1):37–43, 1995 7882872

Compton WM, Cottler LB, Ben-Abdallah A, et al: The effects of psychiatric comorbidity on response to an HIV prevention intervention. Drug Alcohol Depend 58(3):247–257, 2000 10759035

Cunningham MD, Reidy TJ: Antisocial personality disorder and psychopathy: diagnostic dilemmas in classifying patterns of antisocial behavior in sentencing evaluations. Behav Sci Law 16(3):333–351, 1998 9768465

Cunradi CB, Todd M, Duke M, et al: Problem drinking, unemployment, and intimate partner violence among a sample of construction industry workers and their partners. J Fam Violence 24(2):63–74, 2009 22096270

Darke S, Williamson A, Ross J, et al: Borderline personality disorder, antisocial personality disorder and risk-taking among heroin users: findings from the Australian Treatment Outcome Study (ATOS). Drug Alcohol Depend 74(1):77–83, 2004 15072810

Delain SL, Stafford KP, Ben-Porath YS: Use of the TOMM in a criminal court forensic assessment setting. Assessment 10(4):370–381, 2003 14682483

DeLisi M, Reidy D, Heirigs M, et al: Psychopathic costs: a monetization study of the fiscal toll of psychopathy features among institutionalized delinquents. Journal of Criminal Psychology 8(2):112–124, 2018

Dickens GL, Sugarman PA: Adult firesetters: prevalence, characteristics, and psychopathology, in Firesetting and Mental Health: Theory, Research, and Practice. Edited by Dickens GL, Sugarman PA, Gannon TA. London, Royal College of Psychiatrists, 2012, pp 3–27

Dickey B, Normand SL, Weiss RD, et al: Medical morbidity, mental illness, and substance use disorders. Psychiatr Serv 53(7):861–867, 2002 12096170

Dixon-Gordon KL, Turner BJ, Chapman AL: Psychotherapy for personality disorders. Int Rev Psychiatry 23(3):282–302, 2011 21923228

Dom G, De Wilde B, Hulstijn W, et al: Decision-making deficits in alcohol-dependent patients with and without comorbid personality disorder. Alcohol Clin Exp Res 30(10):1670–1677, 2006 17010134

Douglas KS, Lilienfeld SO, Skeem JL, et al: Relation of antisocial and psychopathic traits to suicide-related behavior among offenders. Law Hum Behav 32(6):511–525, 2008 18080733

Dowling NA, Cowlishaw S, Jackson AC, et al: The prevalence of comorbid personality disorders in treatment-seeking problem gamblers: a systematic review and meta-analysis. J Pers Disord 29(6):735–754, 2015 25248010

Dudley MG, Rostosky SS, Korfhage BA, et al: Correlates of high-risk sexual behavior among young men who have sex with men. AIDS Educ Prev 16(4):328–340, 2004 15342335

Dumais A, Lesage AD, Boyer R, et al: Psychiatric risk factors for motor vehicle fatalities in young men. Can J Psychiatry 50(13):838–844, 2005 16483118

El Chliaoutakis J, Demakakos P, Tzamalouka G, et al: Aggressive behavior while driving as predictor of self-reported car crashes. J Safety Res 33(4):431–443, 2002 12429101

Erbelding EJ, Hutton HE, Zenilman JM, et al: The prevalence of psychiatric disorders in sexually transmitted disease clinic patients and their association with sexually transmitted disease risk. Sex Transm Dis 31(1):8–12, 2004 14695951

Evenden JL: Varieties of impulsivity. Psychopharmacology (Berl) 146(4):348–361, 1999 10550486

Evren C, Kural S, Erkiran M: Antisocial personality disorder in Turkish substance dependent patients and its relationship with anxiety, depression and a history of childhood abuse. Isr J Psychiatry Relat Sci 43(1):40–46, 2006 16910384

Farrer TJ, Frost RB, Hedges DW: Prevalence of traumatic brain injury in intimate partner violence offenders compared to the general population: a meta-analysis. Trauma Violence Abuse 13(2):77–82, 2012 22467643

Farrington DP: Childhood aggression and adult violence: early precursors and later life outcomes, in The Development and Treatment of Childhood Aggression. Edited by Pepler DJ, Rubin KH. New York, Lawrence Erlbaum, 1991, pp 5–29

Frances A, Ross R: DSM-IV-TR Case Studies: A Clinical Guide to Differential Diagnosis. Washington, DC, American Psychiatric Publishing, 2001

Frankenburg FR, Zanarini MC: Personality disorders and medical comorbidity. Curr Opin Psychiatry 19(4):428–431, 2006 16721176

Freeman A, Rosenfield B: Modifying therapeutic homework for patients with personality disorders. J Clin Psychol 58(5):513–524, 2002 11967877

Freestone M, Howard R, Coid JW, et al: Adult antisocial syndrome co-morbid with borderline personality disorder is associated with severe conduct disorder, substance dependence and violent antisociality. Pers Ment Health 7(1):11–21, 2013 24343921

French DC, Conrad J: School dropout as predicted by peer rejection and antisocial behavior. J Res Adolesc 11:225–244, 2001

Fulop G, Strain JJ, Fahs MC, et al: Medical disorders associated with psychiatric comorbidity and prolonged hospital stay. Hosp Community Psychiatry 40(1):80–82, 1989 2912843

Furlanetto LM, da Silva RV, Bueno JR: The impact of psychiatric comorbidity on length of stay of medical inpatients. Gen Hosp Psychiatry 25(1):14–19, 2003 12583922

Galovski T, Blanchard EB, Veazey C: Intermittent explosive disorder and other psychiatric comorbidity among court-referred and self-referred aggressive drivers. Behav Res Ther 40(6):641–651, 2002 12051483

Garno JL, Goldberg JF, Ramirez PM, et al: Bipolar disorder with comorbid Cluster B personality disorder features: impact on suicidality. J Clin Psychiatry 66(3):339–345, 2005 15766300

Genovese T, Dalrymple K, Chelminski I, et al: Subjective anger and overt aggression in psychiatric outpatients. Compr Psychiatry 73:23–30, 2017 27855338

Gerring J, Vasa R: Head injury and externalizing behavior, in The Oxford Handbook of Externalizing Spectrum Disorders. Edited by Beauchaine T, Hinshaw SP. New York, Oxford University Press, 2014, pp 403–415

Gibson TB, Jing Y, Smith Carls G, et al: Cost burden of treatment resistance in patients with depression. Am J Manag Care 16(5):370–377, 2010 20469957

Gill K, Nolimal D, Crowley TJ: Antisocial personality disorder, HIV risk behavior and retention in methadone maintenance therapy. Drug Alcohol Depend 30(3):247–252, 1992 1396106

Ginsberg Y, Lindefors N: Methylphenidate treatment of adult male prison inmates with attention-deficit hyperactivity disorder: randomised double-blind placebo-controlled trial with open-label extension. Br J Psychiatry 200(1):68–73, 2012 22075648

Gobin RL, Reddy MK, Zlotnick C, et al: Lifetime trauma victimization and PTSD in relation to psychopathy and antisocial personality disorder in a sample of incarcerated women and men. Int J Prison Health 11(2):64–74, 2015 26062658

Goldstein RB, Powers SI, McCusker J, et al: Gender differences in manifestations of antisocial personality disorder among residential drug abuse treatment clients. Drug Alcohol Depend 41(1):35–45, 1996 8793308

Goodwin RD, Hamilton SP: Lifetime comorbidity of antisocial personality disorder and anxiety disorders among adults in the community. Psychiatry Res 117(2):159–166, 2003 12606017

Grillo J, Brown RS, Hilsabeck R, et al: Raising doubts about claims of malingering: implications of relationships between MCMI-II and MMPI-2 performances. J Clin Psychol 50(4):651–655, 1994 7983217

Grima N, Ponsford J, Rajaratnam SMW, et al: Sleep disturbances in traumatic brain injury: a meta-analysis. J Clin Sleep Med 12(3):419–428, 2016 26564384

Gvion Y, Apter A: Aggression, impulsivity, and suicide behavior: a review of the literature. Arch Suicide Res 15(2):93–112, 2011 21541857

Havens JR, Cornelius LJ, Ricketts EP, et al: The effect of a case management intervention on drug treatment entry among treatment-seeking injection drug users with and without comorbid antisocial personality disorder. J Urban Health 84(2):267–271, 2007 17334939

Hibbard MR, Bogdany J, Uysal S, et al: Axis II psychopathology in individuals with traumatic brain injury. Brain Inj 14(1):45–61, 2000 10670661

Hodgins S, De Brito SA, Chhabra P, et al: Anxiety disorders among offenders with antisocial personality disorders: a distinct subtype? Can J Psychiatry 55(12):784–791, 2010 21172099

Holmes SE, Slaughter JR, Kashani J: Risk factors in childhood that lead to the development of conduct disorder and antisocial personality disorder. Child Psychiatry Hum Dev 31(3):183–193, 2001 11196010

Hong V, Pirnie L, Shobassy A: Antisocial and borderline personality disorders in the emergency department: conceptualizing and managing "malingered" or "exaggerated" symptoms. Curr Behav Neurosci Rep 6(2):127–132, 2019

Howard RC, Khalifa N, Duggan C: Antisocial personality disorder comorbid with borderline pathology and psychopathy is associated with severe violence in a forensic sample. Journal of Forensic Psychiatry and Psychology 25(6):658–672, 2014

Hurley AD, Sovner R: Six cases of patients with mental retardation who have antisocial personality disorder. Psychiatr Serv 46(8):828–831, 1995 7583487

Jones D, Hollin CR: Managing problematic anger: the development of a treatment program for personality disordered patients in high security. Int J Forensic Ment Health 3(2):197–210, 2004

Kessler RC, Foster CL, Saunders WB, et al: Social consequences of psychiatric disorders, I: educational attainment. Am J Psychiatry 152(7):1026–1032, 1995 7793438

Klonsky ED, May A: Rethinking impulsivity in suicide. Suicide Life Threat Behav 40(6):612–619, 2010 21198330

Knop J, Penick EC, Nickel EJ, et al: Childhood ADHD and conduct disorder as independent predictors of male alcohol dependence at age 40. J Stud Alcohol Drugs 70(2):169–177, 2009 19261228

Kotov R, Krueger RF, Watson D, et al: The Hierarchical Taxonomy of Psychopathology (HiTOP): a dimensional alternative to traditional nosologies. J Abnorm Psychol 126(4):454–477, 2017 28333488

Kotov R, Krueger RF, Watson D: A paradigm shift in psychiatric classification: the Hierarchical Taxonomy of Psychopathology (HiTOP). World Psychiatry 17(1):24–25, 2018 29352543

Krawczyk N, Feder KA, Saloner B, et al: The association of psychiatric comorbidity with treatment completion among clients admitted to substance use treatment programs in a U.S. national sample. Drug Alcohol Depend 175:157–163, 2017 28432939

Lahey BB, Loeber R, Burke JD, et al: Predicting future antisocial personality disorder in males from a clinical assessment in childhood. J Consult Clin Psychol 73(3):389–399, 2005 15982137

Ledgerwood DM, Weinstock J, Morasco BJ, et al: Clinical features and treatment prognosis of pathological gamblers with and without recent gambling-related illegal behavior. J Am Acad Psychiatry Law 35(3):294–301, 2007 17872548

Magidson JF, Blashill AJ, Wall MM, et al: Relationship between psychiatric disorders and sexually transmitted diseases in a nationally representative sample. J Psychosom Res 76(4):322–328, 2014 24630184

Marmorstein NR: Adult antisocial behaviour without conduct disorder: demographic characteristics and risk for cooccurring psychopathology. Can J Psychiatry 51(4):226–233, 2006 16629347

Marshall AD, Martin EK, Warfield GA, et al: The impact of antisocial personality characteristics on anger management treatment for veterans with PTSD. Psychol Trauma 2:224–231, 2010

Martens WHJ: Multidimensional model of trauma and correlated personality disorder. J Loss Trauma 10:115–129, 2006

Maughan B, Gray G, Rutter M: Reading retardation and antisocial behaviour: a follow-up into employment. J Child Psychol Psychiatry 26(5):741–758, 1985 4044719

McAllister TW, Flashman LA, McDonald BC, et al: Mechanisms of working memory dysfunction after mild and moderate TBI: evidence from functional MRI and neurogenetics. J Neurotrauma 23(10):1450–1467, 2006 17020482

McCoul MD, Haslam N: Predicting high risk sexual behaviour in heterosexual and homosexual men: the roles of impulsivity and sensation seeking. Pers Individ Dif 31(8):1303–1310, 2001

McCutcheon VV, Heath AC, Edenberg HJ, et al: Alcohol criteria endorsement and psychiatric and drug use disorders among DUI offenders: greater severity among women and multiple offenders. Addict Behav 34(5):432–439, 2009 19167170

McGonigal P, Dixon-Gordon KL: Anger and emotion regulation associated with borderline and antisocial personality features within a correctional sample. J Correct Health Care 26(3):215–226, 2020 32787624

McGonigal P, Kerr S, Morgan T, et al: Should childhood conduct disorder be necessary to diagnose antisocial personality disorder in adults? Ann Clin Psychiatry 31(1):36–44, 2019 30699216

Miranda A, Presentación MJ: Efficacy of cognitive-behavioral therapy in the treatment of children with ADHD, with and without aggressiveness. Psychology in the Schools 37(2):169–182, 2000

Modesto-Lowe V, Kranzler HR: Diagnosis and treatment of alcohol-dependent patients with comorbid psychiatric disorders. Alcohol Res Health 23(2):144–149, 1999 10890809

Moeller FG, Dougherty DM: Antisocial personality disorder, alcohol, and aggression. Alcohol Res Health 25(1):5–11, 2001 11496966

Morrissey C, Hollin C: Antisocial and psychopathic personality disorders in forensic intellectual disability populations: what do we know so far? Psychology, Crime, and Law 17(2):133–149, 2010

Mueser KT, Crocker AG, Frisman LB, et al: Conduct disorder and antisocial personality disorder in persons with severe psychiatric and substance use disorders. Schizophr Bull 32(4):626–636, 2006 16574783

Najt P, Perez J, Sanches M, et al: Impulsivity and bipolar disorder. Eur Neuropsychopharmacol 17(5):313–320, 2007 17140772

Nelson KG, Oehlert ME: Psychometric exploration of the sexual addiction screening test in veterans. Sex Addict Compulsivity 15(1):39–58, 2008

Ng TH, Burke TA, Stange JP, et al: Personality disorder symptom severity predicts onset of mood episodes and conversion to bipolar I disorder in individuals with bipolar spectrum disorder. J Abnorm Psychol 126(3):271–284, 2017 28368159

Niesten IJM, Nentjes L, Merckelbach H, et al: Antisocial features and "faking bad": a critical note. Int J Law Psychiatry 41:34–42, 2015 25843907

Ogloff JRP, Talevski D, Lemphers A, et al: Co-occurring mental illness, substance use disorders, and antisocial personality disorder among clients of forensic mental health services. Psychiatr Rehabil J 38(1):16–23, 2015 25799303

Ozkan M, Altindag A: Comorbid personality disorders in subjects with panic disorder: do personality disorders increase clinical severity? Compr Psychiatry 46(1):20–26, 2005 15714190

Perry JC, Lavori PW, Pagano CJ, et al: Life events and recurrent depression in borderline and antisocial personality disorders. J Pers Disord 6:394–407, 1992

Petry NM: Substance abuse, pathological gambling, and impulsiveness. Drug Alcohol Depend 63(1):29–38, 2001 11297829

Pietrzak RH, Petry NM: Antisocial personality disorder is associated with increased severity of gambling, medical, drug and psychiatric problems among treatment-seeking pathological gamblers. Addiction 100(8):1183–1193, 2005 16042649

Poythress NG, Edens JF, Watkins MM: The relationship between psychopathic personality features and malingering symptoms of major mental illness. Law Hum Behav 25(6):567–582, 2001 11771635

Ralevski E, Ball S, Nich C, et al: The impact of personality disorders on alcohol-use outcomes in a pharmacotherapy trial for alcohol dependence and comorbid Axis I disorders. Am J Addict 16(6):443–449, 2007 18058408

Raymond NC, Coleman E, Miner MH: Psychiatric comorbidity and compulsive/impulsive traits in compulsive sexual behavior. Compr Psychiatry 44(5):370–380, 2003 14505297

Reichborn-Kjennerud T, Czajkowski N, Ystrøm E, et al: A longitudinal twin study of borderline and antisocial personality disorder traits in early to middle adulthood. Psychol Med 45(14):3121–3131, 2015 26050739

Reidy DE, Kearns MC, DeGue S, et al: Why psychopathy matters: implications for public health and violence prevention. Aggress Violent Behav 24:214–225, 2015 29593448

Repo-Tiihonen E, Virkkunen M, Tiihonen J: Mortality of antisocial male criminals. Journal of Forensic Psychiatry 12(3):677–683, 2010

Retz W, Retz-Junginger P: Prediction of methylphenidate treatment outcome in adults with attention-deficit/hyperactivity disorder (ADHD). Eur Arch Psychiatry Clin Neurosci 264 (suppl 1):S35–S43, 2014 25231833

Robins LN, Tipp J, Przybeck T: Antisocial personality, in Psychiatric Disorders in America. Edited by Robins LN, Regier DA. New York, Free Press, 1991, pp 258–290

Rowe JB, Sullivan PF, Mulder RT, et al: The effect of a history of conduct disorder in adult major depression. J Affect Disord 37(1):51–63, 1996 8682978

Roy A, Garner AA, Epstein JN, et al: Effects of childhood and adult persistent attention-deficit/hyperactivity disorder on risk of motor vehicle crashes: results from the Multimodal Treatment Study of Children With Attention-Deficit/Hyperactivity Disorder. J Am Acad Child Adolesc Psychiatry 59(8):952–963, 2020 31445873

Saravay SM, Pollack S, Steinberg MD, et al: Four-year follow up of the influence of psychological comorbidity on medical rehospitalization. Am J Psychiatry 153(3):397–403, 1996 8610829

Scott LN, Stepp SD, Pilkonis PA: Prospective associations between features of borderline personality disorder, emotion dysregulation, and aggression. Pers Disord 5(3):278–288, 2014 24635753

Semiz UB, Basoglu C, Oner O, et al: Effects of diagnostic comorbidity and dimensional symptoms of attention-deficit-hyperactivity disorder in men with antisocial personality disorder. Aust N Z J Psychiatry 42(5):405–413, 2008 18473259

Shacham E, Önen NF, Donovan MF, et al: Psychiatric diagnoses among an HIV-infected outpatient clinic population. J Int Assoc Provid AIDS Care 15(2):126–130, 2016 25348798

Shea MT, Widiger TA, Klein MH: Comorbidity of personality disorders and depression: implications for treatment. J Consult Clin Psychol 60(6):857–868, 1992 1460149

Sheehan L, Nieweglowski K, Corrigan P: The stigma of personality disorders. Curr Psychiatry Rep 18(1):11, 2016 26780206

Sher L, Siever LJ, Goodman M, et al: Gender differences in the clinical characteristics and psychiatric comorbidity in patients with antisocial personality disorder. Psychiatry Res 229(3):685–689, 2015 26296756

Shiroma EJ, Ferguson PL, Pickelsimer EE: Prevalence of traumatic brain injury in an offender population: a meta-analysis. J Correct Health Care 16(2):147–159, 2010 20339132

Simonoff E, Elander J, Holmshaw J, et al: Predictors of antisocial personality: continuities from childhood to adult life. Br J Psychiatry 184:118–127, 2004 14754823

Skodol AE, Clark LA, Bender DS, et al: Proposed changes in personality and personality disorder assessment and diagnosis for DSM-5 part I: description and rationale. Pers Disord 2(1):4–22, 2011 22448687

Slutske WS, Eisen S, Xian H, et al: A twin study of the association between pathological gambling and antisocial personality disorder. J Abnorm Psychol 110(2):297–308, 2001 11358024

Sokal J, Messias E, Dickerson FB, et al: Comorbidity of medical illnesses among adults with serious mental illness who are receiving community psychiatric services. J Nerv Ment Dis 192(6):421–427, 2004 15167405

Soloff PH, Fabio A, Kelly TM, et al: High-lethality status in patients with borderline personality disorder. J Pers Disord 19(4):386–399, 2005 16178681

Stephens DB, Havens JR: Predictors of alcohol use among rural drug users after disclosure of hepatitis C virus status. J Stud Alcohol Drugs 74(3):386–395, 2013 23490567

Storebø OJ, Simonsen E: The association between ADHD and antisocial personality disorder (ASPD): a review. J Atten Disord 20(10):815–824, 2016 24284138

Swann AC, Lijffijt M, Lane SD, et al: Antisocial personality disorder and borderline symptoms are differentially related to impulsivity and course of illness in bipolar disorder. J Affect Disord 148(2–3):384–390, 2013 22835849

Trzesniewski KH, Moffitt TE, Caspi A, et al: Revisiting the association between reading achievement and antisocial behavior: new evidence of an environmental explanation from a twin study. Child Dev 77(1):72–88, 2006 16460526

Tyrer P, Reed GM, Crawford MJ: Classification, assessment, prevalence, and effect of personality disorder. Lancet 385(9969):717–726, 2015 25706217

Ullrich S, Coid J. Antisocial personality disorder: co-morbid Axis I mental disorders and health service use among a national household population. Personal Ment Health 164(3):151–164, 2009

van Impelen A, Merckelbach H, Jelicic M, et al: Antisocial features are not predictive of symptom exaggeration in forensic patients. Legal Criminol Psychol 23(2):135–147, 2018

Verdejo-García A, Lawrence AJ, Clark L: Impulsivity as a vulnerability marker for substance-use disorders: review of findings from high-risk research, problem gamblers and genetic association studies. Neurosci Biobehav Rev 32(4):777–810, 2008 18295884

Verona E, Patrick CJ, Joiner TE: Psychopathy, antisocial personality, and suicide risk. J Abnorm Psychol 110(3):462–470, 2001 11502089

Watson DC, Sinha BK: Comorbidity of DSM-IV personality disorders in a nonclinical sample. J Clin Psychol 54(6):773–780, 1998 9783656

Weiss NH, Tull MT, Viana AG, et al: Impulsive behaviors as an emotion regulation strategy: examining associations between PTSD, emotion dysregulation, and impulsive behaviors among substance dependent inpatients. J Anxiety Disord 26(3):453–458, 2012 22366447

Westermeyer J, Thuras P: Association of antisocial personality disorder and substance disorder morbidity in a clinical sample. Am J Drug Alcohol Abuse 31(1):93–110, 2005 15768573

Widiger TA, Livesley WJ, Clark LA: An integrative dimensional classification of personality disorder. Psychol Assess 21(3):243–255, 2009 19719338

Winstanley CA, Eagle DM, Robbins TW: Behavioral models of impulsivity in relation to ADHD: translation between clinical and preclinical studies. Clin Psychol Rev 26(4):379–395, 2006 16504359

Yates WR, Noyes R Jr, Petty F, et al: Factors associated with motor vehicle accidents among male alcoholics. J Stud Alcohol 48(6):586–590, 1987 3682833

Young S, Thome J: ADHD and offenders. World J Biol Psychiatry 12 (suppl 1):124–128, 2011 21906010

Yovtcheva SP, Rifai MA, Moles JK, et al: Psychiatric comorbidity among hepatitis C-positive patients. Psychosomatics 42(5):411–415, 2001 11739908

Yu R, Geddes JR, Fazel S: Personality disorders, violence, and antisocial behavior: a systematic review and meta-regression analysis. J Pers Disord 26(5):775–792, 2012 23013345

Zimmerman M, Pfohl B, Coryell W, et al: Diagnosing personality disorder in depressed patients: a comparison of patient and informant interviews. Arch Gen Psychiatry 45(8):733–737, 1988 3395201

Zimmerman M, Chelminski I, Young D: The frequency of personality disorders in psychiatric patients. Psychiatr Clin North Am 31(3):405–420, vi, 2008 18638643

Zimmerman M, Chelminski I, Young D, et al: Which DSM-IV personality disorders are most strongly associated with indices of psychosocial morbidity in psychiatric outpatients? Compr Psychiatry 53(7):940–945, 2012 22497671

CHAPTER 5

Clinical Symptoms and Assessment of Antisocial Personality Disorder

Donald W. Black, M.D.
Nancee Blum, M.S.W.

Antisocial personality disorder (ASPD) is a lifelong disorder that begins early and continues through adulthood. The misbehaving child receives the diagnosis of conduct disorder, depending on the frequency and severity of the symptoms. If the symptoms persist past age 18 years, the diagnosis changes to ASPD. Symptoms are age appropriate and reflect advancing age and opportunity but may vary from person to person.

Conduct Disorder

If the child has significant behavioral disturbances, he or she might meet criteria for conduct disorder, defined in DSM-5 as "a repetitive and persistent pattern of behavior in which the basic rights of others or major age-appropriate societal norms or rules are violated" (American Psychiatric Association 2013, p. 469). Conduct disorder occurs mainly in boys, many of whom are also diagnosed with ADHD or oppositional defiant disorder. Evident even at a very young age, conduct disorder affects 5%–15% of all children (Robins 1987).

In DSM-5, conduct disorder was moved to the "Disruptive, Impulse-Control, and Conduct Disorders" chapter (Black and Grant 2014). The diagnosis requires that at least 3 of 15 problematic behaviors be present in the previous 12 months, with at least 1 criterion present in the past 6 months. Although the diagnosis can be made in adults, the symptoms usually emerge in childhood or adolescence, and onset is rare after age

16 years. The criteria specify a childhood-onset type (prior to age 10 years) and an adolescent-onset type (after age 10 years), in recognition of the fact that early onset is one of the strongest predictors of poor outcome. Using data from the National Epidemiologic Survey on Alcohol and Related Conditions (NESARC), Goldstein et al. (2006b) reported that childhood-onset conduct disorder was more likely than adolescent-onset conduct disorder to be associated with violent behaviors, including against persons, animals, and property.

When considering the diagnosis, clinicians should note behavioral disturbances in four main categories: aggression toward people or animals, destruction of property, deceitfulness or theft, and serious violations of rules (American Psychiatric Association 2013). Symptoms include fights with peers, conflicts with parents and other authority figures, stealing, vandalism, fire setting, and cruelty to animals or other children. School-related behavior problems are common, as is poor academic performance. In addition, many of these children have a history of running away from home. These problem behaviors must significantly impair the child's social, academic, or occupational functioning. Boys with conduct disorder are more likely to exhibit physical aggression, whereas girls are more likely to show relational aggression (i.e., behavior that harms social relationships). Conduct disorder is discussed further in Chapter 21, "The Antisocial Child."

Aggression

Most childhood aggression is relatively benign, with bullying epitomizing the aggressive tendencies of some children. Research shows that men who were bullied in childhood are more likely to commit criminal acts as adults and to engage in domestic violence (Falb et al. 2011; Loeber and Stouthammer-Loeber 1987). For others, mostly boys, fist fights, intimidation, and milder acts of aggression can escalate depending on age and opportunity. Children gradually take up weapons in their fights, and their crimes may increasingly involve physical intimidation or assault. Cruelty to animals is another form of childhood aggression linked with adult violence (Hellman and Blackman 1966). Many antisocial adults and children with conduct disorder have histories of abusing, torturing, or killing pets. Children who become antisocial as adults often are sexually active before their peers, engaging in early masturbation and sex play, sometimes forcing others to perform sexual acts. In some cases, childhood sexual activity is motivated by abuse from adults, leading to an intergenerational cycle of abuse (Pomeroy et al. 1981).

Damaging Property

Destruction of property, ranging from petty vandalism to starting fires, is symptomatic of conduct disorder and can lead to significant major property damage (e.g., from a fire) or even death. Like animal cruelty, fire setting is an especially alarming behavior that correlates highly with adult violence (Hellman and Blackman 1966).

Lying and Stealing

Deceitfulness is the third major feature of the conduct disorder diagnosis. Lying comes naturally to many of these children who use deceit to cover up bad behavior or to gain rewards. They become adept at lying to parents, teachers, and others. Theft is also common in conduct disorder and may involve shoplifting or breaking into cars, homes, and businesses—crimes in which juvenile offenders often get their start. Some young thieves use stolen credit cards and keep pace with technology by turning to computers and electronic crime (e.g., hacking). Children with conduct disorder can be extremely adaptable, jumping at any opportunity to make mischief to get what they want.

Breaking the Rules

Serious violations of rules, the fourth area of major problem behaviors, often are noted in schools, if not at home. The structure and demands of learning provide ample opportunity for troubled children to rebel, and teachers may be the first to identify "problem" kids with severe behavior disorders. Rule violations and poor school performance—often worse than predicted by measures of intelligence—lead to high rates of failure, truancy, suspension, and permanent expulsion (Black 2013). These problems are of enormous importance because they stunt educational achievement, contribute to future job difficulties, and set the stage for low income and social status in adulthood.

The home, too, is the setting for rule violations like missed curfews, running away, or simply ignoring parental instructions. Children with conduct disorder test the patience, will, and courage of even the most competent parents, especially as they grow older and become more difficult to control. In many cases, however, parents themselves contribute to their children's bad behavior through abuse or neglect.

Antisocial Personality Disorder

A history of conduct disorder is one of four necessary criteria for the diagnosis of adult ASPD (American Psychiatric Association 2013). The criteria require that a person have at least three of seven maladaptive personality traits that include failure to conform to social norms, deceitfulness, impulsivity, irritability or aggressiveness, reckless disregard for others, irresponsibility, and lack of remorse. The person must be age 18 years or older, and there is evidence of conduct disorder with onset before age 15. By requiring that the diagnosis be applied only to those older than 18, DSM-5 discourages diagnosing young people with a serious diagnosis that could remain a troublesome aspect of their medical records even if later proven wrong or if their problems subside (Black and Grant 2014). Schizophrenia and bipolar disorder must be ruled out as a cause of the antisocial behavior. Schizophrenia, for example, can cause personality changes, hallucinations and delusions, and bizarre behavior. Mania causes irritability, aggression, excessive sexual impulses, and hyperactivity, leading people to behave foolishly and make impulsive decisions.

Clinical symptoms of ASPD in 1,422 men and women assessed in the NESARC are shown in Table 5–1.

Failure to Conform

Most individuals with ASPD eventually have trouble with the law because they are unable to conform to the lawful expectations of society. Offenses can range from non-violent property offenses to acts of extreme violence, such as sodomy, rape, or mur-

TABLE 5–1.   **Symptoms of antisocial personality disorder in 1,422 persons participating in the National Epidemiologic Survey on Alcohol and Related Conditions**

Symptoms	Percentage
Childhood criteria	
Bullying	47
Starting fights	26
Using dangerous weapons	28
Cruelty to people	35
Cruelty to animals	15
Stealing with confrontation	2
Forcing someone into sexual activity	0.2
Deliberate fire setting	13
Deliberate vandalism	32
Breaking into someone else's property	32
Frequent lying	43
Nonconfrontational stealing	76
Staying out all night	29
Running away	30
Frequent truancy	41
Adulthood criteria	
Repeated unlawful behaviors	83
Deceitfulness	49
Impulsivity or failure to plan	54
Irritability and aggressiveness	73
Recklessness	71
Consistent irresponsibility	87
Lack of remorse	51

Source.   Adapted from Goldstein et al. 2006b.

der. More often, however, their criminal records are notable not for their violence but for their sheer length and variety. Because so many individuals with ASPD are addicted to drugs or alcohol, their crimes often revolve around substance abuse, whether committed while intoxicated or in the pursuit of a drug. Such behaviors are often behind the individual's arrests, convictions, and incarceration.

Data from the NESARC show that 53% of individuals with ASPD have been incarcerated at some point in their lives, more so for men (58%) than for women (40%) (R.B. Goldstein, S.P. Chou, unpublished data, February 2020). In clinical samples, the percentage of antisocial persons who have been incarcerated is much higher. In Robins' (1966) follow-up study, nearly 75% of individuals with ASPD spent 1 or more years behind bars, with nearly 40% being incarcerated for 5 years or more. Black et al. (1995) also reported in their longitudinal follow-up that 75% of formerly hospitalized antisocial men were arrested multiple times, with 48% having been convicted of a felony.

Deceit

Deceit is another significant way in which antisocial persons show their disregard for others, and for some, lying becomes a way of life. The term *pathological lying* is often used to describe those whose lying is chronic and habitual. An antisocial man might falsify his work record when seeking a better job; another might lie to his wife about a 5-day absence. Or, an antisocial person might concoct a story for his own amusement, in order to impress friends, relatives, or drinking companions.

The use of an alias is common and often appears to be an understandable response to the individual's criminal or legal problems. Motivations underlying the name change are varied but can include escaping responsibility from past obligations or evading law enforcement, creditors, or former spouses.

Impulsiveness

Impulsivity is a common symptom, with the individual making quick decisions without adequate reflection or consideration of possible outcomes. *Wanderlust* is an apt descriptor for many of these individuals because they move from place to place without any goal or destination in mind. Some antisocial persons thrive on the excitement of escape. Whether called hoboes, vagrants, or nomads, some antisocial men prefer their peripatetic lives to the workaday drudgery of maintaining a job, home, and responsibility to family.

Aggression

Aggression and violence are perhaps the most disturbing symptoms of ASPD. The aggressive antisocial person can be dangerous and his or her actions sudden and unpredictable. In mild cases, the antisocial individual is simply irritable and hostile, occasionally lashing out at family, coworkers, or strangers. In other cases, minor disputes can lead to brutality. Domestic violence is commonplace in the families of these men, creating a climate of terror for spouses and children who live in fear of the next outburst, knowing that the attacks often stem from no apparent cause. Violent antisocial persons often end up incarcerated because of the nature of the crime.

Reckless Disregard for the Rights of Others

People with ASPD often have a pervasive disregard for the rights of others. Antisocial individuals' disregard for others and for themselves is expressed in subtler ways as well. Many show a symptomatic recklessness, such as driving too fast or while drunk, practicing unsafe sex, or taking countless other risks. People with ASPD are also more likely to have motor vehicle and other accidents or even to be murdered, reflecting their overall degree of recklessness.

Irresponsibility

General irresponsibility can take many forms. Job histories are replete with periods of unemployment, frequent job changes, and poor performance. Lack of dependability (e.g., being late, unexcused absences) can lead to being fired. Arguments or fights with coworkers or supervisors are not uncommon. If the antisocial person is not fired, his or her lack of interest or frustration with the demands of employment may drive him or her to quit abruptly, often without any alternative source of support. Irresponsibility combined with work problems create difficult financial situations, and many antisocial persons end up on public assistance or receive charity. Robins (1966) suggested that antisocial persons might do better in jobs with little direct supervision or with self-employment.

Antisocial persons who join the armed forces often have unsatisfactory experiences because of their inability to accept military discipline. They are more likely than others to be absent without leave, court-martialed, or dishonorably discharged (Robins 1966). In a follow-up study of 36 men with ASPD who joined the armed forces, 35 had disciplinary or other problems, and they were much more likely than control participants to be absent without leave, court-martialed, or dishonorably discharged (Fiedler et al. 2004).

Personal relationships and family life are another area where irresponsibility is manifested. Early marriage is common, and these marriages are characterized by infidelity, separation, and divorce. Domestic violence is common. Furthermore, antisocial persons often make incompetent parents and are more likely than others to abuse or neglect their children (Egami et al. 1996). Some of these problems might be due in part to the antisocial person's tendency to become involved with equally unstable partners. A study of female felons found that 75% had married antisocial men, providing evidence of assortative mating, at least in the case of antisocial persons (Guze et al. 1970).

Consistent irresponsibility also contributes to a lack of social relationships among antisocial persons. Relationships that develop tend to be shallow, perhaps based on shared affinities for alcohol or drugs rather than anything more meaningful. They rarely join community organizations, volunteer agencies, or church groups, although some attend Alcoholics Anonymous meetings or other recovery groups, especially when motivated by a court order.

Lack of Remorse

Related to irresponsibility is the antisocial person's seeming inability to feel regret or remorse for his or her actions. His or her lack of conscience can lead to emotional isolation and a disregard for all standards of behavior. Many antisocial persons see themselves as the true victims, not those whom they betray or hurt. They hold a perpetual grudge against the social order and inspire outrage when they divulge the contorted logic that, in their eyes, absolves them of all responsibility. Research confirms that lack of remorse is particularly common with more severe and violent forms of ASPD (Goldstein et al. 1996, 2006a).

The following vignette shows many of the typical symptoms of ASPD and how they affected one of our patients over a lifetime. The patient had been admitted to the University of Iowa Psychopathic Hospital (now Psychiatric Hospital) in the 1950s and was followed up over 30 years later in the 1980s (Black and Andreasen 2020).

> Burton, age 18 years, was admitted for evaluation of antisocial behavior at the request of his adoptive parents. His early childhood had been chaotic and abusive. His alcoholic father had married five times and abandoned his family when Burton was 6. Because his mother had a history of incarceration and was unable to care for him, Burton was placed in foster care until he was adopted at age 8. As a child, Burton lied, cheated at games,

shoplifted, and stole money from his mother's purse. He was sent to a juvenile reformatory at age 16. While there, he slashed another boy with a razor blade in a fight.

In the hospital, the psychiatrists interviewed Burton and his adoptive parents, conducted an encephalogram (deemed normal), and measured his IQ at 112. He showed no interest in psychotherapy, insulted staff members, and left abruptly after a 16-day stay. He was described as "unimproved" on discharge.

Burton was followed up 30 years later at age 48. Burton, appearing old and haggard, was living in an impoverished neighborhood in a nearby community. He admitted to more than 20 arrests and 5 felony convictions on charges ranging from attempted murder and armed robbery to driving while intoxicated. He had spent more than 17 years in prison. Burton reported having nine hospitalizations for alcohol detoxification, the most recent occurring earlier that year.

Burton had never held a full-time job and had lived in six different states; he had moved more than 20 times in 10 years. Burton's common-law marriage was described as unsatisfactory, and he admitted committing spousal abuse. He occasionally attended Alcoholics Anonymous meetings but otherwise did not socialize. When asked, Burton admitted that he had not yet settled down and still got a "charge out of doing dangerous things."

Care Seeking in Antisocial Persons

Few people with ASPD seek mental health care for their disorder, yet in the Epidemiologic Catchment Area survey, nearly 20% of antisocial persons had sought such care within the past year (Shapiro et al. 1984). A similar survey in the United Kingdom showed that nearly 25% had sought care within the last year (Ullrich and Coid 2009). Accompanying problems, not ASPD per se, are typically responsible for their care seeking. Problems that lead to care seeking include co-occurring depression, substance misuse, or difficulties relating to marital maladjustment, anger dyscontrol, or suicidal behavior (Black and Braun 1998). Other antisocial persons are brought for evaluation by concerned family members or the courts.

Typically, the antisocial person will be evaluated in an outpatient setting where an array of services is available if needed, such as case management, psychological assessment, medication management, and psychotherapy. Hospitalization is rarely needed unless the patient is suicidal or homicidal or needs medically monitored alcohol or drug withdrawal. Treatment of ASPD is further discussed in Chapter 17, "Psychosocial Treatment of Antisocial Personality Disorder," and Chapter 18, "Pharmacological Treatment of Antisocial Personality Disorder."

Assessing the Antisocial Person

The patient's history is the most important basis for diagnosing ASPD. The diagnosis rests on the patient's history of chronic and repetitive behavior problems beginning in childhood or early adolescence that continue into adulthood (American Psychiatric Association 2013). The patient will be the best source of information.

Taking the History

With the diagnosis of ASPD in mind, the clinician's first step is to construct an accurate history. The goal of the interview is to assess the breadth of the individual's problematic behaviors and distorted thinking patterns that underlie the disorder. For general screening purposes, a clinician might ask

- Did you ever get into fights as a child?
- When in trouble, do you blame others?
- Have you ever been arrested or jailed?
- Do you tend to disregard laws you don't like, such as those against speeding?
- Have you ever failed to follow through on financial or other obligations?

Positive responses should be followed up with more specific inquiries to flesh out the extent of the person's misbehavior. Antisocial individuals may come across as proud of their manipulations and cons rather than feeling embarrassed or ashamed.

The clinician should identify the patient's chief complaint—that is, what motivates him or her to seek care. Common chief complaints for antisocial individuals tend to center around depression or anxiety, substance abuse, aggression, or disturbed relationships.

After obtaining the individual consents, family members and friends can be helpful informants. They are often more accurate in describing their relatives' antisocial behavior than are the patients themselves (Andreasen et al. 1986), who may have little motivation to be truthful. Medical records for previous clinic or hospital visits can provide additional diagnostic information. Legal records can help substantiate an ASPD diagnosis.

Medical History

The patient's history of illness, surgical procedures, and medical treatment is important to assess. Use of alcohol, prescription medications, illicit drugs, and cigarette smoking warrants specific questions because of their potential for significant physical and psychological effects, and all are commonly used by antisocial persons. This information can help rule out several diagnostic possibilities and can be helpful in developing recommendations for lifestyle modifications (e.g., reducing the intake of caffeine or other stimulants to counter anxiety).

The medical history is important because of the antisocial person's tendency to engage in impulsive or risky behavior that places him or her at risk for accidental injuries. Patients should be asked about traumatic injuries and other events that could suggest a reckless lifestyle as well as sexually transmitted diseases. Many antisocial patients will have a history of head injury or motor vehicle and other accidents (Woodruff et al. 1971). Prompted by their impulsiveness, antisocial persons are prone to leave hospitals against medical advice and so should be asked about such behaviors (Brook et al. 2006).

Family History

ASPD is strongly familial, and the disorder tends to coaggregate with mood disorders (major depression, bipolar disorder), substance abuse, and ADHD (Slutske 2001). If family history identifies a history consistent with ASPD in a relative, then that should raise the level of suspicion of ASPD in the patient. The clinician should inquire about the emotional and psychiatric health of parents, grandparents, aunts, uncles, and other relatives. Because a disproportionate percentage of antisocial individuals are adoptees, many will be unfamiliar with their biological background (Schechter 1989).

Personal and Social History

The inquiry begins with anything the patient has been told about his or her birth, including difficulties with delivery, and continues through early development and childhood problems such as bed-wetting. In their study of juvenile delinquents, Glueck and Glueck (1950) reported that 28% of delinquent youths were bed-wetters compared with 15% of nondelinquent youths. The significance of bed-wetting remains unclear, but it could reflect a lag in brain or CNS maturation, a problem also linked to learning disorders and ADHD. The interviewer should explore early family life, including details about the home, the community, and any history of abuse or neglect. Educational background and troubles at school are important to understand. The sexual history will note when the patient became sexually active, frequency of sexual relations, and sexual orientation.

Major areas where ASPD symptoms tend to emerge—work and job history, personal relationships, military service, and arrests or convictions—are explored through the patient interview plus details from family members, friends, and official records. It is important to identify the number and type of jobs patients have held, periods of unemployment, relationships with coworkers, and trouble complying with job requirements. Questions about marriage and relationships trace how they were initiated, what the mental status of partners has been, and whether domestic abuse has occurred. Reports of military service history, criminal behavior, arrests, convictions, and incarceration can be compared with official documents when available.

Living arrangements, finances, and children are additional aspects of the personal history that help fill out the overall image of the patient's life, especially when ASPD is a possibility. Frequency of moves, homelessness, and home ownership enter the picture, as do stability of income, credit history, and receipt of public assistance. If the patient has children, their number, ages, and health status are noted, along with whether the patient takes an active parental role. Further questions ask about abuse and neglect and about whether the patient, if male, could have fathered additional children of whom he is unaware.

Formal Assessments

Psychological testing is usually unnecessary but can be helpful when a patient is not forthcoming in his or her responses or if informants are unavailable. The Minnesota Multiphasic Personality Inventory (MMPI), and subsequent revisions, yields a broad profile of personality functioning. Antisocial persons often show peaks on Scale 4 (psychopathic deviance) and Scale 9 (hypomania), referred to as the "4–9 profile" (Butcher et al. 1989; Dahlstrom et al. 1972; Tellegen et al. 2003). Projective tests, such as the Rorschach ("ink blot test"), aim to reveal insights about the person's "inner world" by asking him or her to respond to ambiguous stimuli. For example, responses of those with ASPD might show evidence of emotional detachment, chronic anger, or fantasies of omnipotent control (Meloy and Gacano 2003).

The Psychopathy Checklist—Revised can be helpful in measuring the severity of the individual's psychopathic traits. In prison populations, the scale appears to predict recidivism and parole violations. For example, in a study of 231 male prison inmates categorized as psychopaths (Psychopathy Checklist score ≥34) or nonpsychopaths (score ≤24), 65% of the psychopaths violated their release conditions compared with

24% of the nonpsychopaths (Hart et al. 1988). The parent instrument is relatively lengthy and requires special training to administer, but a shorter version is available.

Several structured interviews are available to help diagnose ASPD. Mainly used in research, several instruments have been shown to be reliable and valid, including the Alcohol Use Disorder and Associated Disabilities Interview Schedule, DSM-5 Version (Hasin et al. 2015); Structured Interview for DSM-IV Personality Disorders (Pfohl et al. 1997); Structured Clinical Interview for DSM-5 Personality Disorders (First et al. 2016); and ICD-10 International Personality Disorder Examination (Loranger et al. 1997). These interviews require training and are usually administered by clinicians. The Personality Diagnostic Questionnaire-IV also can be used to diagnose ASPD and has the advantage of being self-administered (Hyler 1994). Of note, the criteria set for ASPD did not change from DSM-IV (American Psychiatric Association 1994) to DSM-5, which is important to understand if using these instruments.

Standardized questionnaires can be used to assess traits or problems of interest to the clinician or researcher, including mood and anxiety, aggression and hostility, impulsiveness, substance use, and suicidality. For example, the Beck Depression Inventory (Beck 1978) can be used to assess depressive symptoms such as sadness, apathy, or suicidal behavior. The Michigan Alcoholism Screening Test (Teitelbaum and Mullen 2000) can be used to measure a patient's use of alcohol. The Buss-Durkee Hostility Inventory (Velicer et al. 1985) can help assess aggressive tendencies. The Barratt Impulsiveness Scale (Barratt 1959) can be used to assess the person's potential for impulsive acting out. The choice of questionnaires should be tailored to the needs of the clinician or researcher.

Cognitive and intellectual testing can be helpful in selected individuals particularly because many antisocial persons have borderline intellectual functioning or a diagnosable learning disorder (Moffitt 1993; Raine 2018). Understanding the patient's specific learning disabilities can help inform goals for therapy or rehabilitation services. A qualified neuropsychologist should be consulted regarding the choice and administration of specific cognitive tests.

Mental Status Examination

The mental status examination in people with ASPD is generally unrevealing. Some antisocial persons might display a sullen, angry, or hostile demeanor during an interview, but these affects are not unique to the disorder. Orientation and sensorium are typically normal in the absence of intoxication or neurocognitive disorders. The presence of a thought disorder, hallucinations, or delusions is unexpected unless the person has an associated psychotic disorder (e.g., a drug-induced psychosis). Tests of memory and calculation are likely unremarkable.

Because antisocial persons are at increased risk for suicide attempts and completed suicide, they should be asked about current suicidal thoughts and past suicidal behaviors, particularly if they endorse depressed mood or have a depressed affect. More worrisome, occasional patients will endorse thoughts of harming or even killing another person. If so, the clinician should make further inquiries to determine whether an intended victim needs to be notified in fulfillment of the *Tarasoff* rule regarding third-party warnings (Knoll 2015; McNiel et al. 1998).

Curiously, antisocial persons typically lack insight into their ASPD and often blame others for their problems. Their lack of insight led Cleckley (1976) to write: "[The] psychopath lacks insight more consistently than some schizophrenic patients.

He has absolutely no capacity to see himself as others see him" (p. 383). His comment would apply equally to people with ASPD.

Physical Examination and Laboratory Tests

A patient presenting with symptoms of ASPD should receive a physical examination including a neurological examination. The physical examination might detect evidence of past injuries from fights or accidents, knife or gunshot wounds, scars from self-injurious behaviors (e.g., cutting), or even nail-biting (Walker and Ziskind 1977). Physical signs of alcohol or drug abuse could be present depending on the patient's pattern of misuse; for example, an enlarged liver, a Dupuytren's contracture, or track marks from repeated injection drug use.

The presence of tattoos has been associated with ASPD (Newman 1982). Even as their frequency in the general population has increased in men and women, tattoos continue to be associated with risk-taking behaviors, such as greater use of alcohol or other drugs and criminality (Laumann and Derick 2006). Tattoos are especially common in prison populations, where they might have special significance by indicating individual or group identity. One prison-based study found that persons with ASPD had more tattoos and more total body surface area tattooed than did those without ASPD (Cardasis et al. 2008).

The choice of laboratory tests, if any, will be prompted by the patient's medical history or presenting symptoms, such as a blood alcohol test or urine drug screen, or liver enzyme tests for those who abuse alcohol. Perhaps reflecting their tendency to engage in impulsive or risky behaviors, persons with ASPD are at increased risk for sexually transmitted diseases, including HIV and hepatitis C infections, and motor vehicle and other accidents that can result in fractures, lacerations, and closed head injuries (Brooner et al. 1993; Woodruff et al. 1971).

Routine structural or functional brain scans are unnecessary in the absence of localizing neurological signs. Electroencephalograms (EEGs) are appropriate in antisocial persons when a seizure disorder is suspected but are otherwise not indicated. Many antisocial persons have abnormal EEG results compared with nonantisocial persons, but they have little diagnostic significance (Dolan 1994).

Differential Diagnosis

The differential diagnosis of ASPD includes other personality disorders (e.g., borderline personality disorder, narcissistic personality disorder), substance use disorders, psychotic and mood disorders, intermittent explosive disorder, and medical conditions such as temporal lobe epilepsy (Black 2013). ASPD needs to be distinguished from borderline personality disorder, a syndrome characterized by the presence of unstable moods, relationships, and behaviors (e.g., self-harm) diagnosed predominantly in women. Although ASPD and borderline personality disorder are often comorbid, they are fundamentally distinct (Paris et al. 2013).

Chronic or intermittent alcohol or drug use can contribute to the development of antisocial behavior, either as a direct consequence of the intoxication itself or as a result of a drug habit that needs financial support. Psychoses or bipolar disorder also can lead to violent or assaultive behavior and should be ruled out as a cause of antisocial behavior. Psychotic patients occasionally commit criminal offenses, but such behavior typically results from psychotic thought processes. Intermittent explosive disorder involves isolated episodes of assaultive or destructive behavior, but the patient usually has no history of childhood conduct disorder or other features of ASPD, such as a pattern of chronic irresponsibility or failure to honor obligations.

Medical explanations for antisocial behavior that need ruling out include temporal lobe epilepsy, which can cause random outbursts of violence, and tumors or strokes, which could lead to personality changes (Anderson et al. 1999).

Key Points

- The symptoms of antisocial personality disorder (ASPD) can be roughly divided among those associated with childhood (or adolescence) and those associated with adulthood. They often reflect the individual's age and degree of opportunity for misconduct.

- Symptoms occur along a spectrum of severity. More severe cases tend to be associated with aggression or violence and lack of remorse.

- Diagnosis of ASPD is driven by the individual's history because there are no diagnostic tests.

- The individual's mental status examination is likely to be unremarkable unless there is evidence of intoxication, depression, suicidality, or expressions of violence. Antisocial persons often have a profound lack of insight regarding their ASPD.

- The differential diagnosis should be broad. The ASPD diagnosis will be excluded if antisocial behaviors are present only during the course of mania or schizophrenia.

References

American Psychiatric Association: Diagnostic and Statistical Manual of Mental Disorders, 4th Edition. Washington, DC, American Psychiatric Association, 1994

American Psychiatric Association: Diagnostic and Statistical Manual of Mental Disorders, 5th Edition. Arlington, VA, American Psychiatric Association, 2013

Anderson SW, Bechara A, Damasio H, et al: Impairment of social and moral behavior related to early damage in human prefrontal cortex. Nat Neurosci 2(11):1032–1037, 1999 10526345

Andreasen NC, Rice J, Endicott J, et al: The family history approach to diagnosis: how useful is it? Arch Gen Psychiatry 43(5):421–429, 1986 3964020

Barratt ES: Anxiety and impulsiveness related to psychomotor efficiency. Percept Mot Skills 9:191–198, 1959

Beck AT: Depression Inventory. Philadelphia, PA, Philadelphia Center for Cognitive Therapy, 1978

Black DW: Bad Boys, Bad Men: Confronting Antisocial Personality Disorder (Sociopathy), Revised and Updated. New York, Oxford University Press, 2013

Black DW, Andreasen NC: Interviewing and assessment, in Introductory Textbook of Psychiatry, 7th Edition. Washington, DC, American Psychiatric Association Publishing, 2020

Black DW, Braun D: Antisocial patients: a comparison of those with and those without childhood conduct disorder. Ann Clin Psychiatry 10(2):53–57, 1998 9669536

Black DW, Grant JE: DSM-5 Guidebook: The Essential Companion to the Diagnostic and Statistical Manual of Mental Disorders, Fifth Edition. Washington, DC, American Psychiatric Publishing, 2014

Black DW, Baumgard CH, Bell SE: A 16- to 45-year follow-up of 71 men with antisocial personality disorder. Compr Psychiatry 36(2):130–140, 1995 7758299

Brook M, Hilty DM, Liu W, et al: Discharge against medical advice from inpatient psychiatric treatment: a literature review. Psychiatr Serv 57(8):1192–1198, 2006 16870972

Brooner RK, Greenfield L, Schmidt CW, et al: Antisocial personality disorder and HIV infection among intravenous drug abusers. Am J Psychiatry 150(1):53–58, 1993 8417580

Butcher JN, Dahlstrom WG, Graham JR, et al: The Minnesota Multiphasic Personality Inventory-2 (MMPI-2): Manual for Administration and Scoring. Minneapolis, University of Minnesota, 1989

Cardasis W, Huth-Bocks A, Silk KR: Tattoos and antisocial personality disorder. Personality and Mental Health 2(3):171–182, 2008

Cleckley H: The Mask of Sanity: An Attempt to Clarify Some Issues About the So-Called Psychopathic Personality, 5th Edition. St. Louis, MO, CV Mosby, 1976

Dahlstrom WG, Welsh GS, Dahlstrom LE: An MMPI Handbook. Minneapolis, University of Minnesota Press, 1972

Dolan M: Psychopathy—a neurobiological perspective. Br J Psychiatry 165(2):151–159, 1994 7953028

Egami Y, Ford DE, Greenfield SF, et al: Psychiatric profile and sociodemographic characteristics of adults who report physically abusing or neglecting children. Am J Psychiatry 153(7):921–928, 1996 8659615

Falb KL, McCauley HL, Decker MR, et al: School bullying perpetration and other childhood risk factors as predictors of adult intimate partner violence perpetration. Arch Pediatr Adolesc Med 165(10):890–894, 2011 21646570

Fiedler ER, Oltmanns TF, Turkheimer E: Traits associated with personality disorders and adjustment to military life: predictive validity of self and peer reports. Mil Med 169(3):207–211, 2004 15080240

First MB, William JBW, Benjamin LS, et al: Structured Clinical Interview for DSM-5 Personality Disorders. Washington, DC, American Psychiatric Publishing, 2016

Glueck S, Glueck E: Unraveling Juvenile Delinquency. New York, Commonwealth Fund, 1950

Goldstein RB, Powers SI, McCusker J, et al: Lack of remorse in antisocial personality disorder among drug abusers in residential treatment. J Pers Disord 10(4):321–334, 1996

Goldstein RB, Grant BF, Huang B, et al: Lack of remorse in antisocial personality disorder: sociodemographic correlates, symptomatic presentation, and comorbidity with Axis I and Axis II disorders in the National Epidemiologic Survey on Alcohol and Related Conditions. Compr Psychiatry 47(4):289–297, 2006a 16769304

Goldstein RB, Grant BF, Ruan WJ, et al: Antisocial personality disorder with childhood- vs. adolescence-onset conduct disorder: results from the National Epidemiologic Survey on Alcohol and Related Conditions. J Nerv Ment Dis 194(9):667–675, 2006b 16971818

Guze SB, Goodwin DW, Crane JB: A psychiatric study of the wives of convicted felons: an example of assortative mating. Am J Psychiatry 126(12):1773–1776, 1970 5441731

Hart SD, Kropp PR, Hare RD: Performance of male psychopaths following conditional release from prison. J Consult Clin Psychol 56(2):227–232, 1988 3372830

Hasin DS, Greenstein E, Aivadyan C, et al: The Alcohol Use Disorder and Associated Disabilities Interview Schedule-5 (AUDADIS-5): procedural validity of substance use disorders modules through clinical re-appraisal in a general population sample. Drug Alcohol Depend 148:40–46, 2015 25604321

Hellman DS, Blackman N: Enuresis, firesetting and cruelty to animals: a triad predictive of adult crime. Am J Psychiatry 122(12):1431–1435, 1966 5929498

Hyler SE: PDQ-4 and PDQ-4t: Instructions for Use. New York, New York State Psychiatric Institute, 1994

Knoll JL: The psychiatrist's duty to protect. CNS Spectr 20(3):215–222, 2015 25712614

Laumann AE, Derick AJ: Tattoos and body piercings in the United States: a national data set. J Am Acad Dermatol 55(3):413–421, 2006 16908345

Loeber R, Stouthammer-Loeber M: Prediction, in Handbook of Juvenile Delinquency. Edited by Quay HC. New York, Wiley, 1987, pp 325–382

Loranger AW, Janca A, Sartorius N: The ICD-10 International Personality Disorder Examination. Cambridge, UK, Cambridge University Press, 1997

McNiel DE, Binder RL, Fulton FM: Management of threats of violence under California's duty-to-protect statute. Am J Psychiatry 155(8):1097–1101, 1998 9699700

Meloy JR, Gacano CB: The internal world of the psychopath, in Psychopathy: Antisocial, Criminal, and Violent Behavior. Edited by Millon T, Simonsen E, Birket-Smith M, et al. New York, Guilford, 2003, pp 95–109

Moffitt T: The neuropsychology of conduct disorder. Dev Psychopathol 5:135–151, 1993

Newman G: The implications of tattooing in prisoners. J Clin Psychiatry 43(6):231–234, 1982 7085576

Paris J, Chenard-Poirier MP, Biskin R: Antisocial and borderline personality disorders revisited. Compr Psychiatry 54(4):321–325, 2013 23200574

Pfohl B, Zimmerman M, Blum N: A Structured Interview for DSM-IV Personality Disorders (SIDP-IV). Washington, DC, American Psychiatric Press, 1997

Pomeroy JC, Behar D, Stewart MA: Abnormal sexual behaviour in pre-pubescent children. Br J Psychiatry 138:119–125, 1981 7260490

Raine A: Antisocial personality as a neurodevelopmental disorder. Annu Rev Clin Psychol 14:259–289, 2018 29401045

Robins L: Deviant Children Grown Up. Baltimore, MD, Williams & Wilkins, 1966

Robins LN: The epidemiology of antisocial personality disorder, in Psychiatry, Volume 3. Edited by Michels RO, Cavenar JO. Philadelphia, PA, Lippincott, 1987, pp 1–14

Schechter MD: Adoption, in Comprehensive Textbook of Psychiatry, 5th Edition. Edited by Kaplan HI, Sadock BJ. Baltimore, MD, Williams & Wilkins, 1989, pp 1958–1962

Shapiro S, Skinner EA, Kessler LG, et al: Utilization of health and mental health services: three Epidemiologic Catchment Area sites. Arch Gen Psychiatry 41(10):971–978, 1984 6477055

Slutske WS: The genetics of antisocial behavior. Curr Psychiatry Rep 3(2):158–162, 2001 11276412

Teitelbaum L, Mullen B: The validity of the MAST in psychiatric settings: a meta-analytic integration. Michigan Alcoholism Screening Test. J Stud Alcohol 61(2):254–261, 2000 10757136

Tellegen A, Ben-Porath YS, McNulty JL, et al: The MMPI-2 Restructured Clinical Scales: Development, Validation, and Interpretation. Minneapolis, University of Minnesota, 2003

Ullrich S, Coid J: Antisocial personality disorder: co-morbid Axis I mental disorders and health service use among a national household population. Personal Ment Health 164(3):151–164, 2009

Velicer WF, Govia JM, Cherico NP, et al: Item format and the structure of the Buss-Durkee Hostility Inventory. Aggressive Behavior 11:65–82, 1985

Walker BA, Ziskind E: Relationship of nailbiting to sociopathy. J Nerv Ment Dis 164(1):64–65, 1977 830804

Woodruff RA Jr, Guze SB, Clayton PJ: The medical and psychiatric implications of antisocial personality (sociopathy). Dis Nerv Syst 32(10):712–714, 1971 5146430

PART III

Etiology and Pathophysiology

CHAPTER 6

Natural History and Course of Antisocial Personality Disorder

Donald W. Black, M.D.
Risë B. Goldstein, Ph.D., M.P.H.

Antisocial personality disorder (ASPD) is a lifelong disorder with an onset in childhood that is fully expressed by the late teens or early 20s. Antisocial behaviors typically have their onset around the ninth year of life (Robins 1987). Nearly 80% of future patients have developed their first symptom by age 11 years (Robins 1987; Robins et al. 1991). Robins (1966) has observed that a child who makes it to age 15 without showing antisocial behaviors (i.e., conduct disorder) will not develop ASPD. This finding, however, was based on a cohort ascertained through a child guidance clinic, among whom 82% of boys and 69% of girls were age 15 years

The National Epidemiologic Survey on Alcohol and Related Conditions (NESARC) and the National Epidemiologic Survey on Alcohol and Related Conditions-III (NESARC-III) were funded by the National Institute on Alcohol Abuse and Alcoholism (NIAAA) with supplemental support from the National Institute on Drug Abuse, National Institutes of Health (NIH), Bethesda, MD. This work was supported in part by the Intramural Program of the NIH, NIAAA, and *Eunice Kennedy Shriver* National Institute of Child Health and Human Development. Data from the NESARC-III were analyzed using a limited access data set obtained from NIAAA. The NIH had no further role in study design; in the collection, analysis, and interpretation of data; in the writing of the chapter; or in the decision to submit the chapter for publication.

The views, opinions, and assertions expressed in this chapter are those of the authors and should not be construed to represent the views or the official policy or position of any of the sponsoring organizations or agencies or the U.S. government.

or younger at referral. In addition, 73% were male and two-thirds were referred to the clinic for serious childhood antisocial behavior (Robins 1966; Tweed et al. 1994). It would therefore have been difficult for Robins (1966) to identify a substantial prevalence of later-onset antisociality (Tweed et al. 1994), which has been found in some but not all studies to be overrepresented among girls and women. Nevertheless, based in substantial part on Robins' (1966) finding, diagnostic classifications since the criteria of Feighner et al. (1972) have required evidence of both conduct disorder before age 15 years and severe, versatile antisocial behavior through (and, in most instances, beyond) age 18 years.

An estimated 40% of male and 25% of female respondents in the St. Louis, Missouri, Epidemiologic Catchment Area (ECA) sample who endorsed at least three DSM-III (American Psychiatric Association 1980) conduct problems before age 15 met criteria for ASPD (Robins 1987). More recent epidemiological samples based on DSM-IV (American Psychiatric Association 1994), DSM-IV-TR (American Psychiatric Association 2000), and DSM-5 (American Psychiatric Association 2013) criteria identified much higher progression rates. In the National Epidemiologic Survey on Alcohol and Related Conditions (NESARC; Compton et al. 2005), 79% of male and 73% of female respondents diagnosed with conduct disorder with onset before age 15 met criteria for ASPD. In the National Epidemiologic Survey on Alcohol and Related Conditions-III (NESARC-III), the parallel estimates were 91% of male and 88% of female respondents (R.B. Goldstein, S.P. Chou, unpublished data, July 2019).

In this chapter, we focus on studies based on general population, clinical, and correctional samples that describe the course and continuity of serious antisocial behavior from childhood through adulthood, the duration and persistence of such behavior, outcomes of antisocial behavior, and factors associated with its remission or clinical improvement.

Course and Continuity of Antisocial Behavior From Childhood to Adulthood

Early Follow-up Studies: the Gluecks and Robins

Contemporaneous research conducted in the 1940s and 1950s by Glueck and Glueck (1950) at Harvard University with a sample of boys identified through the Massachusetts correctional system and Robins (1966) and her colleagues at Washington University in St. Louis with former child guidance clinic patients independently showed the continuity between behavior problems in childhood and adulthood. Glueck and Glueck (1950), among the first researchers to observe this continuity, followed up 500 boys between ages 10 and 17 judged "officially delinquent." These boys were studied intensively and were reinterviewed at ages 25, 32, and 45 years. Severe antisocial behavior in childhood remained strongly linked to adult crime and deviance. Arrests between ages 17 and 32 years were three to four times more likely to occur among men who had been delinquent boys than among their nondelinquent peers. Childhood antisocial behavior also predicted educational achievement, economic status, employment, and family life in adulthood. Based on their reanalyses of the

Gluecks' data, Sampson and Laub (1993) concluded that the Gluecks' research showed "a stable tendency toward criminality and other troublesome behavior…. From this viewpoint, the varied outcomes correlated with childhood behavior are all expressions of the same underlying trait or propensity" (p. 136).

More influential was the work of Robins (1966) and her colleagues who studied 524 subjects seen in a child guidance clinic between 1922 and 1932 and followed up in the 1950s. The children were on average 13 years old when seen at the clinic; 73% were boys, most of whom had been referred from juvenile court, mainly for serious antisocial behaviors as noted previously.

Of the 524 subjects, 94 were retrospectively rediagnosed as "sociopathic" in adulthood, 82 of whom were interviewed an average of 30 years later. Robins found that in these subjects at a mean age of 45 years, 12% had remitted (i.e., no evidence of antisocial behavior), 27% had improved but not remitted, and 61% were unimproved or worse. The fact that a subject had improved, however, did not mean that the disorder was no longer a problem. She writes:

> The finding that more than one-third of the sociopathic group had given up much of the antisocial behavior…does not mean that at present they are strikingly well-adjusted and agreeable persons. Many of them report interpersonal difficulties, irritability, hostility toward wives, neighbors, and organized religion. They are in many cases no longer either a threat to the life and property of others nor a financial drain on society. (p. 236)

More Recent Youth Follow-up Studies

Late twentieth and early twenty-first century follow-up studies of the continuity and course of childhood antisocial behavior include the Developmental Trends Study (Lahey et al. 2005; Loeber et al. 2002a, 2002b). Beginning in 1987, this study involved 177 boys in Pennsylvania and Georgia ages 7–12 years who were followed up at regular intervals into early adulthood. The purpose of the study was to document the course of disruptive behavior over time and its interaction with co-occurring disorders (e.g., anxiety disorders). The boys were recruited from university clinics to which they had been referred because of disruptive behavior disorders such as ADHD or conduct disorder. The investigators showed that boys with an early onset of symptoms had a faster progression to more serious problems than boys whose problems emerged at a later age; physical fighting predicted the onset of conduct disorder more than any other symptoms; oppositional defiant disorder appeared to be a developmental precursor to conduct disorder in some boys; and conduct disorder was predictive of syndromal levels of antisocial behavior in early adulthood (ages 18 and 19 years; Loeber et al. 2002a).

The Pittsburgh Youth Study (Loeber et al. 1993, 2002b) also began in 1987. Its aim was to trace the development of antisocial and delinquent behavior from childhood to early adulthood. The investigators screened 1,517 boys in the first, fourth, and seventh grades in the Pittsburgh, Pennsylvania, public schools, and the 30% most antisocial boys were selected for follow-up along with 30% of the remainder as a comparison group. The boys ranged in age from 7 to 13 years at intake. In this study, the researchers showed that problem behaviors occurred along a developmental trajectory from childhood to adolescence. The onset of minor covert acts, such as lying and shoplifting, tended to occur before the onset of property damage, which occurred before the onset of moderate to serious forms of delinquency.

Outcomes of Antisocial Personality Disorder Among Clinically Referred and General Population Adults

The Iowa Antisocial Follow-up

Black and coworkers (1995a) followed up 71 men who had been psychiatrically hospitalized as adults at the University of Iowa between 1945 and 1970 and who were retrospectively diagnosed with ASPD according to DSM-III criteria. After a mean of 29 years of follow-up, the research team was able to trace more than 90% of the men and had enough information to rate outcomes in 45. At follow-up, the mean age of the men was 56 years. Using ratings of antisocial symptomatology and measures of social and occupational adjustment like those used by Robins, Black et al. concluded that 27% of the subjects had remitted, 31% had improved but not remitted, and 42% were unimproved or worse.

Black et al. (1995a) concluded that many of the antisocial behaviors present at index evaluation were still present at follow-up:

> Although most of our subjects were no longer having frequent confrontations with the police, they continued to have enduring problems with poor occupational performance, social isolation, marital discord, poor family relations, and substance abuse. (p. 138)

Black et al. (1995b) later compared the course of the antisocial men with that of persons with schizophrenia or depression, as well as with control subjects, based on previously published data from the "Iowa 500" study. All subjects had been hospitalized at the same facility. Antisocial men fared less well than depressed subjects and control subjects in their marital, occupational, and psychiatric adjustment. Antisocial men functioned better than patients hospitalized with schizophrenia in their marital status and housing but not in their occupational status or aggregate psychiatric symptoms. In other words, they were more likely than schizophrenic persons to be married and to have their own housing, but they were as likely to perform poorly in the workplace and to have disabling psychiatric symptoms, although the specific symptoms differed (e.g., schizophrenic subjects had delusions, the antisocial men were violent).

The case of Mr. C, one of the antisocial men enrolled in the Iowa Antisocial Follow-up, shows that some antisocial persons "improve" with advancing age, which means that they are no longer regularly misbehaving or that some antisocial symptoms have remitted. In contrast, Burton, whose case was presented in Chapter 5, "Clinical Symptoms and Assessment of Antisocial Personality Disorder," was considered unimproved.

> Mr. C, age 28, was admitted to the University of Iowa Psychiatric Hospital for evaluation of "lack of drive and ambition" and inability to find security and happiness, but the doctors quickly noted his history of stealing, absenteeism from work, and inability to hold a job as suggestive of an underlying ASPD. Mr. C grew up in a two-parent, sol-

idly middle-class home. His father was described as domineering and ill-tempered and would often criticize Mr. C for his shiftlessness, whereas his mother was overprotective, often ignoring his misbehaviors. His two sisters were socially adept and academically gifted, but they had little interest in their troubled brother.

Mr. C's misbehaviors started around age 5 years, when he first ran away from home. At age 6, he started a fire in a shed, and by age 11, he was regularly stealing money from his mother's purse. Mr. C managed to finish high school with middling grades and started college, but he would skip classes and eventually dropped out. At age 20, he broke into a local drugstore but tripped an alarm and was caught. A guilty plea led to his first jail sentence.

Mr. C joined the army and was sent to the European front. He served 6 years but was court-martialed for stealing money from a superior officer's trousers and was dishonorably discharged from the service. After the discharge, he returned home and married after a brief courtship. His wife knew nothing of his past. The family moved to California (he and his wife had one child by then) seeking new opportunities but failed to find work, and in a quixotic move, he stole a car with the plan to drive back to Iowa. He was quickly apprehended, pleaded guilty, and received probation. His criminal career continued, mainly involving breaking and entering, to supplement, he said, his meager income from his work as an unskilled laborer. He often was fired or would quit without having another job lined up.

At the hospital, a physical examination showed only obesity and mild hypertension, and Mr. C's mental status was deemed normal. He reported being anxious and made critical remarks about the doctors. He declined to talk about his criminal past. He was offered individual and group psychotherapy, a standard approach at the time, and remained 5 months. At discharge, he was thought to have a "poor" prognosis.

Mr. C was followed up at age 65. By then, he was living in a small apartment in a small rural community. He reported that he was lonely, as his wife had passed away, and he was estranged from his three children. One daughter had a history of antisocial behavior during adolescence and had been psychiatrically hospitalized. He had a part-time job with an insurance agency and had worked there for 25 years. He admitted to having had severe temper outbursts when younger but said that those had subsided, and he no longer got into arguments or fights. He was ashamed of his earlier court-martial but claimed that his stealing had always been motivated by poor money management. In the intervening decades, Mr. C claimed only an additional two arrests, but his "rap sheet," which was public information, revealed a much different story, with multiple arrests with incarceration for mainly minor nonviolent offenses.

Mr. C felt that the lengthy psychiatric hospitalization had helped him grow as a person and that he had genuinely improved, attributing much of that to the influence of his loving wife. He reported regular church attendance and socialized with his neighbors.

Mr. C meets the criteria for ASPD but has a relatively mild disorder. He had both childhood and adult manifestations, but by age 65, they had mostly subsided. By that age, he was a steady employee and was engaged with his community. He was no longer actively antisocial, but he still never took full responsibility for his criminal conduct and chalked it up to poor budgeting rather than any underlying disorder.

The collective work of Robins (1966) and Black et al. (1995a, 1995b) showed that most dangerous and destructive behaviors associated with ASPD may improve or remit, yet other troublesome problems remain. Older people with ASPD are less likely to commit crimes or become violent, but many remain troublesome to their families and the community (Epstein et al. 1970). Some fail to improve at all. When improvement occurs, it typically follows many years of antisocial behavior that has stunted the individual's educational and work achievement, thus limiting his or her potential achievement.

Follow-up of Antisocial Adults in the General Population

Goldstein and colleagues (Goldstein and Grant 2009; Goldstein et al. 2012) conducted what is, to our knowledge, the only prospective follow-up of antisocial adults in the general population. Goldstein and Grant (2009) used data from Waves 1 and 2 of the NESARC and found that 52.8% of adult respondents (53.8% of men, 47.5% of women) diagnosed with ASPD at Wave 1 reported no antisocial symptoms at all during the 3-year follow-up period between Waves 1 and 2. Considering "more serious" anti-social behaviors, 78.8% (78.5% of men, 79.8% of women) reported no major violations of the rights of others, defined as any of the following: vandalism, fire setting, stealing with or without confrontation of a victim, forgery, illegal occupation, forcing another person into sexual activity, repeated initiation of fights, swapping blows with inti-mates, use of a dangerous weapon, hitting someone and causing injury, harassment or blackmail, hurting another person on purpose, and hurting an animal on purpose. An even larger majority, 86.5% (87.0% of men, 85.2% of women), reported no violent symptoms, defined as any of the following: bullying, pushing around, or intimidat-ing others; vandalism; fire setting; robbing, mugging, or snatching someone's purse; forcing sexual activity; repeated initiation of fights; swapping blows with intimates; use of a dangerous weapon; hitting someone and causing injury; hurting another per-son on purpose; and hurting an animal on purpose. Whether the final remission of symptoms actually began during the 3-year follow-up period or earlier, however, could not be determined from the available data.

Despite the substantial prevalence of symptomatic remission over follow-up, a broad range of quality-of-life outcomes among antisocial NESARC respondents paint a relatively bleak picture consistent with the findings of Black et al. (1995a, 1995b) and Robins (1966). After adjustment for sociodemographic characteristics and comorbid lifetime psychiatric disorders ascertained at baseline, respondents with ASPD were less likely than those who had no lifetime history of syndromal antisociality to report at 3-year follow-up that they were employed in the past year, felt close to any rela-tives, had any close friends, or saw or talked to relatives or close friends at least every 2 weeks. Conversely, respondents with ASPD were more likely than those who were never antisocial to report past-year dependency on public financial support. Those with ASPD also reported poorer physical health–related quality of life, an association especially pronounced among those oldest at baseline; in addition, women with ASPD reported higher perceived stress. Although statistical significance was fre-quently lost, these patterns generally held among antisocial respondents who re-ported no antisocial symptoms over follow-up (Goldstein et al. 2012). Like Black et al. (1995a, 1995b), Goldstein et al. (2012) interpreted these findings as reflecting per-sistent "scars" left by lengthy durations of severe and versatile antisocial behavior that constrained subsequent life chances.

Duration, Persistence, and Remission

The follow-up studies reviewed earlier confirm both the continuity of serious anti-social behavior over the life course and its chronicity. Several cross-sectional epidemi-ological studies also documented the lengthy duration and persistence of ASPD.

Robins et al. (1991) found that ECA respondents had a mean duration of ASPD (defined as time from first to last symptom) of 19 years. In the NESARC-III, duration was defined among remitted respondents as the time from age at onset of "some" (two or more) symptoms to the age at occurrence reported by respondents who answered affirmatively to the question: "Was there EVER a time when you NO LONGER had ANY of the experiences you just mentioned, that is, a time when NONE of the experiences EVER happened again?" Mean duration was 12.4 years and, as might be expected, positively associated with respondent age at interview, ranging from 7.3 years among those ages 18–29 to 17.2 years among those age 65 and older (R.B. Goldstein, S.P. Chou, unpublished data, June 2019).

Conditional prevalence estimates covering "recent" periods among individuals with lifetime diagnoses provide further cross-sectional evidence of the chronicity of ASPD. Past-year prevalence of ASPD symptomatology among general population respondents with a lifetime diagnosis ranged from 0% in Taiwan (Hwu et al. 1989) to more than 40% in the NESARC-III (R.B. Goldstein, S.P. Chou, unpublished data, June 2019) and ECA (Robins et al. 1991) and 66% in Edmonton, Alberta (Swanson et al. 1994). Proportions of general population respondents with lifetime ASPD who were symptomatic during the preceding 6 months ranged from 29% in Christchurch, New Zealand (Oakley-Browne et al. 1989), to 49% in Edmonton (Swanson et al. 1994).

Despite ASPD's substantial duration and persistence, the studies of both clinical and general population samples reviewed previously demonstrate that remission or substantial clinical improvement of ASPD is also the rule (Black et al. 1995a; Goldstein and Grant 2009; Oakley-Browne et al. 1989; Robins et al. 1991; Swanson et al. 1994). In both cross-sectional and prospective studies of general population and clinical samples, remission or improvement typically begins around the fourth or fifth decade of life (Black et al. 1995a; Goldstein and Grant 2009; Robins 1966; Robins et al. 1991; Swanson et al. 1994). However, as noted by Robins (1966), there was "no age beyond which improvement seemed impossible" (p. 222). In the NESARC-III (R.B. Goldstein, S.P. Chou, unpublished data, June 2019), respondents with lifetime ASPD who remitted reported doing so at a mean age of 24.4 years. Reported age at remission was positively associated with current age, ranging from 19.6 among respondents ages 18–29 years to 29.8 among those age 65 and older.

Trajectories of Antisocial Personality Disorder

Moffitt and colleagues (Moffitt 1993; Odgers et al. 2008) have suggested that ASPD is highly stable in a relatively small percentage of men and women whose behavior problems are "life-course persistent." As part of the Dunedin Multidisciplinary Health and Development Study in New Zealand, Moffitt and coworkers traced the outcome of 1,037 children born between April 1, 1972, and March 31, 1973, from age 3 years to 32 years. At age 32, 10.5% of male and 7.5% of female cohort members showed a life-course-persistent trajectory (Odgers et al. 2008). Approximately twice as many, 19.6% of male and 17.4% of female subjects, were categorized as having an "adolescence-onset" form of antisocial behavior, described as less severe and typically arising in the context of teenage peer group pressure. In addition, 24.3% of male and 20.0% of female cohort members had childhood-limited antisociality. Individuals with trajectories other than life-course persistent improve substantially although not completely on their own (Odgers et al. 2008; Rivenbark et al. 2018), accounting for the fact that the prospectively observed clinical course of most children diagnosed with conduct disorder does not evolve into ASPD. For both men and women, the life-course-persistent group showed an early onset of antisocial behavior, developed more severe behavior problems, and had a greater variety of problems in adulthood compared with the adolescence-onset and childhood-limited individuals.

Outcome Predictors in Antisocial Personality Disorder

Robins (1966) found that most of the children improved as they grew older and did not become antisocial adults. She concluded that variety and severity of childhood behavior problems were the single best predictors of adult antisocial behavior. Robins wrote that

> No patient without moderately severe antisocial behavior, as measured by having six or more kinds of antisocial behavior, four or more episodes of antisocial behavior, or an episode of such behavior serious enough that it might have led to a court appearance, was diagnosed with sociopathic personality as [an] adult. (p. 157)

Among the few variables predictive of long-term adjustment, Robins (1966) observed that greater improvement occurred in those older than 40 years at follow-up. These findings are consistent with data reported by Black et al. (1997) in which improvement in antisocial men was positively associated with increasing age.

In addition, Black et al. (1997) found that antisocial men having a better outcome were more likely to have low initial severity, were not currently alcohol dependent, and had a longer duration of follow-up. Broadly consistent with these findings, Goldstein and Grant (2009) found that persistent antisocial behavior (i.e., lack of symptomatic remission) over 3-year follow-up was independently predicted in the NESARC by male sex, age younger than 45 years at Wave 1, and more antisocial symptoms reported from age 15 years to Wave 1. Additional independent predictors of persistent antisociality in the NESARC follow-up included comorbid lifetime diagnoses up to Wave 1 of drug use disorders, ADHD, and additional personality disorders (Goldstein and Grant 2009). Inasmuch as evidence-based treatments are available for these comorbid conditions, their associations with persistence of antisocial symptomatology raise the clinically urgent question of whether treating the comorbid disorders might hasten its desistance.

Another prognostic variable is incarceration. Robins (1966) found that men incarcerated less than a year had a higher rate of remission than did those who were never incarcerated or those who were incarcerated for a longer time. This latter finding suggests that a brief incarceration could act as a deterrent to further antisocial behavior.

Marriage is an additional factor associated with a relatively favorable prognosis. Robins (1966) found that more than half of married antisocial persons, but few unmarried persons, improved. Similarly, Goldstein and Grant (2009) found that marital status other than currently married or cohabiting at baseline independently predicted persistent antisocial behavior over the 3-year NESARC follow-up. Spouses, partners, and others close to the antisocial person can play an important role in urging therapy, and improvement often comes when one has a source of personal support and motivation. Antisocial individuals who remitted had stronger family ties, were more involved in their communities, and were more likely to live with their spouses. These findings are largely consistent with the Gluecks' (Glueck and Glueck 1950) findings that linked job stability and marital attachment with improvement. Nevertheless, each of these situations—from brief incarceration to relative success with marriage and family life—could easily be the *result* of improvement rather than its cause.

One might expect that antisocial persons who stay happily married, or who have not faced lengthy periods of incarceration, simply have milder cases of ASPD to begin with or are otherwise predisposed to getting better. There is some evidence for this, at least with regard to marriage. In a study of male twins followed up from age 17 to 29 years, the researchers discovered that men with *less* severe forms of antisocial behavior were more likely to marry than their more antisocial twin (Burt et al. 2010). Severe antisocial symptoms may hinder marriage because they interfere with forming intimate relationships.

Another characteristic that may portend more favorable outcomes is degree of childhood socialization, defined as the child's tendency to form relationships and internalize social norms. Jenkins and Glickman (1946) identified two types of children with conduct disorder: the socialized and the undersocialized. They observed that the ability to develop group loyalty is crucial and marks a fundamental division among children with conduct disorder. Socialized children, regardless of their behavior, form strong ties to a familiar group of friends, whereas undersocialized children tend to be loners. In a 10-year follow-up study, Henn et al. (1980) found that socialized juvenile delinquents were less likely to have been convicted of crimes or imprisoned as adults.

Other Studies

Three additional studies are relevant to any review of the natural history of ASPD: the follow-up studies of Maddocks (1970), Gibbens et al. (1959), and Tong (1964), all conducted in the United Kingdom in the 1950s and 1960s. The subjects in each study were considered "psychopaths," a rough equivalent of ASPD.

Maddocks (1970) reported a 5-year follow-up study of patients seen in an outpatient department between 1961 and 1963. The men were considered "psychopaths," and the inclusion criteria included impulsivity, trouble with the law, several spouses or sexual partners, trouble at school, and unreliability. Maddocks traced 52 of 59 men; 10 (19%) had "settled down," 39 (75%) had not settled down, and 3 (6%) had committed suicide. He defined "settled down" as having shown a reduction of impulsiveness, enabling the man to stay in the same job, stay with the same partner, and have "generally a reduction in symptoms that placed him in the category in the first place" (p. 511). Although there was no clear distinction between those who had settled and those who had not, 15 (38%) of those who had not settled down drank excessively or were "frank alcoholics."

Gibbens and coworkers (1959) reported on an 8-year follow-up of 72 incarcerated "criminal psychopaths" whose course was compared with that of 59 "ordinary criminals." The psychopaths were considered severe cases and were selected with the assistance of "experienced prison medical officers." The psychopaths had more subsequent convictions than did the control criminals, yet 24% had only one or no convictions. Of note, the psychopaths were more likely than the control criminals to have an abnormal electroencephalogram result. Gibbens et al. (1959) concluded that psychopathic personality "does not inevitably portend as hopeless a prognosis as is usually implied" (p. 109). Psychopaths considered "aggressive" had a worse prognosis compared with the "inadequate" psychopaths. They had more reconvictions and were committed for aggressive offenses such as willful damage and drunken assault. They wrote: "It seems probable that the aggressive psychopath is so crippled in all his social relations that he is only able to live by crime and his record therefore consists very largely of acquisitive offences" (p. 112).

Tong (1964) reported on the outcome of "criminal psychopaths." They had been legally classified as psychopaths in the United Kingdom and incarcerated between 1954 and 1961 at Rampton Hospital, a special "close security psychiatric hospital" that catered to offenders considered dangerous or to have "violent propensities." Tong defined "psychopathic behavior" as "criminal behavior characterised by extreme callousness, brutality, disregard for others, on the one hand, and/or criminal behavior which is not necessarily violent or serious, but is repeated over and over again." (p. 104). The men were a mean age of 29 years at follow-up and had been incarcerated nearly 9 years. Of the 587 men, 171 (29%) relapsed, from which Tong (1964) concluded that the "prognosis is far from hopeless." Few admitted at later ages relapsed, and "Both age on discharge and length of stay in hospital correlated positively with success" (p. 105), findings that are about similar to what Black et al. (1995a) had reported in their follow-up study.

The Case of Stanley, the Jack-Roller, and Other Personal Accounts

The natural history of ASPD is starkly illustrated in a more personal way by examining the true life of Stanley ("the Jack-Roller"), as portrayed in the books *The Jack-Roller: A Delinquent Boy's Own Story* by Clifford Shaw (1930/1966) and *The Jack-Roller at Seventy* by Jack-Roller et al. (1982). Stanley was a chronic runaway at age 6 years, truant by age 8, and in custody 26 times before age 10 and 38 times by age 17, including 3 terms at a home for incorrigible boys and 1 year each in 2 reformatories. Through a great deal of ingenuity, Snodgrass found and reinterviewed Stanley when he was 70 years old. No longer involved in any significant criminal activity, Stanley continued to have trouble keeping jobs, was constantly on guard against assault by others, and took little responsibility for his own problems. He clearly had all the earmarks of ASPD despite his advanced age.

Shaw also edited *Brothers in Crime* published in 1938 (Shaw 1938), which describes the five Martin boys and their progression from juvenile delinquents to adult criminals, who together spent a total of 55 years in prison. At the time of publication, the brothers ranged in age from 25 to 35 years; four of the five were considered improved and were engaged in "self-supporting" activities, but the oldest, John, was actively alcoholic, and the youngest, Carl, was incarcerated. The stories of their misbehavior intertwine but also show the familial nature of ASPD.

Conclusion

The natural history of ASPD is better understood than other personality disorders because of the many case reports and longitudinal studies that have been published over the past 80 years. Based on this body of work, ASPD should be considered a chronic disorder with an onset in early childhood or early adolescence that continues throughout adulthood. Although antisocial persons may improve with advancing age, problems usually continue on a lesser scale, such as poor job performance, financial dependency, strained family and social networks, and impaired health-related quality of life. Improvement can occur at any age, but it typically starts between the mid-30s and the early 40s. Last, more severe syndromes at the onset and comorbid externalizing pathology, including alcohol use, drug use, and ADHD, appear to predict more severe and persistent antisociality at follow-up. Antisocial individuals with earlier onset tend to have a worse outcome, whereas favorable prognostic factors include marriage, family and community ties, early incarceration (or adjudication in childhood), and degree of socialization.

Key Points

- Follow-up studies show that antisocial personality disorder (ASPD) is a chronic disorder that begins in childhood or early adolescence and is associated with a range of behavioral disturbances.

- Most antisocial persons experience gradual improvement with advancing age, with some appearing to remit altogether.

- Better outcome is associated with lower initial severity, greater duration of follow-up, marriage, positive family and community ties, and the ability to internalize social norms.

- Comorbid personality disorder diagnoses and externalizing psychopathology such as substance misuse and ADHD are associated with worse outcome.

References

American Psychiatric Association: Diagnostic and Statistical Manual of Mental Disorders, 3rd Edition. Washington, DC, American Psychiatric Association, 1980

American Psychiatric Association: Diagnostic and Statistical Manual of Mental Disorders, 4th Edition. Washington, DC, American Psychiatric Association, 1994

American Psychiatric Association: Diagnostic and Statistical Manual of Mental Disorders, 4th Edition, Text Revision. Washington, DC, American Psychiatric Association, 2000

American Psychiatric Association: Diagnostic and Statistical Manual of Mental Disorders, 5th Edition. Arlington, VA, American Psychiatric Association, 2013

Black DW, Baumgard CH, Bell SE: A 16- to 45-year follow-up of 71 men with antisocial personality disorder. Compr Psychiatry 36(2):130–140, 1995a 7758299

Black DW, Baumgard CH, Bell SE: The long-term outcome of antisocial personality disorder compared with depression, schizophrenia, and surgical conditions. Bull Am Acad Psychiatry Law 23(1):43–52, 1995b 7599370

Black DW, Monahan P, Baumgard CH, et al: Predictors of long-term outcome in 45 men with antisocial personality disorder. Ann Clin Psychiatry 9(4):211–217, 1997 9511944

Burt SA, Donnellan MB, Humbad MN, et al: Does marriage inhibit antisocial behavior? An examination of selection vs causation via a longitudinal twin design. Arch Gen Psychiatry 67(12):1309–1315, 2010 21135331

Compton WM, Conway KP, Stinson FS, et al: Prevalence, correlates, and comorbidity of DSM-IV antisocial personality syndromes and alcohol and specific drug use disorders in the United States: results from the National Epidemiologic Survey on Alcohol and Related Conditions. J Clin Psychiatry 66(6):677–685, 2005 15960559

Epstein LJ, Mills C, Simon A: Antisocial behavior of the elderly. Compr Psychiatry 11(1):36–42, 1970 5411213

Feighner JP, Robins E, Guze SB, et al: Diagnostic criteria for use in psychiatric research. Arch Gen Psychiatry 26(1):57–63, 1972 5009428

Gibbens TCN, Pond DA, Staffordclark D: A follow-up study of criminal psychopaths. J Ment Sci 105(438):108–115, 1959 13641961

Glueck S, Glueck E: Unraveling Juvenile Delinquency. Cambridge, MA, Harvard University Press, 1950

Goldstein RB, Grant BF: Three-year follow-up of syndromal antisocial behavior in adults: results from the Wave 2 National Epidemiologic Survey on Alcohol and Related Conditions. J Clin Psychiatry 70(9):1237–1249, 2009 19538901

Goldstein RB, Dawson DA, Smith SM, et al: Antisocial behavioral syndromes and 3-year quality-of-life outcomes in United States adults. Acta Psychiatr Scand 126(2):137–150, 2012 22375904

Henn FA, Bardwell R, Jenkins RL: Juvenile delinquents revisited: adult criminal activity. Arch Gen Psychiatry 37(10):1160–1163, 1980 7425800

Hwu H-G, Yeh E-K, Chang L-Y: Prevalence of psychiatric disorders in Taiwan defined by the Chinese Diagnostic Interview Schedule. Acta Psychiatr Scand 79(2):136–147, 1989 2923007

Jack-Roller, Snodgrass J, Gilbert G, et al: The Jack-Roller at Seventy: a 50-Year Follow-up. Lexington, MA, Lexington Books, 1982

Jenkins RL, Glickman S: Common syndromes in child psychiatry. Am J Orthopsychiatry 16:244–261, 1946 21024324

Lahey BB, Loeber R, Burke JD, et al: Predicting future antisocial personality disorder in males from a clinical assessment in childhood. J Consult Clin Psychol 73(3):389–399, 2005 15982137

Loeber R, Wung P, Keenan K, et al: Developmental pathways in disruptive child behavior. Dev Psychopathol 5:103–133, 1993

Loeber R, Burke JD, Lahey BB: What are adolescent antecedents to antisocial personality disorder? Crim Behav Ment Health 12(1):24–36, 2002a 12357255

Loeber R, Stouthamer-Loeber M, Farrington DP, et al: Editorial introduction: three longitudinal studies of children's development in Pittsburgh: the Developmental Trends Study, the Pittsburgh Youth Study, and the Pittsburgh Girls Study. Crim Behav Ment Health 12(1):1–23, 2002b 12357254

Maddocks PD: A five year follow-up of untreated psychopaths. Br J Psychiatry 116(534):511–515, 1970 5449136

Moffitt TE: Adolescence-limited and life-course-persistent antisocial behavior: a developmental taxonomy. Psychol Rev 100(4):674–701, 1993 8255953

Oakley-Browne MA, Joyce PR, Wells JE, et al: Christchurch Psychiatric Epidemiology Study, Part II: six month and other period prevalences of specific psychiatric disorders. Aust N Z J Psychiatry 23(3):327–340, 1989 2803145

Odgers CL, Moffitt TE, Broadbent JM, et al: Female and male antisocial trajectories: from childhood origins to adult outcomes. Dev Psychopathol 20(2):673–716, 2008 18423100

Rivenbark JG, Odgers CL, Caspi A, et al: The high societal costs of childhood conduct problems: evidence from administrative records up to age 38 in a longitudinal birth cohort. J Child Psychol Psychiatry 59(6):703–710, 2018 29197100

Robins LN: Deviant Children Grow Up. Baltimore, MD, Williams & Wilkins, 1966

Robins LN: The epidemiology of antisocial personality disorder, in Psychiatry, Volume 3. Edited by Michels RO, Cavenar JO. Philadelphia, PA, Lippincott, 1987, pp 1–14

Robins LN, Tipp J, Przybeck T: Antisocial personality disorder, in Psychiatric Disorders in America: The Epidemiologic Catchment Area Study. Edited by Robins LN, Regier DA. New York, Free Press, 1991, pp 258–290

Sampson R, Laub J: Crime in the Making: Pathways and Turning Points Through Life. Cambridge, MA, Harvard University Press, 1993

Shaw CR (ed): Brothers in Crime. Chicago, IL, University of Chicago Press, 1938

Shaw CR: The Jack-Roller: A Delinquent Boy's Own Story (1930). Chicago, IL, University of Chicago Press, 1966

Swanson MC, Bland RC, Newman SC: Epidemiology of psychiatric disorders in Edmonton: antisocial personality disorders. Acta Psychiatr Scand Suppl 376:63–70, 1994 8178687

Tong JE: Studies of the psychopathic offender. N Z Med J 63:103–107, 1964 14124237

Tweed JL, George LK, Blazer D, et al: Adult onset of severe and pervasive antisocial behavior: a distinct syndrome? J Pers Disord 8(3):192–202, 1994

CHAPTER 7

Family, Twin, and Adoption Studies in Antisocial Personality Disorder and Antisocial Behavior

Wendy S. Slutske, Ph.D.

Christal N. Davis, M.A.

Antisocial personality disorder (ASPD) runs in families. One of the most robust risk factors for engaging in antisocial behaviors is being from a family in which there is a father, mother, or sibling with a history of committing antisocial acts. In the classic Cambridge Study in Delinquent Development of 411 South London families, half of the criminal convictions that had occurred over the course of the family members' lives were attributable to only 6% of the families (Farrington et al. 1996). In a total population study of Sweden, there was evidence for substantial familial aggregation of convictions for interpersonal violence, with correlation coefficients of 0.29 between parents and offspring and 0.37 between siblings (Frisell et al. 2011). Studies such as these provide convincing evidence for the contribution of familial factors in the etiology of antisocial behavior. But genetically informative research designs, such as those used in twin and adoption studies, are required to disentangle the extent to which the etiology of antisocial behavior is explained by shared genes or shared environments.

Before proceeding to the topic of twin and adoption studies, it is worth highlighting the substantial assortative mating for criminal behavior that was observed in the London and Sweden studies (Farrington et al. 1996; Frisell et al. 2011). That is, men and women who engaged in criminal and antisocial behavior were more likely to partner with each other. In the Sweden study, the correlation between mating partners ($r=0.38$) was as large as the correlation between biologically related siblings ($r=0.37$; Frisell et al. 2011). This finding has implications for the intergenerational transmission of genetic risk factors for antisocial behavior because with each successive generation, the susceptibility genes will become more concentrated in such families (Krueger et al. 1998; Moffitt 2005). It also may have longer-term implications for an even broader reach of such genetic risk factors. Because antisocial parents have more children on average than do nonantisocial parents (Moffitt et al. 2002), it has been suggested that increasing levels of assortative mating for antisocial behavior might eventually lead to an increased population prevalence of ASPD by influencing the gene pool in future generations (Moffitt 2005).

Contribution of Genes and Environment to Antisocial Personality Disorder

Logic of the Twin Study

In a twin study, one compares the similarity of monozygotic (MZ) twins, who share 100% of their genetic information, with the similarity of dizygotic (DZ) twins, who share on average 50% of their genetic information (specifically, the genetic information that varies in the population). (Two unrelated humans share about 99.9% of their genetic information; studies of individual differences are concerned with the 0.1% that varies.) When MZ twin pairs are more similar than DZ twin pairs, one can infer that there is a contribution of genetic factors to a trait. This represents the cumulative aggregated influence of all genes that contribute to trait variation. If the DZ twin similarity is greater than half the MZ twin similarity, then one can infer that common environmental influences contribute to individual differences in a trait. That is, factors other than the sharing of genetic information are contributing to the similarity of twins. A contribution of unique (individual-specific) environmental influences is inferred when the MZ twin similarity is less than 1.0 (this also includes measurement error). This represents the contribution to individual differences that is not shared by twins and cannot be explained by genes or common environments.

Interestingly, of all the medical and psychological traits or disorders that have been the focus of a twin study, conduct disorder is the second most commonly studied, with only personality and temperament being the subject of more extensive twin research (Polderman et al. 2015). In a meta-analysis of all the twin studies published between 1958 and 2012, Polderman et al. (2015) identified 155 studies, including 304,885 twin pairs from 10 different countries[1] (Figure 7–1). The aggregated MZ and DZ twin correlations for conduct disorder were 0.66 and 0.41, which are consistent with significant genetic (MZ>DZ), common environmental (DZ>½ MZ), and unique environmental influences (MZ<1.0). (Unfortunately, there were far fewer studies of ASPD in this meta-analysis.)

Logic of the Adoption Study

In an adoption study, one compares the similarity of biological relative dyads (e.g., biological parent–adoptee) who share 50% of their genetic information and none of

---

[1] All of the results from this meta-analysis can be viewed at the MaTCH interactive website (http://match.ctglab.nl/#/home).

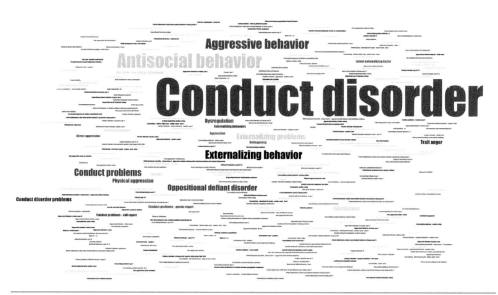

FIGURE 7–1. Word cloud of traits included in the conduct disorder meta-analysis of Polderman et al. (2015).

their environment with the similarity of nonbiological relative dyads (e.g., adoptive parent–adoptee) who share environments but none of their genetic information. Because there is a relatively clean separation of genetic and environmental factors in a parent-offspring adoption study, one can infer the importance of genetic factors when the similarity of biological relative dyads is significantly greater than zero and the importance of common environmental factors when the similarity of nonbiological relative dyads is significantly greater than zero.

Previous Reviews of Twin and Adoption Studies of Antisocial Behavior

There have been many qualitative (Baker et al. 2006; Moffitt 2005; Slutske 2001; Viding et al. 2008) and quantitative (Rhee and Waldman 2002) literature reviews focused specifically on twin and adoption studies of antisocial behavior.[2] Although two decades old, the meta-analysis of Rhee and Waldman (2002) of 41 twin and 10 adoption studies is still the most widely cited and definitive review. After combining the results of all 51 studies, they found that there were significant contributions of genetic factors (32%), common environment (9%), and unique environment (43%) to variation in antisocial behavior (Table 7–1). The results based on the twin and adoption studies significantly differed, with larger estimates of genetic and common environmental factors in the twin compared with the adoption studies. Without the inclusion of the adoption data, the estimates from the 2002 meta-analysis of Rhee and Waldman are reassuringly similar to the estimates of the contributions of genetic (51%), common

---

[2] Other reviews have focused on twin and adoption studies of conduct disorder (Salvatore and Dick 2018), crime (Odgers and Russell 2017), and all personality disorders (Reichborn-Kjennerud and Kendler 2018).

environmental (15%), and unique environmental factors (25%) to variation in conduct disorder in the more recent meta-analysis of the worldwide twin literature (Polderman et al. 2015).

Note on the Measurement of Antisocial Personality Disorder

The methods that have been used to assess antisocial behaviors in the extant literature (and included in the reviews) have varied considerably. In addition to diagnostic assessments based on the *Diagnostic and Statistical Manual of Mental Disorders* (DSM) criteria for ASPD, there are studies based on official records or self-reports of delinquent or criminal behavior and self-reports of the personality trait of aggression. In fact, there are few twin or adoption studies of ASPD per se—that is, studies meeting both the child and the adult criteria for the DSM disorder (e.g., Slutske et al. 2001), because studies that have used diagnostic assessments have tended to individually focus on the childhood criteria (i.e., conduct disorder) or the adult criteria (i.e., adult antisocial behavior).

A handful of studies, including the Rhee and Waldman (2002) meta-analysis, empirically evaluated whether lumping together different approaches to conceptualizing and measuring antisocial behavior is appropriate. In the Rhee and Waldman meta-analysis, there were significantly greater estimates of genetic influences for crime than for diagnoses of antisocial behavior disorders (see Table 7–1). However, these disparate estimates came from different studies.

When antisocial behavior is assessed using different approaches within the same study, one can make a more direct comparison and also evaluate the extent to which they are tapping the same genetic and environmental risk factors. For example, in a Swedish study of adolescent male twins, five self-report measures of antisocial behavior were compared with official government records of criminal behaviors in a multivariate genetic analysis (Kendler et al. 2013). Although the contributions of genetic factors to the self-reported and official records of behavior were similar (e.g., the heritabilities of self-reported delinquency and recorded criminality were 42% and 48%, respectively), only about one-third of the genetic variation in recorded criminality was tapped by the five self-report measures. In a study of Norwegian adult twins, interview and questionnaire measures of ASPD yielded heritability estimates of 31% and 46%, respectively; about two-thirds of the genetic variation in the questionnaire measure of ASPD was tapped by the interview measure (Torgersen et al. 2012). An interesting result of this study was the finding of a heritability of 69% for a latent ASPD factor that was estimated from a joint analysis of the two measures. In summary, there is reason to believe that the various operationalizations of antisocial behavior may be differentially heritable and, perhaps more importantly, are tapping different genetic and environmental sources of variation. The most progress might be made by the use of multiple measures of antisocial behavior within a study. These multiple measures could then be combined (as in the Torgersen et al. 2012 study) as fallible indicators of an underlying latent ASPD construct. Unfortunately, in this chapter, we often have no choice but to treat the different operationalizations of antisocial behavior as equivalent.

TABLE 7–1. **Selected results from the meta-analytic review of twin and adoption studies of antisocial behavior of Rhee and Waldman (2002)**

	Number of samples	Percentage of variation explained by		
		Genetic factors	Common environment	Unique environment
All studies	52	32	9	43
Operationalization				
Diagnosis	14	44	11	45
Crime	5	75	0	25
Study design				
Twin	42	45	12	43
Adoption	10	32	5	63
Sex				
Male	21	38	17	45
Female	19	41	19	40
Sex[a]				
Male	17	43	19	38
Female	17	41	20	39
Age				
Child	15	46	20	34
Adolescent	11	43	16	41
Adult	17	41	9	50

Note. There were significant differences for operationalization, study design, sex, and age.
[a]Limited to studies that included both males and females; no longer significant differences.

Sex Differences

Men are much more likely to be diagnosed with ASPD than women (Coid et al. 2006; Compton et al. 2005). For example, in a nationally representative epidemiological survey, 5.7% of the men, compared with 1.9% of the women, met the DSM-IV-TR (American Psychiatric Association 2000) diagnostic criteria for ASPD (Trull et al. 2010). This sex difference may provide an important clue into the etiology of ASPD (Rutter et al. 2003).

Genetically informed studies have the potential to yield valuable insights into two types of sex differences in the causes of variation in a trait. Studies that include both men and women can examine whether the magnitude of genetic or environmental effects differs (i.e., quantitative sex differences). Studies that include opposite-sex relative dyads (e.g., male/female DZ twin pairs, father/daughter) can also test whether the genetic risk factors (and family environmental risk factors) are distinct or overlapping by comparing the similarity of opposite-sex with that of same-sex relative dyads (i.e., qualitative sex differences).

We can return to the massive meta-analysis of the world twin literature on conduct disorder (Polderman et al. 2015) to see whether there is any evidence for quantitative or qualitative sex differences. With respect to quantitative sex differences, the estimates of genetic and common environmental influences were 42% and 20% in men, respectively, and 51% and 16% in women, respectively. Given the extremely large sample sizes of 175,721 male and 118,250 female twin pairs, these differences were significant—conduct disorder was slightly more heritable among females than among males, and there was a slightly larger contribution of the common environment in males than in females. In the Rhee and Waldman (2002) meta-analysis, the estimates of genetic and common environmental influences were also significantly higher among women than among men when all studies were included, but they were no longer significant when the analyses were limited to those studies that included both men and women (see Table 7–1). As with evaluating the potential differences due to operationalization of antisocial behavior, the most incisive test is from a within-study comparison (Slutske 2001). It is probably safest to conclude that there is no convincing evidence for quantitative sex differences in the contributions of genetic and common environmental factors to antisocial behaviors.

With respect to evidence for qualitative sex differences culled from the massive conduct disorder meta-analysis (Polderman et al. 2015), the correlation coefficient in the opposite-sex DZ twins was 0.39 compared with 0.44 among same-sex DZ pairs. Again, given the very large sample sizes of 87,738 opposite-sex and 105,608 same-sex twin pairs, this was a significant difference. This finding suggests that there may be slight differences in the genetic or common environmental risk factors for conduct disorder among males than among females (see also Meier et al. 2011).

Aside from providing insights into qualitative sex differences, opposite-sex twin pairs provide an elegant (and underused) "natural experiment" for evaluating whether higher rates of antisociality among men than among women can be explained by differential exposure or differential vulnerability of men and women to risk factors for antisociality, after between-family confounding factors are taken into account (Meier et al. 2009). For example, Meier et al. (2009) showed that brothers were more likely to be harshly punished than their twin sisters and that this partially explained the higher rate of conduct disorder symptoms in the boys compared with the girls (although the possibility that boys were more harshly punished than girls because of their higher rates of conduct disorder could not be ruled out). In contrast, brothers were not more vulnerable to the effect of harsh discipline than their sisters—that is, the correlation between harsh discipline and conduct disorder was not higher in boys than in girls. Despite the massive differences in the prevalence of antisocial behavior disorders between boys and girls and men and women, the results of behavioral genetic studies suggest that the genetic and environmental risk factors are largely overlapping.

Are Twin and Adoption Studies Obsolete?

After nearly a century of twin research (Rende et al. 1990), it has become increasingly clear that genes contribute to individual differences for virtually all human behavioral traits (Plomin et al. 2016; Turkheimer 2000), including ASPD. With the availability (thanks to the Human Genome Project) of informative genetic markers across the entire genome, scientists are better equipped than ever before to identify the individual susceptibility genes contributing to the risk for complex disorders such as ASPD. Recent advances in molecular genetic methods may lead one to question whether twin studies may be obsolete. However, twin studies are still invaluable beyond merely estimating the relative contributions of genetic and environmental factors. In the remainder of this chapter, we focus on four areas in which twin and adoption studies continue to make important contributions to science in general, and our understanding of antisocial behavior in particular: 1) multivariate twin studies of developmental change, 2) multivariate twin studies of comorbidity, 3) studies of gene-environment interplay, and 4) studies of twin pairs discordant for a putative environmental risk or protective factor.

Developmental Changes

Behavioral genetics research can help to answer the question of whether there are developmental changes in the contribution of genetic and environmental factors to antisocial behavior disorders. In a cross-sectional research design, this is accomplished by comparing the heritability estimates for samples at different ages. In the Rhee and Waldman (2002) meta-analysis, the estimates of both genetic and common environmental influences for antisocial behaviors decreased from childhood to adolescence to adulthood (see Table 7–1); these results were presented with the caveat that age may have been confounded with other important differences between the studies, such as operationalization or method of assessment.

Three cross-sectional studies have made within-study comparisons across these developmental stages by obtaining retrospective reports of child and adolescent behaviors in adult samples of twins (Jacobson et al. 2002; Lyons et al. 1995; Meier et al. 2011). In all three "quasi-longitudinal" twin studies, the relative contribution of genetic factors was greater in adulthood than in childhood, and the relative contribution of common environmental factors was greater in childhood than in adulthood.

By obtaining measures of antisocial behavior in both childhood and adulthood within the same study, one can analyze the data in much the same way that one would analyze data from a bivariate twin study with the measures obtained for the two developmental epochs representing the two variables. The logic of bivariate twin modeling is similar to that of univariate twin modeling (the analysis of a single trait). With bivariate twin modeling, one is interested in the cross-trait as well as the within-trait similarity. For example, one might examine the similarity of a diagnosis of conduct disorder in one twin with adult antisocial behavior in the other twin. If the MZ cross-age, cross-twin similarity is greater than the DZ cross-age, cross-twin similarity, then one infers that genetic factors are contributing to the association between conduct disorder and adult antisocial behavior. In other words, there is at least one gene that is a risk factor for both conduct disorder and adult antisocial behavior. If the DZ cross-age, cross-twin similarity is greater than half the MZ cross-age, cross-twin similarity, then one infers that shared environmental factors are contributing to the association between conduct disorder and adult antisocial behavior. Unique environmental factors are implicated when the MZ cross-age, cross-twin similarity is less than the cross-age, within-twin correlation between conduct disorder and adult antisocial behavior.

Bivariate twin analyses of the three "quasi-longitudinal" twin studies showed that the genetic influences on childhood and adult antisocial behavior overlapped either partially (Jacobson et al. 2002) or completely (Lyons et al. 1995; Meier et al. 2011). When there was evidence for common environmental influences on adult antisocial behavior, two studies found that common environmental influences overlapped completely with the influences on child antisocial behavior (Jacobson et al. 2002; Lyons et al. 1995), and the other found that these environmental influences were specific to adulthood (Meier et al. 2011). All three studies found that there were persisting effects of the unique environment from child to adult antisocial behavior but that there was a stronger influence of adult-specific unique environmental influences in adulthood. In summary, these three studies support the premise that genes are related to the persistence of antisocial behavior from childhood to adulthood, whereas environments are related to changes.

Of course, the best research design for studying developmental change is a longitudinal study in which antisocial behaviors are repeatedly assessed over time. A recent 27-year longitudinal twin study from the Netherlands Twin Register examined the contributions of genetic and environmental factors to antisocial behaviors assessed by maternal report in childhood (at ages 9–10) and by self-report in adolescence (at ages 13–18) and adulthood (at a mean age of 30; Wesseldijk et al. 2018). The results were consistent with results from the quasi-longitudinal studies in demonstrating that nearly all of the stability in antisocial behavior from childhood to adulthood was explained by genetic factors. This is evident from the patterns of correlations obtained across the developmental epochs. For example, the cross-age, within-twin correlation between child and adult antisocial behavior was 0.22, and the cross-age, cross-twin correlations were 0.22 and 0.11 among MZ and DZ twins, respectively.

To our knowledge, only one study has examined the stability of the contribution of genetic and environmental factors to antisocial behavior across adulthood. This was a 10-year longitudinal twin study from the Norwegian Twin Register that assessed ASPD from early to middle adulthood, when the twins were ages 28 and 38 years, on average (Reichborn-Kjennerud et al. 2015). Similar to the results spanning childhood to adulthood, the results of this study suggested that the genetic influences on ASPD were persistent across this 10-year period from early to middle adulthood, whereas the unique environmental influences were more transient.

In summary, longitudinal twin research has consistently shown that the relative importance of genetic and environmental factors for explaining individual differences in antisocial behavior disorders shifts from childhood to adulthood, with genetic factors increasing in importance and common environmental factors decreasing. But despite this shift in relative importance, the sets of genes that are on board early in life and that are associated with conduct disorder in childhood are the same genes that continue to exert an influence on risk for adult ASPD.

Causes of Antisocial Personality Disorder Comorbidity

ASPD rarely occurs in isolation. Nearly 75% of individuals with a history of ASPD in a large epidemiological survey met the diagnostic criteria for an Axis I psychiatric disorder in the past year (Lenzenweger et al. 2007). It is, therefore, not surprising that significant associations have been observed between ASPD and every other DSM-IV and DSM-IV-TR (American Psychiatric Association 1994, 2000) Axis I and Axis II[3] disorder assessed in large epidemiological surveys, with especially strong associations with drug dependence (Trull et al. 2010), dysthymia and bipolar disorder (Lenzenweger et al. 2007), gambling disorder (Petry et al. 2005), and dependent and histrionic personality disorders (Grant et al. 2005; Trull et al. 2013). Multivariate twin studies have yielded important insights into the underlying causes of ASPD comorbidity that may have implications for the diagnosis of psychiatric disorders.

Previously, we described the logic of bivariate twin modeling as applied to measures of child and adult antisocial behaviors to address questions of persistence and change. Bivariate twin modeling is also extremely useful for examining the causes of comorbidity between two disorders, and multivariate twin modeling is useful for examining the causes of comorbidity between more than two disorders. For example, with bivariate twin modeling one might examine the causes of the comorbidity between ASPD and borderline personality disorder (BPD), whereas with multivariate twin modeling, one might examine whether there are common genetic and environmental underpinnings of DSM-IV Cluster A, B, and C personality disorders (Kendler et al. 2008) and whether there are common genetic and environmental underpinnings for sets of disorders considered to reflect "externalizing" and "internalizing" psychopathology (Kendler et al. 2003).

Comorbidity With Other Personality Disorders

The best genetically informed research on ASPD Axis II comorbidity comes from a series of papers based on data from the Norwegian Institute of Public Health Twin Panel (Kendler et al. 2008; Reichborn-Kjennerud et al. 2015; Torgersen et al. 2008). A multivariate twin study that focused on the comorbidity of DSM-IV-TR (American Psychiatric Association 2000) Cluster B disorders (borderline, antisocial, histrionic, and narcissistic personality disorders) found evidence for one genetic factor that influenced all four Cluster B personality disorders, one genetic factor that influenced only ASPD and BPD, and genetic factors specific to each personality disorder; these three sources accounted for about 30%, 30%, and 40%, respectively, of the genetic variation in ASPD (Torgersen et al. 2008). The authors concluded that ASPD and BPD "may share genetic and environmental risk factors above and beyond that due to the genetic and environmental factors common to all four cluster B personality disorders" (Reichborn-Kjennerud 2008, p. 425).

A more comprehensive study included all 10 DSM-IV personality disorders in a biometric model (Kendler et al. 2008). The covariation between the 10 disorders was best explained by a model that included three common genetic factors and three common unique environmental factors (and no familial environmental factors). The three genetic factors did not correspond with the A, B, and C clusters in DSM-IV. ASPD significantly loaded on only one of the three common genetic factors, and there was no residual genetic variation included in a disorder-specific genetic factor for ASPD. The

---

[3] We use the now-outdated terms "Axis I" and "Axis II" as a shorthand way to refer to the major mental disorders and the personality disorders, respectively.

common genetic factor on which ASPD loaded included substantial loadings from only two disorders—ASPD and BPD—and explained 97% of the genetic variation in ASPD. The unique environmental structure of the 10 disorders more closely corresponded to the A, B, and C clusters in DSM, with high loadings of the first environmental factor on all four Cluster B disorders (as well as obsessive-compulsive and paranoid personality disorders). This common factor explained 42% of the unique environmental influences on ASPD, with the remainder explained by a disorder-specific environmental factor.

The results of this more comprehensive analysis are consistent with one of the conclusions drawn from the earlier analysis that was restricted to the Cluster B disorders (Reichborn-Kjennerud 2008), namely, that ASPD and BPD share genetic risk factors above what is shared by all four Cluster B personality disorders. Where it departs from the previous conclusions is that the unique environmental risk factors are about equally shared across all four of the Cluster B disorders. In summary, this study suggests that the genetic risk for ASPD mostly overlaps with the genetic risk for BPD, whereas environmental risk factors for ASPD are about evenly split between factors that contribute to the risk for all four of the Cluster B personality disorders and factors that are unique to ASPD.

Comorbidity With Other Psychiatric Disorders

A similar multivariate twin study based on data from the Virginia Twin Registry examined the causes of the comorbidity of conduct disorder and adult antisocial behavior with five other common Axis I psychiatric disorders (major depression, generalized anxiety disorder, phobia, alcohol dependence, and drug abuse/dependence) (Kendler et al. 2003). Consistent with the concepts of "internalizing" and "externalizing" disorders (Krueger 1999), most of the genetic variation in major depression, generalized anxiety disorder, and phobia was explained by one factor, and most of the genetic variation in conduct disorder, adult antisocial behavior, alcohol dependence, and drug abuse/dependence was explained by another. In contrast, environmental contributions to conduct disorder and adult antisocial behavior were not shared with any of the other psychiatric disorders.

Returning to the Norwegian Institute of Public Health Twin Panel data set, an ambitious multivariate twin study examined the genetic and environmental overlap between 12 psychiatric disorders (the 7 included in the previous study of Kendler et al. [2003], plus dysthymia, social phobia, agoraphobia, eating disorders, and somatoform disorder) and the 10 personality disorders (Kendler et al. 2011). Even when 12 psychiatric and all of the personality disorders were included in the model, there was still evidence for a genetic factor that primarily explained variation in conduct disorder, ASPD, alcohol abuse/dependence, and drug abuse/dependence (and to a lesser extent BPD)—similar to the "externalizing factor" identified in the previous study that did not include all 10 of the personality disorders (Kendler et al. 2003).

The robustness of the externalizing factor highlights important genetic risk factors that are shared between the antisocial and the addictive disorders. A handful of studies have examined the genetic overlap between specific illicit drug use or disorders and personality disorders (Gillespie et al. 2018a, 2018b) rather than a composite "other drug abuse or dependence" measure used in previous research (Kendler et al. 2003, 2011). ASPD was the personality disorder that was most strongly associated with cannabis use, cocaine use, and cannabis use disorder; genetic influences on ASPD explained 56%, 72%, and 43% of the genetic risk for cannabis use, cocaine use, and cannabis use disorder, respectively (Gillespie et al. 2018a, 2018b). To our knowledge, there have not been similar studies that have examined the genetic overlap between ASPD and the use or abuse of other illicit drugs, such as stimulants, opioids, and hallucinogens. However, it has been suggested that the genetic factors that link ASPD and drug use or drug use disorders are related to the general risk for initiation and maintenance of substance use rather than to the pharmacological properties of any given substance (Gillespie et al. 2018b). If this is the case, it is anticipated that similar genetic overlap with ASPD would be found for the entire panoply of illicit substances.

Genetic influences on ASPD also appear to be associated with those for non-substance-related "behavioral addictions." Genetic influences on conduct disorder, adult antisocial behavior, and ASPD explained 22%, 18%, and 16% of the variation in genetic liability for disordered gambling, respectively (Slutske et al. 2001). Gambling disorder is currently the only behavioral addiction that has been formally defined in DSM-5 (American Psychiatric Association 2013) or been scrutinized from a behavioral genetic perspective. It is hypothesized that other behavioral addictions, such as internet addiction (Grant et al. 2010), gaming disorder (recently included in the 11th revision of ICD; World Health Organization 2018), and compulsive sexual behavior (Kraus et al. 2016), will also share genetic risk factors with ASPD. It will be interesting to see whether the genetic overlap is as strong as that observed for cocaine use (72%) or more on the order of that observed for gambling disorder (16%).

There are several take-away messages from the multivariate twin studies of ASPD comorbidity. One is the unsurprising conclusion that the main causes of comorbidity between ASPD and psychiatric and addictive disorders are shared genetic risk factors. This is unsurprising because it is consistent with a robust finding in the behavioral genetic literature that the correlations between psychiatric disorders are usually at least partially genetically mediated: "More than 100 twin studies have addressed the key question of comorbidity in psychopathology, and this body of research also consistently shows substantial genetic overlap between common disorders" (Plomin et al. 2016, p. 7).

Multivariate twin studies of ASPD have led to at least two less anticipated findings relevant to psychiatric diagnosis. First, although it may make intuitive sense, there does not appear to be strong empirical support for the hypothesis that ASPD shares many genetic and environmental risk factors with DSM-IV Cluster B personality disorders other than BPD. Second, consistent with the removal of the distinction between Axis I and II disorders in DSM-5, there is not strong empirical support for assigning ASPD to a different axis than the other psychiatric and addictive disorders. From a behavioral genetic perspective, ASPD has as much (or more) in common with the Axis I disorders as it does with the other Axis II disorders.

Gene-Environment Interplay

Genes and environments do not operate in isolation. This is why heritability is not a fixed property of a trait; rather, it is an estimate of the sources of individual differences for a particular population, at a particular time, and in a particular circumstance (Knopik et al. 2017). As the situation changes, the heritability estimate can change.

Gene-Environment Interaction

Gene-environment interaction is the process by which one's genetic predisposition affects one's sensitivity to environmental risks (Dick 2011; Manuck and McCaffery 2014; Shanahan and Hofer 2005). That is, one's genotype may influence the effect of an environmental risk factor. There have arguably been more replicated findings of gene-environment interaction for antisocial behavior disorders than for any other psychiatric disorder. Early evidence came from three adoption studies conducted in the United States (Cadoret et al. 1983), Sweden (Cloninger et al. 1982), and Denmark (Mednick et al. 1984).

One way that gene-environment interaction is inferred in an adoption study is when there is an increased risk to adoptees with both an affected biological parent (indexing genetic risk) and an adoptive parent (indexing environmental risk), compared with the risk associated with either one in isolation. For example, in more than 6,000 male adoptees in the Danish Adoption Study, 14% were convicted of a crime when neither their biological parents nor their adoptive parents had been convicted, 15% were convicted when their adoptive parent alone had been convicted, 20% were convicted when their biological parent alone had been convicted, and 25% were convicted when both their biological parents and their adoptive parents had been convicted (Mednick et al. 1984). Although the interaction was not statistically significant, this pattern illustrates how the effect of genetic and environmental risk in combination is greater than the effect of either genetic or environmental risk in isolation.

A more recent study of more than 18,000 adoptees that used data from Swedish national registers had a different approach to studying gene-environment interaction. Rather than inferring genetic and environmental risk from the criminal histories of the biological and adoptive parents, genetic and environmental risk scores were created on the basis of a host of characteristics of biological and adoptive parents and siblings (including a history of criminal conviction, but also alcohol and drug abuse, psychiatric disorder, [maternal] age, [maternal] divorce, [parental] educational attainment, medical hospitalizations, and death), which were used to predict adoptee criminal behavior (Kendler et al. 2014). There were significant effects of the genetic and environmental risk scores, but not of their interaction, in predicting adoptee criminal offending. The environmental risk factors for criminal behavior had a similar effect on those who were at high genetic risk as they did for those who were at low genetic risk for criminal behavior.

A gene-environment interaction in a twin study would be reflected in differences in the heritability of an outcome observed in different environments. In Table 7–2, we summarize the results of selected studies that have examined gene-environment interactions for antisocial behaviors in adolescent and young adult twin samples. As Table 7–2 illustrates, there was a relatively consistent pattern indicating that the contribution of genetic and unique environmental influences to variation in antisocial behavior was amplified in high-risk compared with low-risk environments (this is reflected by "↑A" and "↑E" under the column titled "Effect of high-risk environment"), although it should be noted that all of these findings came from the landmark Minnesota Twin Family Study (MTFS; Iacono and McGue 2002). In one study, this pattern

TABLE 7–2. Selected twin studies of environmental mediation and moderation of genetic influences on antisocial outcomes

Outcome	Environmental moderator	rGE?	Effect of high-risk environment	Age	Study
Antisocial behavior	Parental negativity	NA	↑A	Child/adolescent	Feinberg et al. 2007
Antisocial behavior	Neighborhood disadvantage	NA	↓A ↑C	Adolescent	Tuvblad et al. 2006
Aggression	Neighborhood disadvantage	NA	↑C	Adolescent	Cleveland 2003
Externalizing	Antisocial peers	✓	↑E ↑A	Adolescent	Hicks et al. 2009
Antisocial behavior	Academic performance	✓	↑E ↑A	Adolescent/young adult	Johnson et al. 2009
Externalizing	Parent-child problems	✓	↑E ↑A	Adolescent/young adult	Samek et al. 2015
Antisocial behavior	Antisocial peers	✓	↑E ↑A	Adolescent	Samek et al. 2017
Antisocial behavior	Antisocial peers	✓	↑E	Adult	Samek et al. 2017

Note. A=genetic variation; C=common environmental variation; E=unique environmental variation; NA=not applicable; rGE=gene-environment correlation. Five other environmental moderators were included in the Hicks et al. 2009 article, with similar findings.

held across six environmental risk factors, including academic achievement, antisocial peers, parent-child relationship problems, and stressful life events, such that genetic vulnerability for a latent externalizing variable (including adult antisocial behavior and substance use) was increased in high-risk environments at age 17 years (Hicks et al. 2009). The same result was also obtained when the study authors focused specifically on adult ASPD symptom counts rather than on an externalizing composite (Johnson et al. 2009). Genetic and environmental variation in antisocial behavior was greater among adolescents with lower grade point averages than among their peers with higher grade point averages. However, parental socioeconomic status and adolescent IQ did not moderate genetic and environmental influences on antisocial behavior, suggesting that school performance was uniquely important as a moderator, rather than academic ability or intelligence (Johnson et al. 2009).

The previous twin studies showing a consistent pattern of gene-environment interaction for antisocial and externalizing behaviors were limited to adolescence. These findings were extended, again by means of data from the MTFS, by examining whether antisocial peer involvement moderated genetic and environmental influences on DSM-III-R (American Psychiatric Association 1987) externalizing disorders (ASPD and substance use disorders) at ages 17, 20, 24, and 29 years (Samek et al. 2017). Genetic variation for externalizing disorders was greater among those with more antisocial peers at age 17 years, but this effect did not persist into adulthood (Samek et al. 2017). Similarly, genetic influences on externalizing disorders were higher among those adolescents who had more problems with their parents at age 17 years, but by age 24 years, this moderation effect was no longer observed (Samek et al. 2015). These findings suggest that adolescence may be a window of vulnerability within which environmental risk factors exert their effect on those at heightened genetic risk for antisociality.

These selected findings from the twin and adoption literature on gene-environment interaction for antisocial behavior reinforce the notion that, much like the estimate of heritability, the presence of gene-environment interaction is not a fixed property of a trait. Whether or not a gene-environment interaction for antisocial behavior is detected appears to depend on the developmental stage of the participants and the characterization of the high-risk environment. Much research remains to be done to map the environmental terrain across the life course that moderates the genetic risk for antisocial behavior.

Gene-Environment Correlation

Gene-environment correlation is the process by which one's genetic predisposition affects the likelihood of being exposed to environmental risks (Rutter 2006; Scarr and McCartney 1983). One way that this occurs early in life is when we inherit from our birth parents both our genes and our rearing environments. Gene-environment correlation makes the interpretation of associations between parental behavior and offspring outcomes ambiguous because genes and environments are confounded with each other. For example, one can simultaneously inherit from one's parents a genetic predisposition to develop ASPD along with an environment in which there is abuse or neglect (Jaffee et al. 2006; Rutter 1997). An adoption study is a useful natural experiment in which genes and environments are "un-confounded" because birth parents provide genes and adoptive parents provide postnatal environments. (However, because of the phenomenon of selective placement, these can sometimes be correlated; see, e.g., Kendler et al. 2014.)

Gene-environment correlation can also occur later in life through a more active process whereby one seeks out or creates environments based on genetic propensities; this can apply to whom we choose as friends, whom we marry, activities that we select, and where we choose to live. In a twin study, active gene-environment correlation can be examined in a bivariate twin analysis, with one variable being the outcome of interest and the other being the putative environment. This is the same approach that was described earlier in exploring the causes of comorbidity between two disorders. As Table 7–2 illustrates, there was consistent evidence for gene-environment correlation (this is reflected by a check mark in the column titled "*r*GE?"). For example, those who had a genetic propensity for ASPD were more likely to have friends who were also antisocial (Hicks et al. 2009; Samek et al. 2017). Moving into adulthood (and coming full circle in this chapter), antisocial individuals often go on to marry others who are also antisocial (Farrington et al. 1996; Frisell et al. 2011; Krueger et al. 1998). Not only do genes influence one's exposure to an environment that is conducive to antisocial behavior, such as pairing with an antisocial partner, but also antisocial behavior may influence the gene pool in future generations—that is, when pairing with an antisocial partner results in having more than the average number of offspring with a heightened genetic susceptibility to become antisocial (Moffitt 2005).

Testing the Causal Significance of Putative Risk and Protective Factors

Because genes influence the environments that we encounter and shape our responses to the environment, many putative risk and protective factors for engaging in antisocial behaviors are partially heritable (Kendler and Baker 2007; Plomin et al. 2016; Slutske et al. 2015). In observational, nonexperimental studies (as in life), environments are not randomly assigned to people. Establishing that a risk factor is truly environmental requires more sophisticated research designs than have typically been used in studies of ASPD. This is a question that is of critical importance to public health (Kendler 2017). Establishing that a risk factor is truly environmental is synonymous with establishing that the association between the risk factor and the outcome is causal.

The discordant twin design is a "natural experiment" or "quasi-experimental" method (D'Onofrio et al. 2013; Lahey and D'Onofrio 2010; McGue et al. 2010; Rutter 2007a, 2007b), in which an unexposed twin serves as the control for an exposed co-twin in examining potentially causal[4] associations. It is based on the knowledge that MZ twins are perfectly correlated for genetic and family environmental background factors, and DZ twins are perfectly correlated for family environmental background fac-

---

[4] The phrase "potentially causal" is used because causality cannot be definitively established using observational data. For example, in the discordant twin design, the underlying reason for twin discordance can never be known with certainty, thereby making it impossible to rule out alternative noncausal explanations.

tors and correlated 0.5 (on average) for genetic factors. A comparison of ASPD among MZ twins who are discordant for an exposure such as neighborhood disadvantage allows one to control completely for genetic and family environmental background factors (i.e., between-family risk factors), and a comparison among discordant DZ twins allows one to partially control for genetic and completely control for family environmental background factors. This type of control is more powerful than the standard statistical controls that are commonly used in the behavioral sciences because it controls for a whole host of possible confounds—including those that we know about and even those that we do not.

A potentially causal effect of neighborhood disadvantage on ASPD, for example, would be implicated when the twin living in a more disadvantaged neighborhood has a greater likelihood of developing ASPD than the co-twin living in a less disadvantaged neighborhood (i.e., there is a within-family difference). If there are no differences between the twin living in a more disadvantaged neighborhood and the co-twin living in a less disadvantaged neighborhood in the likelihood of ASPD, then the association between neighborhood disadvantage and ASPD is more likely to be due to between-family differences that are related to both living in a disadvantaged neighborhood and ASPD. These two scenarios are not mutually exclusive, and neighborhood disadvantage could be a causal factor as well as noncausally associated via between-family differences.

The elegance of the discordant twin study is illustrated by the groundbreaking NASA Twins Study (Garrett-Bakelman et al. 2019). MZ twin astronauts Mark and Scott Kelly participated in a historical experiment in which one twin (Scott) spent an entire year aboard the International Space Station in orbit, while his co-twin (Mark) remained on Earth. NASA was especially interested in understanding the effects of space travel on the human body by comparing Scott and Mark. Because they were genetically identical and had similar family background characteristics, any differences between Scott and Mark could be more unequivocally attributed to the effects of space travel. The use of the discordant twin design uncovered numerous largely transitory effects of space travel on epigenetic, immune, and cognitive functioning, concluding that maintaining human health over longer periods of time in space was possible.

Of course, in the study of ASPD, one is not at the liberty of assigning twins to discordant environments such as living aboard the International Space Station versus remaining on Earth, or living in a more disadvantaged versus a more advantaged neighborhood. Instead, we are limited to identifying naturally occurring discordant twin pairs. This is why this design is considered a "natural" or "quasi-experiment." In Table 7–3, we summarize the results of selected studies that have examined antisocial outcomes among twins discordant for a putative risk or protective environmental factor. As Table 7–3 illustrates, in many cases the results of discordant twin studies have shown that putative environmental risk or protective factors are not actually causal. In the following subsections, we discuss two examples of studies that focused on adult antisocial outcomes that reached different conclusions.

Childhood Maltreatment

Experiencing maltreatment as a child appears to have far-reaching effects in adulthood (Teicher and Samson 2013), including the development of ASPD (Afifi et al. 2011; Luntz and Widom 1994). The maltreatment of children is obviously unaccept-

TABLE 7–3.   **Selected findings from studies of twins discordant for a putative environmental risk or protective factor**

Exposure	Outcome	Correlation?	Causation?	Study
Space travel	Comprehensive set of health and biological metrics		✓	Garrett-Bakelman et al. 2019
Exposure to smoking during pregnancy	Conduct problems	✓		D'Onofrio et al. 2008
Father antisocial	Son cognitive ability	✓		Latvala et al. 2015
Childhood sexual abuse	Conduct disorder	✓	✓	Nelson et al. 2002
Child maltreatment	Adult crime	✓		Forsman and Långström 2012
Marriage	Antisociality	✓	✓	Burt et al. 2010
Marriage	Antisociality		✓	Jaffee et al. 2013

Note.   Causation?=associated at the within-family level; Correlation?=associated at the between-family level.

able and inhumane and in a perfect world would be eradicated. At the same time, however, it is important to understand the mechanisms by which it exerts its effects. If child maltreatment has causal effects on antisocial behavior, then preventing it should decrease the likelihood that maltreated children would grow up to become antisocial. By contrast, if child maltreatment and adult antisocial behavior are associated through shared genetic and common environmental background factors, then eradicating maltreatment may not necessarily lead to decreases in antisocial behavior.

In a study of 18,083 adult Swedish twins, the association between childhood maltreatment and adult criminal offending was examined in order to adjudicate between these two possibilities (Forsman and Långström 2012). Five types of childhood maltreatment (emotional neglect, physical neglect, exposure to family violence, physical abuse, and sexual abuse) were assessed by self-report questionnaire. Convictions for offenses were obtained from the Swedish Crime Register. There was a significant association between at least one form of childhood maltreatment and having an adult criminal conviction (OR=1.28), which remained significant after adjustment for age, sex, and educational attainment (OR=1.44). After adjustment for genetic and environmental background factors in a discordant twin analysis, however, the association was no longer significant (OR=0.84). This suggests that child maltreatment did not have a causal effect on criminal offending.

Marriage

Consistent evidence indicates that being in a stable marriage is associated with reductions in criminal behavior, at least among men, a phenomenon that has become known as "the marriage effect" (Craig et al. 2014). An important question is whether this is because criminal or antisocial individuals are less likely to enter into marriage (a selection effect) or because marriage actually has a protective influence on criminal and antisocial behavior (a causal effect). Two studies have used data from twins or twins and siblings to adjudicate between these possible explanations (Burt et al. 2010; Jaffee et al. 2013).

In the MTFS, assessments of DSM-III-R (American Psychiatric Association 1987) adult antisocial behavior symptoms completed at ages 17, 20, 24, and 29 years were predicted by marital status at age 29 years among 289 male twin pairs (Burt et al. 2010). At all four ages, those who were unmarried at age 29 years endorsed more symptoms of adult antisocial behavior than did those who were married at all previous assessments. Discordant twin analyses suggested that marriage had both a causal protective and a noncausal selection effect on adult antisocial behaviors. After genetic and common environmental factors were controlled for, the twins who were married had fewer symptoms of adult antisocial behaviors than did their co-twins who were unmarried, but a residual association remained that could not be explained by this potentially causal influence. This suggests that the association between marital status and adult antisocial behaviors is also due to between-family differences that are related to both being unmarried and engaging in antisocial behaviors.

There was also evidence for a causal protective effect (but not a selection effect) of marriage on antisocial behavior among 618 male sibling pairs (including MZ and DZ twin pairs) from Wave 4 of the National Longitudinal Study of Adolescent to Adult Health (Add Health; Jaffee et al. 2013). The outcome of interest was antisocial behaviors assessed when the participants were, on average, 29 years old. Marital status was based on transitioning from unmarried (at Wave 3) to married 6 years later (at Wave 4 of the Add Health study). Of the sibling pairs, 42% were discordant for marital status at Wave 4; within the 160 discordant sibling pairs, the unmarried participants endorsed more antisocial behaviors at Waves 3 and 4 than did the married participants. After adjustment for a host of covariates such as employment, income, educational attainment, and physical health in discordant twin models, the causal protective effect persisted. In summary, the results of both the MTFS and the Add Health studies suggest that marriage has a causal protective effect on antisocial behavior among men. Neither study addressed the issue of assortative mating described earlier in this chapter—that is, that antisocial men are more likely to marry antisocial women. Although most of the men would have married women who were not engaged in antisocial behaviors (given the massive sex differences in antisocial behavior), we expect that the protective effect of marriage probably would not apply to the minority of cases in which an antisocial man married an antisocial woman.

Conclusion

Many important insights about antisocial behavior disorders have come from family, twin, and adoption studies. It has long been known that antisocial behavior disorders run in families; we also now know that there is substantial assortative mating for antisocial behavior disorders. That is, families enriched for antisocial behavior disorders tend to become linked with other antisocial behavior disorder–enriched families through the coupling of antisocial individuals.

There have been many cross-sectional univariate twin and adoption studies that have documented the relative contributions of genetic and environmental influences to antisocial behavior disorders. When informative within-study comparisons are made, the contributions of genetic and environmental factors to antisocial behavior disorders among males and females are similar. Within-study comparisons have also firmly established that there is a greater contribution of genetic factors to adult than to child antisocial behavior disorders and a greater contribution of common environmental factors to child than to adult antisocial behavior disorders. The results of multivariate twin studies suggest that, despite a shift in their relative importance, the sets of genes that are on board early in life and that are associated with conduct disorder in childhood are the same genes that continue to exert an influence on risk for adult antisocial behaviors. Multivariate twin studies of antisocial behavior disorder comorbidity also confirm that the main cause of the co-occurrence with other disorders is overlapping genetic risk factors. The stability of genetic risk factors for antisocial behavior disorders across the life course and the substantial genetic overlap of the antisocial behavior disorders with other psychiatric disorders (especially other externalizing disorders and BPD) have important implications for molecular genetic investigations (as reviewed in Chapter 6, "Natural History and Course of Antisocial Personality Disorder," in this volume).

Twin and adoption studies are essential for understanding the role of the environment in the development of antisocial behavior disorders, because they allow one to home in on the potential effect of the environment while controlling for genetic factors. As our selected reviews illustrate, most putative environmental risk factors are genetically correlated with antisocial outcomes (Table 7–2), and most putative causal environmental risk factors are actually noncausally associated with antisocial outcomes via correlated genetic and common environmental background factors (Table 7–3). As Moffitt (2005, p. 88) noted, "[R]esearch that does not attack the co-occurrence of genetic and environmental risks will have only limited relevance for prevention. As such, research into gene–environment interplay will continue to prove critical in the future of research into antisocial behavior." There is much work left to be done to document across the life course the environmental risks that may be causally associated with antisocial behavior disorders and may moderate the genetic susceptibility to develop an antisocial behavior disorder.

Key Points

- Family studies have confirmed that antisocial behavior not only runs in (within) families but also runs across families through the coupling of antisocial individuals.

- Twin studies have confirmed that the contribution of genetic and environmental factors to antisocial behavior shifts in importance from childhood to adulthood.

- Twin studies have demonstrated that the main causes of comorbidity between antisocial behavior disorders and psychiatric and addictive disorders are shared genetic risk factors.

- Twin and adoption studies provide examples of how genetic risk for antisocial behavior is associated with both greater exposure to a high-risk environment and greater sensitivity to a high-risk environment.

- Twin studies of pairs discordant for a putative environmental risk or protective factor have provided incisive tests about whether a risk or protective factor might potentially be causally related to antisocial behavior.

References

Afifi TO, Mather A, Boman J, et al: Childhood adversity and personality disorders: results from a nationally representative population-based study. J Psychiatr Res 45(6):814–822, 2011 21146190

American Psychiatric Association: Diagnostic and Statistical Manual of Mental Disorders, 3rd Edition, Revised. Washington, DC, American Psychiatric Association, 1987

American Psychiatric Association: Diagnostic and Statistical Manual of Mental Disorders, 4th Edition. Washington, DC, American Psychiatric Association, 1994

American Psychiatric Association: Diagnostic and Statistical Manual of Mental Disorders, 4th Edition, Text Revision. Washington, DC, American Psychiatric Association, 2000

American Psychiatric Association: Diagnostic and Statistical Manual of Mental Disorders, 5th Edition. Arlington, VA, American Psychiatric Association, 2013

Baker LA, Bezdjian S, Raine A: Behavioral genetics: the science of antisocial behavior. Law Contemp Probl 69(1–2):7–46, 2006 18176636

Burt SA, Donnellan MB, Humbad MN, et al: Does marriage inhibit antisocial behavior?: An examination of selection vs causation via a longitudinal twin design. Arch Gen Psychiatry 67(12):1309–1315, 2010 21135331

Cadoret RJ, Cain CA, Crowe RR: Evidence for gene-environment interaction in the development of adolescent antisocial behavior. Behav Genet 13(3):301–310, 1983 6615382

Cleveland HH: Disadvantaged neighborhoods and adolescent aggression: behavioral genetic evidence of contextual effects. J Res Adolesc 13(2):211–238, 2003

Cloninger CR, Sigvardsson S, Bohman M, et al: Predisposition to petty criminality in Swedish adoptees, II: cross-fostering analysis of gene-environment interaction. Arch Gen Psychiatry 39(11):1242–1247, 1982 7138224

Coid J, Yang M, Tyrer P, et al: Prevalence and correlates of personality disorder in Great Britain. Br J Psychiatry 188:423–431, 2006 16648528

Compton WM, Conway KP, Stinson FS, et al: Prevalence, correlates, and comorbidity of DSM-IV antisocial personality syndromes and alcohol and specific drug use disorders in the United States: results from the National Epidemiologic Survey on Alcohol and Related Conditions. J Clin Psychiatry 66(6):677–685, 2005 15960559

Craig JM, Diamond B, Piquero AR: Marriage as an intervention in the lives of criminal offenders, in Effective Interventions in the Lives of Criminal Offenders. Edited by Humphrey JA, Cordella P. New York, Springer, 2014, pp 19–37

Dick DM: Gene-environment interaction in psychological traits and disorders. Annu Rev Clin Psychol 7:383–409, 2011 21219196

D'Onofrio BM, Van Hulle CA, Waldman ID, et al: Smoking during pregnancy and offspring externalizing problems: an exploration of genetic and environmental confounds. Dev Psychopathol 20(1):139–164, 2008 18211732

D'Onofrio BM, Lahey BB, Turkheimer E, et al: Critical need for family based, quasi-experimental designs in integrating genetic and social science research. Am J Public Health 103 (suppl 1):S46–S55, 2013 23927516

Farrington DP, Barnes GC, Lambert S: The concentration of offending in families. Leg Criminol Psychol 1:47–63, 1996

Feinberg ME, Button TM, Neiderhiser JM, et al: Parenting and adolescent antisocial behavior and depression: evidence of genotype x parenting environment interaction. Arch Gen Psychiatry 64(4):457–465, 2007 17404122

Forsman M, Långström N: Child maltreatment and adult violent offending: population-based twin study addressing the 'cycle of violence' hypothesis. Psychol Med 42(9):1977–1983, 2012 22236772

Frisell T, Lichtenstein P, Långström N: Violent crime runs in families: a total population study of 12.5 million individuals. Psychol Med 41(1):97–105, 2011 20334717

Garrett-Bakelman FE, Darshi M, Green SJ, et al: The NASA Twins Study: a multidimensional analysis of a year-long human spaceflight. Science 364(6436):eaau8650, 2019 30975860

Gillespie NA, Aggen SH, Neale MC, et al: Associations between personality disorders and cannabis use and cannabis use disorder: a population-based twin study. Addiction 113(8):1488–1498, 2018a 29500852

Gillespie NA, Aggen SH, Gentry AE, et al: Testing genetic and environmental associations between personality disorders and cocaine use: a population-based twin study. Twin Res Hum Genet 21(1):24–32, 2018b 29369040

Grant BF, Hasin DS, Stinson FS, et al: Co-occurrence of 12-month mood and anxiety disorders and personality disorders in the US: results from the National Epidemiologic Survey on Alcohol and Related Conditions. J Psychiatr Res 39(1):1–9, 2005 15504418

Grant JE, Potenza MN, Weinstein A, et al: Introduction to behavioral addictions. Am J Drug Alcohol Abuse 36(5):233–241, 2010 20560821

Hicks BM, South SC, Dirago AC, et al: Environmental adversity and increasing genetic risk for externalizing disorders. Arch Gen Psychiatry 66(6):640–648, 2009 19487629

Iacono WG, McGue M: Minnesota Twin Family Study. Twin Res 5(5):482–487, 2002 12537881

Jacobson KC, Prescott CA, Kendler KS: Sex differences in the genetic and environmental influences on the development of antisocial behavior. Dev Psychopathol 14(2):395–416, 2002 12030698

Jaffee SR, Belsky J, Harrington H, et al: When parents have a history of conduct disorder: how is the caregiving environment affected? J Abnorm Psychol 115(2):309–319, 2006 16737395

Jaffee SR, Lombardi CM, Coley RL: Using complementary methods to test whether marriage limits men's antisocial behavior. Dev Psychopathol 25(1):65–77, 2013 23398753

Johnson W, McGue M, Iacono WG: School performance and genetic and environmental variance in antisocial behavior at the transition from adolescence to adulthood. Dev Psychol 45(4):973–987, 2009 19586174

Kendler KS: Causal inference in psychiatric epidemiology. JAMA Psychiatry 74(6):561–562, 2017 28467524

Kendler KS, Baker JH: Genetic influences on measures of the environment: a systematic review. Psychol Med 37(5):615–626, 2007 17176502

Kendler KS, Prescott CA, Myers J, et al: The structure of genetic and environmental risk factors for common psychiatric and substance use disorders in men and women. Arch Gen Psychiatry 60(9):929–937, 2003 12963675

Kendler KS, Aggen SH, Czajkowski N, et al: The structure of genetic and environmental risk factors for DSM-IV personality disorders: a multivariate twin study. Arch Gen Psychiatry 65(12):1438–1446, 2008 19047531

Kendler KS, Aggen SH, Knudsen GP, et al: The structure of genetic and environmental risk factors for syndromal and subsyndromal common DSM-IV Axis I and all Axis II disorders. Am J Psychiatry 168(1):29–39, 2011 20952461

Kendler KS, Patrick CJ, Larsson H, et al: Genetic and environmental risk factors in males for self-report externalizing traits in mid-adolescence and criminal behavior through young adulthood. Psychol Med 43(10):2161–2168, 2013 23369621

Kendler KS, Larsson Lönn S, Morris NA, et al: A Swedish national adoption study of criminality. Psychol Med 44(9):1913–1925, 2014 24180693

Knopik VS, Neiderhiser JM, DeFries JC, et al: Behavioral Genetics. New York, Worth Publishers, 2017

Kraus SW, Voon V, Potenza MN: Should compulsive sexual behavior be considered an addiction? Addiction 111(12):2097–2106, 2016 26893127

Krueger RF: The structure of common mental disorders. Arch Gen Psychiatry 56(10):921–926, 1999 10530634

Krueger RF, Moffitt TE, Caspi A, et al: Assortative mating for antisocial behavior: developmental and methodological implications. Behav Genet 28(3):173–186, 1998 9670593

Lahey BB, D'Onofrio BM: All in the family: comparing siblings to test causal hypotheses regarding environmental influences on behavior. Curr Dir Psychol Sci 19(5):319–323, 2010 23645975

Latvala A, Kuja-Halkola R, Långström N, et al: Paternal antisocial behavior and sons' cognitive ability: a population-based quasiexperimental study. Psychol Sci 26(1):78–88, 2015 25425060

Lenzenweger MF, Lane MC, Loranger AW, et al: DSM-IV personality disorders in the National Comorbidity Survey Replication. Biol Psychiatry 62(6):553–564, 2007 17217923

Luntz BK, Widom CS: Antisocial personality disorder in abused and neglected children grown up. Am J Psychiatry 151(5):670–674, 1994 8166307

Lyons MJ, True WR, Eisen SA, et al: Differential heritability of adult and juvenile antisocial traits. Arch Gen Psychiatry 52(11):906–915, 1995 7487339

Manuck SB, McCaffery JM: Gene-environment interaction. Annu Rev Psychol 65:41–70, 2014 24405358

McGue M, Osler M, Christensen K: Causal inference and observational research: the utility of twins. Perspect Psychol Sci 5(5):546–556, 2010 21593989

Mednick SA, Gabrielli WF Jr, Hutchings B: Genetic influences in criminal convictions: evidence from an adoption cohort. Science 224(4651):891–894, 1984 6719119

Meier MH, Slutske WS, Heath AC, et al: The role of harsh discipline in explaining sex differences in conduct disorder: a study of opposite-sex twin pairs. J Abnorm Child Psychol 37(5):653–664, 2009 19280334

Meier MH, Slutske WS, Heath AC, et al: Sex differences in the genetic and environmental influences on childhood conduct disorder and adult antisocial behavior. J Abnorm Psychol 120(2):377–388, 2011 21319923

Moffitt TE: Genetic and environmental influences on antisocial behaviors: evidence from behavioral-genetic research. Adv Genet 55:41–104, 2005 16291212

Moffitt TE, Caspi A, Harrington H, et al: Males on the life-course-persistent and adolescence-limited antisocial pathways: follow-up at age 26 years. Dev Psychopathol 14(1):179–207, 2002 11893092

Nelson EC, Heath AC, Madden PA, et al: Association between self-reported childhood sexual abuse and adverse psychosocial outcomes: results from a twin study. Arch Gen Psychiatry 59(2):139–145, 2002 11825135

Odgers CL, Russell MA: What can genetically informed research tell us about the causes of crime?, in Measuring Crime & Criminality: Advances in Criminological Theory, Vol 17. Edited by MacDonald J. New York, Routledge, 2017, pp 141–160

Petry NM, Stinson FS, Grant BF: Comorbidity of DSM-IV pathological gambling and other psychiatric disorders: results from the National Epidemiologic Survey on Alcohol and Related Conditions. J Clin Psychiatry 66(5):564–574, 2005 15889941

Plomin R, DeFries JC, Knopik VS, et al: Top 10 replicated findings from behavioral genetics. Perspect Psychol Sci 11(1):3–23, 2016 26817721

Polderman TJ, Benyamin B, de Leeuw CA, et al: Meta-analysis of the heritability of human traits based on fifty years of twin studies. Nat Genet 47(7):702–709, 2015 25985137

Reichborn-Kjennerud T: Genetics of personality disorders. Psychiatr Clin North Am 31(3):421–440, vi–vii, 2008 18638644

Reichborn-Kjennerud T, Kendler KS: Genetics of personality disorders, in Neurobiology of Personality Disorders. Edited by Schmahl C, Phan KL, Friedel RO. New York, Oxford University Press, 2018, pp 57–73

Reichborn-Kjennerud T, Czajkowski N, Ystrøm E, et al: A longitudinal twin study of borderline and antisocial personality disorder traits in early to middle adulthood. Psychol Med 45(14):3121–3131, 2015 26050739

Rende RD, Plomin R, Vandenberg SG: Who discovered the twin method? Behav Genet 20(2):277–285, 1990 2191648

Rhee SH, Waldman ID: Genetic and environmental influences on antisocial behavior: a meta-analysis of twin and adoption studies. Psychol Bull 128(3):490–529, 2002 12002699

Rutter M: Nature–nurture integration: the example of antisocial behavior. Am Psychol 52(4):390–398, 1997

Rutter M: Genes and Behavior: Nature-Nurture Interplay Explained. Malden, MA, Blackwell, 2006

Rutter M: Gene-environment interdependence. Dev Sci 10(1):12–18, 2007a 17181693

Rutter M: Proceeding from observed correlation to causal inference: the use of natural experiments. Perspect Psychol Sci 2(4):377–395, 2007b 26151974

Rutter M, Caspi A, Moffitt TE: Using sex differences in psychopathology to study causal mechanisms: unifying issues and research strategies. J Child Psychol Psychiatry 44(8):1092–1115, 2003 14626453

Salvatore JE, Dick DM: Genetic influences on conduct disorder. Neurosci Biobehav Rev 91:91–101, 2018 27350097

Samek DR, Hicks BM, Keyes MA, et al: Gene-environment interplay between parent-child relationship problems and externalizing disorders in adolescence and young adulthood. Psychol Med 45(2):333–344, 2015 25066478

Samek DR, Hicks BM, Keyes MA, et al: Antisocial peer affiliation and externalizing disorders: evidence for gene×environment×development interaction. Dev Psychopathol 29(1):155–172, 2017 27580681

Scarr S, McCartney K: How people make their own environments: a theory of genotype greater than environment effects. Child Dev 54(2):424–435, 1983 6683622

Shanahan MJ, Hofer SM: Social context in gene-environment interactions: retrospect and prospect. J Gerontol B Psychol Sci Soc Sci 60(Spec No 1):65–76, 2005 15863711

Slutske WS: The genetics of antisocial behavior. Curr Psychiatry Rep 3(2):158–162, 2001 11276412

Slutske WS, Eisen S, Xian H, et al: A twin study of the association between pathological gambling and antisocial personality disorder. J Abnorm Psychol 110(2):297–308, 2001 11358024

Slutske WS, Deutsch AR, Statham DJ, et al: Local area disadvantage and gambling involvement and disorder: evidence for gene-environment correlation and interaction. J Abnorm Psychol 124(3):606–622, 2015 26147321

Teicher MH, Samson JA: Childhood maltreatment and psychopathology: a case for ecophenotypic variants as clinically and neurobiologically distinct subtypes. Am J Psychiatry 170(10):1114–1133, 2013 23982148

Torgersen S, Czajkowski N, Jacobson K, et al: Dimensional representations of DSM-IV Cluster B personality disorders in a population-based sample of Norwegian twins: a multivariate study. Psychol Med 38(11):1617–1625, 2008 18275631

Torgersen S, Myers J, Reichborn-Kjennerud T, et al: The heritability of Cluster B personality disorders assessed both by personal interview and questionnaire. J Pers Disord 26(6):848–866, 2012 23281671

Trull TJ, Jahng S, Tomko RL, et al: Revised NESARC personality disorder diagnoses: gender, prevalence, and comorbidity with substance dependence disorders. J Pers Disord 24(4):412–426, 2010 20695803

Trull TJ, Vergés A, Wood PK, et al: The structure of DSM-IV-TR personality disorder diagnoses in NESARC: a reanalysis. J Pers Disord 27(6):727–734, 2013 23718818

Turkheimer E: Three laws of behavior genetics and what they mean. Curr Dir Psychol Sci 9:160–164, 2000

Tuvblad C, Grann M, Lichtenstein P: Heritability for adolescent antisocial behavior differs with socioeconomic status: gene-environment interaction. J Child Psychol Psychiatry 47(7):734–743, 2006 16790008

Viding E, Larsson H, Jones AP: Quantitative genetic studies of antisocial behaviour. Philos Trans R Soc Lond B Biol Sci 363(1503):2519–2527, 2008 18434281

Wesseldijk LW, Bartels M, Vink JM, et al: Genetic and environmental influences on conduct and antisocial personality problems in childhood, adolescence, and adulthood. Eur Child Adolesc Psychiatry 27(9):1123–1132, 2018 28638947

World Health Organization: ICD-11 for Mortality and Morbidity Statistics. 2018. Available at: http://icd.who.int/browse11/l-m/en. Accessed June 29, 2020.

CHAPTER 8

Molecular Genetics of Antisocial Personality Disorder

Christopher Adanty, B.Sc.
Zhuoran Ma, B.S.
Anvesh Roy, M.D.
Anil Srivastava, M.D.
Nasia Dai, B.Sc.
Vincenzo De Luca, M.D., Ph.D.

Antisocial personality disorder (ASPD) is a psychiatric condition that is detailed in DSM-5 (American Psychiatric Association 2013), which describes symptoms such as lack of empathy, disregard of others' rights, and impulsive or aggressive behavior (Ellis 1982; Glenn et al. 2013; Verona et al. 2012).

As in other psychiatric disorders, in ASPD, there is an interplay between genes and the environment. To examine this relationship in more detail, one has to look at the mechanisms that have been investigated in regard to these interactions. A review of the family psychiatric history of ASPD patients often shows a large number of family members who have been diagnosed with similar behavioral issues (Baker et al. 2006). It is believed that heredity accounts for 30%–50% of the risk for acquiring ASPD. A specific DNA sequence is polymorphic if it varies between individuals, and the different sequence variants are alleles. Several genetic polymorphisms have been discovered that are associated with an increased risk for ASPD. To account for the risk of ASPD, we need to consider not only variations in specific genes but also epigenetic factors, which can influence gene expression as a result of environmental influences such as child maltreatment. These epigenetic variations can be transmitted to offspring, accounting for another form of inheritance. As our understanding of the biological mechanisms that underlie ASPD evolves, there are several real-world implications for the ethical, legal, and psychiatric treatment of individuals with ASPD.

The clinician who is tasked with diagnosing and treating ASPD should therefore keep in mind the genetic mechanisms that contribute to ASPD. An understanding of these genetic mechanisms can help one empathize with individuals who appear to be markedly aggressive or manipulative and can also help educate the public about the etiology of characteristic behaviors of ASPD. In the future, one can potentially envision having available several genetic or epigenetic test batteries to help in the diagnosis of ASPD. This strategy could be of potential importance in legal matters and forensic examinations. Finally, as our technologies improve over time, gene therapies targeting the epigenetics and genetics of ASPD may be envisioned. The hope would be to use these targeted therapies to lessen the risk of developing or even prevent ASPD rather than have to rely on the blunt instruments of detention and punishment to control the symptoms of ASPD, and to possibly reintegrate individuals with ASPD into society.

In this chapter, we review the molecular genetics and epigenetic mechanisms that may contribute to the development of ASPD.

Genetic Studies in Antisocial Personality Disorder

DNA segments that are adjacent to each other are often inherited together, and such linkages between genes can be statistically analyzed to track inheritance of specific genetic patterns to study these correlations. Several studies have examined the effect of genes on the structure and function of brain regions, such as the hippocampus and the amygdala; these are regions often associated with emotional control (Martin et al. 2009). Damage to these regions could possibly affect brain activities and connections, resulting in behaviors similar to symptoms of ASPD (Iofrida et al. 2014). Linkage studies conducted in families affected by alcohol use disorder (AUD) have found that individuals with both AUD and ASPD show significantly different allele patterns when compared with individuals who do not have AUD. These individuals are believed to have different genetic variants of the dopamine D_2 receptor gene (*DRD2*) (Hill et al. 1999). These variants can account for substance-seeking behaviors such as those found in AUD that are often seen in ASPD (Blum et al. 1996). *DRD2* polymorphisms are a likely explanation of the inherited comorbidity of AUD and ASPD. One such study used a dimensional model of externalizing behaviors to encompass alcohol and drug dependence, conduct disorder, adult antisocial behavior, novelty seeking, and sensation seeking. The study found a gene via linkage analysis localized to a region on chromosome 7 that broadly predisposes individuals to externalizing behavior. *Genetic association* occurs when one or more genotypes within a population co-occur with a phenotypic trait more often than would be expected by chance occurrence. Association analyses of one candidate gene, *CHRM2*, which codes for a muscarinic acetylcholine receptor, suggest that it is involved in a general externalizing phenotype (Dick et al. 2008).

Dopaminergic Genes and Antisocial Personality Disorder

Dopamine is a key neurotransmitter responsible for transmission of reward signals. Dopaminergic pathways are also involved in many functions, such as executive function, learning, motivation, and neuroendocrine control. The dopaminergic neurons are located in the brain at the substantia nigra and ventral tegmental area, which are both located in the midbrain, as well as the arcuate nucleus of the hypothalamus. Four main pathways in the brain—mesocortical, mesolimbic, tuberoinfundibular, and nigrostriatal—are involved in regulating dopamine flow, which translates to the above functions. The human *DRD2* gene is located on chromosome 11. Dysfunction of the D_2 receptor can often lead to disturbances of dopamine transmission in these pathways. Elevated dopamine levels are also known to mediate aggression. Animal studies show that dopamine levels are increased with aggressive fights in rodents (Hadfield 1983). When one antagonizes dopamine transmission in healthy male volunteers, there is a selective disruption in the recognition of facial expressions of anger. For example, acute administration of the dopamine D_2-class receptor antagonist sulpiride achieves this effect (Lawrence et al. 2002).

DRD2 has been linked to compulsive, impulsive, and addictive behaviors as well as ADHD. The prevalence of a particular gene variant of *DRD2* (the Taq A1 allele) has been associated with violent behavior in addition to school fights and imprisonment for violent crimes as adults (Baker et al. 2006). Therefore, it follows that administration of common D_2 antagonist antipsychotics is used routinely in hospitals for the treatment of aggressive behaviors in a wide range of psychiatric conditions, including personality disorders, psychotic disorders, and mood disorders. The disruption of aggression, however, seems to be independent of the antipsychotic effect of such drugs.

The catechol O-methyltransferase gene (*COMT*) codes for the enzyme COMT, which is responsible for the catabolism of catecholamines; this gene is located on chromosome 22 and plays a crucial role in modulating emotional responses and behaviors by degrading neurotransmitters such as epinephrine, norepinephrine, and dopamine (Hoth et al. 2006). COMT activity has been proposed to play a pivotal role in prefrontal cortical function. The enzyme accounts for most of the degradation of dopamine in the prefrontal cortex (PFC) (Winterer and Goldman 2003). A common functional polymorphism of *COMT* results in a three- to fourfold variation in enzyme activity. This variation, in turn, affects the ability of *COMT* to inactivate dopamine (Hallikainen et al. 2000).

COMT polymorphisms have been linked to several psychiatric disorders, such as depression, anxiety, schizophrenia, bipolar disorder, and substance use disorders, all of which are common comorbidities of ASPD (Bilder et al. 2002; Hallikainen et al. 2000; Hoth et al. 2006; Iofrida et al. 2014; Vevera et al. 2009). The most commonly identified single nucleotide polymorphism (SNP) of *COMT* is *COMT*Val158Met, a SNP that replaces the methionine (Met) with valine (Val) at codon 158, which results in a high-activity form of COMT (Thapar et al. 2005). Evidence indicates that this allele is associated with higher impulsivity and violent behaviors, which correspond with ASPD symptomatology (Hallikainen et al. 2000; Hirata et al. 2013; Thapar et al. 2005; Vevera et al. 2009). More research is needed to investigate the role of COMT activity in ASPD (Iofrida et al. 2014).

A study conducted by Thapar and colleagues (2005) investigated whether the functional *COMT* variant would be associated with antisocial behavior. This study provided insight on the potential importance of gene-environment interactions—specifically the main effects of the *COMT* variant and birth weight (Thapar et al. 2005). As a result, evidence from the study reported that the *COMT*Val/Val genotype and lower birth weight were linked to increased symptoms of conduct disorder, which holds promise as a predictor of early-onset antisocial behavior (Thapar et al. 2005).

Individuals can be homozygous for the high-activity *COMT* allele (HH genotype), homozygous for the low-activity *COMT* allele (LL genotype), and heterozygous for intermediate activity (LH genotype) (Hallikainen et al. 2000). Empirical evidence has shown a link between the LL*COMT* allele and psychiatric disorders, such as velocardiofacial syndrome and schizophrenia (Hallikainen et al. 2000). For humans, it is unknown whether variation in COMT enzyme level encoded by the 158 polymorphism affects brain dopamine metabolization. Low COMT activity also affects dopamine transmission in the frontal cortex (Hallikainen et al. 2000). Others have identified a relation between the LL*COMT* allele and violence in schizophrenia, as well as aggressive behavior in *COMT* knockout mice with reduced COMT activity (Hallikainen et al. 2000). Hallikainen and colleagues hypothesized that reduced COMT activity may contribute to violent behavior associated with alcoholism. Specifically, they studied *COMT* polymorphisms in subjects with Type II (early-onset and habitual impulsive violent behavior) alcoholism. Results indicated no association between *COMT* and subjects with Type II alcoholism; however, a link between subjects with Type I (late onset without prominent antisocial behavior) alcoholism and LL*COMT* was identified (Hallikainen et al. 2000). These findings provide tentative evidence that *COMT* polymorphisms may influence aggressive behavior in psychiatric disorders. However, the effect of *COMT* polymorphisms is potentially dependent on whether a central deficit in catecholamine transmission exists (Hallikainen et al. 2000). Therefore, it appears that low COMT activity increases violent behavior in individuals who have schizophrenia with abnormal dopamine transmission but does not affect individuals with Type II alcoholism with potential serotonin (5-HT) transmission deficits (Hallikainen et al. 2000).

Currently, the etiology of childhood-onset aggression is poorly understood, and this is relevant because childhood-onset aggression is often a precursor to full-blown ASPD in adulthood. Callous-unemotional (CU) traits are used to classify aggression in children based on lack of empathy, lack of guilt, shallow emotions, and severe antisocial behavior. CU traits were proposed by Frick and Morris (2004) as traits that lead to a developmental model of aggressive and antisocial behavior; individuals with high levels of CU traits have had more severe patterns of aggressive behavior. These individuals have also shown earlier contact with juvenile justice systems. Researchers considered that it was important to include CU traits as a subtype of child-onset aggression in genetic research to find preventive treatments for aggressive behavior. The literature indicates that the dopaminergic system is important in relation to pathological aggression and problems in children and adolescents. Hirata and colleagues studied *COMT* in children with high aggression to examine four *COMT* polymorphisms, one being Val158Met (Hirata et al. 2013). This study found some evidence from one of the first studies to investigate the role of *COMT* variants in child aggression and in CU traits that child aggression is associated with two markers of *COMT*: rs6269 and rs4818 (Hirata et al. 2013). However, more studies are required to further understand the relationship between rs6269 and rs4818 polymorphisms and CU scores.

Serotonergic Genes and Antisocial Personality Disorder

Serotonergic pathways are also often disrupted in ASPD as in many other psychiatric disorders. Studies have found serotonergic transmission to be important in the comorbidity of ASPD and AUD (Ficks and Waldman 2014). Chronic consumption of alcohol can reduce 5-HT levels. If an individual already has a low-activity 5-HT polymorphism, then chronic alcohol consumption can further suppress serotonergic activity, resulting in behaviors such as impulsive aggression (Kranzler et al. 2002). Serotonin 5-HT$_3$ receptors are also believed to modulate ethanol response and 5-HT release. There are currently two identified subunits, 5-HT$_{3A}$ and 5-HT$_{3B}$ (encoded by *HTR3A* and *HTR3B* genes, respectively). A homomer consists of two similar subunits, whereas a heteromer has two different subunits. It is believed that depending on the combination of either the 5-HT$_{3A}$ homomer or the 5-HT$_{3A}$/5-HT$_{3B}$ heteromer, receptor activity can be altered (Ducci et al. 2009). A whole-genome linkage investigation[1] concluded that genetic variation within *HTR3B* can potentially influence AUD vulnerability with comorbid ASPD. In comparison, Arias and colleagues (2011) aimed to identify and characterize high-order gene-to-gene interactions in ASPD. Results identified epistatic interaction with serotonergic genes and polymorphisms relating to the disorder. Epistatic relations were found for *COMT*, tryptophan hydroxylase gene, and *HTR2A*. Genetic polymorphisms, therefore, affect 5-HT receptors and low COMT enzyme activity (Arias et al. 2011). As a result, susceptibility to ASPD is affected, and these aforementioned gene interactions may be associated with ASPD (Arias et al. 2011). These interactions may also influence the dopamine reward pathways and modulate 5-HT levels (Arias et al. 2011). Another study investigated the role of both 5-HTTLPR and 5-HTTVNTR polymorphisms of the gene *SLC6A4* (Garcia et al. 2010). Garcia and colleagues found that within a sample of 147 male inmates, those presenting with both 5-HTTLPR S/S+S/L and 5-HTTVNTR 12/12 had a higher risk of being classified as having ASPD (Garcia et al. 2010). The results of this study highlighted the potential for the 5-HTTVNTR polymorphism to be a candidate for association studies with ASPD because of its prominence in the study sample (Garcia et al. 2010). Further studies regarding the 5-HT$_3$ receptor gene would be very beneficial in understanding its effect on increasing vulnerability toward acquiring ASPD (Ducci et al. 2009).

Genetic variation in candidate genes such as those that modulate neurotransmitter levels or regulate cognitive function is hypothesized to be associated with alteration of brain connections in ASPD patients. Many studies have focused on the investigation of these candidate genes in the hopes of better understanding the underlying molecular mechanisms of ASPD. The serotonin transporter (5-HTT), for example, is responsible for 5-HT reuptake and 5-HT regulation (Douglas et al. 2011). It, therefore, acts as a crucial regulatory element for stress response (Chaouloff 2000). 5-HT neurotransmission modulation is very important for emotion control (Kobiella et al. 2011). One study has found an association of a 5-HTT gene polymorphism with ASPD (Douglas et al. 2011). This study

---

[1] A linkage study of the entire genome as opposed to a certain region of a chromosome. This type of study is increasingly easier to perform as costs pertaining to genetic sequencing decrease.

examined genetic and environmental determinants of ASPD in a sample of individuals who had substance use disorders. The study looked at different ethnic populations in the United States, comprising Caucasian or European Americans and African Americans. These groups were further classified by gender. The study investigated adverse childhood experiences (ACEs) and their effect on moderating the risk for developing ASPD. The gene coding for 5-HTT is located on the long arm of chromosome 17 (17q11.1–q12). 5-HTT gene polymorphisms have resulted from the functional insertion or deletion of the 5′ promoter region (5-HTTLPR) of *SLC6A4* (chromosome 17, location 17q11.1–q12), which encodes for the 5-HTT protein. As a result, there are three main variants of the transporter: a short allele (S allele) and two long alleles (L allele), which differ by a SNP of A/G, denoted here as L_G and L_A (Douglas et al. 2011). It is believed that the L_A allele has great translational efficiency, while the S allele underexpresses the 5-HTT protein. The L_G allele has a similar translation efficacy as the S allele (Douglas et al. 2011). Low 5-HTT gene expression is often associated with anxiety and negative mood, and S allele individuals are at increased risk for ASPD and are more likely to display impulsivity (Douglas et al. 2011; Kobiella et al. 2011). Other stress-reactive phenotypic expressions such as depression and substance use are often comorbid with ASPD and are also associated with S allele expression (Douglas et al. 2011). In Caucasian or European Americans, logistic regression analysis showed that only male sex and the number of types of ACEs were significantly associated with an ASPD diagnosis. In African Americans, the three-way interaction of sex and number of S alleles and ACE was significantly associated with an ASPD diagnosis. For African American men, each additional ACE significantly increased the odds of ASPD irrespective of the number of 5-HTTLPR S alleles. However, among African American women, the effect of ACE score on ASPD was significant only for those with two S alleles. There are limitations of this study, including a small sample size (Douglas et al. 2011). There have been other studies that rebut this hypothesis, such as an investigation by Sakai et al. (2007), who studied 1,736 Caucasian adolescents and found no significant relationship between the low-activity 5-HTTLPR genotype and measures of conduct problems.

MRI studies have discovered smaller amygdala structures and higher amygdala activations in the S allele individuals. It is likely that the 5-HTTLPR polymorphism is associated with structural alteration of the amygdala during early neurodevelopment. This study was carried out in 54 healthy volunteers and emphasizes the structural influence of the genotype rather than the actual availability of 5-HTT (Kobiella et al. 2011). Results also indicated that mutations or variations of the serotonergic system genes were strongly associated with impulsivity and aggression, as 5-HT level is an important modulating element for the amygdala and frontal cortex (Ficks and Waldman 2014).

As discussed previously, *SLC6A4* is a gene responsible for the 5-HTT protein; another example of a gene involved in 5-HT regulation is the monoamine oxidase A gene (*MAOA*). *MAOA* encodes the MAOA enzyme that catabolizes monoamine transmitters such as 5-HT, dopamine, and norepinephrine. It is located on the X chromosome (Xp11.23). As discussed below, a deficiency in this enzyme is associated with aggressive behaviors, which are relevant to the genetic etiology of ASPD (Kolla and Bortolato 2020).

Two studies have reported a Dutch family in which eight males were affected by a syndrome characterized by borderline mental retardation and impulsive behavior, including serious violence and aggression. The syndrome was thought to be due to a stop-codon variant in the eighth exon of *MAOA*, leading to complete and selective deficiency of monoamine oxidase A activity (Brunner et al. 1993a, 1993b).

A polymorphism was found upstream of the gene for monoamine oxidase A. This was a promoter region for this gene. This promoter region polymorphism is thought to be a genetic marker for MAOA function. The polymorphism, which is located 1.2 kb upstream of *MAOA*, consists of a 30–base pair repeated sequence present in 3, 3.5, 4, or 5 copies. The polymorphism displays significant variations in allele frequencies across ethnic groups. The polymorphism has been shown to affect the transcriptional activity of the monoamine oxidase A gene promoter. Alleles with 3.5 or 4 copies of the repeat sequence are transcribed 2–10 times more efficiently than those with 3 or 5 copies of the repeat (Sabol et al. 1998).

A landmark study that elucidated the significance of *MAOA* in combination with environmental influences was performed by Caspi et al. in 2003, and it has spawned meta-analyses examining this intriguing area in detail. The investigators hypothesized that the *MAOA* genotype can moderate the influence of childhood maltreatment on neurological systems that are implicated in antisocial behavior. They aimed to determine whether this gene in combination with environmental effects would lead to antisocial behavior in adults. They genotyped the polymorphism in the promoter region described earlier (Sabol et al. 1998) in the Dunedin Study cohort, which consisted of 1,037 children (52% male and 48% female). These children were assessed at various points during their growth until age 26 years. They were classified as those with either low *MAOA* activity or high *MAOA* activity genotypes. The children, who were all male in this study, were categorized by the amount of childhood mistreatment they had experienced; 8% had experienced "severe maltreatment," 28% had experienced "probable maltreatment," and 64% reported no maltreatment. The main finding was that those males who were maltreated and possessed the low *MAOA* genotype were more likely to develop conduct disorder or a conviction for a violent crime. On the other hand, those males who were maltreated and had the high *MAOA* genotype did not have increased risk for conduct disorder or a violent crime conviction as adults. These results provided compelling evidence for a gene×environment interaction. Subsequent meta-analyses have also examined this phenomenon. A study of 975 boys, as well as a meta-analysis of studies, examining this interaction confirmed the original finding (Kim-Cohen et al. 2006). Moreover, the meta-analysis demonstrated that the association between early maltreatment and mental health problems was significantly stronger for the group of males with the low *MAOA* genotype. Another meta-analysis, which contained 27 studies and 20 different male cohorts, confirmed the same finding (Byrd and Manuck 2014). However, the finding was mixed and inconclusive among females, and 11 such cohorts were included (Byrd and Manuck 2014). Subsequent studies have shown some mixed results; however, the meta-analyses cited earlier are fairly conclusive for the relationship in males. The interested reader is referred to an excellent review article summarizing the field by Nilsson et al. (2018), who proposed that the variation in study results may lie in the type of maltreatment experienced by affected children and the timing of early maltreatment in relation to developing violent or antisocial behavior.

Epigenetics is also an intriguing mechanism of the gene×environment interactions; we discuss possible epigenetic mechanisms implicated in ASPD later in this chapter.

Genome-Wide Association Studies of Antisocial Personality Disorder

In addition to specific candidate gene investigations, more general and wide-scale approaches have been implemented in the study of the molecular genetics of ASPD. By conducting genome-wide association studies (GWASs), large amounts of raw genomic information can be generated and compared more conveniently. The association of different genetic polymorphisms can be presented together, allowing the genomic analysis to be more thorough and efficient. This method is also able to identify potential genotype-phenotype associations that have not been studied (Tam et al. 2019). However, GWASs have several limitations. They are very costly, and the result can be essentially uninformative; moreover, not all results lead to a viable causation (Tam et al. 2019). Depending on the sample size, it is easy to receive a false-negative or false-positive result, and confounding effects also must be accounted for during data analysis. Regardless, GWAS is still a very powerful research method (Need and Goldstein 2010). A GWAS in ASPD patients performed by Rautiainen et al. (2016) found a strong variant association at 6p21.2. The best identified gene, *rs4714329*, had a strong connection with the expression of the genes *LINC00951*, *LRFN2*, and *TDRG1*. All three genes are closely associated with brain regions such as the cerebellum and the frontal cortex. *LINC00951* and *LRFN2* are both expressed in the frontal cortex, a brain region involved in modulating behavior and cognitive control, and reduced overall gray matter in that region has been reported in ASPD patients (Rautiainen et al. 2016). As noted throughout this textbook, the PFC appears especially relevant for biological research related to ASPD (Raine 2002; Rautiainen et al. 2016; Thapar et al. 2005). Moreover, the gene discussed here is a promising target for future gene-specific investigations. Another GWAS focused on antisocial behaviors, which are closely related to ASPD (Tielbeek et al. 2017). The study concluded that polygenic risk (which is often described as a polygenic risk score that informs how a person's risk compares with the risk of others with a different genetic constitution) is likely to be at play, given that no specific genetic variant passed the threshold for significance. However, several loci did seem to provide promising results; these results suggest that heterogeneous genetic effects can combine and produce different degrees of effects. For example, many genes with small effects can combine cumulatively to produce a certain phenotype, such as aggressive behavior (Tielbeek et al. 2017). Several studies that focused on the effects of gene-gene interactions also support the idea of additive polygenic effects (Ducci et al. 2008; Tielbeek et al. 2012).

Imaging Genetics Studies of Antisocial Personality Disorder

As previously discussed, behavioral disorders such as ASPD are often due to dysregulation of brain connections or structural changes of brain regions responsible for emotion and cognition control. Imaging studies often use technologies such as MRI to investigate and compare brain structures to answer questions such as whether a genetic variation of a candidate gene can alter the structure or activation of certain brain regions or whether it affects neural connections (Greene et al. 2016). It is believed that cognition and adaptive emotional responding are highly associated with neural activation, especially in the amygdala and prefrontal, temporal, and parietal regions of the brain (Abu-Akel and Shamay-Tsoory 2011). Using functional MRI (fMRI), Kolla et al. (2017) investigated the association of *MAOA* variants with morphological changes in brain regions such as the orbitofrontal cortex and the amygdala. As discussed previously, low-activity *MAOA* is associated with higher vulnerability of ASPD and an increased likelihood of violent behaviors (Glenn et al. 2013; Kolla and Vinette 2017). Consequently, the current imaging study also found associations of low-activity *MAOA* variants with morphological changes of the brain. ASPD individuals who possessed the low-activity *MAOA* genotype were found to have reduced surface area of the right anterior cortical amygdaloid nucleus. This finding suggests that *MAOA* variation may contribute to the morphological changes of the amygdala in ASPD cases. Further investigation of this association could potentially discover a novel mechanism that explains the morphological alteration. It was hypothesized that because the low-activity *MAOA* genotype correlates with higher 5-HT accumulation, excess 5-HT could disrupt the developing amygdala and affect the integrity of the amygdala nucleus (Kolla et al. 2017). Further support of this hypothesis could have larger implications, such as for development of novel diagnostic markers and potential therapeutic targets. Another imaging study by Kolla and colleagues (2018) found associations of *MAOA* polymorphisms with differences in brain functional connectivity. ASPD individuals with the high-activity *MAOA* variant were found to have higher caudate functional connectivity of the right frontal pole and the anterior cingulate cortex compared with individuals without ASPD, which suggests that increased caudate functional connectivity of the frontal pole and the anterior cingulate cortex could play a role in the pathophysiology of ASPD. Individuals with the low-activity *MAOA* genotype were also found to express higher levels of aggression when compared with high-activity *MAOA* individuals, and a corresponding increase in corticostriatal connectivity between the precuneus and the angular gyrus also was detected (Kolla et al. 2018). Given that the precuneus and the angular gyrus are modules linked to moral judgment and control of aggression, the association of *MAOA* variants with the connectivity of these modules is biologically plausible (Lou et al. 2004; Seghier 2013). Imaging genetic studies represent an opportunity to better understand how genetic polymorphisms influence brain functionality and connectivity in ASPD.

Role of Epigenetics in Antisocial Personality Disorder

Epigenetics is a relatively new addition to the field of genetics. Certain effects such as phenotype discordance in monozygotic twins, late age at onset of an illness, and fluctuating disease course have not been adequately explained by strictly studying the genome at the DNA sequence level. Epigenetics is the regulation of DNA by certain nonsequence chemical alterations, where these modifications can alter gene expression. In some cases, these alterations can turn the gene on or off, markedly affecting the phenotype. DNA methylation is a common form of epigenetic modification. There have been other biochemical mechanisms. Epigenetic changes can occur by interaction with the environment in an individual's lifetime; they can also be inherited by the offspring, thereby serving as a mechanism of genetic transmission of a certain disease or characteristic.

Environmental stressors such as early life adversity can contribute to the epigenetic alteration of gene expression (Weder et al. 2009). Individuals who experience childhood sexual abuse show evidence of hypermethylated *SLC6A4* and are found to be more prone to aggressive behaviors. Childhood sexual abuse was found to be particularly associated with ASPD in women (Beach et al. 2010a, 2010b). The degree of *SLC6A4* methylation is found to be associated with childhood maltreatment and also with the development of major depressive disorder. Individuals with higher degrees of methylation had altered emotional processing of negative or positive visual stimuli correlating with brain structures on fMRI scans. Individuals without *SLC6A4* methylation did not show this effect. The individuals with *SLC6A4* methylation and major depressive disorder were also unable to judge stimuli as positive or neutral, which highlighted altered emotional processing in these individuals compared with the control group (Frodl et al. 2015). In the only known epigenetics study of ASPD, it was reported that hypermethylation in the *MAOA* promoter regions was present in a sample of incarcerated males with ASPD. Hypermethylation affects the regulation of monoamine oxidase A activity by downregulating gene expression, which dysregulates 5-HT availability. In particular, 5-HT activity is increased, which is associated with increased aggression. This study showcases another mechanism of altered monoamine oxidase A activity that may be associated with ASPD. This finding could help clarify why some of the studies, purely at the genetic level as opposed to the epigenetic level, have shown mixed results. Epigenetic mechanisms may also explain associated psychopathology, such as mood disorders and suicide risk (Checknita et al. 2015). Another vista is the intergenerational transmission of epigenetics, which modulates neurobiology. Studies in humans are still in their infancy; however, animal studies and small human epigenetic studies show compelling evidence for this methodology (Scorza et al. 2019). This methodology could explain another mechanism accounting for the clustering of ASPD within families intergenerationally. Further evidence of these effects could have effects for population-level public policy planning and potential therapeutics.

Epigenetics is an important aspect of future research; however, the investigation of posttranslational modification is still, as of this writing, in a nascent stage.

Conclusion

The molecular genetics of ASPD represent the interplay between several factors, including genetics, environmental factors, and epigenetics. A comprehensive understanding of the molecular genetics of ASPD and the etiological basis for this disorder requires surveying each of the aforementioned factors.

With heritability already accounting for 30%–50% of the ASPD risk, current molecular genetics investigations of ASPD have reported important findings. Overall, the current GWAS investigations of ASPD are few but do show good evidence of polygenic effects. Alterations in candidate genes involved in the serotonergic system, such as *MAOA* and *SLC6A4*, have been shown to be associated with ASPD symptoms, such as impulsivity and violent aggression. Alternatively, nonserotonergic gene polymorphisms in *COMT* also have been highly noted for their association with ASPD symptomatology across the life span.

Environmental factors, especially childhood adversity, could be mediated by epigenetic mechanisms in influencing disease severity. Indeed, evidence has emerged that childhood adversity, especially in the form of sexual abuse, has been linked to hypermethylation of serotonergic genes, which are already implicated in the development of ASPD. Long-term epigenetic changes associated with childhood adversity and their subsequent influence on brain functionality in ASPD patients are of high research priority. Moreover, future research focusing on the effects of aberrant posttranslational modifications in ASPD can similarly yield high-impact results.

Genetics play an important role in ASPD symptoms, and the continuation of further investigations in this field can be extremely beneficial for the understanding of the molecular mechanisms of the disorder. A thorough understanding of genetic, epigenetic, and environmental factors, along with elucidation of their interplay in ASPD, should ultimately lead to the development of better diagnostic modalities, which may contribute to new pharmacological interventions and other novel treatments.

Key Points

- Accumulating evidence suggests that genetic factors contribute to the pathogenesis of antisocial personality disorder (ASPD).

- The monoamine oxidase A gene (*MAOA*), particularly the low-activity genotype, shows the strongest relationship to ASPD and violent and aggressive behaviors.

- Epigenetic regulation of *MAOA* highlights another mechanism of altered monoamine oxidase A functioning that may be related to ASPD.

References

Abu-Akel A, Shamay-Tsoory S: Neuroanatomical and neurochemical bases of theory of mind. Neuropsychologia 49(11):2971–2984, 2011 21803062

American Psychiatric Association: Diagnostic and Statistical Manual of Mental Disorders, 5th Edition. Arlington, VA, American Psychiatric Association, 2013

Arias JMC, Palacio Acosta CA, Valencia JG, et al: Exploring epistasis in candidate genes for antisocial personality disorder. Psychiatr Genet 21(3):115–124, 2011 21519306

Baker LA, Bezdjian S, Raine A: Behavioral genetics: the science of antisocial behavior. Law Contemp Probl 69(1–2):7–46, 2006 18176636

Beach SRH, Brody GH, Gunter TD, et al: Child maltreatment moderates the association of MAOA with symptoms of depression and antisocial personality disorder. J Fam Psychol 24(1):12–20, 2010a 20175604

Beach SRH, Brody GH, Todorov AA, et al: Methylation at SLC6A4 is linked to family history of child abuse: an examination of the Iowa Adoptee sample. Am J Med Genet B Neuropsychiatr Genet 153B(2):710–713, 2010b 19739105

Bilder RM, Volavka J, Czobor P, et al: Neurocognitive correlates of the COMT Val(158)Met polymorphism in chronic schizophrenia. Biol Psychiatry 52(7):701–707, 2002 12372660

Blum K, Sheridan PJ, Wood RC, et al: The D2 dopamine receptor gene as a determinant of reward deficiency syndrome. J R Soc Med 89(7):396–400, 1996 8774539

Brunner HG, Nelen M, Breakefield XO, et al: Abnormal behavior associated with a point mutation in the structural gene for monoamine oxidase A. Science 262(5133):578–580, 1993a 8211186

Brunner HG, Nelen MR, van Zandvoort P, et al: X-linked borderline mental retardation with prominent behavioral disturbance: phenotype, genetic localization, and evidence for disturbed monoamine metabolism. Am J Hum Genet 52(6):1032–1039, 1993b 8503438

Byrd AL, Manuck SB: MAOA, childhood maltreatment, and antisocial behavior: meta-analysis of a gene-environment interaction. Biol Psychiatry 75(1):9–17, 2014 23786983

Caspi A, Sugden K, Moffitt TE, et al: Influence of life stress on depression: moderation by a polymorphism in the 5-HTT gene. Science 301(5631):386–389, 2003 12869766

Chaouloff F: Serotonin, stress and corticoids. J Psychopharmacol 14(2):139–151, 2000 10890308

Checknita D, Maussion G, Labonté B, et al: Monoamine oxidase A gene promoter methylation and transcriptional downregulation in an offender population with antisocial personality disorder. Br J Psychiatry 206(3):216–222, 2015 25497297

Dick DM, Aliev F, Wang JC, et al: Using dimensional models of externalizing psychopathology to aid in gene identification. Arch Gen Psychiatry 65(3):310–318, 2008 25497297

Douglas K, Chan G, Gelernter J, et al: 5-HTTLPR as a potential moderator of the effects of adverse childhood experiences on risk of antisocial personality disorder. Psychiatr Genet 21(5):240–248, 2011 21399568

Ducci F, Enoch MA, Hodgkinson C, et al: Interaction between a functional MAOA locus and childhood sexual abuse predicts alcoholism and antisocial personality disorder in adult women. Mol Psychiatry 13(3):334–347, 2008 17592478

Ducci F, Enoch MA, Yuan Q, et al: HTR3B is associated with alcoholism with antisocial behavior and alpha EEG power—an intermediate phenotype for alcoholism and co-morbid behaviors. Alcohol 43(1):73–84, 2009 19185213

Ellis PL: Empathy: a factor in antisocial behavior. J Abnorm Child Psychol 10(1):123–134, 1982 7108052

Ficks CA, Waldman ID: Candidate genes for aggression and antisocial behaviour: a meta-analysis of association studies of the 5HTTLPR and MAOA-uVNTR. Behav Genet 44(5):427–444, 2014 24902785

Frick PJ, Morris AS: Temperament and developmental pathways to conduct problems. J Clin Child Adolesc Psychol 33(1):54–68, 2004 15028541

Frodl T, Szyf M, Carballedo A, et al: DNA methylation of the serotonin transporter gene (SLC6A4) is associated with brain function involved in processing emotional stimuli. J Psychiatry Neurosci 40(5):296–305, 2015 25825812

Garcia LF, Aluja A, Fibla J, et al: Incremental effect for antisocial personality disorder genetic risk combining 5-HTTLPR and 5-HTTVNTR polymorphisms. Psychiatry Res 177(1–2):161–166, 2010 20363030

Glenn AL, Johnson AK, Raine A: Antisocial personality disorder: a current review. Curr Psychiatry Rep 15(12):427, 2013 24249521

Greene DJ, Black KJ, Schlaggar BL: Considerations for MRI study design and implementation in pediatric and clinical populations. Dev Cogn Neurosci 18:101–112, 2016 26754461

Hadfield MG: Dopamine: mesocortical vs nigrostriatal uptake in isolated fighting mice and controls. Behav Brain Res 7(3):269–281, 1983 6682330

Hallikainen T, Lachman H, Saito T, et al: Lack of association between the functional variant of the catechol-O-methyltransferase (COMT) gene and early onset alcoholism associated with severe antisocial behavior. Am J Med Genet 96(3):348–352, 2000 10898913

Hill SY, Zezza N, Wipprecht G, et al: Linkage studies of D2 and D4 receptor genes and alcoholism. Am J Med Genet 88(6):676–685, 1999 10581489

Hirata Y, Zai CC, Nowrouzi B, et al: Study of the catechol-O-methyltransferase (COMT) gene with high aggression in children. Aggress Behav 39(1):45–51, 2013 22972758

Hoth KF, Paul RH, Williams LM, et al: Associations between the COMT Val/Met polymorphism, early life stress, and personality among healthy adults. Neuropsychiatr Dis Treat 2(2):219–225, 2006 19412467

Iofrida C, Palumbo S, Pellegrini S: Molecular genetics and antisocial behavior: where do we stand? Exp Biol Med (Maywood) 239(11):1514–1523, 2014 24764243

Kim-Cohen J, Caspi A, Taylor A, et al: MAOA, maltreatment, and gene-environment interaction predicting children's mental health: new evidence and a meta-analysis. Mol Psychiatry 11(10):903–913, 2006 16801953

Kobiella A, Reimold M, Ulshöfer DE, et al: How the serotonin transporter 5-HTTLPR polymorphism influences amygdala function: the roles of in vivo serotonin transporter expression and amygdala structure. Transl Psychiatry 1(8):e37, 2011 22832611

Kolla NJ, Bortolato M: The role of monoamine oxidase A in the neurobiology of aggressive, antisocial, and violent behavior: a tale of mice and men. Prog Neurobiol 194:101875, 2020 32574581

Kolla NJ, Vinette SA: Monoamine oxidase A in antisocial personality disorder and borderline personality disorder. Curr Behav Neurosci Rep 4(1):41–48, 2017 29568721

Kolla NJ, Patel R, Meyer JH, et al: Association of monoamine oxidase-A genetic variants and amygdala morphology in violent offenders with antisocial personality disorder and high psychopathic traits. Sci Rep 7(1):9607, 2017 28851912

Kolla NJ, Dunlop K, Meyer JH, et al: Corticostriatal connectivity in antisocial personality disorder by MAO-A genotype and its relationship to aggressive behavior. Int J Neuropsychopharmacol 21(8):725–733, 2018 29746646

Kranzler HR, Hernandez-Avila CA, Gelernter J: Polymorphism of the 5-HT1B receptor gene (HTR1B): strong within-locus linkage disequilibrium without association to antisocial substance dependence. Neuropsychopharmacology 26(1):115–122, 2002 11751038

Lawrence AD, Calder AJ, McGowan SW, et al: Selective disruption of the recognition of facial expressions of anger. Neuroreport 13(6):881–884, 2002 11997706

Lou HC, Luber B, Crupain M, et al: Parietal cortex and representation of the mental self. Proc Natl Acad Sci USA 101(17):6827–6832, 2004 15096584

Martin EI, Ressler KJ, Binder E, et al: The neurobiology of anxiety disorders: brain imaging, genetics, and psychoneuroendocrinology. Psychiatr Clin North Am 32(3):549–575, 2009 19716990

Need AC, Goldstein DB: Whole genome association studies in complex diseases: where do we stand? Dialogues Clin Neurosci 12(1):37–46, 2010 20373665

Nilsson KW, Åslund C, Comasco E, et al: Gene-environment interaction of monoamine oxidase A in relation to antisocial behaviour: current and future directions. J Neural Transm (Vienna) 125(11):1601–1626, 2018 29881923

Raine A: Annotation: the role of prefrontal deficits, low autonomic arousal, and early health factors in the development of antisocial and aggressive behavior in children. J Child Psychol Psychiatry 43(4):417–434, 2002 12030589

Rautiainen MR, Paunio T, Repo-Tiihonen E, et al: Genome-wide association study of antisocial personality disorder. Transl Psychiatry 6(9):e883, 2016 27598967

Sabol SZ, Hu S, Hamer D: A functional polymorphism in the monoamine oxidase A gene promoter. Hum Genet 103(3):273–279, 1998 9799080

Sakai JT, Lessem JM, Haberstick BC, et al: Case-control and within-family tests for association between 5HTTLPR and conduct problems in a longitudinal adolescent sample. Psychiatr Genet 17(4):207–214, 2007 17621163

Scorza P, Duarte CS, Hipwell AE, et al: Research review: intergenerational transmission of disadvantage: epigenetics and parents' childhoods as the first exposure. J Child Psychol Psychiatry 60(2):119–132, 2019 29473646

Seghier ML: The angular gyrus: multiple functions and multiple subdivisions. Neuroscientist 19(1):43–61, 2013 22547530

Tam V, Patel N, Turcotte M, et al: Benefits and limitations of genome-wide association studies. Nat Rev Genet 20(8):467–484, 2019 31068683

Thapar A, Langley K, Fowler T, et al: Catechol O-methyltransferase gene variant and birth weight predict early onset antisocial behavior in children with attention-deficit/hyperactivity disorder. Arch Gen Psychiatry 62(11):1275–1278, 2005 16275815

Tielbeek JJ, Medland SE, Benyamin B, et al: Unraveling the genetic etiology of adult antisocial behavior: a genome-wide association study. PLoS One 7(10):e45086, 2012 23077488

Tielbeek JJ, Johansson A, Polderman TJC, et al: Genome-wide association studies of a broad spectrum of antisocial behavior. JAMA Psychiatry 74(12):1242–1250, 2017 28979981

Verona E, Sprague J, Sadeh N: Inhibitory control and negative emotional processing in psychopathy and antisocial personality disorder. J Abnorm Psychol 121(2):498–510, 2012 22288907

Vevera J, Stopkova R, Bes M, et al: COMT polymorphisms in impulsively violent offenders with antisocial personality disorder. Neuroendocrinol Lett 30(6):753–756, 2009 20038933

Weder N, Yang BZ, Douglas-Palumberi H, et al: MAOA genotype, maltreatment, and aggressive behavior: the changing impact of genotype at varying levels of trauma. Biol Psychiatry 65(5):417–424, 2009 18996506

Winterer G, Goldman D: Genetics of human prefrontal function. Brain Res Brain Res Rev 43(1):134–163, 2003 14499466

CHAPTER 9

Social Theories of Causation

Joel Paris, M.D.
Donald W. Black, M.D.

Antisocial personality disorder (ASPD) is best considered a "multiple-hit" illness like cancer, diabetes, or cardiovascular disease. Although individuals might carry a genetic predisposition, the vulnerability is not "released" unless other factors intervene. Many of these risk factors are of psychological or social origin and are reviewed in this chapter.

Definitional Problems

Numerous studies reporting on the origins of antisocial behavior were published before DSM-III provided an operational definition (American Psychiatric Association 1980). They pertain to earlier concepts of antisocial behavior that may not fully align with recent definitions. Also, some of the more recent studies concern *psychopathy*, a psychological construct that could be either a more severe form of ASPD (Coid and Ullrich 2010) or a related but separate disorder (Ogloff 2006). Often, older studies use the word *sociopathy* instead of ASPD, although the terms are interchangeable. Regarding younger persons, some studies might use the terms *delinquent* or *juvenile delinquent*. Finally, relatively few current investigations have examined the role of psychosocial risk factors in the development of ASPD because the field has focused on neurobiological correlates.

Interactions Between Predispositions and Environmental Stressors

Biologically rooted temperamental variations are necessary conditions for the development of ASPD, but they are not sufficient (Tremblay et al. 2018). Rather, the disorder may develop only when both types of risk are present. There is good evidence for the role of environmental risks, with the strongest data coming from longitudinal studies in which stressors can be accurately measured prior to the development of the full disorder (Jaffee 2017; Moffitt 2005).

As shown in Robins' (1966) classic follow-up study of child guidance clinic patients in the 1950s, having a father who is sociopathic, whether living with the family or not, is the strongest predictor of antisocial behavior in offspring. But if parents have similar behavioral disorders, transmission of traits to children could be largely genetic. We need a method to separate correlations between a stressful environment and the partially heritable traits underlying ASPD. This is difficult to do, even in longitudinal prospective studies that follow up children at risk into adulthood (Tremblay et al. 2018). Thus, research needs to examine these relationships in twin samples, allowing us to control for genetic risk.

Behavior genetic studies use twin samples to determine the influence of heritability, shared environment, and unshared environment. Application of this procedure yields results that are unique to ASPD (Jaffee 2017). Unlike most mental disorders, shared environmental variance plays a major role in ASPD. This suggests that nonheritable psychosocial factors are critical for the development of ASPD. The shared variance can come from families, from neighborhoods, or from both.

To account for a complex developmental pathway, we need to apply a biopsychosocial model to ASPD (Paris 2020; Tremblay et al. 2018). This means building a model that considers interfaces and interactions between inherited predispositions and environmental stressors.

Evidence for Environmental Effects Coming From Families

Evidence suggests that children who develop conduct disorder and as adults are diagnosed with ASPD come from dysfunctional families (Jaffee et al. 2003; Moffitt et al. 2001). But antisocial parents have a greater tendency to have antisocial children, and these children are more likely to elicit negative reactions to their behavior from their families (Rutter 2006). As Moffitt (2005) pointed out in a systematic review, until it cannot be shown that relationships are truly causal, research will be "stuck" at a stage of identifying risk factors rather than truly causal pathways.

Nonetheless, twin studies that examine both heritable and nonheritable factors show that about half the variance affecting antisocial behavior is driven by shared environment. In the Environmental Risk (E-Risk) Longitudinal Twin Study, an epidemiological study of 1,116 twin pairs in the United Kingdom, environmental factors had a large and separate contribution to the variance (Jaffee et al. 2003). These risks were primarily related to abusive parenting and highly dysfunctional families. Moreover, although the presence of an antisocial father greatly increased the risk for antisocial behavior in children, the risk increased when the father stayed and lived with the family. Finally, the mothers of antisocial children were often depressed, further increasing psychosocial risk. Studies of adoption registers (Cadoret et al. 1983; Cloninger et al. 1982) have long established that genetic and environmental risks for antisocial behavior tend to be separate but additive. These findings have stood the test of time and were later confirmed by the E-Risk study (Jaffee et al. 2004).

The mechanisms through which genes and environment interact remain unclear. *Epigenetics* is the study of processes that can turn genes off and on without altering the genome (Allis and Jenuwein 2016). Using these methods might be one strategy, but this new technology has not always produced consistent findings. For example, a study examining epigenetic variation in blood related to childhood victimization found only weak evidence of an association (Marzi et al. 2018). Drawing on findings from the Dunedin study, a longitudinal follow-up of a birth cohort in New Zealand, as well as the E-Risk study, Wertz et al. (2018) reported that polygenetic risk scores (in which the effects of many genes are summed) were associated with lower school performance, which was a major predictor of antisocial behavior.

As shown years ago, antisocial behavior in children has a different outcome depending on age at onset (Moffitt et al. 2001). Those with an early onset of antisocial behavior and callous-unemotional traits (a marker for psychopathy) are most likely to develop ASPD in adulthood. In contrast, those with an adolescent onset of antisocial behavior and an absence of callous-unemotional traits have a much better prognosis and do not typically develop adult ASPD. Button et al. (2005) reported that in twin samples, the first group had symptoms that were more heritable, whereas the second group showed more influence of shared environment.

Family Factors

Parents of antisocial persons are often significantly troubled themselves and show high levels of antisocial behavior, addictions, and other mental illnesses. An early study conducted in the 1940s (Glueck and Glueck 1950) was one of the first to show the connection between antisocial behavior and the family. The Gluecks compared 500 delinquent and 500 nondelinquent boys who were roughly matched for age and socioeconomic standing. Parents of delinquent boys more often had alcoholism or engaged in criminal behavior, and their homes were more frequently broken by divorce, separation, or absence of a parent than were the parents of nondelinquent boys. Parents of delinquent boys were often hostile and more likely to reject their children, were inconsistent and erratic in their discipline, and were more likely to use physical punishment than were the parents of nondelinquent boys.

Systematic family studies later confirmed these observations. Robins (1966) found that approximately one-third of fathers of children seen in a child guidance clinic and later diagnosed as sociopathic and 10% of the mothers either had sociopathy themselves or had alcoholism. In a study of male felons, half of whom were sociopathic, 20% of first-degree relatives were sociopathic (Guze et al. 1967). Dinwiddie and Reich (1993) reported that 29% of 364 first-degree relatives of people with ASPD had alcoholism, 29% had depression, 25% had drug dependence, 15% had ASPD, and 4% had somatization disorder. Black (2013) found that of 81 first-degree relatives of 13 antisocial patients, 17% had ASPD and 26% had alcoholism, rates much higher than what would be expected in the general population; broken down by sex, 24% of the male relatives and 12% of the female relatives were antisocial.

Broken Homes

Individuals with ASPD often come from broken homes that experience high rates of divorce and separation. The effect of either on a child's behavior depends on the initial quality of the parental relationship (Raine 1993). When parents cannot get along, their children may have little opportunity to observe normal affection and communication and instead come to see fights and arguments as appropriate ways to solve disputes. In some instances, children may be better off after a separation or divorce, especially when the split saves them from a violent or an abusive parent (Rutter and Smith 1995). Unhappy intact families may produce more delinquency than relatively happy but broken homes (Lykken 2018). Remarriage is no panacea either, because it depends on the quality of stepparenting, and many children have difficult and conflict-ridden relationships with stepparents (Cassoni and Caldana 2012).

Parental Separation or Absence

An important factor in the development of antisocial behavior is the absence of one or both parents during the child's formative years (Lykken 2018). Although prolonged separation from the mother was implicated by psychologist John Bowlby (1946) in his study of juvenile thieves, later research (Rutter 1982) suggested that the critical link was not the maternal bond, but the child's need to bond with *any* significant adult, regardless of that person's relationship with the child. A grandparent, for example, could fill the role, so long as he or she provided an instructive model for interpersonal relationships. Depriving young children of a significant emotional bond damages their ability to form intimate and trusting relationships later in life or to feel guilt when another person is wronged.

Poor Parenting

Parents of antisocial persons are often described as neglectful, incompetent, or abusive (Farrington 1993; Robins 1966, 1987; Snyder 2015). An important aspect of parenting is the ability to provide consistent and appropriate discipline. In contrast, parents of antisocial children are described as providing erratic or inappropriate discipline (Reti et al. 2002) and showing a tendency to rely on harsh punishment. Because inconsistent discipline rapidly becomes ineffective, parents escalate the intensity of punishment to regain control. They alternate between permissiveness and harshness until discipline becomes irrelevant. If a child is verbally abused or beaten regardless of his or her behavior, the punishment loses its power, and the child sees no advantage to being good. This could be why many people with ASPD are not affected by punishment or social sanctions and are unable to consider consequences unless they are immediate. As children, they never learned the connection between breaking the rules and paying the penalty.

Parents of antisocial persons also provide inadequate supervision (Loeber et al. 1991; Reti et al. 2002), failing to effectively monitor their child's behavior, set rules and ensure that they are obeyed, check on the child's whereabouts, or steer him or her away from troubled playmates. Parents who provide adequate supervision take an interest in activities and schooling that help promote appropriate social behavior, making adequate parental supervision a vital component of a child's social development. Adequate supervision is less likely in broken homes because parents may not be available and antisocial parents may lack the motivation to keep an eye on their children. However, having an antisocial child also can induce negative, neglectful responses in parents (Bell and Chapman 1986). The irony is that parents whose child is difficult to manage are often the least emotionally and financially able to cope constructively with their child's behavior problems.

Teenage Parents

Being born to an unmarried mother or to a mother younger than 18 years increases the risk for developing antisocial behavior (Conseur et al. 1997; Kolvin et al. 1990). This association could merely reflect the characteristics of those who have children at a very young age. Follow-up studies show that girls who become teenage parents often display antisocial behavior and engage in impulsive liaisons. These features are associated with a breakdown of the cohabiting relationship and with poor parenting. The Dunedin Multidisciplinary Health and Development Study (Moffitt et al. 2001) similarly showed that those who had become parents by age 21 were more likely to have a history of delinquency (OR=6.3) and to be a perpetrator of domestic violence (OR=3.2) (Rutter et al. 1998). Teenage parenthood is also associated with a host of other risk factors, including poverty, low levels of education, and inability to provide adequate parenting. Much of the risk for a child's antisocial behavior may result from these associated risk factors and not the mother's age (Rutter et al. 1998).

Large Families

Being reared in a large family—often defined as a family with at least four children—has been linked with delinquency, crime, and violence (Derefinko and Widiger 2018; Ellis 1988; Rutter and Giller 1983). Why large family size increases risk for antisocial behavior is uncertain, but there are several possibilities. It could be that in large families each child receives proportionately less attention and, therefore, less parental supervision. It could be that there is a "contagion" effect from the influence of having a delinquent sibling (Offord 1982). Offord (1982) also found that delinquency risk was associated with the number of brothers in the family and not the number of sisters. Another possibility is that risk derives from the tendency of antisocial individuals to have large families, with the risk genetically mediated in part (Rutter et al. 1998).

Abuse and Neglect

People with ASPD are more likely than others to report histories of childhood maltreatment (Finkelhor et al. 2005; Jaffee 2017; Luntz and Widom 1994; Trickett and McBride-Chang 1995). Maltreatment tends to be associated with physical abuse and serious neglect (Van Zomeren-Dohm et al. 2016). Whether the presence of abuse and neglect causes the antisocial behavior or is merely a marker of overall family chaos is unclear. In some cases, abuse might become a learned behavior that formerly abused adults perpetuate with their own children, contributing to an intergenerational cycle of abuse (Widom 2017). In fact, in one study antisocial individuals were 7 times more likely to abuse their children than were individuals with no antisocial behavior and more than 12 times more likely to neglect them (Egami et al. 1996).

Adoption Status

Adoptees are at increased risk for antisocial behavior (Moffitt 2005; Peters et al. 1999). As Schechter (1989) pointed out, although 1%–2% of the general public are adoptees, the figure among people with ASPD is closer to 15%. Adoptees are also more likely than nonadoptees to have behavior problems in general. There are several possible explanations. The finding could reflect the characteristics of mothers who put their child up for adoption—that is, they are often young, unmarried women who are themselves at risk for antisocial behavior. Or, the finding could result from the failure to develop emotional attachments to adult figures, because the adoptee might move from one caregiver to another before a final adoption.

Peer Relationships

Disturbed peer relationships are an important and often overlooked factor associated with the development of antisocial behavior. Glueck and Glueck (1950) found that 98% of 500 delinquent boys had delinquent friends compared with 7% of 500 nondelinquent peers. The delinquent boys also were more likely to have been gang members (56% vs. 1%). This finding has been confirmed by later research (Mann et al. 2016).

This "birds of a feather" pattern of association often begins during the elementary school years, when peer group acceptance and the need for belonging first become important. Loeber et al. (1991) showed that children with behavior problems prior to reaching school age—and before they have an opportunity to associate with similarly troubled children—are more likely to become delinquent than their better-behaved peers.

Aggressive children are among the most likely to be rejected by their peers, and this rejection drives social outcasts to form bonds with one another (Dodge et al. 1990). Socially rejected children tend to "hang out" together and form relationships that can encourage and reward aggression and other antisocial behaviors. In a study of 200 middle-school children, Juvonen and Ho (2008) found that youths who were attracted to antisocial peers engaged in antisocial behavior themselves to gain acceptance.

Media Influence

Media depictions of violence have long been thought to foster the development of antisocial behavior. Research suggests that exposure to media violence is related to the development of violent behavior (Huesmann and Taylor 2006; Huesman et al. 1997). One recent meta-analysis of prospective studies found a relationship between violent video game play and aggression in preadolescent and adolescent samples (Prescott et al. 2018).

Although such exposure is common, other data suggest that those who act out are otherwise predisposed to doing so (Ferguson et al. 2008). Youths may become desensitized to violence and learn to accept a more hostile view of the world. Those most vulnerable to the media onslaught appear to be those who already live in a "culture of violence" where there are few curbs against aggressive behavior. This relationship has been confirmed by a meta-analysis (Martins and Weaver 2019).

General Societal Factors

Many children who become antisocial endure poverty, substandard housing, bad neighborhoods, parental abuse and neglect, and inadequate nutrition and medical care. In a large-scale longitudinal study of children raised in families marked by socioeconomic deprivation, Farrington (1993) documented how childhood antisocial behavior and a constellation of adversities, including poverty, large families, ineffective child rearing, antisocial parents, parental disharmony, and separation, predicted antisocial behaviors at age 18 years. The most frequent outcomes in adolescence were violence, dishonesty, heavy drinking, drug abuse, reckless driving, sexual promiscuity, and an unstable job record. Farrington and Welsh (2008) extended the follow-up to age 30 and noted the persistence of antisocial behavior.

Another important social factor for the development of antisocial behavior derives from the neighborhood in which children are raised (Jennings and Fox 2016). A related risk factor for antisocial behavior is poverty (Mcleod and Shanahan 1996). One possibility is that people with limited opportunities are more likely to turn to crime. Another possibility is that adolescents who join gangs commit many offenses. However, most children raised in poverty do not embrace these options. One reason can be the protective effects of family support (Schofield et al. 2012). Robins (1966) showed that poor children whose family lives are otherwise normal are unlikely to become antisocial. The association of ASPD with socioeconomic status is further explored in Chapter 3, "Epidemiology of Antisocial Personality Disorder."

Conclusion

Psychosocial factors do not fully determine the emergence of antisocial behavior, and neither do biological factors. The antisocial syndrome has a complex etiology, involving genetic and environmental interactions. Thus, a dysfunctional family, parental maltreatment, and a dangerous neighborhood might increase the risk for antisocial behavior but are not fully predictive of the disorder. Children with antisocial traits might react with aggressive behavior to any or all of these stressors, but children with a different trait profile (e.g., one marked by introversion) might not. As Lykken (1995) once suggested, an antisocial child who retains the same traits in adulthood is a bit like a pit bull—dangerous when stressed or deprived, yet capable of companionship when the environment is stable, predictable, and sympathetic. That said, children with a genetic predisposition who experience serious environmental adversities are primed to develop ASPD. Although neither ingredient is determinative, it is the combination that "cooks" the disorder.

Key Points

- Antisocial personality disorder (ASPD) is the result of interactions between genetic-temperamental vulnerability and environmental risks.

- The conduct disorder that precedes ASPD is related to shared environment, particularly dysfunctional families associated with poor parenting.

- Parents of children who go on to develop ASPD often have histories of antisocial behavior and/or substance use.

- Peer groups that support antisocial behavior play a major role in the development of ASPD.

- Poverty and problematic neighborhoods also increase the risk for developing ASPD.

References

Allis CD, Jenuwein T: The molecular hallmarks of epigenetic control. Nat Rev Genet 17(8):487–500, 2016 27346641

American Psychiatric Association: Diagnostic and Statistical Manual of Mental Disorders, 3rd Edition. Washington, DC, American Psychiatric Association, 1980

Bell RQ, Chapman M: Child effect in studies using experimental or brief longitudinal approaches to socialization. Dev Psychol 22(8):595–603, 1986

Black DW: Bad Boys, Bad Men: Confronting Antisocial Personality Disorder (Sociopathy), Revised and Updated. New York, Oxford University Press, 2013

Bowlby J: Forty-Four Juvenile Thieves: Their Character and Home-Life. Baillere, UK, Tindall & Cox, 1946

Button TMM, Scourfield J, Martin N: Family dysfunction interacts with genes in the causation of antisocial symptoms. Behav Genet 35(8):115–120, 2005 15685425

Cadoret RJ, Cain CA, Crowe RR: Evidence for gene-environment interaction in the development of adolescent antisocial behavior. Behav Genet 13(3):301–310, 1983 6615382

Cassoni C, Caldana RH: Parenting style and practices in stepfamilies. Psychol Res Behav Manag 5:105–111, 2012 22977315

Cloninger CR, Sigvardsson S, Bohman M, et al: Predisposition to petty criminality in Swedish adoptees, II: cross-fostering analysis of gene-environment interaction. Arch Gen Psychiatry 39(11):1242–1247, 1982 7138224

Coid J, Ullrich S: Antisocial personality disorder is on a continuum with psychopathy. Compr Psychiatry 51(4):426–433, 2010 20579518

Conseur A, Rivara FP, Barnoski R, et al: Maternal and perinatal risk factors for later delinquency. Pediatrics 99(6):785–790, 1997 9164769

Derefinko KJ, Widiger TA: Antisocial personality disorder, in The Medical Basis of Psychiatry. Edited by Hosseini SH, Clayton P. New York, Springer, 2018, pp 229–245

Dinwiddie SH, Reich T: Attribution of antisocial symptoms in coexistent antisocial personality disorder and substance abuse. Compr Psychiatry 34(4):235–242, 1993 8348801

Dodge KA, Price JM, Bachorowski JA, et al: Hostile attributional biases in severely aggressive adolescents. J Abnorm Psychol 99(4):385–392, 1990 2266213

Egami Y, Ford DE, Greenfield SF, et al: Psychiatric profile and sociodemographic characteristics of adults who report physically abusing or neglecting children. Am J Psychiatry 153(7):921–928, 1996 8659615

Ellis L: The victimful-victimless crime distinction and seven universal demographic correlates of victimful crime behavior. Pers Individ Dif 9(3):528–548, 1988

Farrington DP: Childhood origins of teenage antisocial behaviour and adult social dysfunction. J R Soc Med 86(1):13–17, 1993 8423566

Farrington DP, Welsh BC: Saving Children From a Life of Crime: Early Risk Factors and Effective Intervention. Oxford, UK, Oxford University Press, 2008

Ferguson CJ, Rueda SM, Cruz AM, et al: Violent video games and aggression: causal relationship or byproduct of family violence and intrinsic violence motivation? Criminal Justice and Behavior 35(3):311–332, 2008

Finkelhor D, Ormrod R, Turner H, et al: The victimization of children and youth: a comprehensive, national survey. Child Maltreat 10(1):5–25, 2005 15611323

Glueck S, Glueck E: Unraveling Juvenile Delinquency. Cambridge, MA, Harvard University Press, 1950

Guze SB, Wolfgram ED, McKinney JK, et al: Psychiatric illness in the families of convicted criminals: a study of 519 first-degree relatives. Dis Nerv Syst 28(10):651–659, 1967 6051292

Huesmann LR, Taylor LD: The role of media violence in violent behavior. Annu Rev Public Health 27:393–415, 2006 16533123

Huesman LR, Moise JF, Podolski CL: The effects of media violence on the development of antisocial behavior, in Handbook of Antisocial Behavior. Edited by Stoff DM, Breiling J, Maser J. New York, Wiley, 1997, pp 181–193

Jaffee SR: Child maltreatment and risk for psychopathology in childhood and adulthood. Annu Rev Clin Psychol 13:525–551, 2017 28375720

Jaffee SR, Moffitt TE, Caspi A, et al: Life with (or without) father: the benefits of living with two biological parents depend on the father's antisocial behavior. Child Dev 74(1):109–126, 2003 12625439

Jaffee SR, Caspi A, Moffitt TE, et al: Physical maltreatment victim to antisocial child: evidence of an environmentally mediated process. J Abnorm Psychol 113(1):44–55, 2004 14992656

Jennings WG, Fox BH: Neighborhood risk and development of antisocial behavior, in The Oxford Handbook of Externalizing Spectrum Disorders. Edited by Beauchaine TP, Hinshaw SP. New York, Oxford University Press, 2016, pp 313–322

Juvonen J, Ho A: Social motives underlying antisocial behavior across middle school grades. J Youth Adolesc 37:747–756, 2008

Kolvin I, Miller FJW, Scott DM, et al: Continuities of Deprivation: The Newcastle Thousand Family Survey. Brookfield, VT, Avebury, 1990

Loeber R, Stouthamer-Loeber M, Green SM: Age at onset of problem behavior in boys and later disruptive and delinquent behaviors. Criminal Behavior and Mental Health 1(3):229–246, 1991

Luntz BK, Widom CS: Antisocial personality disorder in abused and neglected children grown up. Am J Psychiatry 151(5):670–674, 1994 8166307

Lykken D: The Antisocial Personalities. Hillsdale, NJ, Erlbaum, 1995

Lykken D: Psychopathy, sociopathy, and antisocial personality disorder, in Handbook of Psychopathy, 2nd Edition. Edited by Patrick C. New York, Guilford, 2018, pp 22–32

Mann FD, Patterson MW, Grotzinger AD, et al: Sensation seeking, peer deviance, and genetic influences on adolescent delinquency: evidence for person-environment correlation and interaction. J Abnorm Psychol 125(5):679–691, 2016 27124714

Martins N, Weaver A: The role of media exposure on relational aggression: a meta-analysis. Aggression and Violent Behavior 47:90–99, 2019

Marzi SJ, Sugden K, Arseneault L, et al: Analysis of DNA methylation in young people: limited evidence for an association between victimization stress and epigenetic variation in blood. Am J Psychiatry 175(6):517–529, 2018 29325449

Mcleod JD, Shanahan MJ: Trajectories of poverty and children's mental health. J Health Soc Behav 37(3):207–220, 1996 8898493

Moffitt TE: The new look of behavioral genetics in developmental psychopathology: gene-environment interplay in antisocial behaviors. Psychol Bull 131(4):533–554, 2005 16060801

Moffitt TE, Caspi A, Rutter M, et al: Sex effects in risk predictors for antisocial behaviour: are males more vulnerable than females to risk factors for antisocial behaviour?, in Sex Differences in Antisocial Behavior. Edited by Moffitt TE. Cambridge, UK, Cambridge University Press, 2001, pp 90–108

Offord DR: Family backgrounds of male and female delinquents, in Abnormal Offenders: Delinquency and the Criminal Justice System. Edited by Gunn J, Farrington DR. Chichester, UK, Wiley, 1982, pp 129–151

Ogloff JR: Psychopathy/antisocial personality disorder conundrum. Aust N Z J Psychiatry 40(6–7):519–528, 2006 16756576

Paris J: Social Factors in the Personality Disorders: Finding a Niche, 2nd Edition. Cambridge, UK, Cambridge University Press, 2020

Peters BR, Atkins MS, McKay MM: Adopted children's behavior problems: a review of five explanatory models. Clin Psychol Rev 19(3):297–328, 1999 10097873

Prescott AT, Sargent JD, Hull JG: Metaanalysis of the relationship between violent video game play and physical aggression over time. Proc Natl Acad Sci U S A 115(40):9882–9888, 2018 30275306

Raine A: The Psychopathology of Crime. New York, Academic Press, 1993

Reti IM, Samuels JF, Eaton WW, et al: Adult antisocial personality traits are associated with experiences of low parental care and maternal overprotection. Acta Psychiatr Scand 106(2):126–133, 2002 12121210

Robins LN: Deviant Children Grown Up. Baltimore, MD, Williams & Wilkins, 1966

Robins LN: The epidemiology of antisocial personality disorder, in Psychiatry, Vol 3. Edited by Michels RO, Cavenar JO. Philadelphia, PA, Lippincott, 1987, pp 1–14

Rutter M: Maternal Deprivation Reassessed, 2nd Edition. Harmondsworth, UK, Penguin, 1982

Rutter M: Genes and Behavior: Nature-Nurture Interplay Explained. London, Blackwell, 2006

Rutter M, Giller H: Juvenile Delinquency: Trends and Perspectives. Harmondsworth, UK, Penguin, 1983

Rutter M, Smith DJ: Psychosocial Problems in Young People. Cambridge, UK, Cambridge University Press, 1995

Rutter M, Giller H, Hagell A: Antisocial Behavior by Young People. New York, Cambridge University Press, 1998

Schechter MD: Adoption, in Comprehensive Textbook of Psychiatry, 5th Edition. Edited by Kaplan HI, Sadock BJ. Baltimore, MD, Williams & Wilkins, 1989, pp 1958–1962

Schofield TJ, Conger RD, Conger KJ, et al: Neighborhood disorder and children's antisocial behavior: the protective effect of family support among Mexican American and African American families. Am J Community Psychol 50(1–2):101–113, 2012 22089092

Snyder J: Coercive family processes in the development of externalizing behavior: incorporating neurobiology into intervention research, in The Oxford Handbook of Externalizing Spectrum Disorders. Edited by Beauchaine TP, Hinshaw SP. New York, Oxford University Press, 2015, pp 286–302

Tremblay RE, Vitaro F, Cote SM: Developmental origins of chronic physical aggression: a biopsychosocial model for the next generation of preventive interventions. Ann Rev Psychol 69:383–407, 2018 29035692

Trickett A, McBride-Chang C: The developmental impact of different forms of child abuse and neglect. Developmental Review 15(3):311–337, 1995

Van Zomeren-Dohm K, Xu X, Thibodeau E, et al: Child maltreatment and vulnerability to externalizing spectrum disorders, in The Oxford Handbook of Externalizing Spectrum Disorders. Edited by Beauchaine TP, Hinshaw SP. New York, Oxford University Press, 2016, pp 267–285

Wertz J, Agnew-Blais J, Caspi A, et al: From childhood conduct problems to poor functioning at age 18 years: examining explanations in a longitudinal cohort study. J Am Acad Child Adolesc Psychiatry 57(1):54–60.e4, 2018 29301670

Widom CS: Long-term impact of childhood abuse and neglect on crime and violence. Clinical Psychology: Science and Practice 24(2):186–202, 2017

CHAPTER 10

Biological Risk Factors for Antisocial Personality Disorder

Jaeger Lam, M.A.

Anthony C. Ruocco, Ph.D.

Diverse risk factors are implicated in the etiology of antisocial personality disorder (ASPD). Theories on the development of ASPD underscore the relevance of several biological factors and their interactions with environmental conditions and social contexts. In particular, the emergence of ASPD appears to be influenced by a multitude of biological risk factors that arise during different developmental periods, beginning during the prenatal and postnatal periods and continuing into childhood, adolescence, and early adulthood. A range of biological risk factors has been studied in relation to ASPD.[1] In this chapter, we focus on a subset of these potential biological risk factors: prenatal substance exposure, pregnancy and childbirth complications, psychophysiological factors, hormonal influences, and neurological insults.

Most of the research on these risk factors has centered on antisocial behavior (ASB), which can include a range of indicators, such as inadequate behavioral control, criminal acts, and delinquency and behavior problems early in life (Hare 2003). Historically, ASB was included in Robins' (1966) description of sociopathy in juvenile delinquents, which influenced the diagnostic criteria for ASPD provided by Feighner et al. (1972). In DSM-5 (American Psychiatric Association 2013), ASB, including unlawful acts and impulsive behaviors and aggressiveness, remains a core component

---

[1] A detailed review of neuroimaging studies falls outside of the scope of this chapter. Please see Chapter 13, "Structural MRI Studies of Antisocial Personality Disorder," Chapter 14, "Functional MRI Studies of Antisocial Personality Disorder," and Chapter 15, "SPECT and PET Studies of Antisocial Personality Disorder and Aggression."

of the ASPD diagnosis, and we use the term to capture the broader construct of exter-nalizing problem behaviors. As might be expected, ASB has been operationalized in various ways across biological studies, and we provide an integrative summary of these research findings to advance understanding of the potential biological risk fac-tors for ASPD. Similarly, research on biological influences during early development frequently centers on conduct disorder, which is a prerequisite for a diagnosis of ASPD in adulthood in DSM-5. Although conduct disorder is a robust predictor of the progression to ASPD (Loeber et al. 2002), not all youths with this disorder go on to develop ASPD in adulthood. This chapter incorporates biological studies of conduct disorder because of the strong developmental ties of the diagnosis to ASPD and the potential relevance of these findings to biological risk factors for the ASPD diagnosis.

Prenatal Substance Exposure

The question of whether prenatal exposure to alcohol and other recreational sub-stances predisposes the child to ASPD and related problem behaviors has been stud-ied for decades. Maternal smoking during pregnancy is perhaps the most highly studied and intensely debated topic in this area. Several studies have found an asso-ciation of maternal smoking during pregnancy with a range of offspring externalizing behavior problems in childhood. For example, among children diagnosed with ADHD, maternal smoking during pregnancy is linked to hyperactive-impulsive symptoms of ADHD, as well as symptoms of conduct disorder and oppositional de-fiant disorder (Langley et al. 2007). In a systematic literature review, Latimer et al. (2012) synthesized evidence from studies examining the associations of prenatal and early life risk factors with disruptive behavior disorders, including ADHD, conduct disorder, oppositional defiant disorder, and other related symptoms. They concluded that there was evidence for a relationship between maternal smoking during preg-nancy and disruptive behavior disorders in offspring. However, the causal direction of the relationship could not be established based on the type of evidence available. More recently, Sutin et al. (2017) found an association between maternal smoking during pregnancy and childhood externalizing behaviors, including problems with conduct and peer relationships. Meta-analytic research suggests an overall (not dose-dependent) relationship of maternal smoking during pregnancy with offspring con-duct problems, which appears to be magnified in clinical samples of conduct disorder compared with the general population (Ruisch et al. 2018).

Beyond childhood outcomes, maternal smoking during pregnancy also appears to be a risk factor for ASB in adulthood. A study of a subset of adult offspring of women enrolled in the Collaborative Perinatal Project set out to examine adolescent and adult ASB assessed by means of a combination of self-report measures and official records of criminal behaviors (Paradis et al. 2017). Maternal smoking during pregnancy was significantly associated with self-reported aggressive behavior and nonviolent of-fenses during adolescence. Additionally, prenatal smoking was related to ASPD symp-toms, nonaggressive ASB, and violent offenses during adulthood. Paradis et al. (2015) found that a combination of risk factors, including maternal smoking during preg-nancy, lower childhood IQ, and childhood aggressive and impulsive behavior, was associated with ASPD symptoms and an arrest record in adulthood. Similarly, maternal smoking during the third trimester of pregnancy (data from the first and second trimesters were not available to the researchers) showed a dose-response relationship with both adolescent-limited and adulthood criminal behavior in a perinatal birth cohort study of 4,129 males in Denmark (Brennan et al. 1999).

Precisely how maternal smoking during pregnancy might lead to ASB in offspring has been studied less frequently despite the public health significance of the potential causal association. Fergusson (1999) argued that two primary issues need to be resolved to elucidate this relationship: first, neurobiological mechanisms of the association between prenatal smoking and offspring ASB outcomes need to be identified; and second, more research is required to determine whether the links "reflect a genetic process in which the offspring of mothers who smoke during pregnancy are more likely to inherit genotypes that are associated with increased risk of later externalizing behaviors" (p. 224). Potential neurobiological mechanisms include the direct toxic effects of a substance on the developing fetus, hypoxia, effects on the functioning of the placenta, and immunological and inflammatory mechanisms (Rice et al. 2018). One suggested neurobiological pathway from maternal smoking during pregnancy to conduct disorder is through the inhibitory effects of cigarette smoking on brain monoamine oxidase during fetal development, possibly in conjunction with polymorphisms in the MAO-A gene (*MAOA*) that produce lower brain enzyme concentrations (Baler et al. 2008). These factors require further study, but multiple investigations have made progress in disentangling how genetic and familial influences might affect the association of prenatal smoking on ASB in offspring.

A systematic review of studies on maternal smoking during pregnancy and severe ASB in offspring concluded that evidence is consistent for an association that is independent of several confounders, such as sociodemographic and parental psychiatric factors (Wakschlag et al. 2002). However, multiple studies using a variety of sophisticated research designs have yielded more nuanced findings across childhood, adolescent, and adulthood offspring samples. A recent systematic review concluded that nearly all identified studies "based on appropriate genetically informative designs reported no association between maternal smoking during pregnancy and offspring antisocial behavior during childhood, adolescence, and adulthood once familial/genetic confounding had been controlled" (Rice et al. 2018, p. 1122). Using data from the National Longitudinal Survey of Youth 1979, D'Onofrio et al. (2012) determined that even though maternal smoking during pregnancy was associated with a range of adolescent offspring ASB, when genetic and environmental factors that correlated with prenatal smoking across families were controlled between siblings, there was no evidence of a causal relationship. Ellingson et al. (2012) used multivariate genetic models in a population-based sample of full- and half-sister pairs from Sweden and suggested that "the intergenerational transmission of genes conferring risk for ASB and substance misuse, at least partially, influence the associations between maternal [smoking during pregnancy] and adverse offspring outcomes" (p. 1555). Their findings indicate that genetic factors that jointly influence a mother's criminal behavior, substance use problems, and offspring rearing environment also influence prenatal smoking. Maughan et al. (2004) studied 1,116 twin pairs at ages 5–7 years and found that maternal smoking during pregnancy was strongly associated with conduct problems in a dose-response pattern. Approximately half of this association was attributable to correlated genetic effects. Importantly, mothers who smoked during pregnancy differed from other mothers in that they reported more depressive episodes since the time of their twins' birth, endorsed more antisocial behaviors, described the father of their offspring as more antisocial, and reported greater family socioeconomic disadvantage. When the researchers controlled for these variables and genetic risk, the observed effects of maternal smoking were substantially attenuated. These results suggest that the observed relationship between maternal smoking during pregnancy and childhood conduct problems is confounded by several other risk factors and that an independent causal association cannot be inferred.

Research has also linked prenatal alcohol exposure to externalizing problem behaviors in children (Sood et al. 2001), conduct disorder in adolescents (Disney et al. 2008), and ASPD in adults (Langbehn and Cadoret 2001). Fetal alcohol spectrum disorder is also associated with an increased risk of ASPD (and other psychiatric disorders, especially substance use disorders) in adults (Chudley et al. 2007). Beyond alcohol use, a range of other substances has been studied in relation to ASB; however, a detailed review of the research literature on the consequences of these other substances is beyond the scope of this chapter. Nevertheless, given the findings pertaining to cigarette smoking, it is important to consider that there may also be genetic factors that influence the intergenerational transmission of maternal substance use more broadly (i.e., across different substances) and that other familial factors (e.g., parental psychopathology, rearing environment) also should be considered in relation to offspring ASB and related problem behaviors.

In summary, maternal smoking during pregnancy is a risk factor for a range of ASB and related outcomes in childhood, adolescence, and adulthood. The evidence for an independent, direct causal influence of prenatal exposure to smoking on ASB, however, is obscured by multiple genetic and familial effects. Rather, studies employing genetically informative research designs suggest that correlated genetic factors may at least partially explain the association between maternal smoking during pregnancy and ASB in offspring. Whether similar genetic and environmental factors influence the association between prenatal substance exposure, use of other substances (e.g., alcohol), and ASB in offspring has yet to be determined and has important implications for public health policy and the prevention of ASPD in adulthood.

Pregnancy and Childbirth Complications

Pregnancy and childbirth complications refer to a range of conditions that can occur prenatally (e.g., gestational hypertension, diabetes), perinatally (e.g., breech birth, forceps or cesarean delivery, fetal distress), and postnatally (e.g., cyanosis [blue or purple discoloration of the skin due to low oxygen saturation]) (Liu et al. 2009). These complications may affect neurobiology, consequently disrupting neurodevelopment in ways that can increase the likelihood of developing ASB and personality disorders more generally. For example, a nested case-control and population-based control study found that the risk of developing any personality disorder is increased in children born preterm or with a low birth weight (Fazel et al. 2012).

Few studies have focused on pregnancy and childbirth complications and the risk for ASPD in adulthood. In an early study of 46 Danish men who had committed a serious criminal offense by age 36, Kandel (1989) compared perinatal and childbirth complications between men who had a diagnosis of ASPD and those who did not. Only 12 of the men had ASPD, and two-thirds of them were classified as having had high perinatal complications, a rate that was not significantly different from the rate in a non-ASPD group and a third group of men without a serious criminal history. Similarly, there were no differences between the groups in birth complications. In a separate prospective study of participants studied prenatally until 7 years old and then recontacted between 18 and 27 years old, the likelihood of receiving an ASPD diagnosis was not elevated in individuals with a history of pregnancy or childbirth complications compared with persons with a normal pregnancy and delivery (Buka et al. 1993). The results of these initial studies suggest that such complications do not increase the likelihood of an ASPD diagnosis in adulthood, although more research is needed to determine whether such findings are replicable in other larger and more diverse samples.

Rather than directly leading to ASPD in adulthood, complications during pregnancy and childbirth might instead increase the likelihood of ASB in childhood. Liu et al. (2009) investigated the association between birth complications and childhood externalizing behavior problems in a longitudinal birth cohort study of 3-year-old children in Mauritius, an island nation in the Indian Ocean. Children with birth complications were more likely to have externalizing behavior problems at age 11 years. This relationship was mediated by IQ, suggesting that birth complications might affect cognitive ability (potentially because of disrupted brain function) and promote the development of ASB later in childhood. A range of maternal medical risks during pregnancy also appears to predispose children to externalizing behavior problems in childhood. As part of the Early Childhood Longitudinal Study, Birth Cohort, Jackson and Vaughn (2018) investigated a nationally representative sample of American children born in 2001. While the mothers of both males and females experienced a similar frequency of medical risks during their pregnancy, greater medical risk was associated with higher childhood externalizing behavior problems across settings during kindergarten—however, the relationship was evident only among male offspring. Several individual medical risks were independently associated with externalizing behavior, including hypertension/preeclampsia, prenatal diabetes, previous preterm delivery, incompetent cervix, uterine bleeding, and prenatal obesity.

Other research indicates that low birth weight is not significantly associated with conduct disorder symptoms in children ages 6 to 16 years who have a diagnosis of ADHD (Langley et al. 2007). In an individual-participant-data meta-analysis, adults with a history of preterm birth and with a very low birth weight (≤1,500 g) reported less externalizing, rule breaking, and antisocial personality problems than did a control group of adults who had been born at term (Pyhälä et al. 2017).

To investigate potential interactions between biological and social factors, van Hazebroek et al. (2019) performed a systematic review of studies examining a combination of perinatal and prenatal complications and social risk factors as they relate to ASB. They found some evidence that pregnancy and delivery complications were more strongly associated with aggressive and violent delinquent behavior for individuals with higher familial adversity. For example, Beck and Shaw (2005) reported the results of a 10-year longitudinal study of boys from low-income homes followed up from birth and assessed for perinatal complications, social risk factors, and externalizing behavior problems. They determined that boys with a combination of risk factors—high perinatal complications, high rejecting parenting, and high familial adversity—had greater externalizing behavior than boys with high scores on two of the risk factors. Notably, perinatal complications and rejecting parenting were not associated with internalizing problems.

In summary, complications during pregnancy and childbirth increase the risk for ASB in early to middle childhood, possibly because of the effects of such events on brain development and cognition. Importantly, these complications interact with social factors, especially rejecting parenting and familial adversity, to increase the likelihood of developing ASB in childhood. Preterm birth and a very low birth weight may be associated with a lower risk for externalizing behavior problems in adulthood. Limited extant research on ASPD itself does not provide evidence for an association with pregnancy and childbirth complications.

Psychophysiological Factors

Theories on the psychophysiology of ASB can be conceptualized as involving an interaction between psychosocial variables and physiological processes. The physiological mechanisms that are most researched and implicated in relation to adolescent and adult ASB and ASPD are the skin conductance response (SCR) and resting heart rate (RHR) (Gao et al. 2015; Pour Ashouri et al. 2017). Although these biological factors are associated with ASB, they most likely contribute to personality and behavioral dispositions that interact with the environment to increase the risk of ASB (Pour Ashouri et al. 2017). We review theories that have been put forward to explain the relation between psychophysiological factors and ASB, with implications for understanding the role of psychophysiology in ASPD.

Social Push Perspective

The Social Push Perspective suggests that biological risk factors exert a greater effect on the expression of ASB in individuals who are not exposed to social risk factors (e.g., low socioeconomic status [SES]) (Mednick and Christiansen 1977; Raine and Venables 1981). This perspective lends itself to an antithetical hypothesis that children who live in environments that are high in antisocial risk factors, such as an adverse early home environment or in the presence of criminal parental figures, are more affected by environmental influences than biological influences. If this hypothesis is true, then the association between psychophysiological factors that predispose individuals to developing ASB should be weaker in high- than in low-risk environments.

Evidence supporting this perspective comes from studies on physiological arousal. RHR appears to be lower in adolescent males who exhibit ASB, and this association is strongest in individuals who come from a high SES class and/or a family in which the parents were separated (Raine and Venables 1984b; Wadsworth 1976). Similarly, Farrington (1997) found that low RHR was more predictive of youths becoming violent offenders if they were exposed to high-risk childhood conditions (e.g., low SES or separation from their parents). However, some studies have found evidence against the Social Push Perspective. Raine et al. (1997) found that the strength of RHR in 3-year-old children in predicting aggression in 11-year-old children was not moderated by environmental risk factors. Similarly, Scarpa et al. (1997) did not find any moderating effects of the environment on biological risk factors for ASB.

In terms of SCR, ASPD-prone adolescents (e.g., individuals who scored high on measures of antisocial or delinquent acts) display a lowered SCR to conditioned stimuli, which has been observed as a distinct marker of antisocial psychopathology (Fung et al. 2005; Raine et al. 2000). In a longitudinal study by Gao et al. (2015), lower SCR during childhood was directly associated with proactive or premeditated aggression at age 18 years. A prediction of the Social Push Perspective is that individuals who have higher arousal during resting states may be at a lower risk for ASB, even if they are exposed to an impoverished environment (Brennan and Raine 1997; Raine et al. 1995). Accordingly, some evidence suggests that higher electrodermal SCR at rest in 15-year-old boys who exhibit ASB reduces their risk for ASB in adulthood (Brennan and Raine 1997; Raine et al. 1995). One study, however, found that RHR was predictive of severe ASB, even after environmental factors, such as parental influences, were controlled (Armstrong et al. 2009).

The association between SCR and ASB appears to be stronger in individuals from high SES classes (Buikhuisen et al. 1984; Raine and Venables 1981) and criminals without adverse childhood experiences (Hemming 1981), which provides evidence of a potential interaction between psychophysiology and environment. Some studies, however, have found that the relationship between reduced SCR and ASB is not mediated by differences in environmental variables (Raine et al. 1990). Overall, the findings suggest that autonomic arousal is a valid and reproducible predictor of ASB; however, the moderating influence of environmental factors is unclear. Some studies have found that this relationship is influenced by environmental variables, such as SES (Buikhuisen et al. 1984; Hemming 1981; Raine et al. 1990), whereas others have failed to detect a moderating effect of the environment on autonomic arousal and ASB (Raine et al. 1990; Scarpa et al. 1997). Future research into the moderating effects of the environment on psychophysiological mechanisms of ASB is necessary to determine both risk and protective qualities of resting arousal states.

Fearlessness Theory

Fearlessness theory suggests that low levels of arousal indirectly correspond to low levels of fear (Raine and Scerbo 1991). This theory posits that recorded autonomic activity in individuals at risk for ASB while they are at "rest" (e.g., in the absence of any applied stressors) reflects reduced anticipatory fear to mild-to-moderate stressors. It should be remembered that while the studies mentioned in the previous subsection recorded heart rate in a "resting" state, this measurement period frequently preceded a series of other procedures or experiments (e.g., medical examination, exposure to aversive tone stimuli). As such, low heart rate may be viewed as reflecting a lack of an anticipatory fear to mild-to-moderate stressors. According to this model, individuals at risk for ASB experience these routine procedures as stressful (Raine 1993). When mild-to-moderate stressors are subsequently applied in a given study, their autonomic activity appears similar to that recorded during the resting state. Under this theory, measurements of low arousal are suggestive of a lack of an anticipatory fear toward mild-to-moderate stressors. In other words, low arousal during "rest" is indicative of reduced fear and anxiety, which predisposes these individuals to ASB. The rationale of this theory is that low levels of fear or anxiety are a prerequisite to the initiation of ASB. More specifically, low levels of fear and anxiety may allow individuals to perform ASB. As further support of this contention, measures of fearlessness have been shown to predict ASB (Raine et al. 1998).

This theory is grounded in traditional conceptualizations positing that individuals who engage in ASB have a reduced fear concept (Mednick and Christiansen 1977; Trasler 1978). These conceptualizations have been substantiated in a meta-analysis finding lower recognition of fear in faces in antisocial populations (i.e., ASPD, psychopathy, conduct disorder, and disorders marked by ASB) (Marsh and Blair 2008), "fear blindness" in children with psychopathic traits (Dadds et al. 2008), and reduced fear startle response in ASPD (Anton et al. 2012). This theory also helps explain poor socialization in ASPD, in which low fear would reduce the effectiveness of social conditioning. This theory posits that autonomic underarousal is a characteristic of an uninhibited or fearless temperament in infancy and childhood (Fowles 2000; Jerome 1994; Scarpa et al. 1997), which may be predictive of ASB in adulthood (Barker et al. 2011; Waller et al. 2013). Recent research in adults has found that callous-unemotional traits of psychopathy, but not impulsive-irresponsible or grandiose-manipulative traits, are associated with lower activation in fear-processing areas of the brain during fear conditioning (Cohn et al. 2013). In addition, individuals with high levels of psychopathic traits show a specific impairment in the recognition of fearful facial expressions (Blair et al. 2004) and fear-inducing behaviors (Marsh and Cardinale 2012). Furthermore, lower SCR is positively correlated with fearlessness, but not impulsive traits, on measures of psychopathy (Dindo and Fowles 2011). Additionally, the fearlessness aspect of psychopathic personality is significantly correlated with proactive and reactive aggression scores (Cima and Raine 2009). Proactive aggression can be conceptualized as instrumental, meaning that the behavior is intended to achieve a goal, with little autonomic arousal (Dodge 1991; Meloy 1988; Mirsky and Siegel 1994). In contrast, reactive aggression is typically impulsive, immediate, and directed (Berkowitz 1993).

Taken together, a large body of research substantiates the fearlessness theory of ASB. Several fear-related constructs—for example, startle response and facial recognition of fear—are affected in individuals who engage in ASB and those who have a diagnosis of ASPD. However, the most convincing evidence supporting the theory comes from research on psychophysiology, showing a direct association of lower SCR and fearlessness (but not impulsivity) with psychopathic traits and aggression (Cima and Raine 2009; Dindo and Fowles 2011).

Sensation-Seeking Theory

Another theory that explains lower arousal in individuals who have ASPD has been termed the *sensation-seeking theory* (Raine 1993; Raine et al. 1997). Sensation seeking is a personality trait defined by the search for novel and intense sensations (Zuckerman 2009; Zuckerman and Kuhlman 2000). Individuals who score high on trait sensation seeking may be more prone to ASB. For example, high sensation seeking and impulsivity have been associated with substance use (Hamdan-Mansour et al. 2018). The rationale of the theory is that the low arousal observed in antisocial populations is an unpleasant physiological state that motivates an individual to seek stimulation to increase his or her arousal to a comfortable level. In this lens, ASB is carried out in the service of increasing arousal.

This theory is supported by multiple investigations. Behavioral measures of stimulation seeking taken at age 3 years predict aggressive behavior at 11 years (Raine et al. 1998). In adolescents, higher scores on trait sensation seeking have been associated with higher levels of childhood conduct problems and other ASB (Maneiro et al. 2017; Mann et al. 2017). It also has been shown that the association between RHR and rule breaking is mediated by sensation seeking in male adolescents (Sijtsema et al. 2010) and that low levels of delinquency and high levels of sensation seeking are associated with low SCR (Gatzke-Kopp et al. 2002). Interestingly, sensation seeking contributes less to adolescent conduct problems when compared with other impulsive components (Vitacco and Rogers 2001). In adults, sensation seeking accounts for a large portion of genetic variance in ASB over and above other personality traits (Mann et al. 2017) and modestly contributes to the expression of externalizing disorders more generally (Khan et al. 2005). Also, adult men with ASPD score higher on sensation seeking and other components of impulsivity when compared with control subjects without ASPD (Hesselbrock and Hesselbrock 1992). In men with ASPD, levels of sensation seeking are also positively correlated with psychopathy (Basoglu et al. 2011). Physiologically, the relation between RHR and ASB appears to be mediated by sensation seeking (Hammerton et al. 2018).

The sensation-seeking theory has been posited to work in tandem with the fearlessness theory—that is, individuals with low levels of arousal may have a predisposition to commit crime because of their fearlessness but may also commit a crime because of sensation seeking (Raine 2002). Indeed, measures of both sensation seeking and fearlessness at age 3 years predict aggression 8 years later (Raine et al. 1998). Sensation seeking may act as the motivator for individuals with low arousal to seek stimulation, with their predisposition to fearlessness guiding them toward ASB. In combination, these two theories explain the relation between ASB, fearlessness, and sensation seeking that may underlie underarousal observed in antisocial populations. In the previous section, we reviewed studies on the relationships among ASB, autonomic arousal, and sensation-seeking behavior (Gatzke-Kopp et al. 2002; Maneiro et al. 2017; Mann et al. 2017), as well as fearlessness (Cima and Raine 2009; Waller et al. 2013). However, to our knowledge, research has yet to directly and jointly examine fearlessness and sensation seeking as moderators of each other in the context of ASB, although some studies found a negative association between sensation seeking, fearlessness, and anxiety (Franken et al. 1992; Lissek et al. 2005). While intuitive, the merit of combining the fearlessness and sensation seeking theory is not as substantiated by research as either theory in isolation. Accordingly, it will be important to conduct research on how sensation seeking and fearlessness might moderate the relation between autonomic arousal and ASB.

Hormonal Influences

Several hormones are thought to influence specific psychological and behavioral symptom components of ASPD. Of particular relevance to this discussion are the ASPD symptoms related to aggression and behavioral dyscontrol, such as irritability, physical altercations or assaults, impulsivity, and unlawful acts. There are multiple potential biological influences of these symptoms and behaviors, including genetics and direct neurological insults to brain regions involved in emotional and behavioral control. However, two hormones have frequently been studied in reference to ASPD and related symptoms: testosterone and cortisol.

According to Bancroft (2012), the sex hormone testosterone has been inconsistently related to aggression in males, and the effects may be exerted indirectly through multiple interrelated psychological constructs, such as irritability, frustration tolerance, interpersonal dominance, and impulsivity. However, a meta-analysis of 45 independent studies found a weak relationship ($r=0.14$) between testosterone levels and aggression (Book et al. 2001). Rather than conceptualizing testosterone as broadly related to aggressive behaviors, the "challenge hypothesis" (Archer 2006) also considers the physiological and behavioral costs of maintaining high levels of testosterone. This hypothesis predicts that it is more adaptive to maintain low levels of testosterone in adulthood until an increase is necessary to facilitate competition relevant to reproduction. In his influential paper, Archer (2006) concluded that research largely supports the notion that testosterone is associated with "aggression-based dominance" and "that challenges and status matters [sic] more to high testosterone people, and influences [sic] their behavior" (p. 340). A recent meta-analysis (Geniole et al. 2017) found support for the challenge hypothesis, determining that the winners of competitive interactions have higher increases in testosterone than losers and that this effect is magnified in studies of males that are conducted outside of the laboratory. Thus, the relation between testosterone levels and aggression is a complex one that requires consideration of the social and competitive context.

Given that aggression is associated with ASPD, several studies have investigated the relation between testosterone and related personality traits and behaviors. A review of studies examining the relation between testosterone and persistent ASB across the life span determined that there is a small-to-moderate association during childhood (ages 3–12 years) and a small association during adolescence (ages 12–20 years) (Yildirim and Derksen 2012a). Adults ages 20–40 years with ASPD had higher testosterone levels compared with control subjects who did not have ASPD, and greater severity of ASB was associated with higher testosterone levels in these adults, even after aggression-related items were removed from relevant measures (Yildirim and Derksen 2012a). Overall, there appeared to be a consistent finding of higher testosterone levels in groups with more severe or violent ASB (see Yildirim and Derksen 2012a for a review). Yildirim and Derksen (2012b) concluded that there is only limited evidence for an association of testosterone with the interpersonal-affective components of psychopathy and perhaps a more consistent relationship with the antisocial lifestyle factor. Finally, a meta-analysis of seven studies detected no difference between sex offenders and non–sex offenders in basal testosterone levels measured through blood or saliva (Wong and Gravel 2018).

Cortisol is a hormone that has been studied as a biomarker of the body's stress response. States of chronic stress can lead to adaptation wherein the body becomes glucocorticoid receptor resistant and insensitive to cortisol, which can have important physiological and psychological consequences (Marino and Teague 2019). One study of boys ages 10–12 years and their parents found that lower cortisol levels were related to higher conduct disorder symptoms among boys and ASPD symptoms among fathers (Vanyukov et al. 1993). Similar findings were obtained in a study of adolescent and young adult male offenders with ASPD and a history of violence in which lower cortisol levels were associated with higher psychopathy scores, notably Psychopathy Checklist—Revised (Hare 2003) factor 1 (affective-interpersonal) scores but not factor 2 (antisocial lifestyle) scores (Holi et al. 2006). Contrary findings have also been reported; for example, Welker et al. (2014) found a positive correlation between cortisol level and psychopathy in males. Importantly, this research group also determined that cortisol moderated the relation between testosterone and psychopathy: the correlation was positive when cortisol levels were high, whereas an inverse relation was observed when cortisol levels were low. Indeed, the relation between cortisol and ASB has frequently been investigated in combination with testosterone, forming what is known as the "dual-hormone hypothesis," which predicts that testosterone is associated with ASB (particularly behaviors in the service of dominance) when cortisol levels are low (Mehta and Josephs 2010). A recent meta-analysis, however, provided only minimal support for the dual-hormone hypothesis in relation to a broad set of outcome measures relevant to ASB, which also included status- and dominance-relevant behaviors (Dekkers et al. 2019). The effect size for the interaction between cortisol and testosterone was small ($r=0.06$) and statistically significant; however, none of the specific outcome measures (e.g., aggression or psychopathy) showed a significant result.

In summary, testosterone may share a specific relationship with aggressive behaviors that occurs in the context of competitive interactions. The hormone appears to show a generally positive relationship with ASB across childhood, adolescence, and adulthood. Studies investigating the association between cortisol and ASB are mixed; however, relations between testosterone and cortisol are essential to consider because the hormones may interact in nuanced ways to influence ASB over development. Nevertheless, research support is only marginal for the dual-hormone hypothesis, suggesting that more research is needed to understand the complex interplay between these hormones and how they might lead to the behaviors and traits associated with ASPD.

Neurological Insults

For the purpose of this chapter, *neurological insult* refers to a form of brain injury attributable to head trauma, birth complication, or disease, which typically produces a neuropsychological (i.e., cognitive) or neurological deficit. These deficits, especially in executive functioning, are considered risk factors for ASB (Moffitt 1990; Morgan and Lilienfeld 2000; Raine 1993). For example, Lewis et al. (1989) found that among 15-year-old juvenile delinquents, having a neuropsychological deficit was associated with perpetrating 2.1 adult violent offenses, whereas child abuse alone was associated with perpetrating 1.9 adult offenses. Both neuropsychological deficit and child abuse had a synergistic effect as they relate to violent offenses, with individuals with both committing an average of 5.4 violent offenses in adulthood. Similar results have been observed in other studies. Moffitt (1990) found that boys with low neuropsychological performance and high family adversity scored higher on measures of aggression than those with either risk factor alone. Similarly, Raine (1996) reported that early neuromotor deficits and an unstable family environment were associated with increased rates of teenage behavior problems and adult criminal and violent offending compared with either risk factor alone. Several theories have been proposed to explain how neuropsychological deficits resulting from various neurological insults and neurodevelopmental processes may place individuals at risk for ASB, including how such deficits may interact with environmental factors to increase risk.

Social and Executive Functioning Model of Aggression

Raine et al. (2005) proposed a neuropsychological model of ASB that explains the interaction of social factors and executive function demands in adolescence. This theory proposes that individuals with a late-developing prefrontal cortex (PFC) are at an increased risk for ASB. A late-developing PFC would result in lower executive functioning capacity, which affects, among other cognitive functions, inhibitory control. Given that the PFC continues to develop in late adolescence, a time when individuals shift from a highly structured environment in early adolescence to an executive-demanding one, individuals with slow-developing PFC are thought to be more susceptible to everyday dysfunction. During late adolescence, individuals are introduced to more novel challenges related to academic performance, peer and relationship complexities, and future career planning. Executive resources in these individuals with a slow-developing PFC are susceptible to becoming overwhelmed, increasing risk for the expression of antisocial and violent behavior, which typically peak during late adolescence (Raine et al. 2005). The PFC is theoretically most burdened during late adolescence, as life challenges require complex executive functions, such as sustained attention, self-regulation, and abstract thinking.

In individuals with a compromised or later-developing PFC, early damage to PFC areas makes them more susceptible to stress or executive overload, which theoretically may increase the risk for ASB. This theory helps to explain why ASB tends to decrease in adulthood, when the PFC further matures. Individuals with PFC dysfunction may not exhibit ASB in the presence of certain protective factors, such as higher social support or reduced life demands. As well, PFC dysfunction does not necessarily result in ASB isolated to adolescence. For example, individuals with PFC dysfunction may not experience overwhelming cognitive demands until later in adulthood, when life stressors may overload the PFC and produce functional impairments.

Raine's neuropsychological theory conceptualizes ASB as being heavily influenced by PFC dysfunction. This lends itself to several hypotheses (Raine et al. 2005): 1) individuals with PFC dysfunction and lower executive functioning are more likely to exhibit ASB in less-structured or impoverished social environments; 2) individuals with significant executive function deficits who do not exhibit ASB are rooted in well-structured and protective environments or are able to compensate for their executive function deficits through other cognitive processes; and 3) individuals exhibiting adolescent-limited ASB show poorer executive functioning earlier in life but better executive functioning in adulthood.

Several lines of research have supported key components of this theory. Individuals with ASPD, or those who engage in violent behavior, typically have neuropsychological deficits (Henry and Moffitt 1997; Ishikawa and Raine 2002; Morgan and Lilienfeld 2000). Impaired verbal functioning is more prominent than spatial impairments in antisocial populations (Quay 1987; Raine et al. 2005; Wilson and Herrnstein 1998). In addition, neuropsychological impairments are more common in life-course-persistent offenders and childhood-limited offenders compared with adolescence-limited offenders (Donnellan et al. 2000; Fergusson and Woodward 2000; Fergusson et al. 2000), although one study did not report this finding (Aguilar et al. 2000). Life-course-persistent offenders also tend to have both neuropsychological impairments and a history of abuse and neglect (Raine et al. 2005). Interestingly, Raine et al. (2005) found that childhood-limited offenders were significantly more impaired on neuro-psychological tests compared with life-course-persistent offenders, suggesting that neuropsychological deficits may be more influential in the former group. Notably, life-course-persistent offenders had significantly more head injuries compared with childhood-limited offenders, and this finding was interpreted to suggest that the absence or reduction of head injury may relate to why childhood-limited offenders are less likely to become life-course-persistent offenders.

Attention-Deficit Hypothesis

Raine and Venables (1984a) proposed that antisocial individuals are characterized by a fundamental deficit in allocating attentional resources to appropriate environmental events. This theory has been interpreted through a lens of PFC dysfunction, with reduced SCR and heart rate interpreted as by-products of a dysfunctional PFC (Raine et al. 1997). This theory argues that damage to the PFC leads to psychophysiological disturbances, such as lower SCR and heart rate. Indeed, neuroscience research implicates the frontal lobes in arousal regulation and responsivity to stress (Damasio et al. 1990; Williams et al. 2009). Accordingly, individuals with frontal lobe dysfunction would be more likely to have traits that predispose to ASB, such as sensation seeking and impulsivity.

As such, this theory suggests that ASB is associated with a psychophysiological disturbance that is initially caused by PFC dysfunction, rather than from a specific and independent psychophysiological disturbance. Consequently, and as mentioned previously, reduced autonomic arousal is associated with increased sensation seeking (Gatzke-Kopp et al. 2002; Maneiro et al. 2017; Mann et al. 2017), fearlessness (Gao et al. 2015), and disinhibition (Fowles 2000; Kavish et al. 2017). Patients with damage to the PFC have attenuated SCR (Zahn et al. 1999), reduced anticipatory SCR (Bechara et al. 1996), and greater self-regulatory deficits (Eslinger et al. 2004), all of which overlap with the characteristics of individuals who exhibit ASB (Raine et al. 1998). A meta-analysis by Yang and Raine (2009) investigated functional and structural brain imaging studies in individuals who exhibit ASB (e.g., ASPD, psychopathy, violent offending, conduct disorder, oppositional defiant disorder, criminal offending) and found smaller frontal lobe volumes and lower activation in the dorsolateral PFC, orbitofrontal cortex, and anterior cingulate cortex during rest and during various cognitive tasks. Lower structural integrity in white matter tracts within the frontal lobes also has been observed in adults with ASPD (Sundram et al. 2012). Furthermore, adults with ASPD and psychopathic traits score higher on measures sensitive to orbitofrontal cortex dysfunction (Dinn and Harris 2000) and show deficits on tests of executive functioning (Dolan and Park 2002). Research on individuals with damage to the frontal lobes suggests that these structures relate to autonomic regulation (Bechara et al. 1996; Zahn et al. 1999) and impulsive traits (Eslinger et al. 2004). Overall, these studies associate frontal lobe damage or dysfunction with autonomic dysregulation, attention deficits, and disorders related to ASB. In the future, it will be imperative to test this theory by examining the extent to which damage to the PFC directly or indirectly leads to psychophysiological disturbances, impulsive traits, and ASB.

Frontal Lobe Dysfunction Theory

Studies dating back as far as the 1800s have documented the onset of traits resembling antisocial personality following injury to the frontal lobes (Stuss and Benson 1984). Onset of these traits typically follows damage to the orbitofrontal cortex or ventromedial PFC and has been associated with deficits in executive functioning, including disinhibition, explosive aggression, and inappropriate social etiquette (Blair and Cipolotti 2000; Duffy et al. 2001; Meyers et al. 1992). So-called acquired sociopathy is unique in that minimal impairments are observed in other cognitive domains outside of executive functioning (Eslinger and Damasio 1985).

Systematic studies on cohorts of war veterans have illuminated the personality-relevant sequelae of frontal lobe injury. An association between orbitofrontal lesions and ASB has been observed in studies of war veterans (Brower and Price 2001), with brain damage confined to the frontal lobes associated with commission of crimes and misdemeanors. In contrast, in a retrospective Finnish study of veterans of World War II, fewer than 5% of individuals with frontal lobe injury possessed a history of criminal convictions, and only one individual had committed a violent offense (Virkkunen et al. 1976). A study of Vietnam War veterans found that frontal lobe injuries tended to be associated with the expression of more aggressive and violent behaviors when compared with control veterans who had sustained other head injuries or those without a head injury (Grafman et al. 1996). Although the findings are somewhat mixed, frontal lobe injuries tend to be associated with the emergence of antisocial-like traits (Brower and Price 2001).

An unresolved question concerns the matter of whether frontal lobe dysfunction in antisocial populations is due to head injury, disrupted prenatal development, or other causes, such as neurological illness. A retrospective study by Blake et al. (1995) reported the results of neurological findings in 31 participants in connection with mitigation claims related to murder charges. Overall, 64.5% of the sample had evidence of frontal lobe dysfunction, such as frontal release signs (e.g., snout, suck, and grasp reflexes; reduced word fluency). Three or more signs were observed in 32.3% of the sample, two signs in 9.7%, and one sign in 22.6%. Another retrospective study investigated the predictors of violent episodes in neuropsychiatric hospital units (Heinrichs 1989). They found that a frontal lobe lesion was the best predictor of violent episodes. One study of frontal lobe function in violent psychiatric inpatients with mood and/or psychotic disorders found no significant differences between violent and nonviolent patients on a comprehensive neurological examination using a quantified neurological scale (Krakowski and Czobor 1997). They did, however, detect more indicators of frontal lobe dysfunction in persistently violent patients compared with transiently violent patients. In another study on an inpatient sample, frontal executive dysfunction was associated with a history of community violence but not inpatient assaults (Krakowski and Czobor 1997). Because these studies were retrospective in nature, it is unclear whether ASB occurred after the onset of the frontal lobe injury.

Personality changes are commonly observed following traumatic brain injuries (TBIs) and do not appear to be related to the severity of the injury (Malia et al. 1995; Prigatano 1992). Commonly reported personality changes include irritability, restlessness, unpredictability, moodiness, and impulsivity (Brooks and McKinlay 1983; Kaitaro et al. 1995). When personality changes due to TBI do occur, they are typically characterized as a "frontal lobe syndrome," which is expressed as irritability, suspiciousness, impulsivity, emotional lability, stubbornness, poor judgment, lack of insight, generalized apathy, and distractibility (Stuss and Benson 1984). Hibbard et al. (2000) investigated pre- and postmorbid personality disorders in 100 participants with TBI. The authors found that the presence of a personality disorder increased from 24% to 66%, with the presence of ASPD increasing from 15% to 21%. When a subsample of this group with a premorbid personality disorder was investigated, the most common personality disorder was ASPD, with a cumulative rate of 63% pre- to post-TBI. This study provides evidence to suggest that brain injury may relate to the emergence of ASPD, with ASPD being the most common personality disorder in individuals with a premorbid personality disorder.

Case Example

Mr. D, a 51-year-old Asian married man, sustained a penetrating head injury following an altercation on a public transit bus. During the incident, he became involved in a verbal argument with a young man whose knapsack accidentally knocked a cup of coffee out of Mr. D's hand. The young man, feeling threatened by Mr. D, produced a gun and pointed it at Mr. D, who then charged at him. The young man shot once at Mr. D, and the bullet penetrated the front of his head. Mr. D survived the injury, and a computed tomography scan revealed severe damage mainly to the right frontal lobe. Several months later, after physically recovering from his injury, he returned to his job as a carpenter, only to be fired after a few weeks of work. According to his wife, Mr. D's personality changed drastically after the injury. He was referred for a psychological assessment to evaluate his personality changes since his head injury.

During the clinical interview, Mr. D appeared fidgety and agitated. He described a normal birth and early development. He said that he had a typical childhood and had no behavioral or academic problems. He always worked well with his hands, excelling at woodworking and other practical classes in high school. He attended a trades school and studied general carpentry. He had been employed with a home renovation company for 30 years before his injury. Mr. D's wife accompanied him to the appointment to provide corroborating information. She described his interpersonal style before the injury as kind and gentle but sometimes impatient and quarrelsome if someone annoyed him. He was a diligent worker and very responsible with his money. They communicated well in their marriage and enjoyed spending time together in nature. She acknowledged that Mr. D sometimes drank alcohol on weekends and occasionally "did something stupid" when he drank too much. She said that after the injury he became increasingly "moody," often became enraged at even minor nuisances, and frequently did "risky" things, such as drinking too much, gambling, and speeding. He spent more time alone, lying to her about where he has been, and saying offensive things to her without any apparent concern for having hurt her feelings.

When he was asked about his personality, Mr. D said that he noticed "a bit of a change" since the injury. He used profanities when describing the altercation that resulted in his injury and described a persistent feeling of anger toward the young man who shot him. He sometimes broke things in his garage—occasionally, his expensive carpentry equipment—when dwelling on his angry feelings toward the young man for "ruining" his life. He stated that he used to be polite, friendly, punctual, and hard-working before he was shot. After the injury, he admitted that he was fired from his job for putting his apprentice in danger while they were remodeling a home. He declined to elaborate on the circumstances that led to his firing but blamed the incident on his manager. He also described his apprentice as "stupid" and that it was his own fault for not knowing enough about the job. His wife added that he was not showing up to work on time and had missed several days of work, but she learned about this only when Mr. D's manager called the home to find out why he was absent from work.

Mr. D expressed a desire to return to work but had doubts about whether he had the patience, persistence, and drive to work full-time again. His irritability made it difficult for him to work with other people, and he had a hard time focusing and staying motivated for long periods of time at work. He also had concerns about losing control of his drinking and gambling, including worries about whether he had the financial backing to sustain these "habits." His wife, who expressed empathy for her husband's struggles, said that she only wishes that she could have her "old" husband back.

In summary, damage to the frontal lobe is posited to increase risk for ASB, likely because such damage disrupts emotional equilibrium and impairs the ability to control behavior and emotional expression (Miller 1994). As a consequence of frontal lobe damage, individuals may also be unable to appreciate or express remorse for their actions. It is important to note, however, that not all individuals with frontal lobe damage have ASB, because the expression of antisocial traits depends on the severity, timing, and location of the injury, as well as premorbid disorders or conditions (Hart and Jacobs 1993). Whether frontal lobe damage leads to ASPD and related traits and behaviors requires further examination within a prospective cohort study to disentangle contributing factors and allow clearer factors to emerge.

Conclusion

In this chapter, we identified multiple biological factors that may be implicated in the development of ASPD. Many of these biological variables appear to influence the risk for ASB and related symptoms and traits across development. These biological risk factors emerge early in life during the prenatal and postnatal periods. Whereas pregnancy and childbirth complications may disrupt brain development and lead to ASB in childhood, the risk for ASB conferred by maternal smoking during pregnancy may be influenced by genetic factors that jointly influence offspring ASB and familial factors. Indicators of lower physiological arousal have frequently been associated with specific traits and behaviors related to ASPD (e.g., fearlessness, sensation seeking), although their associations may depend on certain environmental variables (e.g., SES, adverse childhood experiences). The potential effects of testosterone and cortisol on ASPD are complex, in part because of the possible interactions between the two hormones in their association with ASB over development and also because of the contextually dependent nature of the relation between testosterone and aggression. Finally, neurological insults resulting from delayed neurodevelopment, head injury, or disease have been associated with ASB. Frontal lobe dysfunction in particular is considered indicative of risk for ASB and is thought to produce deficits in cognitive functions underlying behavioral control and disruptions in physiological systems regulating arousal. Although we discuss these biological risk factors separately, it is crucial to recognize their interactions as they potentially influence the development and maintenance of ASPD (and ASB more generally), in conjunction with genetic pre-dispositions, early life experiences, familial factors, and social-environmental contexts.

As a clearer picture of the biological risk factors for ASPD emerges, it will be important for future research to determine how these factors might also underlie the pathological personality dimensions core to ASPD, moving beyond the broad behavioral indicators that have formed the basis for most studies on the topic. Ultimately, a more complete understanding of the distal biological risk factors for ASPD can be used to inform preventive strategies, potentially by fostering protective social factors that can effectively curb the development of the disorder earlier in life.

Key Points

- There is a positive association of maternal smoking during pregnancy with disruptive behavior in offspring and antisocial behavior (ASB) in adolescence and adulthood. Approximately half of the association between maternal smoking and ASB is attributable to genetic effects.

- Complications during pregnancy may affect brain development and cognition, which can interact with other social factors, such as parenting style and familial adversity, to increase the risk for ASB. However, some evidence suggests that preterm birth and low birth weight may be associated with a decreased risk of externalizing behavior problems in adulthood.

- Fear-related processes are affected in individuals who engage in ASB or have a diagnosis of antisocial personality disorder. For example, they show differences in startle responses and biases in facial recognition of fear. Evidence also suggests that individuals who engage in ASB may seek stimulation in the form of ASB because of low baseline arousal levels. These two findings may work in tandem, with a lower fear response predisposing an individual to commit ASB, while higher sensation seeking can serve to motivate ASB.

- Testosterone is associated with higher aggressive behavior in the context of competitive interactions across the life span. The relation between cortisol and ASB, however, is mixed. Testosterone and cortisol interact to influence ASB in nuanced ways across development.

- Damage to the frontal lobes and the resulting cognitive deficits are associated with an increased risk for ASB. Higher risk of ASB due to frontal lobe injury appears to be related to disturbances in the regulatory functions of the frontal lobes and their interactions with other neural systems.

References

Aguilar B, Sroufe LA, Egeland B, et al: Distinguishing the early onset/persistent and adolescence-onset antisocial behavior types: from birth to 16 years. Dev Psychopathol 12(2):109–132, 2000 10847620

American Psychiatric Association: Diagnostic and Statistical Manual of Mental Disorders, 5th Edition. Arlington, VA, American Psychiatric Association, 2013

Anton ME, Baskin-Sommers AR, Vitale JE, et al: Differential effects of psychopathy and antisocial personality disorder symptoms on cognitive and fear processing in female offenders. Cogn Affect Behav Neurosci 12(4):761–776, 2012 22886692

Archer J: Testosterone and human aggression: an evaluation of the challenge hypothesis. Neurosci Biobehav Rev 30(3):319–345, 2006 16483890

Armstrong TA, Keller S, Franklin TW, et al: Low resting heart rate and antisocial behavior: a brief review of evidence and preliminary results from a new test. Criminal Justice Behavior 36(11):1125–1140, 2009

Baler RD, Volkow ND, Fowler JS, et al: Is fetal brain monoamine oxidase inhibition the missing link between maternal smoking and conduct disorders? J Psychiatry Neurosci 33(3):187–195, 2008 18592036

Bancroft J: The behavioral correlates of testosterone, in Testosterone: Action, Deficiency, Substitution, 4th Edition. Edited by Nieschlag E, Behre HM. New York, Cambridge University Press, 2012, pp 87–122

Barker ED, Oliver BR, Viding E, et al: The impact of prenatal maternal risk, fearless temperament and early parenting on adolescent callous-unemotional traits: a 14-year longitudinal investigation. J Child Psychol Psychiatry 52(8):878–888, 2011 21410472

Basoglu C, Oner O, Ates A, et al: Temperament traits and psychopathy in a group of patients with antisocial personality disorder. Compr Psychiatry 52(6):607–612, 2011 21397221

Bechara A, Tranel D, Damasio H, et al: Failure to respond autonomically to anticipated future outcomes following damage to prefrontal cortex. Cereb Cortex 6(2):215–225, 1996 8670652

Beck JE, Shaw DS: The influence of perinatal complications and environmental adversity on boys' antisocial behavior. J Child Psychol Psychiatry 46(1):35–46, 2005 15660642

Berkowitz L: Aggression: Its Causes, Consequences, and Control. New York, McGraw-Hill, 1993

Blair RJ, Cipolotti L: Impaired social response reversal: a case of 'acquired sociopathy.' Brain 123(pt 6):1122–1141, 2000 10825352

Blair R, Mitchell D, Peschardt K, et al: Reduced sensitivity to others' fearful expressions in psychopathic individuals. Pers Individ Dif 37(6):1111–1122, 2004

Blake PY, Pincus JH, Buckner C: Neurologic abnormalities in murderers. Neurology 45(9):1641–1647, 1995 7675220

Book AS, Starzyk KB, Quinsey VL: The relationship between testosterone and aggression: a meta-analysis. Aggression and Violent Behavior 6(6):579–599, 2001

Brennan PA, Raine A: Biosocial bases of antisocial behavior: psychophysiological, neurological, and cognitive factors. Clin Psychol Rev 17(6):589–604, 1997 9336686

Brennan PA, Grekin ER, Mednick SA: Maternal smoking during pregnancy and adult male criminal outcomes. Arch Gen Psychiatry 56(3):215–219, 1999 10078497

Brooks DN, McKinlay W: Personality and behavioural change after severe blunt head injury— a relative's view. J Neurol Neurosurg Psychiatry 46(4):336–344, 1983 6842246

Brower MC, Price BH: Neuropsychiatry of frontal lobe dysfunction in violent and criminal behaviour: a critical review. J Neurol Neurosurg Psychiatry 71(6):720–726, 2001 11723190

Buikhuisen W, Bontekoe EH, vd Plas-Korenhoff C, et al: Characteristics of criminals: the privileged offender. Int J Law Psychiatry 7(3–4):301–313, 1984 6537416

Buka SL, Tsuang MT, Lipsitt LP: Pregnancy/delivery complications and psychiatric diagnosis: a prospective study. Arch Gen Psychiatry 50(2):151–156, 1993 8427556

Chudley AE, Kilgour AR, Cranston M, et al: Challenges of diagnosis in fetal alcohol syndrome and fetal alcohol spectrum disorder in the adult. Am J Med Genet C Semin Med Genet 145C(3):261–272, 2007 17640043

Cima M, Raine A: Distinct characteristics of psychopathy relate to different subtypes of aggression. Pers Individ Dif 47(8):835 -840, 2009

Cohn MD, Popma A, van den Brink W, et al: Fear conditioning, persistence of disruptive behavior and psychopathic traits: an fMRI study. Transl Psychiatry 3:e319, 2013 24169638

Dadds MR, El Masry Y, Wimalaweera S, et al: Reduced eye gaze explains "fear blindness" in childhood psychopathic traits. J Am Acad Child Adolesc Psychiatry 47(4):455–463, 2008 18388767

Damasio AR, Tranel D, Damasio H: Individuals with sociopathic behavior caused by frontal damage fail to respond autonomically to social stimuli. Behav Brain Res 41(2):81–94, 1990 2288668

Dekkers TJ, van Rentergem JAA, Meijer B, et al: A meta-analytical evaluation of the dual-hormone hypothesis: does cortisol moderate the relationship between testosterone and status, dominance, risk taking, aggression, and psychopathy? Neurosci Biobehav Rev 96:250–271, 2019 30529754

Dindo L, Fowles D: Dual temperamental risk factors for psychopathic personality: evidence from self-report and skin conductance. J Pers Soc Psychol 100(3):557–566, 2011 21186933

Dinn WM, Harris CL: Neurocognitive function in antisocial personality disorder. Psychiatry Res 97(2–3):173–190, 2000 11166089

Disney ER, Iacono W, McGue M, et al: Strengthening the case: prenatal alcohol exposure is associated with increased risk for conduct disorder. Pediatrics 122(6):e1225–e1230, 2008 19047223

Dodge KA: The structure and function of reactive and proactive aggression, in The Development and Treatment of Childhood Aggression. Edited by Kenneth RH, Debra PJ. Hillsdale, NJ, Erlbaum, 1991, pp 201–218

Dolan M, Park I: The neuropsychology of antisocial personality disorder. Psychol Med 32(3):417–427, 2002 11989987

Donnellan MB, Ge X, Wenk E: Cognitive abilities in adolescent-limited and life-course-persistent criminal offenders. J Abnorm Psychol 109(3):396–402, 2000 11016109

D'Onofrio BM, Van Hulle CA, Goodnight JA, et al: Is maternal smoking during pregnancy a causal environmental risk factor for adolescent antisocial behavior? Testing etiological theories and assumptions. Psychol Med 42(7):1535–1545, 2012 22085725

Duffy JD, Campbell JJ 3rd, Salloway SP, Malloy PF: Regional prefrontal syndromes: a theoretical and clinical overview, in The Frontal Lobes and Neuropsychiatric Illness. Edited by Salloway SP, Malloy PF. Washington, DC, American Psychiatric Publishing, 2001, pp 113–123

Ellingson JM, Rickert ME, Lichtenstein P, et al: Disentangling the relationships between maternal smoking during pregnancy and co-occurring risk factors. Psychol Med 42(7):1547–1557, 2012 22115276

Eslinger PJ, Damasio ARJN: Severe disturbance of higher cognition after bilateral frontal lobe ablation: patient EVR. Neurology 35(12):1731–1741, 1985 4069365

Eslinger PJ, Flaherty-Craig CV, Benton AL: Developmental outcomes after early prefrontal cortex damage. Brain Cogn 55(1):84–103, 2004 15134845

Farrington DP: A critical analysis of research on the development of antisocial behavior from birth to adulthood, in Handbook of Antisocial Behavior. Edited by Stoff DM, Breiling J, Maser JD. New York, Wiley, 1997, pp 234–240

Fazel S, Bakiyeva L, Cnattingius S, et al: Perinatal risk factors in offenders with severe personality disorder: a population-based investigation. J Pers Disord 26(5):737–750, 2012 23013342

Feighner JP, Robins E, Guze SB, et al: Diagnostic criteria for use in psychiatric research. Arch Gen Psychiatry 26(1):57–63, 1972 5009428

Fergusson DM: Prenatal smoking and antisocial behavior. Arch Gen Psychiatry 56(3):223–224, 1999 10078498

Fergusson DM, Woodward LJ: Educational, psychosocial, and sexual outcomes of girls with conduct problems in early adolescence. J Child Psychol Psychiatry 41(6):779–792, 2000 11039690

Fergusson DM, Horwood LJ, Nagin DS: Offending trajectories in a New Zealand birth cohort. Criminology 38:525–552, 2000

Fowles DC: Electrodermal hyporeactivity and antisocial behavior: does anxiety mediate the relationship? J Affect Disord 61(3):177–189, 2000 11163420

Franken RE, Gibson KJ, Rowland GL: Sensation seeking and the tendency to view the world as threatening. Pers Individ Dif 13(1):31–38, 1992

Fung MT, Raine A, Loeber R, et al: Reduced electrodermal activity in psychopathy-prone adolescents. J Abnorm Psychol 114(2):187–196, 2005 15869350

Gao Y, Tuvblad C, Schell A, et al: Skin conductance fear conditioning impairments and aggression: a longitudinal study. Psychophysiology 52(2):288–295, 2015 25174802

Gatzke-Kopp LM, Raine A, Loeber R, et al: Serious delinquent behavior, sensation seeking, and electrodermal arousal. J Abnorm Child Psychol 30(5):477–486, 2002 12403151

Geniole SN, Bird BM, Ruddick EL, Carré JM: Effects of competition outcome on testosterone concentrations in humans: an updated meta-analysis. Horm Behav 92:37–50, 2017 27720891

Grafman J, Schwab K, Warden D, et al: Frontal lobe injuries, violence, and aggression: a report of the Vietnam Head Injury Study. Neurology 46(5):1231–1238, 1996 8628458

Hamdan-Mansour AM, Mahmoud KF, Al Shibi AN, et al: Impulsivity and sensation-seeking personality traits as predictors of substance use among university students. J Psychosoc Nurs Ment Health Serv 56(1):57–63, 2018 28892553

Hammerton G, Heron J, Mahedy L, et al: Low resting heart rate, sensation seeking and the course of antisocial behaviour across adolescence and young adulthood. Psychol Med 48(13):2194–2201, 2018 29310737

Hare RD: Manual for the Revised Psychopathy Checklist, 2nd Edition. Toronto, ON, Canada, Multi-Health Systems, 2003

Hart T, Jacobs HE: Rehabilitation and management of behavioral disturbances following frontal lobe injury. J Head Trauma Rehabil 8(1):1–12: 1993

Heinrichs RW: Frontal cerebral lesions and violent incidents in chronic neuropsychiatric patients. Biol Psychiatry 25(2):174–178, 1989 2930801

Hemming J: Electrodermal indices in a selected prison sample and students. Pers Individ Dif 2(1):37–46, 1981

Henry B, Moffitt TE: Neuropsychological and neuroimaging studies of juvenile delinquency and adult criminal behavior, in Handbook of Antisocial Behavior. Edited by Stoff DM, Breiling J, Maser JD. New York, Wiley, 1997, pp 280–288

Hesselbrock MN, Hesselbrock VM: Relationship of family history, antisocial personality disorder and personality traits in young men at risk for alcoholism. J Stud Alcohol 53(6):619–625, 1992 1434635

Hibbard MR, Bogdany J, Uysal S, et al: Axis II psychopathology in individuals with traumatic brain injury. Brain Inj 14(1):45–61, 2000 10670661

Holi M, Auvinen-Lintunen L, Lindberg N, et al: Inverse correlation between severity of psychopathic traits and serum cortisol levels in young adult violent male offenders. Psychopathology 39(2):102–104, 2006 16424682

Ishikawa SS, Raine A: Psychophysiological correlates of antisocial behavior: a central control hypothesis, in The Neurobiology of Criminal Behavior. Edited by Glicksohn J. Norwell, MA, Kluwer Academic Publishers, 2002, pp 187–229

Jackson DB, Vaughn MG: Maternal medical risks during pregnancy and childhood externalizing behavior. Soc Sci Med 207:19–24, 2018 29727746

Jerome K: Galen's Prophecy: Temperament in Human Nature. New York, Basic Books, 1994

Kaitaro T, Koskinen S, Kaipio M-LJBI: Neuropsychological problems in everyday life: a 5-year follow-up study of young severely closed-head-injured patients. Brain Inj 9(7):713–727, 1995 8680398

Kandel E: Genetic and perinatal factors in antisocial personality in a birth cohort. Journal of Crime and Justice 12(2):61–77, 1989

Kavish N, Vaughn MG, Cho E, et al: Physiological arousal and juvenile psychopathy: is low resting heart rate associated with affective dimensions? Psychiatr Q 88(1):103–114, 2017 27160003

Khan AA, Jacobson KC, Gardner CO, et al: Personality and comorbidity of common psychiatric disorders. Br J Psychiatry 186:190–196, 2005 15738498

Krakowski M, Czobor P: Violence in psychiatric patients: the role of psychosis, frontal lobe impairment, and ward turmoil. Compr Psychiatry 38(4):230–236, 1997 9202880

Langbehn DR, Cadoret RJ: The adult antisocial syndrome with and without antecedent conduct disorder: comparisons from an adoption study. Compr Psychiatry 42(4):272–282, 2001 11458301

Langley K, Holmans PA, van den Bree MBM, et al: Effects of low birth weight, maternal smoking in pregnancy and social class on the phenotypic manifestation of attention deficit hyperactivity disorder and associated antisocial behaviour: investigation in a clinical sample. BMC Psychiatry 7:26, 2007 17584500

Latimer K, Wilson P, Kemp J, et al: Disruptive behaviour disorders: a systematic review of environmental antenatal and early years risk factors. Child Care Health Dev 38(5):611–628, 2012 22372737

Lewis DO, Mallouh C, Webb V: Child abuse, delinquency, and violent criminality, in Child Maltreatment: Theory and Research on the Causes and Consequences of Child Abuse and Neglect. New York, Cambridge University Press, 1989, pp 707–721

Lissek S, Baas JM, Pine DS, et al: Sensation seeking and the aversive motivational system. Emotion 5(4):396–407, 2005 16366744

Liu J, Raine A, Wuerker A, et al: The association of birth complications and externalizing behavior in early adolescents: direct and mediating effects. J Res Adolesc 19(1):93–111, 2009 22485069

Loeber R, Burke JD, Lahey BB: What are adolescent antecedents to antisocial personality disorder? Crim Behav Ment Health 12(1):24–36, 2002 12357255

Malia K, Powell G, Torode S: Personality and psychosocial function after brain injury. Brain Inj 9(7):697–712, 1995 8680397

Maneiro L, Gómez-Fraguela JA, Cutrín O, et al: Impulsivity traits as correlates of antisocial behaviour in adolescents. Pers Individ Dif 104:417–422, 2017

Mann FD, Engelhardt L, Briley DA, et al: Sensation seeking and impulsive traits as personality endophenotypes for antisocial behavior: evidence from two independent samples. Pers Individ Dif 105:30–39, 2017 28824215

Marino JH, Teague TK: The immune system as a sensor and regulator of stress: implications in human development and disease, in Biobehavioral Markers in Risk and Resilience Research. Edited by Harrist AW, Gardner BC. Cham, Switzerland, Springer International Publishing, 2019, pp 1–11

Marsh AA, Blair RJR: Deficits in facial affect recognition among antisocial populations: a meta-analysis. Neurosci Biobehav Rev 32(3):454–465, 2008 17915324

Marsh AA, Cardinale EM: Psychopathy and fear: specific impairments in judging behaviors that frighten others. Emotion 12(5):892–898, 2012 22309726

Maughan B, Taylor A, Caspi A, et al: Prenatal smoking and early childhood conduct problems: testing genetic and environmental explanations of the association. Arch Gen Psychiatry 61(8):836–843, 2004 15289282

Mednick SA, Christiansen KO: Biosocial Bases of Criminal Behavior. New York, Gardner Press, 1977

Mehta PH, Josephs RA: Testosterone and cortisol jointly regulate dominance: evidence for a dual-hormone hypothesis. Horm Behav 58(5):898–906, 2010 20816841

Meloy JR: The Psychopathic Mind: Origins, Dynamics, and Treatment. Lanham, MD, Rowman & Littlefield, 1988

Meyers CA, Berman SA, Scheibel RS, et al: Case report: acquired antisocial personality disorder associated with unilateral left orbital frontal lobe damage. J Psychiatry Neurosci 17(3):121–125, 1992 1390621

Miller L: Traumatic brain injury and aggression. J Offender Rehabil 21(3–4):91–104, 1994

Mirsky AF, Siegel A: The neurobiology of violence and aggression, in Understanding and Preventing Violence, Vol 2. Edited by Reiss AJ, Miczek KA, Roth JA. Washington, DC, National Academies Press, 1994, pp 59–172

Moffitt TE: Juvenile delinquency and attention deficit disorder: boys' developmental trajectories from age 3 to age 15. Child Dev 61(3):893–910, 1990 2364762

Morgan AB, Lilienfeld SO: A meta-analytic review of the relation between antisocial behavior and neuropsychological measures of executive function. Clin Psychol Rev 20(1):113–136, 2000 10660831

Paradis AD, Fitzmaurice GM, Koenen KC, et al: A prospective investigation of neurodevelopmental risk factors for adult antisocial behavior combining official arrest records and self-reports. J Psychiatr Res 68:363–370, 2015 26050211

Paradis AD, Shenassa ED, Papandonatos GD, et al: Maternal smoking during pregnancy and offspring antisocial behaviour: findings from a longitudinal investigation of discordant siblings. J Epidemiol Community Health 71(9):889–896, 2017 28696927

Pour Ashouri F, Hamadiyan H, Parvizpanah A, et al: Associations between resting heart rate and antisocial behavior. International Electronic Journal of Medicine 6(1):33–36, 2017

Prigatano GP: Personality disturbances associated with traumatic brain injury. J Consult Clin Psychol 60(3):360–368, 1992 1619090

Pyhälä R, Wolford E, Kautiainen H, et al: Self-reported mental health problems among adults born preterm: a meta-analysis. Pediatrics 139(4):e20162690, 2017 28283612

Quay HC: Patterns of delinquent behavior, in Handbook of Juvenile Delinquency. Edited by Quay HC. New York, Wiley, 1987, pp 118–138

Raine A: The Psychopathology of Crime: Criminal Behavior as a Clinical Disorder. New York, Academic Press, 1993

Raine A: Autonomic nervous system factors underlying disinhibited, antisocial, and violent behavior: biosocial perspectives and treatment implications. Ann NY Acad Sci 794:46–59, 1996 8853591

Raine A: Biosocial studies of antisocial and violent behavior in children and adults: a review. J Abnorm Child Psychol 30(4):311–326, 2002 12108763

Raine A, Scerbo A: Biological theories of violence, in Neuropsychology of Aggression. Edited by Milner JS. Boston, MA, Kluwer Academic Publishers, 1991, pp 1–25

Raine A, Venables PH: Classical conditioning and socialization—a biosocial interaction. Pers Individ Dif 2:273–283, 1981

Raine A, Venables PHJP: Electrodermal nonresponding, antisocial behavior, and schizoid tendencies in adolescents. Psychophysiology 21(4):424–433, 1984a 6463175

Raine A, Venables PH: Tonic heart rate level, social class and antisocial behaviour in adolescents. Biol Psychol 18(2):123–132, 1984b 6733191

Raine A, Venables PH, Williams M: Relationships between central and autonomic measures of arousal at age 15 years and criminality at age 24 years. Arch Gen Psychiatry 47(11):1003–1007, 1990 2241502

Raine A, Venables PH, Williams M: High autonomic arousal and electrodermal orienting at age 15 years as protective factors against criminal behavior at age 29 years. Am J Psychiatry 152(11):1595–1600, 1995 7485621

Raine A, Venables PH, Mednick SA: Low resting heart rate at age 3 years predisposes to aggression at age 11 years: evidence from the Mauritius Child Health Project. J Am Acad Child Adolesc Psychiatry 36(10):1457–1464, 1997 9334560

Raine A, Reynolds C, Venables PH, et al: Fearlessness, stimulation-seeking, and large body size at age 3 years as early predispositions to childhood aggression at age 11 years. Arch Gen Psychiatry 55(8):745–751, 1998 9707386

Raine A, Lencz T, Bihrle S, et al: Reduced prefrontal gray matter volume and reduced autonomic activity in antisocial personality disorder. Arch Gen Psychiatry 57(2):119–127, discussion 128–129, 2000 10665614

Raine A, Moffitt TE, Caspi A, et al: Neurocognitive impairments in boys on the life-course persistent antisocial path. J Abnorm Psychol 114(1):38–49, 2005 15709810

Rice F, Langley K, Woodford C, et al: Identifying the contribution of prenatal risk factors to offspring development and psychopathology: what designs to use and a critique of literature on maternal smoking and stress in pregnancy. Dev Psychopathol 30(3):1107–1128, 2018 30068414

Robins LN: Deviant Children Grown Up. Baltimore, MD, Williams & Wilkins, 1966

Ruisch IH, Dietrich A, Glennon JC, et al: Maternal substance use during pregnancy and offspring conduct problems: a meta-analysis. Neurosci Biobehav Rev 84:325–336, 2018 28847489

Scarpa A, Raine A, Venables PH, et al: Heart rate and skin conductance in behaviorally inhibited Mauritian children. J Abnorm Psychol 106(2):182–190, 1997 9131838

Sijtsema JJ, Veenstra R, Lindenberg S, et al: Mediation of sensation seeking and behavioral inhibition on the relationship between heart rate and antisocial behavior: the TRAILS study. J Am Acad Child Adolesc Psychiatry 49(5):493–502, 2010 20431469

Sood B, Delaney-Black V, Covington C, et al: Prenatal alcohol exposure and childhood behavior at age 6 to 7 years, I: dose-response effect. Pediatrics 108(2):E34, 2001 11483844

Stuss DT, Benson DF: Neuropsychological studies of the frontal lobes. Psychol Bull 95(1):3–28, 1984 6544432

Sundram F, Deeley Q, Sarkar S, et al: White matter microstructural abnormalities in the frontal lobe of adults with antisocial personality disorder. Cortex 48(2):216–229, 2012 21777912

Sutin AR, Flynn HA, Terracciano A: Maternal cigarette smoking during pregnancy and the trajectory of externalizing and internalizing symptoms across childhood: similarities and differences across parent, teacher, and self reports. J Psychiatr Res 91:145–148, 2017 28359941

Trasler G: Relations between psychopathy and persistent criminality: methodological and theoretical issues, in Psychopathic Behaviour: Approaches to Research. Edited by Hare RD. Chichester, NY, Wiley, 1978, pp 273–298

van Hazebroek BCM, Wermink H, van Domburgh L, et al: Biosocial studies of antisocial behavior: a systematic review of interactions between peri/prenatal complications, psychophysiological parameters, and social risk factors. Aggression and Violent Behavior 47:169–188, 2019

Vanyukov MM, Moss HB, Plail JA, et al: Antisocial symptoms in preadolescent boys and in their parents: associations with cortisol. Psychiatry Res 46(1):9–17, 1993 8464960

Virkkunen M, Nuutila A, Huusko S: Effect of brain injury on social adaptability: longitudinal study on frequency of criminality. Acta Psychiatr Scand 53(3):168–172, 1976 1274641

Vitacco MJ, Rogers R: Predictors of adolescent psychopathy: the role of impulsivity, hyperactivity, and sensation seeking. J Am Acad Psychiatry Law 29(4):374–382, 2001 11785608

Wadsworth ME: Delinquency, pulse rates and early emotional deprivation. Br J Criminol 16:245, 1976

Wakschlag LS, Pickett KE, Cook E Jr, et al: Maternal smoking during pregnancy and severe antisocial behavior in offspring: a review. Am J Public Health 92(6):966–974, 2002 12036791

Waller R, Gardner F, Hyde LW: What are the associations between parenting, callous-unemotional traits, and antisocial behavior in youth? A systematic review of evidence. Clin Psychol Rev 33(4):593–608, 2013 23583974

Welker KM, Lozoya E, Campbell JA, et al: Testosterone, cortisol, and psychopathic traits in men and women. Physiol Behav 129:230–236, 2014 24631306

Williams PG, Suchy Y, Rau HK: Individual differences in executive functioning: implications for stress regulation. Ann Behav Med 37(2):126–140, 2009 19381748

Wilson JQ, Herrnstein RJ: Crime Human Nature: The Definitive Study of the Causes of Crime. New York, Simon & Schuster, 1998

Wong JS, Gravel J: Do sex offenders have higher levels of testosterone? Results from a meta-analysis. Sex Abuse 30(2):147–168, 2018 27000267

Yang Y, Raine A: Prefrontal structural and functional brain imaging findings in antisocial, violent, and psychopathic individuals: a meta-analysis. Psychiatry Res 174(2):81–88, 2009 19833485

Yildirim BO, Derksen JJL: A review on the relationship between testosterone and life-course persistent antisocial behavior. Psychiatry Res 200(2–3):984–1010, 2012a 22925371

Yildirim BO, Derksen JJL: A review on the relationship between testosterone and the interpersonal/affective facet of psychopathy. Psychiatry Res 197(3):181–198, 2012b 22342179

Zahn TP, Grafman J, Tranel D: Frontal lobe lesions and electrodermal activity: effects of significance. Neuropsychologia 37(11):1227–1241, 1999 10530723

Zuckerman M: Sensation seeking, in Handbook of Individual Differences in Social Behavior. Edited by Leary MR, Hoyle RH. New York, Guilford, 2009, pp 455–465

Zuckerman M, Kuhlman DM: Personality and risk-taking: common biosocial factors. J Pers 68(6):999–1029, 2000 11130742

CHAPTER 11

Neurophysiology of Antisocial Personality Disorder

Marijn Lijffijt, Ph.D.

Nithya Ramakrishnan, B.E., M.S.

Nicholas Murphy, Ph.D.

Dylan A. Fall, M.D.

Alan C. Swann, M.D.

At least 4% of U.S. adults have a lifetime history of antisocial personality disorder (ASPD) (Goldstein et al. 2017), a DSM-5 (American Psychiatric Association 2013) Cluster B disorder combining persistent irresponsible, impulsive, deceitful, unlawful, and aggressive behaviors, possibly with a lack of remorse, that starts before age 15 years as a diagnosis of conduct disorder. An additional 20% of U.S. adults have a lifetime history of adult antisocial behavior (Goldstein et al. 2017), which begins after age 15 but can be as clinically severe as ASPD (Goldstein et al. 2017). ASPD and conduct disorder are associated with increased risk of incarceration; lower education and income; increased risk of coexisting mental and behavior disorders, including addictions; and lower self-reported emotional and social functioning (Black et al. 2010; Goldstein et al. 2017). ASPD, therefore, warrants treatment, preferably at a young age because of evidence that young children with problematic disinhibited behaviors are at an increased risk to continue or escalate those behaviors in adolescence and adulthood (White et al. 2001). Insights into neurobiological mechanisms of ASPD and conduct disorder could aid in defining targets for treatment (van Goozen and Fairchild 2008).

Research has generally focused on specific antisocial behaviors (e.g., aggression, criminal behavior) or on psychopathy rather than on the diagnosis of ASPD or conduct disorder. Although antisocial behaviors are an aspect of the diagnosis of ASPD, those behaviors, even when they are persistent, do not themselves constitute ASPD (American Psychiatric Association 2013; Patrick 2014). Similarly, findings from research on psychopathy may not be generalizable to ASPD, even though psychopathy and ASPD share patterns in personality, behavior, and cognitions (Decuyper et al. 2009; Ogloff 2006; Patrick 2014).

ASPD and psychopathy could be two separate conditions or part of a continuum. Psychopathy, and to a lesser extent ASPD, consist of at least two aspects: antisocial/impulsive aspects (factor 2 on some psychopathy scales, such as the Hare Psychopathy Checklist—Revised [PCL-R; Hare 2003]) and emotional/interpersonal aspects (glibness, shallow emotions, lack of remorse or empathy, grandiosity, conning, and deceitful behavior; factor 1 on the PCL-R). ASPD and antisocial/impulsive aspects of psychopathy are associated with higher motor and nonplanning impulsivity on the Barratt Impulsiveness Scale (BIS-11; Patton et al. 1995; Snowden and Gray 2011), especially impulsivity during emotional events (Gray et al. 2019). Emotional/interpersonal aspects of psychopathy, on the other hand, are associated with lower nonplanning impulsivity (Gray et al. 2019). These findings are consistent with a diminished ability to adapt behaviors to contextual demands despite negative consequences in individuals with ASPD irrespective of coexisting psychopathy (De Brito et al. 2013). Other research suggests, by contrast, that psychopathy could represent a more severe illness course of ASPD (Coid and Ullrich 2010). Findings about psychopathy may therefore not be generalizable to ASPD or may be generalizable only to individuals with severe ASPD. In this chapter, we examine neurobiological mechanisms of ASPD by reviewing neurophysiological correlates.

Background

What Is Neurophysiology and How Is It Measured?

Neurophysiological techniques measure rapidly (e.g., tens to hundreds of milliseconds) changing physiological states that define neuronal functioning associated with brain processes (Cohen 2014). Brain processes rely on activation of groups of neurons, which generate electrical and magnetic fields that can be measured noninvasively with electroencephalography (EEG) or magnetoencephalography (MEG), respectively, from sensors distributed evenly over the entire scalp. This chapter focuses on EEG, including event-related potential (ERP) and event-related oscillation (ERO).

Scalp EEG is mostly derived from changes in electrical potentials along the vertical central apical dendrites of cortical pyramidal neurons (Kirschstein and Köhling 2009). Cortical pyramidal neurons are aligned in parallel columns perpendicular to the cortical surface, which is itself folded. The perpendicular alignment permits spatial summation of electrical potentials when neuronal clusters are synchronously active. The summated EEG activity can be represented as a field with a positive and negative pole (i.e., dipole) (Kirschstein and Köhling 2009). A dipole can be visualized best as a battery with a positive and negative pole. The pole depends on where along the apical dendrite the neuron is being engaged. The activity of dipoles can be measured on the scalp as small changes in voltage. Depending on the orientation of the dipole(s), changes in dipole activity can be detected by sensors positioned over the frontal, central, parietal, occipital, and/or temporal cortex.

Neuronal activity has sinusoidal characteristics when neurons are at relative rest and when they are activated. Neurons engage in synchronized rhythmic cycling (oscillations) between excitatory and inhibitory states mediated by neurotransmitters that depolarize or polarize neurons, respectively. Synchronized rhythmic cycling underlies information processing and information transfer (Fries 2015). The EEG is a composite of faster and slower cycling signals. Changes in synchronization can be visualized as changes in EEG band power. The EEG can be decomposed with spectral analyses into its frequency band content at rest or time-locked to an event such as a stimulus or a response (ERP, ERO).

Different brain processes rely on activation of neuronal groups that cycle at different rhythms, including at delta (0.5–3 Hz), theta (3–8 Hz), alpha (8–12 Hz), beta (12–30 Hz), and gamma (30–80 Hz) frequencies. Lower frequencies are involved in governing long-range communication between neurons; higher frequencies are implicated in local communication between neurons (Buzsáki and Draguhn 2004; von Stein et al. 2000). Broadly speaking, gamma oscillations appear to be involved in the processing of sensory information; alpha-beta oscillations appear to be involved in prefrontal control functions in part by influencing gamma oscillations; alpha oscillations appear to be involved in the blocking of neuronal communication that characterizes the natural state of the brain during rest; theta oscillations appear to be involved in attentional sampling of information carried by the other frequency bands; and delta oscillations appear to be involved in control of interference among types of information or responses. Information processing and transfer, and associated cognitive functioning, deteriorate with dysfunctional synchronization within or between neuronal groups (Fries 2015).

ERPs are a small part of the composite EEG that is time-locked to stimulus presentation or a response. For analysis, ERPs are generally summed and averaged across trials to obtain a personalized signal and averaged across subjects to obtain a group signal that is used to analyze group differences. Figure 11–1 shows a typical ERP. Note that ERPs are sinusoidal waveforms with positive and negative components. The direction and strength of brain signals depend on the relative locations of active dipoles, the location of the sensors that measure the neurophysiological signals, and the location of the sensor that serves as a baseline reference. The ERPs that are used to examine group differences or relationships with behavior are generally obtained from the sensor(s) with the most pronounced signal. The characteristics of the ERP that are analyzed most frequently are the peak amplitude in microvolts from baseline or from a prior peak (peak-to-peak amplitude), and the peak latency as the time between the stimulus and the peak amplitude.

ERPs are named based on the polarity of the wave and on the time at which the individual component peaks. In Figure 11–1, the positive peak around 300–400 ms after the presentation of a stimulus is therefore called a *P300* (or P3) ERP. Only a few signals flaunt that convention and are named for a condition that elicits the signal, for example, error-related negativity (ERN) or feedback-related negativity (FRN). ERO is a separation of the ERP by frequency band.

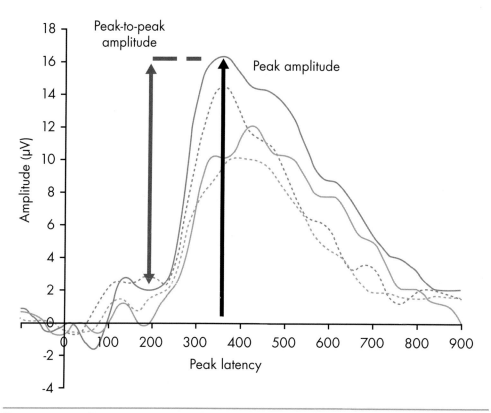

FIGURE 11–1.   Example of a P300 (P3) event-related potential (ERP).

To view this figure in color, see Plate 1 in Color Gallery.

An ERP is a small part of electroencephalography (EEG) that is time-locked to an event (e.g., a stimulus or a response). The ERP reflects multiple stages of information processing before and after an event. The time before the event serves as baseline. The most frequently used measures of the ERP are the amplitude of an ERP component (wave) that is measured from either baseline or a prior peak and the time (latency) of the peak. The amplitude is measured in microvolt (µV), and the latency is measured in milliseconds (ms). This shows that neuronal activity measured by EEG sensors placed on the scalp is very small and that the dynamics of neuronal processes related to information processing are very fast.

Source.   Adapted from Lijffijt M, Swann AC, Moeller FG: "Biological Substrate of Personality Traits Associated With Aggression," in *The SAGE Handbook of Personality Theory and Assessment: Volume 1—Personality Theories and Models.* Edited by Boyle GJ, Matthews G, Saklofske DH. Thousand Oaks, CA, Sage, 2008, pp. 334–356. Used with permission.

Neurophysiology and the Hypoarousal Theory of Antisocial Personality Disorder

A leading theory of externalizing disorders postulates that individuals with relative hypoarousal seek stimulation to compensate for that state. Externalizing disorders are characterized by a pattern of behaviors with real or potential negative consequences and include ASPD. The hypoarousal theory of antisocial behaviors has been proposed to explain the pattern of electrophysiological activity observed in antisocial and ADHD literatures (Quay 1965). Satterfield and Dawson (1971) found evidence for hypoarousal through measurements of heart rate and skin conductance in hyperactive children. Using EEG, several studies found that externalizing behavior is associated with more slow-wave oscillations (delta, theta, alpha frequencies) and less fast-wave activity (beta and gamma frequencies) (Rudo-Hutt 2015). Lower frequencies represent lower physiological arousal; higher frequencies represent higher physiological arousal.

Organization of This Chapter

In this chapter, we review studies that have used EEG or ERPs to examine brain processes in relation to ASPD, conduct disorder, antisocial traits (e.g., antisocial/impulsive aspects of psychopathy), and conduct problems assessed with clinical or self-report scales. We have excluded studies that focused exclusively on psychopathy without differentiating between emotional/interpersonal and antisocial/impulsive aspects; studies that focused exclusively on offenders if there was no diagnosis of ASPD; or studies that focused exclusively on violence, aggression, theft, use of controlled substances, or other examples of discrete antisocial behaviors without assessment of ASPD.

This chapter is divided roughly by physiological state or hypothesized stage of information processing: resting state, filtering of information, executive functions, and emotion and motivation. For outcomes, we rely primarily on meta-analyses if they are available. Meta-analyses summarize the existing literature by quantifying differences between groups or conditions on any given measure as effect sizes. Effect sizes include OR (the likelihood of an event occurring in one group compared with another group), Cohen's *d* or Hedges' *g* (the difference in means between two groups divided by the [pooled] SD), and *r* (correlation). Meta-analyses take into account random errors between individual studies, providing a more generalizable outcome than is obtained in individual studies. This approach is important for a field that frequently relies on small samples to obtain generalizable outcomes. When appropriate, we contrast findings in ASPD with findings in psychopathy.

Resting Electroencephalography

Brain processes rely on synchronized activity within or across clusters of pyramidal neurons to transfer information. Baseline or tonic synchronized activity can be measured as oscillations during rest, whereas reactive or phasic changes in activity can be measured in response to a stimulus or other event. At rest, neural oscillations provide insight into the general framework for local and distal communication patterns, while in response to an event, we can observe changes in the biological mechanisms required to coordinate more dynamic communication (Honda et al. 2020).

A meta-analysis across 62 studies examined resting EEG across externalizing disorders, including studies on antisocial (disruptive) behaviors (Rudo-Hutt 2015). The meta-analysis revealed significantly higher resting delta and theta power but lower alpha, beta, and gamma power across externalizing disorders compared with healthy control subjects (Rudo-Hutt 2015). This is consistent with findings from individual studies in ASPD or conduct disorder: compared with healthy adult control subjects (Reyes and Amador 2009) and with violent offenders without ASPD (Calzada-Reyes et al. 2012), violent offenders with ASPD had increased delta and theta power during rest. For children ages 9–13 years, parental or teacher reports of delinquent behavior, conduct problems, and emotional problems correlated significantly with higher frontal theta power during eyes closed, and conduct problems correlated negatively with frontal alpha power (Knyazev et al. 2002a). Increased resting delta and theta activity correlated with higher scores on impulsivity scales, although only at parietal sites (Knyazev et al. 2002b). Individuals with psychopathy may share decreased alpha activity with individuals who score high on measures of ASPD or conduct disorder, whereas beta activity was increased and decreased for individuals with psychopathy and ASPD, respectively (Calzada-Reyes et al. 2013, 2017).

In general, elevated power of delta and theta, and lower power of alpha, beta, and gamma, oscillations in ASPD appear consistent with the theory of physiological hypoarousal of ASPD and could be related to impulsivity. These outcomes indicate disruption of long range and in local communication between neurons (Buzsáki and Draguhn 2004; von Stein et al. 2000). Lower alpha and beta activity could be a biomarker of diminished prefrontal control with subsequent impaired modulation of gamma oscillations involved in sensory processing. Enhanced theta oscillations could indicate a change in attentional sampling of information, although it is uncertain if it relates to under- or oversampling of information. Finally, increased resting delta and theta activity and decreased resting alpha activity have been related to low inhibitory control (Knyazev 2006, 2007), an important aspect of decision-making and impulsive behaviors. This suggests that hypoarousal could be associated with poor decision-making because of widespread cognitive difficulties in ASPD. Psychopathy could be marked with a compensatory mechanism indicated by increased beta activity.

Filtering of Information

Early processes are engaged in the processing of sensory information as well as in the filtering of information. Early filtering of information prioritizes more extensive processing of more relevant sensory information, such as auditory or visual information; it restricts resources to less relevant information. Early filtering of information has not been extensively researched in ASPD or conduct disorder, in part because it was believed for a long time that these two disorders were related mostly to changes in higher-order cognitive functions (Raine 2019; Yang and Raine 2009) without recognizing that higher-order functions can be influenced by very early sensory processes (Lijffijt et al. 2009).

Passive listening to a simple click stimulus activates the auditory sensory cortex (Blenner and Yingling 1994; Röhl and Uppenkamp 2010; Thaerig et al. 2008). This elicits the P50, a positivity wave peaking between 40 and 80 ms poststimulus at central or frontocentral electrodes with a reversed pattern at temporal electrodes, reflecting preattentional auditory information processing; the N100 (N1), a central negativity peaking around 100 ms poststimulus, reflecting early attention orienting; and the P200 (P2), a central positivity peaking around 200 ms, reflecting early attentional processing and initial conscious awareness (Näätänen 1992; Rinne et al. 2006). The amplitude of the P50, N1, and P2 are smaller when an initial stimulus is rapidly followed by a second stimulus (prepulse inhibition; P50 sensory gating). The N1 and P2 amplitude increase when stimuli get louder or brighter but plateau or diminish in amplitude when stimuli get too intense (N1 and P2 intensity sensitivity function). Suppression of the P50, N1, and P2 is thought to reflect the restriction of resources to process repetitive and more intense information, potentially protecting resources for higher-order information processing of more relevant stimuli (Wan et al. 2008).

P50-N1-P2 Sensory Gating

Sensory gating can be measured with a paired-click paradigm. The paired-click paradigm presents pairs of identical click stimuli, S1 and S2, separated by about 500 ms; the period between pairs can be 5–10 seconds. Figure 11–2 shows that auditory stimuli (S1) evoke a P50-N1-P2 complex. Rapid repetition of the same stimulus (S2) elicits the same complex but with reduced amplitudes. The suppression following S2 is interpreted as filtering, or gating, of information (Freedman et al. 1991). P50, N1, and P2 gating can be measured as the absolute S1–S2 difference or an S2/S1 relative difference (Fruhstorfer et al. 1970): a smaller S2/S1 ratio is taken to signify more efficient sensory gating.

Our group has studied P50, N1, and P2 auditory sensory gating in healthy individuals and individuals with ASPD recruited from the local community. We found no differences between the two groups in P50, N1, and P2 sensory gating or in P50-N1-P2 S1 or S2 amplitudes (Lijffijt et al. 2012). However, within the ASPD group, higher DSM-IV (American Psychiatric Association 1994) conduct disorder and ASPD symptom counts, as well as higher trait impulsivity scores on all the subscales of the BIS-11 (Patton et al. 1995), correlated significantly with weaker P50 and N1 sensory gating measured as a higher S2/S1 ratio or smaller S1–S2 difference. By contrast, the healthy control subjects had better P50 and P2 sensory gating with elevated BIS-11 scores (Lijffijt et al. 2012). Group differences in the BIS-11–P50 gating relationship were associated with a larger S2 amplitude with higher BIS-11 nonplanning and attentional impulsivity scores for ASPD but a smaller S2 amplitude with elevated BIS-11 nonplanning and attentional impulsivity scores for control subjects. These findings suggest that ASPD and conduct disorder are associated with changes in early preattentional filtering of information, as well as with changes in filtering of information by early attentional processes. These relationships could perhaps be mediated by impulsivity, or they could mediate impulsivity. Control subjects, on the other hand, had improved preattentional gating with elevated impulsivity. These outcomes raise the question of what "impaired" gating means when relationships between elevated impulsivity and P50 gating are reversed in subjects with ASPD and control subjects. It is likely that similarities in elevated P50 ratios with high impulsivity in ASPD and low impulsivity in control subjects are related to a different physiological or cognitive mechanism that is directly or indirectly related to gating mechanisms.

Prepulse Inhibition

Prepulse inhibition (PPI) measures neuronal activity indirectly as inhibition of the eye blink startle reflex in reaction to acoustic startle cues (e.g., loud sounds) preceded 30–150 ms earlier by a milder acoustic stimulus (e.g., prepulse). The PPI measures changes in muscle activity from sensors placed around the eye. The eye blink is stronger for louder startle cues. Suppression of this automatic and preattentional response is thought to involve frontal cortical areas, the hippocampus, the amygdala, the thalamus, and the basal ganglia (Kumari et al. 2005). Group comparisons showed that the PPI did not differ between control subjects and individuals with antisocial traits (Fuertes-Saiz et al. 2019; Kumari et al. 2005; Sedgwick et al. 2018). However, higher scores on measures of antisocial traits correlated negatively with PPI (Fuertes-Saiz et al. 2019; Kumari et al. 2005; Sedgwick et al. 2018), indicating diminished suppression of the blink response despite presentation of a prepulse. This outcome is similar to that found for P50 gating.

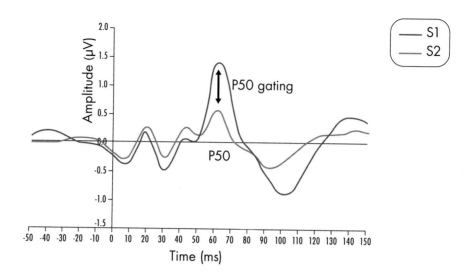

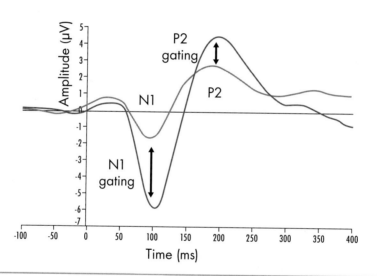

FIGURE 11–2. Sensory gating of the auditory P50 (*top graph*) and the N100 (N1) and P200 (P2) (*bottom graph*).

To view this figure in color, see Plate 2 in Color Gallery.

P50 rides on top of the beginning of N1 and is therefore more difficult to analyze. To better visualize and analyze the P50, researchers often filter the data between 10 and 50 Hz (band-pass filter with zero-phase shift). This significantly diminishes the influence of the N1 and P2 on the P50. To visualize and analyze the N1 and P2, the signal can be analyzed by applying a band-pass filter set between 1 and 30 Hz. The figure shows the P50-N1-P2 auditory evoked potential to S1 of the paired-click paradigm. A small P50-N1-P2 auditory event-related potential is evoked by S2. The difference between the amplitudes of S1 and S2 is interpreted as sensory gating.

Source. Adapted from Lijffijt M, Lane SD, Meier SL, et al.: "P50, N100, and P200 Sensory Gating: Relationships With Behavioral Inhibition, Attention, and Working Memory." *Psychophysiology* 46(5):1059–1068, 2009. Copyright © 2009 John Wiley and Sons. Used with permission.

N1 and P2 Intensity Sensitivity Function

Louder or brighter stimuli produce larger N1 and P2 amplitudes. This increase levels off or reverses when stimuli become more intense (Prescott et al. 1984). The relation between stimulus intensity and N1, P2, or combined N1-P2 amplitude can be expressed as a linear slope, as shown in Figure 11–3. A steeper slope indicates less suppression at higher intensities, which is hypothesized to reflect deficient inhibitory control of prefrontal control processes (Blenner and Yingling 1994). A steeper slope has been theorized to reflect deficient serotonergic functioning (Juckel and Hegerl 1994), although this theory is actively debated: a steeper slope before treatment could predict a better treatment response of selective serotonin reuptake inhibitors (SSRIs) (Jaworska et al. 2013), even though the slope itself appears to be insensitive to acute changes in serotonin concentrations (O'Neill et al. 2008).

We examined relationships between the intensity sensitivity slope and ASPD. Based on a rich literature of relationships between intensity sensitivity slope and impulsivity or externalizing disorders (Barratt et al. 1987; Lijffijt et al. 2015), we expected to find a steeper slope in individuals with ASPD compared with control subjects, or an increased slope with more ASPD symptoms or higher impulsivity. However, we found no significant differences in slopes between individuals with ASPD and control subjects, and no significant relationships between slopes with ASPD symptom count or with BIS-11 trait impulsivity emerged (Lijffijt et al. 2017). On the other hand, we did find a correlation for each of the two groups between a steeper N1 and P2 slope with more commission errors on the Immediate Memory Task (IMT; Dougherty 1999). The IMT is a complex continuous performance task in which subjects have to press a button as quickly as possible when a 5-digit number exactly matches the 5-digit number presented just before (e.g., 36795–36795). Commission errors are responses to 5-digit numbers that differ from the previous number by only 1 digit (e.g., 36795–38795). These errors are interpreted as impulsive responses associated with diminished response inhibition or with slower processing of a stimulus relative to the generation of the response (Dougherty et al. 2000) and are increased in people with a variety of impulsivity-related problems (Dougherty et al. 2000, 2003; Swann et al. 2009a, 2009b, 2011). This outcome suggests that more impulsive actions could be related to diminished suppression of the processing of more intense stimuli. This appears consistent with elevated impulsive behavior in ASPD during emotional events (Gray et al. 2019).

Conclusion

Deficient preattentional and early attentional filtering of information could be related to aberrant prefrontal top-down control over bottom-up processes. Deficient early filtering of information in more severe ASPD or conduct disorder may decrease the signal-to-noise ratio during information processing and may divert resources from higher-order processing such as response inhibition or attention to the further processing or suppressing of less relevant information. This could translate to additional interference between information, which could result in spurious actions. In addition, the requirement of resources to process irrelevant information also diminishes resources for decision-making or behavioral control in individuals with ASPD.

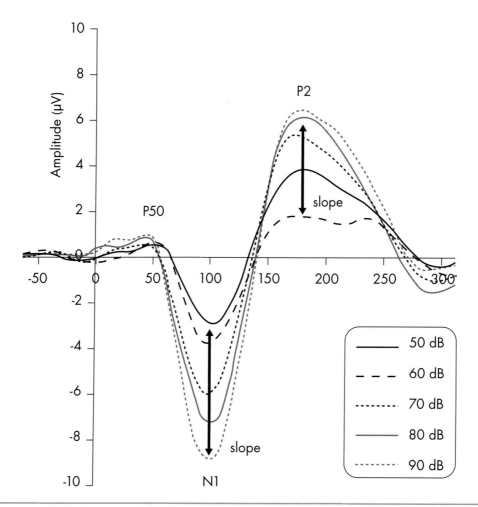

FIGURE 11–3. N100 (N1) and P200 (P2) intensity sensitivity function is expressed as the linear slope for N1 or P2 peak amplitude as a function of stimulus loudness or stimulus brightness.
To view this figure in color, see Plate 3 in Color Gallery.
In this example, N1 and P2 were evoked by auditory stimuli. The N1 and the P2 amplitude can be taken from baseline or from the P50 and N1, respectively.
Source. Adapted from Lijffijt M, Lane SD, Moeller FG, et al: "Trait Impulsivity and Increased Pre-Attentional Sensitivity to Intense Stimuli in Bipolar Disorder and Controls." *Journal of Psychiatric Research* 60:73–80, 2015. Copyright © 2015 Elsevier. Used with permission.

Executive Functions

ASPD has been associated most often with deficient executive functioning because of an early focus on the P3 and contingent negative variation (CNV), which measure allocation of attentional resources and of preparatory processes, respectively.

P300 (P3)

The P3 is a positive wave that peaks between 300 and 700 ms after stimulus presentation. The P3 is hypothesized to index allocation of attentional resources for stimulus orienting

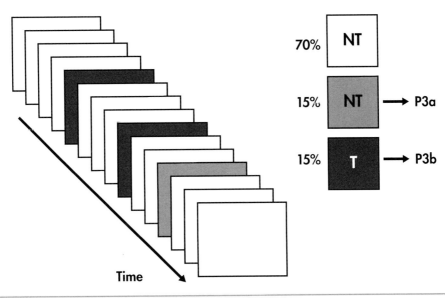

FIGURE 11–4. Oddball task, which is most often used to study the P300 (P3) in antisocial personality disorder.

The oddball task consists of a sequence of pseudo-randomly presented frequent (sometimes called "standard") and infrequent (sometimes called "deviant") stimuli. Some tasks have two or more infrequent stimuli. Stimuli can be of any type but frequently are low-arousing geometric figures, letters, or sounds. The task instruction determines the interpretation of the event-related potential (ERP). Instructing participants to passively listen to or look at stimuli elicits ERP components that reflect automatic detection of differences between stimuli and that reflect automatic attentional processes. Examples of ERPs related to passive oddball tasks are the mismatch negativity and the P3a. Instructing participants to press a button, count, or do any other action when they see an infrequent stimulus elicits ERP components that reflect top-down attentional control measured by the P3b, although the P3b is not the only component that is amplified by an attention manipulation. If there is more than one deviant stimulus, the second stimulus that subjects are not instructed about elicits a P3a. Instructing subjects to press a button when they see a frequent stimulus elicits a no-go P3 to infrequent stimuli that reflects the ability to inhibit a response tendency. NT=nontarget/frequent stimulus; T=target /novel/deviant/infrequent stimulus.

and for developing or updating memory (Polich 2007). The P3 consists of several subcomponents that react differently to task context and task demand. The task that is most often used to study the P3 in ASPD is the oddball task. As illustrated in Figure 11–4, the oddball task consists of sequences of two or more different stimuli. One stimulus is presented frequently (e.g., on 70% of all trials of the task), and one or more stimuli are presented sparingly (e.g., on 15% of all trials). Infrequent stimuli elicit the P3. A larger P3 has been linked to better performance on memory tasks (Polich 2007), faster responses, and higher accuracy (Nieuwenhuis et al. 2005, 2011), indicating improved decision-making.

Research suggests at least two P3 subcomponents (Polich 2007). The P3a peaks relatively early and has a frontocentral distribution. The P3a, elicited by novel, infrequent nontarget stimuli, including those requiring the withholding of a response, is thought to be involved in stimulus-driven allocation of attention and stimulus-orienting carried out primarily by theta oscillations (Bachman and Bernat 2018). The P3b, peaking relatively late with a centroparietal distribution, is a manifestation primarily of delta oscillations and is thought to be involved in top-down stimulus evaluation when one of the infrequent stimuli is designated as a target. Both the P3a and the P3b involve activation of the frontal, temporal, and parietal cortices (Polich 2007), with the P3a perhaps being more dependent on dopamine (Polich 2007), and the P3b being more dependent on norepinephrine (Nieuwenhuis et al. 2005). The amplitude of the P3 is highly heritable and is smaller with lower physiological arousal (Polich 2007).

Two excellent and complementary meta-analyses reviewed the P3 across antisocial populations, including those with ASPD and conduct disorder. In a meta-analysis that reviewed studies until the year 2007, Gao and Raine (2009) showed evidence of a smaller P3 amplitude (Cohen's $d = -0.252$) and a longer P3 latency ($d = 0.130$) in antisocial individuals irrespective of type of P3 (P3a or P3b) or of antisocial psychopathology (ASPD, conduct disorder, psychopathy). This finding, which was confirmed in a review published in 2018 that discussed studies from 2009 through 2016 (Pasion et al. 2018), could reflect diminished allocation of resources to stimuli relevant in decision-making, perhaps associated with physiological hypoarousal.

Both studies showed that P3 amplitudes were similar in psychopathic and nonpsychopathic antisocial populations (Gao and Raine 2009). However, studies consistently find a smaller P3 for populations with ASPD and conduct disorder, whereas studies in psychopathic populations are equally divided between those reporting larger and those reporting smaller P3 amplitudes, perhaps because of variation in impulsivity. A regression analysis revealed that within psychopathic populations, antisocial/impulsive aspects predicted smaller P3 amplitudes, whereas affective/interpersonal aspects predicted larger P3 amplitudes (Pasion et al. 2018).

In summary, these outcomes suggest diminished P3 amplitude for ASPD, which appears to be consistent with hypothesized hypoarousal (Raine 2002) and attenuated frontal functioning (Yang and Raine 2009) in ASPD. The P3 could be increased in relation to affective/interpersonal aspects of psychopathy, and this appears consistent with a better ability to plan actions, potentially resulting in improved decision-making abilities. As we discuss later, this pattern for the P3 could be specific for tasks that use low valence–low arousing stimuli such as geometric figures or numbers. The P3 may also function as a biomarker for a balance between antisocial and psychopathic traits in individuals with ASPD and conduct disorder.

Contingent Negative Variation

The CNV is a slow negative wave that develops during a period before an actionable event. The CNV can be measured with cued reaction time tasks that use a long interval between an initial cue that indicates an upcoming task-relevant stimulus and the task-relevant stimulus. The CNV could reflect expectancy, attention, or action preparation (Fabiani et al. 2007). An increase has been associated with activity in the anterior cingulate cortex (ACC), the supplemental motor area, the thalamus, the pons, and the cerebellum (Nagai et al. 2004). The CNV is made up of at least two overlapping components related to an early orienting response and a later expectancy wave. Quicker development of the CNV and a larger amplitude of what is possibly the orienting response have been related to faster reaction times (Wild-Wall et al. 2007). The CNV is larger when responses can result in a monetary gain or loss (Williams et al. 2018), indicating that the CNV is sensitive to motivation manipulations.

Outcomes for the CNV obtained from antisocial populations have been inconsistent. In patients of a residential substance use clinic who had a substance use disorder with or without comorbid DSM-III-R (American Psychiatric Association 1987) ASPD, the orienting response of the CNV developed faster than it did in control subjects in a 2-second time-estimation task (Bauer 2001). The faster development was especially pronounced in individuals with DSM-III-R ASPD who pressed the button within 1 second to indicate that they thought 2 seconds had elapsed (Bauer 2001). Individuals with psychopathic personality (Forth and Hare 1989; Raine et al. 1990) also had faster development of a CNV, which was related to the emotional/interpersonal aspects of psychopathy (Carlson and Thái 2010; Howard et al. 1984). A weak correlation was found between a lower CNV and higher antisocial/impulsive scores (Howard et al. 1984). Other studies found no significant relationships between CNV and antisocial behaviors in patients residing in a forensic psychiatric hospital (Fenton et al. 1978). Finally, the CNV measured in male high school students when they were 15 years old did not predict a history of criminal behavior at age 24 years (Raine et al. 1990).

These outcomes provide weak evidence of a relation between smaller CNV and more impulsive/antisocial aspects of psychopathy and ASPD. Outcomes suggest faster response preparation related perhaps to faster time estimation, which could relate to a perception that time is going faster than it actually is.

Mismatch Negativity

The mismatch negativity (MMN) is generated during oddball tasks with the instruction to simply perceive stimuli or to read a book during the experiment. This task also generates a P3a. The MMN is a negative wave peaking between 150 and 250 ms after the presentation of an infrequent (deviant) stimulus embedded in a sequence of frequent (standard) stimuli. The MMN is generally visualized by subtracting the ERP of frequently presented "standard" stimuli from the ERP of infrequent "deviant" stimuli (Näätänen et al. 2011). ERPs for standard and deviant stimuli are displayed in Figure 11–5. Subtraction obtains the MMN and P3a. The MMN reflects an involuntary preconscious stimulus-driven call for attention induced by a mismatch between a memory trace composed by preceding stimuli or stimulus contexts (e.g., frequent stimuli) and an actual incoming event (e.g., infrequent stimulus) (Garrido et al. 2009; Näätänen et al. 2011). The MMN could reflect functioning of the neurotransmitter glutamate (de la Salle et al. 2019). The P3a is associated with automatic allocation of attention and stimulus orienting (Näätänen et al. 2011) carried by theta oscillations (Choi et al. 2013; Fuentemilla et al. 2008).

Adults with ASPD or juvenile offenders with conduct disorder had a larger MMN amplitude compared with healthy control subjects (Hung et al. 2013; Liu et al. 2007). Emotionally salient deviants (e.g., fearful voices) appear especially suitable to generate a larger MMN in ASPD; this larger MMN correlated with antisocial/impulsive aspects of psychopathy but not with other aspects of psychopathy (Hung et al. 2013).

We examined relationships among MMN, ASPD symptoms, and impulsivity measured with the BIS-11 and IMT (M. Lijffijt and A.C. Swann, unpublished data, August 2013). In an institutional review board (IRB)–approved study, 11 healthy volunteers, 9 volunteers with bipolar disorder, and 9 volunteers with ASPD performed a passive auditory oddball task. Pearson correlation analyses revealed a significant correlation between a smaller MMN amplitude and more IMT commission errors ($r=-0.50$; $P=0.007$; $r=-0.52$; $P=0.005$ for commission errors corrected for correct detections)

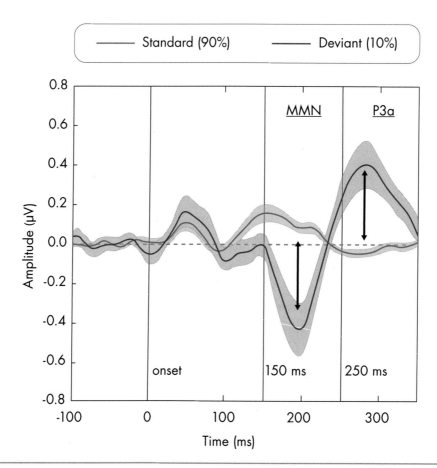

FIGURE 11–5. Mismatch negativity (MMN) evoked in a passive listening task by deviant stimuli presented randomly among standard stimuli.

To view this figure in color, see Plate 4 in Color Gallery.

The deviant stimulus can differ from the standard stimulus in pitch, duration, or any other property. The deviant stimulus elicits a negativity between 100 and 250 ms poststimulus compared with a standard stimulus. Following the MMN is a P3a, which is also enhanced for deviant compared with standard stimuli. The MMN and P3a are studied often as a difference wave by subtracting the event-related potential (ERP) of the standard from the ERP of the deviant stimulus.

across all subjects (Figure 11–6). This relationship is consistent with other reports of a smaller or delayed MMN amplitude and more commission errors on choice reaction time or response inhibition tasks (Elton et al. 2004; Liu et al. 2013), although others did not find this association (Smit 2008). However, we found no difference in MMN amplitude between the ASPD and healthy control subjects and no significant associations between MMN amplitude and ASPD symptom count or BIS-11 trait impulsivity. The latter absence of an association is partially inconsistent with reports of a larger MMN (Franken et al. 2005; Hung et al. 2013; Sawada et al. 2008; Wang et al. 2001) or a smaller MMN (Shimano et al. 2014; Smit 2008, p. 200) and higher scores on a variety of self-report or clinician-administered impulsivity scales.

Our outcomes suggest that impaired response inhibition in ASPD could be associated with diminished detection of new and potentially relevant information reflected

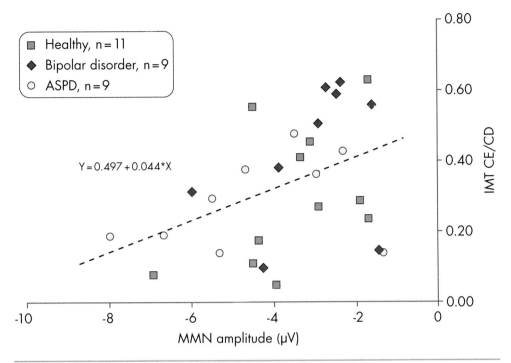

FIGURE 11–6. Association between mismatch negativity (MMN) amplitude and impulsive action.

To view this figure in color, see Plate 5 in Color Gallery.

Significant correlation between MMN amplitude and impulsive action measured as Immediate Memory Task (IMT) commission errors corrected for correct detections (CE/CD ratio) ($r=0.52$; $P=0.005$) across 11 healthy volunteers and 18 patients with impulsivity-related disorders (9 with bipolar disorder; 9 with antisocial personality disorder [ASPD]).

by a diminished MMN. Impaired detection of new information could result in a diminished neuronal representation of the stimulus, contributing to the possible decreased signal-to-noise ratio discussed earlier for filtering mechanisms. In general, the inconsistent outcomes across studies raise questions, including the potential contributions of specific EEG power bands and the contribution of specific brain structures to the MMN and its components in antisocial and control populations.

N200 (N2)

The N2 is a frontocentral negative wave evoked between 200 and 400 ms on tasks demanding attention or response inhibition. The N2 could reflect response conflict or response inhibition related to activation of the ACC (Ridderinkhof et al. 2004b). The N2 could be carried by theta (Huster et al. 2013) and delta (Harmony 2013) oscillations, although delta oscillations could also reflect attention instead of or in conjunction with response inhibition (Kirmizi-Alsan et al. 2006).

A comprehensive meta-analysis reviewed studies that used the N2 as a marker of conflict monitoring or response inhibition in antisocial compared with healthy child, adolescent, and adult populations (Pasion et al. 2019). Pasion and colleagues reported a significantly smaller N2 amplitude for studies that used clinical or inmate samples of individuals with violent behavior (eight studies; Hedges' $g=-1.04$), conduct disorder (one study; $g=-1.19$), and ASPD (three studies; $g=-0.55$) compared with healthy populations (Pasion et al. 2019). Unfortunately, the outcomes for conduct disorder and ASPD are unreliable because they are based on only one and three studies, respectively. Another meta-analysis showed a very small effect size for the N2 across four studies in children or adolescents with conduct disorder or oppositional defiant disorder (ODD) compared with healthy youths ($g=-0.03$) (Hoyniak and Petersen 2019).

Pasion et al. (2019) also reported that the relation between antisocial features and diminished N2 contrasts with nonsignificant differences for studies that used samples of individuals who met criteria for psychopathy (10 studies; $g=-0.01$). The difference in findings of relationships between N2 and antisocial features compared with N2 and psychopathy is likely a result of inconsistencies across studies that use mixed samples, similar to outcomes for the P3. Finally, elevated impulsivity in nonclinical populations was related to a larger N2 (15 studies; $g=0.23$) (Pasion et al. 2019). As we have shown in this chapter, the majority of neurophysiological outcomes in ASPD have been related to impulsivity. However, the relationship between ASPD and a smaller N2 amplitude contrasts with findings of a larger N2 generally associated with impulsivity. Pasion argued that the increased N2 with impulsivity in nonpathological populations could be a compensating mechanism (Pasion et al. 2019) against pathological impulsivity (defined as continued situationally inappropriate behavior despite repeated negative consequences) (Barratt et al. 2005). A similar argument may apply to the difference in impulsivity–P50 gating relationship found in individuals with ASPD compared with control subjects discussed in previous sections.

Additional analyses of antisocial populations found that 1) the most pronounced differences were seen for the inhibition-related N2 evoked during the stop-signal task but not go/no-go tasks, whereas no change was seen for the attention-related or conflict monitoring-related N2, and 2) compensation for study participation or feedback about task performance diminished the difference in N2 between control subjects and antisocial populations (Pasion et al. 2019). This suggests that a smaller N2 in populations with violent behaviors, conduct disorder, or ASPD could be the result of differences in motivation rather than persistent changes in mechanisms underlying the N2.

Thus, conduct disorder and ASPD could be associated with a smaller N2 related to response inhibition, although rewards seem to enhance the N2 in those populations. The N2 could be enhanced with higher impulsivity reflecting compensation against pathological impulsivity. We explore this topic further in the next section concerning error and feedback processing.

Error-Related Negativity

The ERN is a negative wave with a frontocentral distribution that is evoked between 50 and 200 ms following an error. The ERN reflects the detection of outcomes that deviate from predicted outcomes (Falkenstein et al. 2000; Ridderinkhof et al. 2004b) and has been associated with activation of the ACC involved in cognitive and behavioral control (Ridderinkhof et al. 2004a, 2004b). Information processing reflected by the ERN is carried by theta oscillations, with errors increasing theta power (Trujillo and Allen 2007). A stronger ERN and a stronger increase in theta activity following errors have been associated with better adjustment of behaviors to meet task demand, including behavioral slowing on trials that succeed errors (Kalfaoğlu et al. 2018). This mechanism could be closely related to deficient behavioral control and repeated rule-violating behaviors that characterize ASPD, in which behavior is not adjusted despite negative consequences.

A meta-analysis across 160 studies found that externalizing disorders share a smaller ERN on tasks that require inhibiting a response (Pasion and Barbosa 2019) In a high-externalizing population, this decrease was associated with diminished theta (4–7 Hz) oscillations (Hall et al. 2007). A smaller ERN at age 6 years in children who had been irritable since age 3 years predicted the development at age 9 years of an externalizing disorder, whereas an enhanced ERN in the same population could predict the development of an internalizing disorder (Kessel et al. 2016). Finally, a lower ERN was found for adults (Ruchsow et al. 2005) and adolescents but not children (Taylor et al. 2018), who scored high compared with low on trait impulsivity measured with the BIS-11. This suggests that the relation between ASPD and a smaller ERN could be mediated by impulsivity or that a smaller ERN predisposes to pathological impulsivity and ASPD. Scores on antisocial/impulsive aspects of psychopathy were nonsignificantly related to the ERN (Bresin et al. 2014; Maurer et al. 2016a, 2016b), suggesting that the relationship between ASPD and a smaller ERN could also be mediated or modulated by mechanisms unrelated to impulsivity, such as emotion or motivation. A smaller ERN at a young age could provide a basis for interventions focused on disinhibition.

Conclusion

ASPD could be associated with deficient executive functioning as illustrated by a smaller P3a, P3b, CNV, MMN, N2, and ERN. The increase in P3 for emotional stimuli relative to low-arousal stimuli could be mediated by pathological impulsivity, or these changes could underlie pathological impulsivity that is expressed as ASPD. However, as discussed in the next section, the changes do not appear to be static, because emotion and motivation are able to diminish differences between ASPD and control subjects.

Emotion and Motivation

P3

As discussed earlier (see "Executive Functions"), previous studies showed a smaller P3a and P3b for ASPD, conduct disorder, and elevated antisocial traits. However, those studies used low valence–low arousal stimuli such as letters.

The P3 is modulated by emotional content and motivation, consistent with the ability of emotional content to capture attention. Studies using arousing stimuli (e.g., aversive or erotic scenes, startling sounds) reported an elevated P3 for negative emotional words in offenders diagnosed with ASPD (Verona et al. 2012), although another study found no difference in P3 between subjects with and without ASPD (Drislane et al. 2013). These findings are in contrast to a diminished P3 for negative emotional words or to an aversive acoustic stimulus in offenders with psychopathy (Drislane et al. 2013; Verona et al. 2012), which has been related to the affective/interpersonal aspect of psychopathy (Drislane et al. 2013). These outcomes are at odds with the smaller P3 evoked by low valence–low arousal stimuli for ASPD and the stronger P3 for psychopathy. This illustrates the importance of experimental context and shows that it is not the allocation of attentional resources per se that is deficient, but rather the control in allocating those resources. In addition, the increase in P3 for emotional stimuli relative to low-arousal stimuli could be a translational measure in which individuals with ASPD act more impulsively during emotional events.

Late Positive Potential

The late positive potential (LPP) is a positive wave with a central to posterior distribution. The LPP is associated with activation of the amygdala, ACC, anterior insula, parietal cortex, and visual cortex (Liu et al. 2012; Sabatinelli et al. 2007, 2013). The LPP reflects automatic allocation of attentional resources to emotionally salient stimuli (Hajcak et al. 2010), including faces with an emotional expression or pictures from the International Affective Picture System (Lang et al. 2008). In adults, the LPP begins around 300 ms after presentation of an emotionally salient stimulus (Cuthbert et al. 2000; Hajcak et al. 2010; Schupp et al. 2004) and is sustained through the end of stimulus presentation (Hajcak et al. 2009, 2010). The LPP is larger with increased subjective arousal of the stimulus rather than enhanced valence (i.e., more negative or positive) (Cuthbert et al. 2000) and could be a marker of emotion regulation (Dennis and Hajcak 2009).

There has been very limited research on LPP in ASPD or conduct disorder outside of the context of psychopathy. Youths with emotional and behavior problems who had been part of a psychosocial intervention for less than 4 months had smaller LPP amplitudes to negative images, which correlated with higher scores on the Strengths and Difficulties Questionnaire, a self-report of youth antisocial behavior (Pincham et al. 2016). This outcome suggests blunted processing of negative stimuli in youths with more antisocial behavior. Youths with emotional and behavior problems who had been part of a psychosocial intervention for more than 9 months had the opposite relationship between LPP and negative images and scores on the Strengths and Difficulties Questionnaire (Pincham et al. 2016). Outcomes should, therefore, be interpreted with caution. In another study, variation in the severity of externalizing behaviors (substance use disorder, adulthood or childhood rule breaking) among healthy undergraduates was not significantly associated with variation in LPP amplitude in response to emotional or neutral International Affective Picture System images (Rozalski and Benning 2019).

These outcomes provide limited evidence for possible diminished processing of negative stimuli in antisocial populations, which contrasts with findings for the P3 in the context of emotions. However, the smaller LPP may be related to emotional/interpersonal and not to impulsive/antisocial aspects of ASPD or conduct disorder: a meta-analysis showed that individuals with psychopathic traits had a smaller LPP for aversive stimuli than did control subjects, whereas no group differences were found for positive or neutral stimuli (Vallet et al. 2020). This blunted response was indeed related to emotional/interpersonal rather than antisocial/impulsive aspects of psychopathy (Venables et al. 2015).

Feedback-Related Negativity

A task can be made more salient by rewarding correct behavior and punishing incorrect behavior. Responsiveness to reward and punishment can be examined with the FRN (Glazer et al. 2018). The FRN is a negative wave occurring 100–500 ms after negative compared with positive feedback in response to an action. Information processing underlying the FRN is carried by theta oscillations that overlap with slower delta oscillations related to a somewhat later P3 (Bernat et al. 2015). Like the ERN, the FRN originates from the ACC and may also reflect a prediction error (Holroyd and Coles 2002). In contrast to the ERN, which relies on an internal signal of outcomes, the FRN is elicited by an external outcome signal, with a larger FRN to punishment than to reward.

Compared with IQ- and age-matched healthy control subjects, nonpsychopathic juvenile offenders had an enhanced FRN due to increased positivity following positive feedback (Vilà-Balló et al. 2015), which suggests increased sensitivity to reward compared with punishment. This finding would be consistent with continued antisocial behavior despite negative consequences in ASPD. Undergraduates scoring high compared with low on a measure of antisocial traits also had an elevated FRN, related to enhanced negativity following negative feedback, but only when the feedback was numerical (a proxy for monetary loss); the difference between groups was absent when feedback was provided by facial expression (a proxy for social-emotional feedback) (Pfabigan et al. 2011). By contrast, FRN to negative feedback, using a small (5-cent) punishment, was smaller in undergraduate students scoring high compared with low on the BIS-11 (Potts et al. 2006). Finally, no effect was found for FRN in a study using monetary feedback in undergraduates who scored high compared with low on an externalizing questionnaire (Bernat et al. 2015). Therefore, in populations with ASPD and conduct disorder, relationships to diminished reactivity of punishment compared with reward require further investigation but could be a valid measure of continuation of antisocial and impulsive behaviors despite the negative consequences. ASPD and conduct disorder may be related to enhanced sensitivity to reward, whereas high antisocial traits, perhaps outside of the context of ASPD, may be more sensitive to punishment, which could be a protective mechanism against more extreme antisocial behavior.

Feedback also elicits a P3. The feedback P3 was lower in undergraduates scoring high compared with low on an externalizing scale, irrespective of incentive type (Bernat et al. 2015). On the other hand, another study found that the feedback P3 was influenced by type of incentive and not by antisocial traits (Pfabigan et al. 2011). As with the FRN, more research is needed in this field.

Conclusion

We have reviewed neurophysiological correlates of ASPD, conduct disorder, and impulsive/antisocial aspects of psychopathy to come to an understanding of their neurobiological mechanisms. Outcomes have been summarized in Table 11–1.

One of the most replicated findings in the ASPD and conduct disorder literature is a smaller P3 for tasks that use low-arousal stimuli. This difference suggests diminished allocation of attentional resources to salient information, perhaps reflecting physiological hypoarousal. Physiological hypoarousal is also reflected by increased activity in resting state delta and theta band power and diminished activity in alpha, beta, and gamma band power. Increased resting delta and theta and diminished resting alpha have been related to impaired response inhibition (Knyazev 2006, 2007), which is an aspect of impulsivity (Moeller et al. 2001).

TABLE 11–1. Overview of main findings and hypothesized functional significance of neurophysiology in antisocial personality disorder (ASPD), conduct disorder (CD), conduct problems, and the impulsive/antisocial aspect of psychopathy

Electroencephalography (EEG) measure	Source/Location	Measure	Main finding in ASPD	Functional significance
Resting EEG				
Delta, beta, theta, alpha, gamma power			↑ Delta and theta power; ↓ Alpha, beta, and gamma power	Hypoarousal; imbalance between local and distal neuronal communication
Sensory gating				
P50-N1-P2 sensory gating	Frontal lobe, auditory cortex	Smaller decrease in amplitude of P50-N1-P2 response to auditory stimulus S2 relative to S1 in the context of fast S1–S2 stimulus presentation	No difference between ASPD and control group; ↓ P50 gating, ↑ S2 P50, and ↓ N1 gating with ↑ CD/ASPD symptoms and ↑ Barratt Impulsiveness Scale–11 scores	Poor preattentional and early attentional filtering of information
Prepulse inhibition (PPI)	Frontal lobe, hippocampus, amygdala, thalamus, basal ganglia	Suppression of eye blink startle response with mild prepulse	No difference between ASPD and control group; ↓ PPI with ↑ antisocial traits	Poor preattentional filtering of information
N1-P2 intensity sensitivity function	Frontal lobe, auditory cortex	Linear N1 and P2 slopes with increased stimulus loudness	No difference between ASPD and control group; ↑ N1 and P2 slopes with ↑ impulsive commission errors or trait impulsivity	Poor early attentional filtering of information, which could contribute to poor response inhibition

TABLE 11–1. Overview of main findings and hypothesized functional significance of neurophysiology in antisocial personality disorder (ASPD), conduct disorder (CD), conduct problems, and the impulsive/antisocial aspect of psychopathy *(continued)*

Electroencephalography (EEG) measure	Source/Location	Measure	Main finding in ASPD	Functional significance
Executive functions				
P300: P3a, P3b	Frontal, temporal, and parietal	Event-related potential (ERP) peaking between 300 and 700 ms following salient stimuli	↓P3 amplitude and ↑P3 latency for low-arousing stimuli in ASPD or ↑impulsive/antisocial aspects of psychopathy; ↑P3 amplitude with ↑affective/interpersonal aspects of psychopathy	Deficient allocation of attention; possible means to assess a balance between antisocial and psychopathic traits
Contingent negative variation (CNV)	Frontal lobe, thalamus, pons, cerebellum	Wave developing during a wait period of an expected actionable event	↓CNV for ↑impulsive/antisocial aspects of psychopathy; steeper CNV development for ↑affective/interpersonal aspects of psychopathy	Deficient response preparation in ASPD? (evidence is weak but suggestive)
Mismatch negativity (MMN)	Frontal-temporal network	Deviant *vs.* standard ERP negative wave peaking between 150 and 250 ms	↓MMN with ↑impulsive commission errors; perhaps ↑MMN with ASPD or CD	Elevated deviancy detection in ASPD or diminished MMN related to impaired response inhibition
N200/N2	Anterior cingulate cortex	Wave evoked between 200 and 400 ms on stimulus interference or response inhibition tasks	↓N2 for ASPD or CD but smaller or no difference in N2 with motivational manipulation; ↑N2 with ↑impulsivity	Deficient interference or response control in ASPD that could be corrected with motivation
Error-related negativity (ERN)	Anterior cingulate cortex	Negative wave between 50 and 200 ms following an error	↓ERN with ASPD and CD or ↑trait impulsivity; normal ERN in the context of psychopathy	Deficient behavioral control perhaps related to deficient adaptive changes in behaviors

TABLE 11–1. Overview of main findings and hypothesized functional significance of neurophysiology in antisocial personality disorder (ASPD), conduct disorder (CD), conduct problems, and the impulsive/antisocial aspect of psychopathy *(continued)*

Electroencephalography (EEG) measure	Source/Location	Measure	Main finding in ASPD	Functional significance
Emotion and motivation				
P300: P3a, P3b	Frontal, temporal, and parietal	ERP peaking between 300 and 700 ms following salient stimuli	↑ P3 amplitude for high-arousing stimuli in ASPD or ↑ impulsive/antisocial aspects of psychopathy; ↓ P3 amplitude with ↑ affective/interpersonal aspects of psychopathy	Increased allocation of attentional resources to emotionally arousing stimuli in ASPD and decreased allocation with high affective/interpersonal aspects of psychopathy
Late positive potential (LPP)	Anterior cingulate cortex, amygdala, anterior insula, parietal cortex, and visual cortex	Wave starts around 300 ms after an emotional high arousal stimulus and lasts until removal of the stimulus	↓ LPP to negative stimuli in ASPD, which may be related to affective/interpersonal aspects of psychopathy	Decreased allocation of attention to negative emotional stimuli with high affective/interpersonal aspects of psychopathy? (data are inconsistent but suggestive)
Feedback-related negativity (FRN)	Anterior cingulate cortex	Negative wave between 100 and 500 ms after negative outcomes compared with positive outcomes	↑ FRN due to an elevated positivity to reward or negativity following monetary losses in ASPD, but ASPD similar to control subjects for nonmonetary losses; FRN ↓ with increased impulsivity	Enhanced reactivity to monetary reward or losses in ASPD? (data are very preliminary but suggestive)

Hypoarousal may underlie deficits in other executive functions suggested by smaller amplitudes of the CNV, MMN, N2, and ERN with higher impulsivity or antisocial features. These outcomes indicate insufficient preparation for upcoming responses (CNV), insufficient inhibition of competing information or responses (N2), insufficient allocation of attention to contextually salient information (MMN, P3), and insufficient detection of contextually inappropriate information (ERN). These deficiencies may predispose to insufficient protection of eliciting responses to irrelevant information or to events that must not be responded to, such as being cut off in traffic. Insufficient executive functioning may also predispose to insufficient processing of warning signals related to possible negative consequences, including possible serious harm.

In addition to impaired executive functioning, we discussed studies showing that ASPD could be associated with deficient preattentional and early attentional filtering of information. This is suggested by changes in P50 and N1 gating-related ERPs. Interestingly, the studies consistently found no differences between groups with and without ASPD, but they did find more deficient gating with more severe ASPD, antisocial features, or impulsivity. These outcomes suggest that ASPD is a disorder that goes beyond deficient executive functioning and that these deficits in executive functioning could have their origin in deficient preattentional processes. Deficits in early filtering of information could result in increased mental noise in the form of context-irrelevant information and insufficient neuronal gain of context-relevant information. This, in consequence, could consume resources to 1) further suppress irrelevant information, 2) process irrelevant information, and 3) boost neuronal gain for relevant information. A result could be a reduction in resources for other functions and a disposition to continue antisocial actions.

However, changes in executive functioning in ASPD appear to be modulated by the motivational context. In motivational contexts, attentional processes appear unaffected or even amplified in ASPD and conduct disorder as shown by the P3, LPP, and FRN. This may lead to overreactions to emotional events. In both nonemotional and emotional contexts, however, inappropriate actions are not eliminated, although specific mechanisms may differ. This underscores the need to study effects of motivation when examining neurobiological correlates of ASPD. Thus, diminished resources for executive functioning may not be a static state in ASPD but in all likelihood change dynamically depending on context and perhaps change dynamically depending on time of day, sleeping behavior, and other external events.

In summary, ASPD and conduct disorder are related to impaired prefrontal control over sensory, cognitive, and behavioral processes, potentially overcome by engagement of motivation. In addition, there may be a change in the relationship between preconscious and postawareness processes. All these aspects may be related to physiological underarousal, although instead of antisocial or high-risk behaviors being an expression to enhance low arousal, those behaviors could be an expression of underarousal itself independent of possible consequences on arousal state. However, neurophysiological research in the important area of motivational processes in ASPD and conduct disorder outside the context of psychopathy is still at an early stage.

Key Points

- More severe antisocial personality disorder (ASPD) has been associated with deficient preattentional and early attentional filtering of information, perhaps predisposing to extra noise during information processing and difficulty selecting actions.

- ASPD has been associated with deficient higher-order cognitive functioning and impaired feedback from negative consequences, perhaps predisposing to poor attention, response inhibition, and learning.

- Deficient higher-order processing found in ASPD research appears to be related in part to low motivation of research subjects and to low-arousal stimuli; high-arousal events could result in impulsive actions.

- Outcomes appear to confirm in part the hypoarousal theory of ASPD.

References

American Psychiatric Association: Diagnostic and Statistical Manual of Mental Disorders, 3rd Edition, Revised. Washington, DC, American Psychiatric Association, 1987

American Psychiatric Association: Diagnostic and Statistical Manual of Mental Disorders, 4th Edition. Washington, DC, American Psychiatric Association, 1994

American Psychiatric Association: Diagnostic and Statistical Manual of Mental Disorders, 5th Edition. Arlington, VA, American Psychiatric Association, 2013

Bachman MD, Bernat EM: Independent contributions of theta and delta time-frequency activity to the visual oddball P3b. Int J Psychophysiol 128:70–80, 2018 29574233

Barratt ES, Pritchard WS, Faulk DM, et al: The relationship between impulsiveness subtraits, trait anxiety, and visual N100 augmenting/reducing: a topographic analysis. Pers Individ Dif 8:43–51, 1987

Barratt ES, Lijffijt M, Moeller FG: When does impulsivity become pathologic? Psychiatric Times 22:23–26, 2005

Bauer LO: Antisocial personality disorder and cocaine dependence: their effects on behavioral and electroencephalographic measures of time estimation. Drug Alcohol Depend 63(1):87–95, 2001 11297834

Bernat EM, Nelson LD, Baskin-Sommers AR: Time-frequency theta and delta measures index separable components of feedback processing in a gambling task. Psychophysiology 52(5):626–637, 2015 25581491

Black DW, Gunter T, Loveless P, et al: Antisocial personality disorder in incarcerated offenders: psychiatric comorbidity and quality of life. Ann Clin Psychiatry 22(2):113–120, 2010 20445838

Blenner JL, Yingling CD: Effects of prefrontal cortex lesions on visual evoked potential augmenting/reducing. Int J Neurosci 78(3–4):145–156, 1994 7883451

Bresin K, Finy MS, Sprague J, et al: Response monitoring and adjustment: differential relations with psychopathic traits. J Abnorm Psychol 123(3):634–649, 2014 24933282

Buzsáki G, Draguhn A: Neuronal oscillations in cortical networks. Science 304(5679):1926–1929, 2004 15218136

Calzada-Reyes A, Alvarez-Amador A, Galán-García L, et al: Electroencephalographic abnormalities in antisocial personality disorder. J Forensic Leg Med 19(1):29–34, 2012 22152445

Calzada-Reyes A, Alvarez-Amador A, Galán-García L, et al: EEG abnormalities in psychopath and non-psychopath violent offenders. J Forensic Leg Med 20(1):19–26, 2013 23217372

Calzada-Reyes A, Alvarez-Amador A, Galán-García L, et al: QEEG and LORETA in teenagers with conduct disorder and psychopathic traits. Clin EEG Neurosci 48(3):189–199, 2017 27272168

Carlson SR, Thái S: ERPs on a continuous performance task and self-reported psychopathic traits: P3 and CNV augmentation are associated with Fearless Dominance. Biol Psychol 85(2):318–330, 2010 20723576

Choi JW, Lee JK, Ko D, et al: Fronto-temporal interactions in the theta-band during auditory deviant processing. Neurosci Lett 548:120–125, 2013 23769731

Cohen MX: Analyzing Neural Time Series Data: Theory and Practice. Cambridge, MA, MIT Press, 2014

Coid J, Ullrich S: Antisocial personality disorder is on a continuum with psychopathy. Compr Psychiatry 51(4):426–433, 2010 20579518

Cuthbert BN, Schupp HT, Bradley MM, et al: Brain potentials in affective picture processing: covariation with autonomic arousal and affective report. Biol Psychol 52(2):95–111, 2000 10699350

De Brito SA, Viding E, Kumari V, et al: Cool and hot executive function impairments in violent offenders with antisocial personality disorder with and without psychopathy. PLoS One 8(6):e65566, 2013 23840340

de la Salle S, Shah D, Choueiry J, et al: NMDA receptor antagonist effects on speech-related mismatch negativity and its underlying oscillatory and source activity in healthy humans. Front Pharmacol 10:455, 2019 31139075

Decuyper M, De Pauw S, De Fruyt F, et al: A meta-analysis of psychopathy-, antisocial PD- and FFM associations: MA review on PP, APD and FFM. European Journal of Personality 23(7):531–565, 2009

Dennis TA, Hajcak G: The late positive potential: a neurophysiological marker for emotion regulation in children. J Child Psychol Psychiatry 50(11):1373–1383, 2009 19754501

Dougherty DM: IMT/DMT Immediate Memory Task and Delayed Memory Task: A Research Tool for Studying Attention and Memory Processes. Houston, University of Texas Medical Science Center, 1999

Dougherty DM, Bjork JM, Marsh DM, et al: A comparison between adults with conduct disorder and normal controls on a continuous performance test: differences in impulsive response characteristics. The Psychological Record 50:203–219, 2000

Dougherty DM, Bjork JM, Harper RA, et al: Behavioral impulsivity paradigms: a comparison in hospitalized adolescents with disruptive behavior disorders. J Child Psychol Psychiatry 44(8):1145–1157, 2003 14626456

Drislane LE, Vaidyanathan U, Patrick CJ: Reduced cortical call to arms differentiates psychopathy from antisocial personality disorder. Psychol Med 43(4):825–835, 2013 22850322

Elton M, Spaan M, Ridderinkhof KR: Why do we produce errors of commission? An ERP study of stimulus deviance detection and error monitoring in a choice go/no-go task. Eur J Neurosci 20(7):1960–1968, 2004 15380019

Fabiani M, Gratton G, Federmeier KD: Event related brain potentials: methods, theory, and applications, in Handbook of Psychophysiology, 3rd Edition. Edited by Cacioppo J, Tassinary LG, Berntson GG. New York, Cambridge University Press, 2007, pp 53–84

Falkenstein M, Hoormann J, Christ S, et al: ERP components on reaction errors and their functional significance: a tutorial. Biol Psychol 51(2–3):87–107, 2000 10686361

Fenton GW, Fenwick PB, Ferguson W, et al: The contingent negative variation in antisocial behaviour: a pilot study of Broadmoor patients. Br J Psychiatry 132:368–377, 1978 638390

Forth AE, Hare RD: The contingent negative variation in psychopaths. Psychophysiology 26(6):676–682, 1989 2629015

Franken IHA, Nijs I, Van Strien JW: Impulsivity affects mismatch negativity (MMN) measures of preattentive auditory processing. Biol Psychol 70(3):161–167, 2005 16242534

Freedman R, Waldo M, Bickford-Wimer P, et al: Elementary neuronal dysfunctions in schizophrenia. Schizophr Res 4(2):233–243, 1991 1645590

Fries P: Rhythms for cognition: communication through coherence. Neuron 88(1):220–235, 2015 26447583

Fruhstorfer H, Soveri P, Järvilehto T: Short-term habituation of the auditory evoked response in man. Electroencephalogr Clin Neurophysiol 28(2):153–161, 1970 4189933

Fuentemilla L, Marco-Pallarés J, Münte TF, et al: Theta EEG oscillatory activity and auditory change detection. Brain Res 1220:93–101, 2008 18076870

Fuertes-Saiz A, Benito A, Mateu C, et al: Sensorimotor gating in cocaine-related disorder with comorbid schizophrenia or antisocial personality disorder. J Dual Diagn 15(4):243–253, 2019 31287382

Gao Y, Raine A: P3 event-related potential impairments in antisocial and psychopathic individuals: a meta-analysis. Biol Psychol 82(3):199–210, 2009 19576948

Garrido MI, Kilner JM, Stephan KE, et al: The mismatch negativity: a review of underlying mechanisms. Clin Neurophysiol 120(3):453–463, 2009 19181570

Glazer JE, Kelley NJ, Pornpattananangkul N, et al: Beyond the FRN: broadening the time-course of EEG and ERP components implicated in reward processing. Int J Psychophysiol 132(pt B):184–202, 2018 29454641

Goldstein RB, Chou SP, Saha TD, et al: The epidemiology of antisocial behavioral syndromes in adulthood: results from the National Epidemiologic Survey on Alcohol and Related Conditions-III. J Clin Psychiatry 78(1):90–98, 2017 27035627

Gray NS, Weidacker K, Snowden RJ: Psychopathy and impulsivity: the relationship of psychopathy to different aspects of UPPS-P impulsivity. Psychiatry Res 272:474–482, 2019 30611967

Hajcak G, Dunning JP, Foti D: Motivated and controlled attention to emotion: time-course of the late positive potential. Clin Neurophysiol 120(3):505–510, 2009 19157974

Hajcak G, MacNamara A, Olvet DM: Event-related potentials, emotion, and emotion regulation: an integrative review. Dev Neuropsychol 35(2):129–155, 2010 20390599

Hall JR, Bernat EM, Patrick CJ: Externalizing psychopathology and the error-related negativity. Psychol Sci 18(4):326–333, 2007 17470258

Hare RD: Manual for the Revised Psychopathy Checklist, 2nd Edition. Toronto, ON, Canada, Multi-Health Systems, 2003

Harmony T: The functional significance of delta oscillations in cognitive processing. Front Integr Neurosci 7:83, 2013 24367301

Holroyd CB, Coles MGH: The neural basis of human error processing: reinforcement learning, dopamine, and the error-related negativity. Psychol Rev 109(4):679–709, 2002 12374324

Honda S, Matsumoto M, Tajinda K, et al: Enhancing clinical trials through synergistic gamma power analysis. Front Psychiatry 11:537, 2020 32587536

Howard RC, Fenton GW, Fenwick PB: The contingent negative variation, personality and antisocial behaviour. Br J Psychiatry 144:463–474, 1984 6733370

Hoyniak CP, Petersen IT: A meta-analytic evaluation of the N2 component as an endophenotype of response inhibition and externalizing psychopathology in childhood. Neurosci Biobehav Rev 103:200–215, 2019 31201831

Hung A-Y, Ahveninen J, Cheng Y: Atypical mismatch negativity to distressful voices associated with conduct disorder symptoms. J Child Psychol Psychiatry 54(9):1016–1027, 2013 23701279

Huster RJ, Enriquez-Geppert S, Lavallee CF, et al: Electroencephalography of response inhibition tasks: functional networks and cognitive contributions. Int J Psychophysiol 87(3):217–233, 2013 22906815

Jaworska N, Blondeau C, Tessier P, et al: Response prediction to antidepressants using scalp and source-localized loudness dependence of auditory evoked potential (LDAEP) slopes. Prog Neuropsychopharmacol Biol Psychiatry 44:100–107, 2013 23360662

Juckel G, Hegerl U: Evoked potentials, serotonin, and suicidality. Pharmacopsychiatry 27 (suppl 1):27–29, 1994 7984696

Kalfaoğlu Ç, Stafford T, Milne E: Frontal theta band oscillations predict error correction and posterior slowing in typing. J Exp Psychol Hum Percept Perform 44(1):69–88, 2018 28447844

Kessel EM, Meyer A, Hajcak G, et al: Transdiagnostic factors and pathways to multifinality: the error-related negativity predicts whether preschool irritability is associated with internalizing versus externalizing symptoms at age 9. Dev Psychopathol 28(4 pt 1):913–926, 2016 27739383

Kirmizi-Alsan E, Bayraktaroglu Z, Gurvit H, et al: Comparative analysis of event-related potentials during Go/NoGo and CPT: decomposition of electrophysiological markers of response inhibition and sustained attention. Brain Res 1104(1):114–128, 2006 16824492

Kirschstein T, Köhling R: What is the source of the EEG? Clin EEG Neurosci 40(3):146–149, 2009 19715175

Knyazev GG: EEG correlates of personality types. Netherlands Journal of Psychology 62:81–92, 2006

Knyazev GG: Motivation, emotion, and their inhibitory control mirrored in brain oscillations. Neurosci Biobehav Rev 31(3):377–395, 2007 17145079

Knyazev GG, Slobodskaya HR, Aftanas LI, et al: EEG correlates of emotional problems and conduct disorder in schoolchildren. Human Physiology 28:263–268, 2002a

Knyazev GG, Slobodskaya HR, Wilson GD: Psychophysiological correlates of behavioural inhibition and activation. Pers Individ Dif 33(4):647–660, 2002b

Kumari V, Das M, Hodgins S, et al: Association between violent behaviour and impaired prepulse inhibition of the startle response in antisocial personality disorder and schizophrenia. Behav Brain Res 158(1):159–166, 2005 15680203

Lang PJ, Bradley MM, Cuthbert BN: International Affective Picture System (IAPS): Affective Ratings of Pictures and Instruction Manual: Technical Report. Gainesville, University of Florida, 2008

Lijffijt M, Swann AC, Moeller FG: Biological substrate of personality traits associated with aggression, in The SAGE Handbook of Personality Theory and Assessment: Volume 1—Personality Theories and Models. Edited by Boyle GJ, Matthews G, Saklofske DH. Thousand Oaks, CA, Sage, 2008, pp 334–356

Lijffijt M, Lane SD, Meier SL, et al: P50, N100, and P200 sensory gating: relationships with behavioral inhibition, attention, and working memory. Psychophysiology 46(5):1059–1068, 2009 19515106

Lijffijt M, Cox B, Acas MD, et al: Differential relationships of impulsivity or antisocial symptoms on P50, N100, or P200 auditory sensory gating in controls and antisocial personality disorder. J Psychiatr Res 46(6):743–750, 2012 22464943

Lijffijt M, Lane SD, Moeller FG, et al: Trait impulsivity and increased pre-attentional sensitivity to intense stimuli in bipolar disorder and controls. J Psychiatr Res 60:73–80, 2015 25455512

Lijffijt M, Lane SD, Mathew SJ, et al: Heightened early attentional stimulus orienting and impulsive action in men with antisocial personality disorder. Eur Arch Psychiatry Clin Neurosci 267(7):697–707, 2017 27662886

Liu T, Xiao T, Shi J: Response inhibition, preattentive processing, and sex difference in young children: an event-related potential study. Neuroreport 24(3):126–130, 2013 23262505

Liu Y, Shen X, Zhu Y, et al: Mismatch negativity in paranoid, schizotypal, and antisocial personality disorders. Neurophysiol Clin 37(2):89–96, 2007 17540291

Liu Y, Huang H, McGinnis-Deweese M, et al: Neural substrate of the late positive potential in emotional processing. J Neurosci 32(42):14563–14572, 2012 23077042

Maurer JM, Steele VR, Cope LM, et al: Dysfunctional error-related processing in incarcerated youth with elevated psychopathic traits. Dev Cogn Neurosci 19:70–77, 2016a 26930170

Maurer JM, Steele VR, Edwards BG, et al: Dysfunctional error-related processing in female psychopathy. Soc Cogn Affect Neurosci 11(7):1059–1068, 2016b 26060326

Moeller FG, Barratt ES, Dougherty DM, et al: Psychiatric aspects of impulsivity. Am J Psychiatry 158(11):1783–1793, 2001 11691682

Näätänen R: Attention and Brain Function. Hillsdale, NJ, Erlbaum, 1992

Näätänen R, Kujala T, Winkler I: Auditory processing that leads to conscious perception: a unique window to central auditory processing opened by the mismatch negativity and related responses. Psychophysiology 48(1):4–22, 2011 20880261

Nagai Y, Critchley HD, Featherstone E, et al: Brain activity relating to the contingent negative variation: an fMRI investigation. Neuroimage 21(4):1232–1241, 2004 15050551

Nieuwenhuis S, Aston-Jones G, Cohen JD: Decision making, the P3, and the locus coeruleus-norepinephrine system. Psychol Bull 131(4):510–532, 2005 16060800

Nieuwenhuis S, De Geus EJ, Aston-Jones G: The anatomical and functional relationship between the P3 and autonomic components of the orienting response. Psychophysiology 48(2):162–175, 2011 20557480

Ogloff JRP: Psychopathy/antisocial personality disorder conundrum. Aust N Z J Psychiatry 40(6–7):519–528, 2006 16756576

O'Neill BV, Guille V, Croft RJ, et al: Effects of selective and combined serotonin and dopamine depletion on the loudness dependence of the auditory evoked potential (LDAEP) in humans. Hum Psychopharmacol 23(4):301–312, 2008 18213738

Pasion R, Barbosa F: ERN as a transdiagnostic marker of the internalizing-externalizing spectrum: a dissociable meta-analytic effect. Neurosci Biobehav Rev 103:133–149, 2019 31220503

Pasion R, Fernandes C, Pereira MR, et al: Antisocial behaviour and psychopathy: uncovering the externalizing link in the P3 modulation. Neurosci Biobehav Rev 91:170–186, 2018 28342766

Pasion R, Prata C, Fernandes M, et al: N2 amplitude modulation across the antisocial spectrum: a meta-analysis. Rev Neurosci 30(7):781–794, 2019 30954973

Patrick CJ: Physiological correlates of psychopathy, antisocial personality disorder, habitual aggression, and violence. Curr Top Behav Neurosci 21:197–227, 2014 25129139

Patton JH, Stanford MS, Barratt ES: Factor structure of the Barratt impulsiveness scale. J Clin Psychol 51(6):768–774, 1995 8778124

Pfabigan DM, Alexopoulos J, Bauer H, et al: All about the money—external performance monitoring is affected by monetary, but not by socially conveyed feedback cues in more antisocial individuals. Front Hum Neurosci 5:100, 2011 21960967

Pincham HL, Bryce D, Kokorikou D, et al: Psychosocial intervention is associated with altered emotion processing: an event-related potential study in at-risk adolescents. PLoS One 11(1):e0147357, 2016 26808519

Polich J: Updating P300: an integrative theory of P3a and P3b. Clin Neurophysiol 118(10):2128–2148, 2007 17573239

Potts GF, George MRM, Martin LE, et al: Reduced punishment sensitivity in neural systems of behavior monitoring in impulsive individuals. Neurosci Lett 397(1–2):130–134, 2006 16378683

Prescott J, Connolly JF, Gruzelier JH: The augmenting/reducing phenomenon in the auditory evoked potential. Biol Psychol 19(1):31–44, 1984 6478002

Quay HC: Psychopathic personality as pathological stimulation-seeking. Am J Psychiatry 122:180–183, 1965 14313433

Raine A: Annotation: the role of prefrontal deficits, low autonomic arousal, and early health factors in the development of antisocial and aggressive behavior in children. J Child Psychol Psychiatry 43(4):417–434, 2002 12030589

Raine A: The neuromoral theory of antisocial, violent, and psychopathic behavior. Psychiatry Res 277:64–69, 2019 30473129

Raine A, Venables PH, Williams M: Relationships between N1, P300, and contingent negative variation recorded at age 15 and criminal behavior at age 24. Psychophysiology 27(5):567–574, 1990 2274620

Reyes AC, Amador AA: Qualitative and quantitative EEG abnormalities in violent offenders with antisocial personality disorder. J Forensic Leg Med 16(2):59–63, 2009 19134998

Ridderinkhof KR, Ullsperger M, Crone EA, et al: The role of the medial frontal cortex in cognitive control. Science 306(5695):443–447, 2004a 15486290

Ridderinkhof KR, van den Wildenberg WPM, Segalowitz SJ, et al: Neurocognitive mechanisms of cognitive control: the role of prefrontal cortex in action selection, response inhibition, performance monitoring, and reward-based learning. Brain Cogn 56(2):129–140, 2004b 15518930

Rinne T, Särkkä A, Degerman A, et al: Two separate mechanisms underlie auditory change detection and involuntary control of attention. Brain Res 1077(1):135–143, 2006 16487946

Röhl M, Uppenkamp S: An auditory fMRI correlate of impulsivity. Psychiatry Res 181(2):145–150, 2010 20083394

Rozalski V, Benning SD: Divergences among three higher-order self-report psychopathology factors in normal-range personality and emotional late positive potential reactivity. J Res Pers 82:103861, 2019 32863467

Ruchsow M, Spitzer M, Grön G, et al: Error processing and impulsiveness in normals: evidence from event-related potentials. Brain Res Cogn Brain Res 24(2):317–325, 2005 15993769

Rudo-Hutt AS: Electroencephalography and externalizing behavior: a meta-analysis. Biol Psychol 105:1–19, 2015 25528418

Sabatinelli D, Lang PJ, Keil A, et al: Emotional perception: correlation of functional MRI and event-related potentials. Cereb Cortex 17(5):1085–1091, 2007 16769742

Sabatinelli D, Keil A, Frank DW, et al: Emotional perception: correspondence of early and late event-related potentials with cortical and subcortical functional MRI. Biol Psychol 92(3):513–519, 2013 22560889

Satterfield JH, Dawson ME: Electrodermal correlates of hyperactivity in children. Psychophysiology 8(2):191–197, 1971 5089415

Sawada M, Negoro H, Iida J, et al: Pervasive developmental disorder with attention deficit hyperactivity disorder-like symptoms and mismatch negativity. Psychiatry Clin Neurosci 62(4):479–481, 2008 18778448

Schupp HT, Junghöfer M, Weike AI, et al: The selective processing of briefly presented affective pictures: an ERP analysis. Psychophysiology 41(3):441–449, 2004 15102130

Sedgwick O, Young S, Greer B, et al: Sensorimotor gating characteristics of violent men with comorbid psychosis and dissocial personality disorder: relationship with antisocial traits and psychosocial deprivation. Schizophr Res 198:21–27, 2018 28689756

Shimano S, Onitsuka T, Oribe N, et al: Preattentive dysfunction in patients with bipolar disorder as revealed by the pitch-mismatch negativity: a magnetoencephalography (MEG) study. Bipolar Disord 16(6):592–599, 2014 24807680

Smit CM: Automatic detection of visual change: an analysis of visual mismatch and its relation to impulsivity. Doctoral thesis, University of Trier, Germany, 2008

Snowden RJ, Gray NS: Impulsivity and psychopathy: associations between the Barrett Impulsivity Scale and the Psychopathy Checklist Revised. Psychiatry Res 187(3):414–417, 2011 21377739

Swann AC, Lijffijt M, Lane SD, et al: Trait impulsivity and response inhibition in antisocial personality disorder. J Psychiatr Res 43(12):1057–1063, 2009a 19345957

Swann AC, Lijffijt M, Lane SD, et al: Severity of bipolar disorder is associated with impairment of response inhibition. J Affect Disord 116(1–2):30–36, 2009b 19038460

Swann AC, Lijffijt M, Lane SD, et al: Criminal conviction, impulsivity, and course of illness in bipolar disorder. Bipolar Disord 13(2):173–181, 2011 21443571

Taylor JB, Visser TAW, Fueggle SN, et al: The error-related negativity (ERN) is an electrophysiological marker of motor impulsiveness on the Barratt Impulsiveness Scale (BIS-11) during adolescence. Dev Cogn Neurosci 30:77–86, 2018 29353681

Thaerig S, Behne N, Schadow J, et al: Sound level dependence of auditory evoked potentials: simultaneous EEG recording and low-noise fMRI. Int J Psychophysiol 67(3):235–241, 2008 17707939

Trujillo LT, Allen JJB: Theta EEG dynamics of the error-related negativity. Clin Neurophysiol 118(3):645–668, 2007 17223380

Vallet W, Hone-Blanchet A, Brunelin J: Abnormalities of the late positive potential during emotional processing in individuals with psychopathic traits: a meta-analysis. Psychol Med 50(12):2085–2095, 2020 31477196

van Goozen SHM, Fairchild G: How can the study of biological processes help design new interventions for children with severe antisocial behavior? Dev Psychopathol 20(3):941–973, 2008 18606039

Venables NC, Hall JR, Yancey JR, et al: Factors of psychopathy and electrocortical response to emotional pictures: further evidence for a two-process theory. J Abnorm Psychol 124(2):319–328, 2015 25603361

Verona E, Sprague J, Sadeh N: Inhibitory control and negative emotional processing in psychopathy and antisocial personality disorder. J Abnorm Psychol 121(2):498–510, 2012 22288907

Vilà-Balló A, Cunillera T, Rostan C, et al: Neurophysiological correlates of cognitive flexibility and feedback processing in violent juvenile offenders. Brain Res 1610:98–109, 2015 25839762

von Stein A, Chiang C, König P: Top-down processing mediated by interareal synchronization. Proc Natl Acad Sci USA 97(26):14748–14753, 2000 11121074

Wan L, Friedman BH, Boutros NN, et al: P50 sensory gating and attentional performance. Int J Psychophysiol 67(2):91–100, 2008 18036692

Wang W, Zhu SZ, Pan LC, et al: Mismatch negativity and personality traits in chronic primary insomniacs. Funct Neurol 16(1):3–10, 2001 11396269

White HR, Bates ME, Buyske S: Adolescence-limited versus persistent delinquency: extending Moffitt's hypothesis into adulthood. J Abnorm Psychol 110(4):600–609, 2001 11727949

Wild-Wall N, Hohnsbein J, Falkenstein M: Effects of ageing on cognitive task preparation as reflected by event-related potentials. Clin Neurophysiol 118(3):558–569, 2007 17208044

Williams RS, Kudus F, Dyson BJ, Spaniol J: Transient and sustained incentive effects on electrophysiological indices of cognitive control in younger and older adults. Cogn Affect Behav Neurosci 18(2):313–330, 2018 29392645

Yang Y, Raine A: Prefrontal structural and functional brain imaging findings in antisocial, violent, and psychopathic individuals: a meta-analysis. Psychiatry Res 174(2):81–88, 2009 19833485

CHAPTER 12

Central and Peripheral Biomarkers of Antisocial Personality Disorder

Laura Dellazizzo, M.Sc.

Alexandre Dumais, M.D., Ph.D., FRCPC

Antisocial personality disorder (ASPD) is a chronic psychological condition characterized by a disregard for social norms, a short tolerance for frustration, impulsivity, manipulative behavior, and lack of remorse (Mendez 2009). ASPD applies to adults older than 18 years, although it does require the presence of a diagnosis of conduct disorder prior to age 15 years (American Psychiatric Association 2013). As a general developmental trajectory, individuals with ASPD show signs of conduct problems in youth (e.g., disruptive in school, bullying, physically aggressive) (Farrington and Coid 2003; Fergusson et al. 2005; Moffitt and Caspi 2001). Different subtypes of youths who may go on to develop ASPD have been observed, some with more severe behavioral profiles resulting from the presence of comorbidity with other mental health problems, such as psychopathic traits (e.g., callous-unemotional traits), internalizing symptoms (e.g., anxiety, depression), and ADHD symptoms (e.g., hyperactivity, impulsivity) (Fanti and Henrich 2010; Frick et al. 2014; Lynam 1996). Moreover, as some of these young individuals grow older, they will continue on trajectories associated with further adverse antisocial behaviors (e.g., substance use, involvement in criminal activities, violence) (Beauchaine and McNulty 2013; Niemelä et al. 2008). ASPD is thus a diagnosis especially prone to heterogeneity, with several subtypes having been identified that encompass differences in symptomatic severity, patterns of comorbidity (e.g., psychopathy, mood disorders, substance use disorders), and risk factors (e.g., genetics, environmental factors) (Cox et al. 2013; Glenn et al. 2013; Goldstein et al. 2006; Jones and Westen 2010; McKinley et al. 2018). Because of the important societal consequences of ASPD, there has been growing interest in the biological basis of antisocial behavior and ASPD (Portnoy and Farrington 2015).

Several physiological studies of ASPD and related conditions (e.g., psychopathy) have been informative to advance our understanding of potential biomarkers (Frick et al. 2014; Insel et al. 2010). Two main theories of ASPD and physiological markers have been proposed: the fearlessness theory and the sensation-seeking theory. The fearlessness theory states that the neurobiological systems that process information related to threat (e.g., amygdala and prefrontal cortex) function less effectively (van Goozen and Fairchild 2008). Antisocial individuals, who can be considered fearless, are therefore physiologically underaroused and less sensitive to stress as well as punishment (Raine 1996). Moreover, they will be less inhibited toward engaging in aggressive and antisocial behavior (Raine 2013). The sensation-seeking theory suggests that a sufficient level of arousal or stress is required for individuals to feel pleasantness. Low arousal, in this case, implies an aversive state. Individuals with long-lasting underarousal are believed to pursue physiological stimulation through aggressive and antisocial behavior to counter such undesirable states (Zuckerman 2014).

The principal systems involved in processing and regulating stress and negative emotions (e.g., anxiety) are the neuroendocrine hypothalamic-pituitary-adrenal (HPA) axis, with its end-product cortisol, and the autonomic nervous system (ANS), measured, for instance, by skin conductance and heart rate (van Goozen 2015). These physiological systems have implications to potentiate the state of fear, generate sensitivity to punishment, and induce withdrawal behavior (Schulkin et al. 1998). Because antisocial individuals have deficits in these functions, it has been suggested that the HPA axis and the ANS may be hypoactive (Schulkin et al. 1998). Another endocrine system that has shown a relation with antisociality is the hypothalamic-pituitary-gonadal (HPG) axis, with its end-product testosterone (Archer et al. 2005; Dabbs et al. 1991; Daitzman and Zuckerman 1980).

In this chapter, we review findings on the potential biomarkers of ASPD (see Figure 12–1 for a summary of implicated biomarkers). We also specify trait-based outcomes (e.g., callous-unemotional traits, aggression) in addition to related conditions (e.g., conduct problems, psychopathy) because increasing evidence has defined ASPD as being a heterogeneous condition. While there is no optimal way to clarify this heterogeneity, considering patterns/profiles related to more homogeneous variants and clinical features may bring us closer to unraveling the biomarker basis of ASPD rather than viewing biomarkers of an exclusive operationalized diagnosis. We describe evidence not only from adult literature but also from youth literature because abnormalities in physiological biomarkers may be evident early in life in individuals who may later develop a diagnosis of ASPD. This evidence may have the potential to shed light on the developmental mechanisms leading to ASPD as well as aid in the identification of individuals at risk for ASPD.

Endocrine Systems

Hypothalamic-Pituitary-Adrenal Axis

Extensive research on antisociality in youths and adults has been centered on the HPA axis, which is a central component of the stress system. The HPA axis involves a succession of connections with the hypothalamus, pituitary gland, and adrenal glands,

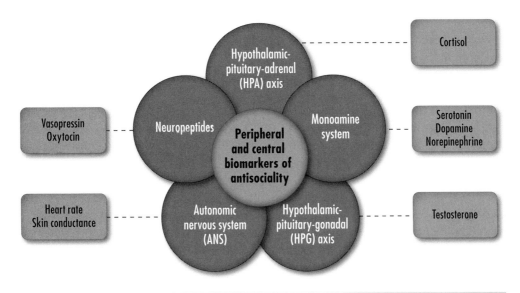

FIGURE 12–1. Summary of potential biomarkers associated with antisocial personality disorder.

which terminates with the secretion of cortisol and other hormones (e.g., epinephrine) (Liening and Josephs 2010). During stressful periods and in certain psychiatric disorders, the paraventricular nucleus of the hypothalamus releases corticotropin-releasing hormone (CRH), which stimulates the anterior pituitary to secrete adrenocorticotropic hormone (ACTH) into the bloodstream. In response to the secretion of ACTH, the adrenal cortex secretes cortisol and other glucocorticoids (Hawes et al. 2009; Kudielka and Kirschbaum 2005). The HPA axis is also controlled by negative feedback regulation to normalize the secretion of cortisol, wherein cortisol secretion inhibits the release of CRH and ACTH (Kudielka and Kirschbaum 2005; Tsigos and Chrousos 2002). Notably, the HPA axis has a diurnal circadian rhythm, with cortisol levels being at their highest in the morning and then diminishing afterward throughout the day (Deuschle et al. 1997). Abnormalities in the HPA axis in relation to ASPD and related conditions have been reported in several studies that are discussed later in this chapter.

Literature has largely focused on salivary measures of cortisol, both basal cortisol and cortisol reactivity to a stressor (see Fairchild et al. 2018 for a review). Given that cortisol is tightly associated with the limbic system and is involved in the potentiation of fear, it is a key biomarker for deficits in stress and fear response (Schulkin 2003). Whereas limited studies have noted increased cortisol levels in antisocial populations (e.g., Barzman et al. 2013; Lopez-Duran et al. 2009; van Bokhoven et al. 2005b), most literature has shown low levels of cortisol associated with several constructs related to ASPD such as total aggression measures (Horn et al. 2014; McBurnett et al. 2000; Platje et al. 2013a, 2013b; Poustka et al. 2010; van de Wiel et al. 2004; Yu and Shi 2009), reactive and proactive aggression (Poustka et al. 2010; Stoppelbein et al. 2014), conduct disorder (Oosterlaan et al. 2005; Pajer et al. 2001), and oppositional defiant disorder (van Goozen et al. 1998). It may be expected that lower levels of cortisol are particularly related to more severe forms of behavior problems (Mitchell et al. 2002; O'Brien and Frick 1996; van Honk et al. 2003). The inconsistencies between studies may, nevertheless, reflect the heterogeneity of antisocial samples and methodological divergences, with studies having different operationalizations of antisocial conduct or disorder as well as methods to measure their constructs, settings (e.g., community samples, clinical samples, forensic samples), age range, and means of assessment of cortisol (e.g., timing, frequency, method) (Feilhauer et al. 2013).

Studies focusing on children and adolescents who may go on to develop ASPD have mainly observed a negative relationship between basal or stress-induced cortisol levels and antisocial behavior, which appears to be strongest in clinically referred samples (Fairchild et al. 2018). A meta-analysis consisting of 82 studies in children and adolescents showed that the association between low basal cortisol levels and antisocial behavior problems was relatively weak but nonetheless significant (Cohen's d=0.10) (Alink et al. 2008). However, cortisol reactivity was not consistently related to externalizing behavior problems (Alink et al. 2008). Basal cortisol secretion and cortisol reactivity to stress may be altered equally in both childhood-onset and adolescent-onset subtypes of conduct disorder (Fairchild et al. 2008; Haltigan et al. 2011). Notably, chronic and more severe aggressive and antisocial behavior has been linked to low cortisol (Matthys et al. 2004; McBurnett et al. 1996, 2000; Popma et al. 2006; van de Wiel et al. 2004). Evidence has suggested that low cortisol was a predictor of persistent antisocial behavior, such as aggression (McBurnett et al. 2000; Platje et al. 2013a; Ruttle et al. 2011; Salis et al. 2016; Shoal et al. 2003). Furthermore, a limited number of studies have examined specific dimensions of antisocial personality traits in youths, such as callous-unemotional traits (see Hawes et al. 2009 for a review). Whereas a general association between these traits and low cortisol levels has been observed in samples from the general population and detained youths (Burke et al. 2007; Holi et al. 2006; Loney et al. 2006; O'Leary et al. 2007, 2010), some authors have failed to find an association between callous-unemotional traits and cortisol levels (Feilhauer et al. 2013; Poustka et al. 2010). These latter authors, however, found that low basal cortisol level was related to impulsivity (Feilhauer et al. 2013; Poustka et al. 2010). As Feilhauer and colleagues (2013) suggested, low basal cortisol levels may be more related to overall deficits in behavioral regulation (i.e., poor impulse-control and aggressive-impulsive behavior) than to callous-unemotional traits. Noteworthy, the relationship between the HPA axis and antisocial traits or behavior may be more complicated and moderated by other factors, such as gender, perinatal risk factors, and comorbidity with internalizing difficulties (Marsman et al. 2008, 2009, 2012). In addition, because individuals with ASPD have frequently experienced traumatic events (e.g., abuse, neglect, violence) early in life (DeLisi et al. 2019), there are indications that such stressful circumstances may have an essential role in defining the HPA axis at an earlier age (Aggarwal 2013; Bremne and Vermetten 2001). Habituation to stressful events may lead to low cortisol release and stress reactivity, which has been found in antisocial youths (van Goozen et al. 2000). Hence, low levels of cortisol in youths may be a contributing biomarker for the development of ASPD in adulthood (Aggarwal 2013).

As for antisocial adults, not all studies have shown consistent findings (van Honk et al. 2003). Some studies have indeed described similar patterns to youth literature with low cortisol levels being associated with antisocial behavior and psychopathy

(Susman 2006; Virkkunen 1985; Woodman et al. 1978). For instance, offenders with psychopathy have shown lower daytime levels of cortisol relative to those without psychopathy (Cima et al. 2008). Men with high psychopathy scores also had lower cortisol reactivity to a typical psychosocial stressor when compared with individuals with low psychopathic traits (O'Leary et al. 2007, 2010; Shirtcliff et al. 2009). These low levels of cortisol in samples with higher psychopathic traits suggest hypoactivity of the HPA axis, which may support neuroimaging literature that shows deficits in brain responding to aversive or stressful stimuli in individuals with high psychopathic traits (e.g., reduced prefrontal, temporal, amygdala, and anterior cingulate activation) (Darby 2018; DeLisi and Vaughn 2014; Raine 2019). This hypoactivity may predispose an individual to be insensitive to punishment (van Honk et al. 2003). Cortisol levels may accordingly be considered a biomarker of stress or emotional reactivity that could aid in predicting future antisocial behavior and help with screening (Loney et al. 2005).

Hypothalamic-Pituitary-Gonadal Axis

The HPG axis may play a role in the psychopathology of ASPD because of its end-product testosterone. Mainly in boys, the latter is an endogenous marker of the degree of pubertal maturation. Activation of the HPG axis at puberty is responsible for the elevation of testosterone and reproductive capacities of gonads, as well as secondary sex features, and it may influence antisocial behavior (Paus et al. 2010). Testosterone is responsible for mediating approach-related behavioral responses to competitive, provocative, socially stressful, or sexually arousing situations (Archer et al. 2005; Buchanan et al. 1992). Moreover, testosterone has been suggested to inhibit the action of the HPA axis and ANS, leading to a certain reduction in punishment sensitivity (Beech et al. 2018).

There are several reviews on the relationship between testosterone levels and different manifestations associated with ASPD (Casto and Edwards 2016; Dabbs and Dabbs 2000; Eisenegger et al. 2011; Montoya et al. 2012; Zilioli and Bird 2017). Meta-analytical literature has shown statistically significant correlations, although generally small (Cohen 1992), between testosterone and risk-taking behavior ($r=0.12$; Kurath and Mata 2018), competition outcome (e.g., higher testosterone rises subsequent to winning; $r=0.10$; Geniole et al. 2017), and aggression ($r=0.08$; Archer et al. 2005). The latter correlation was moderated by factors such as gender, type of sample (general population or offenders), age, and source of testosterone (saliva or blood) (Dekkers et al. 2019).

In youths with antisocial traits and aggressive tendencies, high testosterone levels have been observed, especially in those with conduct disorder (Pajer et al. 2006), as well as in those with externalizing behaviors (Maras et al. 2003) and in offenders (Dabbs et al. 1987, 1991; Kreuz and Rose 1972). It has been proposed that high testosterone levels thus may contribute to the development of antisocial behavior in youths and to the development of a diagnosis of ASPD (Aggarwal 2013). Yildirim and Derksen (2012a) suggested that high levels of testosterone throughout the life span, mostly early on or in response to social stress, could promote the emergence of antisociality. For instance, a longitudinal study showed that high total plasma testosterone levels in boys ages 12–14 years predicted antisocial behavior at age 16 years (Tarter et al. 2009).

More specifically in both youths and adults, several authors have reported that se-rum and salivary testosterone levels correlated significantly with the antisocial/life-style factor (Factor 2) of the Psychopathy Checklist—Revised (PCL-R; Hare 2003) and showed nonsignificant correlations with the constructs associated with interper-sonal/affective factor of psychopathy (Factor 1) (Loney et al. 2006; Stålenheim et al. 1998; Yildirim and Derksen 2012b). Studies also have evaluated differences in testos-terone levels in association with reactive/impulsive and proactive aggression. For in-stance, in studies on adolescent males, one study found that baseline salivary levels of testosterone were positively correlated with reactive as well as proactive aggres-sion (van Bokhoven et al. 2006), whereas another study found that baseline circulat-ing levels of testosterone were positively correlated with only reactive aggression (Olweus et al. 1988). On the other hand, a study examining basal levels of cerebrospi-nal fluid (CSF) testosterone in a group of individuals with personality disorders (16% with a diagnosis of ASPD) found no relationship with aggression or impulsivity. However, there was a relationship between CSF testosterone and sensation-seeking behavior (Coccaro et al. 2007). To better explain the inconsistency between studies, some have proposed that the association between testosterone and antisocial behav-ior is more related to dominance than aggression (Mazur and Booth 1998). Testoster-one may, therefore, increase aggressive and antisocial behavior not in all individuals but in only those with specific behavioral components (e.g., high on dimensions of dominance or low on dimensions of self-control). This highlights the importance of assessing trait behavioral and personality dimensions to better understand the effects of biological compounds (Coccaro 2017). Furthermore, researchers also have sug-gested a biosocial explanation wherein the effects of testosterone on behavior depend on and vary based on social contextual factors (Booth and Osgood 1993; Booth et al. 2003; Sapolsky 2017). Adverse contextual factors early in life, such as high levels of severe disciplining, low quality of parent-child relationships, and presence of more deviant peers, have been shown to increase the probability of finding a positive asso-ciation between testosterone and antisocial behavior (Chen et al. 2018). Additionally, numerous studies have examined various contexts that may alter testosterone con-centration, including competitive exchanges (Carré et al. 2013; Zilioli et al. 2014), so-cial rejection (Geniole et al. 2011), and aggressive provocation (Carré et al. 2014), in addition to contacts with hostile stimuli (Klinesmith et al. 2006). These studies show a consistent association between momentary rises of testosterone and aggression or antisocial behavior (Carré and Olmstead 2015). To summarize, as opposed to leading to the emergence of ASPD, testosterone seems to increase the likelihood that behav-ioral predispositions for aggressive or antisocial tendencies become more readily ex-pressed under suitable contextual situations (Sapolsky 2017).

Autonomic Nervous System

The nervous system consists of the CNS and peripheral nervous system. The CNS in-cludes the brain and spinal cord, whereas the peripheral nervous system contains neurons that directly control the corporal responses and offer feedback to the brain on bodily states. The latter system can be further subdivided into somatic and auto-nomic components (ANS). The hypothalamus controls the functioning of the ANS.

The hypothalamus is a part of the brain that contains small nuclei that have a wide range of functions and links the nervous system to the endocrine system. It is part of the limbic system. The ANS is itself composed of two opposing divisions: the para-sympathetic nervous system (PNS; ensures that the body satisfies its long-term needs) and the sympathetic nervous system (SNS; activated during stressful circumstances when danger is perceived). The SNS involves the release of catecholamines, including norepinephrine, into the blood circulation and is responsible for effects involving elevated cardiovascular tone (Chrousos and Gold 1992). Typical physiological measures of the ANS include elevated heart rate and increased skin conductance (DeLisi and Vaughn 2014). Two aspects of autonomic arousal—that is, resting arousal and reactivity—have been associated with antisocial behavior and have been subsequently explored in relation to antisociality (Lorber 2004; Ortiz and Raine 2004; Portnoy and Farrington 2015). Baseline or resting heart rate and skin conductance levels are suggestive of baseline levels of autonomic activity free of any stimulus, whereas heart rate and skin conductance reactivity are indicative of the level of response of the autonomic system when a stressful stimulus is present. Heart rate is controlled by the opposing effects of the PNS and SNS, whereas skin conductance is primarily controlled by the SNS (Akselrod et al. 1981; Warner and Cox 1962). An adaptive equilibrium between the activities of the SNS and the PNS is thought to reflect the capability to effectively respond to metabolic and behavioral needs (Appelhans and Luecken 2006; Grossman and Taylor 2007). Consequently, aberrations in the activities of these systems are associated with an array of emotional and behavioral regulation problems (Appelhans and Luecken 2006; Grossman and Taylor 2007), including antisocial behavior.

Arousal: Heart Rate and Skin Conductance

Literature suggests an association between diminished ANS responses and conduct disorder, aggression, and antisocial tendencies among youths and adults. Hence, conduct-disordered, oppositional, and aggressive youths, as well as antisocial adults, have tended to have low resting heart rate and skin conductance compared with healthy control subjects (McBurnett et al. 1993; Pitts 1997; Raine 2005). Interestingly, evidence indicates that low heart rate may be diagnostically specific to antisocial conduct and, thereby, ASPD (van Goozen and Fairchild 2008). Low resting heart rate has been associated with numerous antisocial outcomes, including aggression (Portnoy et al. 2014), delinquency (Raine et al. 1997), psychopathy (Gao et al. 2012), and conduct problems and criminality (Armstrong et al. 2009). These relationships appear to persist across the life span (children, adolescents, and adults; Armstrong et al. 2009; Van de Weijer et al. 2017) in both males and females (Moffitt and Caspi 2001). They are also found by means of various measures of antisocial outcomes, such as clinically diagnosed psychopathology (Raine et al. 2014), self-reports (Murray et al. 2016), observational measures (Kindlon et al. 1995), and criminal records (Armstrong et al. 2017; Cauffman et al. 2005; Jennings et al. 2013). Anomalies in skin conductance have been noted in antisocial behavior and related disorders, such as psychopathy. For example, early empirical research conducted in individuals with psychopathy has found that they showed atypical skin conductance in response to aversive stimuli (Hare 1978).

Studies have investigated the association between atypical autonomic activity in children and adolescents and conduct problems. Such information has the potential to elucidate the developmental mechanisms leading to antisocial behavior as well as to identify at-risk individuals who may then go on to receive a diagnosis of ASPD (Beauchaine 2012; Fanti 2018; Raine 2013). Nevertheless, results concerning the physiological activity of children and adolescents with conduct problems have been inconsistent, showing either lower or higher autonomic activity (Fanti 2018). In line with the low arousal theory (Lorber 2004; Ortiz and Raine 2004; Portnoy and Farrington 2015), low resting heart rate and skin conductance, as well as low heart rate and skin conductance reactivity in response to negative emotional stimuli, have been recognized not only in youths with conduct problems but also in adolescents who are later convicted and who engage in violence (Raine et al. 1990, 1997; van Bokhoven et al. 2005a; van Goozen et al. 2000). Furthermore, several meta-analyses have helped to clarify the association and have generally reported that low resting heart rate and skin conductance are important correlates of antisociality in youths. First, a meta-analysis by Ortiz and Raine (2004) of 45 independent effect sizes and a total of 5,868 children reported an effect size (Cohen's d) of –0.44 for the association between resting heart rate and antisocial behavior. Furthermore, the relationship was not moderated by other confounding factors (e.g., age, method of assessment, population). These findings led the authors to suggest that such low resting heart rate seemed to be the best-replicated biological correlate of antisocial behavior in children and adolescents. Second, Lorber (2004) similarly found that conduct problems in children were associated with low resting heart rate. Results for autonomic reactivity have been less consistent. It has been suggested that conduct problems may be associated with higher heart rate reactivity to stressful or threatening stimuli in children (Cohen's $d=0.20$). However, it is noteworthy that there was substantial heterogeneity in effect sizes across studies, ranging from –1.24 to 0.49. Conduct problems were also related to lower levels of skin conductance, both at rest and during activity. Third, Portnoy and Farrington (2015) reported that a low heart rate was related to more aggression and delinquency; an overall effect size of Cohen's $d=-0.20$ was found for antisocial behavior based on 115 effect sizes. They further established that the effect was not moderated by sex, study design, length of follow-up period, sample age, or antisocial behavior type. As in previous studies (Lorber 2004), psychopathy was not associated with heart rate. Fourth, Fanti et al. (2019) conducted a meta-analysis across 66 studies amounting to a total of 10,227 participants on the association between conduct problems and autonomic resting state as well as task-related reactivity. Amid 34 retrieved case-control studies that were based on conduct problem cutoff scores, lower galvanic skin activity (task-related skin conductance and skin conductance reactivity) in response to tasks was found. However, no significant group differences were observed for heart rate or heart rate reactivity or for any baseline measures. On the other hand, amid 32 retrieved studies with correlational designs, the authors noted only significant negative relationships between baseline and task-related heart rate with conduct problems. No significant relationships were found for other physiological measures assessed during tasks and at baseline. On the basis of this meta-analysis and previous work, Fanti et al. (2019) suggested that a reduced heart rate reactivity for youths with conduct problems could not be confirmed. In addition, skin conductance baseline levels were not related to conduct problems. Fanti et al. (2019) suggested that heterogeneity in conduct problems may help explain some of the observed inconsistencies in physiological reactivity, whereas heterogeneous conduct problem profiles may show opposite extremes of physiological arousal.

To improve our understanding of these inconsistencies, it may be pertinent to examine different subgroups of youths and evaluate comorbidity in relation to physiological measures. Hence, some authors have reported that different subgroups of youths with conduct problems may explain these divergences as more homogeneous subgroups display different physiological measures (e.g., heart rate and skin conductance reactivity) (Fanti and Kimonis 2017; Fanti et al. 2019; Frick et al. 2014). Approaches aimed to create more homogeneous groups have thus differentiated youths with conduct problems based on co-occurring psychopathologies, with most being related to ADHD and internalizing disorders (anxiety and depression). Hence, studies differentiating youths with these psychopathologies have yielded interesting findings. Studies have found that children with comorbid conduct problems and ADHD symptoms show physiological dysfunctions (e.g., lower skin conductance and heart rate responses to negative emotional stimuli) similar to those of youths with conduct problems but no ADHD symptoms or that ADHD symptoms do not account for the association between conduct problems and physiological measures (Beauchaine et al. 2001; Herpertz et al. 2001, 2003, 2005; McBurnett et al. 1993; Northover et al. 2016; Posthumus et al. 2009; Raine and Jones 1987; Zahn and Kruesi 1993). Additionally, youths with severe conduct problems also showed less reactivity to negative situations with lower emotional arousal than did youths with comorbid conduct problems and internalizing problems (Garralda et al. 1991; McBurnett et al. 1993). Other methods to classify youths with conduct problems have been based on differentiating youths with levels of callous-unemotional and psychopathic traits. Therefore, in comparison to children with severe conduct problems and callous-unemotional traits, those with only severe conduct problems appeared to have an increased resting heart rate, and in response to negative emotional stimuli, they showed reduced heart rate and skin conductance reactivity (Anastassiou-Hadjicharalambous and Warden 2008; de Wied et al. 2012; Kimonis et al. 2008; Muñoz et al. 2008; Northover et al. 2016).

Notably, such autonomic dysfunctions in youths may be suggested to increase the occurrence of an ASPD diagnosis in adulthood. For instance, a study by Raine and colleagues (1990) found that low arousal at age 15 years as measured using cardiovascular and skin conductance activity was able to predict criminal convictions by age 24 years. Furthermore, another study observed that low heart rate in children at age 3 years was predictive of aggression at age 11 years (Raine et al. 1997). Gao et al. (2010) found that poor skin conductance conditioning at age 3 years was associated with more aggressive behavior at 8 years and appeared to predispose individuals to criminality in early adulthood. Additionally, young individuals with antisocial tendencies, mostly early on in life, have low resting heart rate (Gao et al. 2009; Patrick 2008). Such low heart rate has been proposed to be diagnostically specific to conduct disorder (precursor of ASPD) and is thought to be a childhood predictor of future acts of aggression (Raine et al. 1996, 1997) and persistent offending (Moffitt and Caspi 2001). Although more literature has explored autonomic functioning in adult inmates with higher psychopathy traits and aggression (Benning et al. 2005; Fung et al. 2005; House and Milligan 1976), only a few studies of ASPD have been done (Dinn and Harris 2000; Raine et al. 2000). Consistent with studies exploring the autonomic correlates of men diagnosed with ASPD (Dinn and Harris 2000; Raine et al. 2000), subclinical ASPD has been linked to skin conductance hyporeactivity in anticipation of a threat (Sylvers et al. 2010). Moreover, the relationship between ASPD and skin conductance hyporeactivity was characteristic of ASPD even after the investigators controlled for confounding factors (i.e., features of psychopathy and aggression). When directly examining associations between autonomic arousal or reactivity and psychopathy or psychopathic traits, literature has been relatively mixed. As in the youth literature, examining different subgroups, and thus dimensions of psychopathy, could explain inconsistent results (Fanti et al. 2017). For example, in contrast to findings in aggressive individuals without psychopathy, it has been shown that individuals with psychopathy have diminished rather than increased autonomic reactivity to aversive or stressful stimuli (Hare 1978; Lorber 2004). Aggressive behaviors in those with psychopathy are different from aggression in individuals without psychopathy, with the violent acts perpetrated by individuals with psychopathy being typically more proactive than those perpetrated by individuals with low psychopathic traits or those judged to be high only in the antisocial deviance features of psychopathy (Patrick 2018). An explanation for this disparity has been suggested to lie in the affective-interpersonal features of psychopathy (Factor 1) (Hare and Neumann 2009). Hence, low physiological responsiveness to negative stimuli has been observed in relation to the affective-interpersonal dimensions of psychopathy and associated with grandiosity/callous-unemotional traits, but not with the impulsive-antisocial dimension (Benning et al. 2005; Fanti et al. 2017; Patrick and Bernat 2009). These findings suggest that the affective-interpersonal dimension (Factor 1) may be associated with hypoarousal and low distress. Individuals showing signs of physiological underarousal might engage in more proactive forms of aggression and might also endorse more callous-unemotional and grandiose-manipulative traits. On the other hand, findings suggest that impulsive irresponsibility (Factor 2) is associated with hyperarousal and emotional dysregulation (Fanti et al. 2017; Fowles and Dindo 2006). Thus, individuals who are hypersensitive to threatening/fearful stimuli tend to display emotionally charged and undercontrolled antisocial behaviors, which are associated with features of impulsive irresponsibility, such as emotional and behavioral dysregulation (Frick and Morris 2004; Raine et al. 2014; van Goozen et al. 2007).

Interactions Between Biomarkers

As we have highlighted throughout this chapter, the association between ASPD and related conditions with physiological indicators of stress and emotional responding may be complex, perhaps explaining the divergent findings that have been observed in literature (Alink et al. 2008; Fanti 2018). Elucidating how multiple physiological stress systems and emotional response systems (i.e., ANS, HPA, HPG, neural networks) operate together to affect the emergence and maintenance of antisociality remains a critical line of inquiry (Buss et al. 2018). While most research has focused on a single biomarker or biological system in isolation, incorporating multiple biomarkers may help identify novel mechanisms (Buss et al. 2018). In this next section, we discuss potential interactions between the systems described earlier.

Hypothalamic-Pituitary-Adrenal Axis and Hypothalamic-Pituitary-Gonadal Axis

The HPA and HPG axes are two hormonal axes that both inhibit each other and work in concert to maintain a suitable equilibrium between retreating when perceived fearful or threatening stimuli are present and approaching when rewarding stimuli are present. Much of the literature has connected testosterone and cortisol individually with antisocial behavior, while other authors have suggested that it is critical to consider their association in the context of HPA and HPG functioning, respectively. As a result, there has been interest in the dual-hormone hypothesis, and thereby the testosterone-to-cortisol ratio (Carré and Mehta 2011; Mehta and Josephs 2010; Mehta and Prasad 2015; Terburg et al. 2009).

The testosterone-to-cortisol ratio theory posits that imbalanced levels of testosterone to cortisol may raise the risk of antisocial behavior, such as aggression (Terburg et al. 2009). This dual-hormone model further highlights the central role of cortisol by suggesting that testosterone is predominantly associated with status-relevant behavior (e.g., status itself, dominance, risk taking, aggression, psychopathy) only when cortisol levels are low (Mehta and Beer 2010). Consequently, this model proposes that augmented testosterone-to-cortisol ratios predispose to an increased inclination to confront threat. A higher testosterone-to-cortisol ratio may increase the likelihood that SNS arousal, observed by increased skin conductance in response to stress, will lead to impairments in emotion regulation and aggression (Armstrong et al. 2019). Several studies have been conducted on the dual-hormone interaction on several personality features (e.g., aggression, dominance, risk-taking) associated with antisociality (see Grebe et al. 2019 for a review). Although most empirical work has provided evidence for the dual-hormone theory, mostly for more severe forms of antisociality, other work has nevertheless reported null findings (Geniole et al. 2013; Mazur and Booth 2014) and even opposite patterns (e.g., an association of testosterone with status-relevant behavior at high cortisol levels) (Denson et al. 2013a, 2013b). Overall, a recent meta-analysis by Dekkers et al. (2019) on dual-hormone effects reported a small average effect in the predicted direction ($r=-0.061$ for testosterone×cortisol). However, this finding showed evidence of publication bias and a lack of power in individual studies. Despite its support, the dual-hormone hypothesis remains a fairly novel idea and warrants more examination (Goulter et al. 2019).

Hypothalamic-Pituitary-Adrenal Axis and Monoamine Systems

Dysregulations in neural chemistry have been suggested to contribute to the development of ASPD and have been associated with antisocial behavior such as aggression. Monoamine neurotransmitters, including serotonin (5-HT), dopamine, and norepinephrine, are substances that allow the communication of signals in the brain, and these systems work together and with other systems, including the HPA axis, to inhibit or initiate behaviors (Hagenbeek et al. 2016). These monoamines have implications in self-control. Hence, the dopamine and norepinephrine systems facilitate social dominance and aggressive behavior, whereas the serotonin system inhibits impulsive behavior (van der Vegt et al. 2003; Willner 2015).

Serotonin has cell bodies that reside in the raphe nuclei of the brain stem, and its projections ascend to a diverse group of brain regions including limbic structures (Azmitia and Segal 1978). This monoamine has been more extensively explored in ASPD, with most studies of ASPD having found that 5-HT is downregulated (Aggarwal 2013; Liening and Josephs 2010). Reduced basal levels of 5-HT may diminish the threshold of perceiving threats and of initiating antisocial behavior (Siegel and Douard 2011). Evidence supporting this association stems from reduced levels of the primary 5-HT metabolite, 5-hydroxyindoleacetic acid (5-HIAA). Impulsive violent offenders diagnosed with ASPD have reported lower levels of this metabolite in the CSF (Lidberg et al. 1985), and lower concentrations of 5-HIAA have, in addition, been associated with violent suicide attempts in those with ASPD (Träskman-Bendz et al. 1986). However, such findings have not been observed in all studies, especially in those studies that did not draw participants from the criminal justice system (Coccaro et al. 1997a, 1997b; Hibbeln et al. 2000). For instance, no relationship between CSF 5-HIAA levels and life history of aggression was detected in two distinct samples of participants with personality disorders (12.5% and 4%, respectively, with a diagnosis of ASPD) (Coccaro et al. 1997a, 1997b). Simeon et al. (1992) also observed no relation between 5-HT functioning and life history of aggression or impulsivity in a sample of individuals with personality disorders and a history of self-harm, although none had a diagnosis of ASPD. Nevertheless, a meta-analysis of 20 studies found significantly reduced CSF levels of 5-HIAA in antisocial individuals compared with nonantisocial control groups (Moore et al. 2002). Although several lines of evidence highlight a potential role of 5-HT dysfunction in association with antisocial behavior (Beauchaine et al. 2009; Gunter et al. 2010), serotonergic antidepressants (i.e., selective serotonin reuptake inhibitors), for instance, have only a limited influence on ASPD symptoms, a finding that does not allow us to stipulate that this dysregulation is a leading factor of the disorder (Bandelow and Wedekind 2015).

It should be noted that 5-HT interacts with other systems, including the HPA axis. For example, activation of postsynaptic 5-HT receptors (principally the $5-HT_{1A}$ and $5-HT_{2A}$ subtypes) in the hypothalamus stimulates HPA axis activity and leads to an elevation of ACTH and cortisol levels (Bagdy 1996; Fuller 1992). On the contrary, a disruption of 5-HT neurotransmission by tryptophan depletion impairs regular HPA axis functioning (Sobczak et al. 2002). Aggressiveness also has been shown to be inversely correlated with prolactin (medication used to elevate 5-HT levels) response to buspirone (a selective $5-HT_{1A}$ receptor agonist) (Coccaro et al. 1990), and with cortisol response to ipsapirone (a selective $5-HT_{1A}$ receptor partial agonist) (Coccaro et al. 1995). These findings may have implications for the etiology of antisocial behavior, because it appears that cortisol reactivity is impaired when 5-HT neurotransmission is disrupted (van Goozen and Fairchild 2006). Moreover, low levels of 5-HT with a high testosterone-to-cortisol ratio may facilitate impulsive behavior, such as impulsive aggression (Terburg et al. 2009; van Honk et al. 2010).

Serotonin also influences the activity of the dopaminergic system through the $5-HT_{2C}$ receptor, which reduces dopamine release (De Deurwaerdère et al. 2004) and may be likely involved in the emergence of ASPD symptoms. The dopamine system comprises cell bodies that are localized mainly in the ventral tegmental area of the midbrain and the nucleus accumbens with projections to several brain regions that are implicated in functions, such as cognitive processing, emotion regulation, and neuroendocrine control. Hence, reduced control by 5-HT on the dopamine system may lead to dopamine hyperactivity, which may then increase the tendency toward aggression (Seo et al. 2008; Soderstrom et al. 2003). High levels of the principal dopamine metabolite homovanillic acid (HVA) have been associated with higher levels of aggression in violent forensic samples and males convicted of murder (Lidberg et al. 1985; Soderstrom et al. 2001). Furthermore, an increased HVA–to–5-HIAA ratio, which indicates deficient serotonergic regulation of dopamine activity, has been associated with psychopathy, especially Factor 2 traits of the PCL-R (Soderstrom et al. 2001, 2003). Psychopathy, as suggested by Soderstrom et al. (2003), may be related to a high dopamine turnover in combination with 5-HT dysregulation.

As with the other neural systems, the relationship between norepinephrine and other systems regarding antisocial behavior may be complex. Central norepinephrine is produced in the locus coeruleus, whose cell bodies project to a variety of structures that are implicated in antisocial behavior, including the prefrontal cortex and the amygdala. Preceding literature has notably reported on the associations between several antisocial outcomes and dysregulated HPA axis as well as ANS separately as shown in the previous sections of this chapter, yet less research has examined the responsiveness of these interconnected systems (Del Giudice et al. 2012). Bauer and colleagues (2002) hypothesized that a lack of coordination between the HPA axis and the ANS may predict problem behaviors better than the activity of either individual subsystem on its own. This research has notably implicated measures of cortisol and salivary alpha-amylase (Glenn 2011). The latter is an enzyme produced by the salivary gland and is a biomarker of norepinephrine release/SNS functioning to stress response. These systems have been suggested to interact to maintain homeostasis and allow normal stress response (de Kloet et al. 2005).

With limited literature reporting an association between low cortisol and low alpha-amylase reactivity in relation to higher levels of antisocial behavior, some results (Bendezú and Wadsworth 2018; Chen et al. 2015a; El-Sheikh et al. 2008; Gordis et al. 2006) support the additive model established by Bauer and colleagues (2002), whereby individuals with either hypoactivity or hyperactivity of both SNS and HPA axis may be at greater risk for behavior problems. In contrast, other studies (Bendezú and Wadsworth 2018; Chen et al. 2015b, 2016; Koss et al. 2014) have also lent support for the interactive hypothesis (Bauer et al. 2002), whereas those with asymmetrical profiles may be more vulnerable to behavior problems. Such asymmetrical profiles may signify either SNS hyperactivity with HPA axis hypoactivity or vice versa. Lastly, some authors have found no interaction between alpha-amylase and cortisol (Glenn et al. 2015). Therefore, largely inconsistent results have been observed regarding the interaction of the SNS and HPA axis with antisociality (see Jones et al. 2020 for a review). Discrepancies in these findings are likely due to several methodological inconsistencies (e.g., sampling from different age ranges, assessment of baseline levels vs. reactivity, and heterogeneity in externalizing or aggressive samples) (Glenn et al. 2015).

Hypothalamic-Pituitary-Adrenal Axis and Neuropeptides

Other types of molecules that may be implicated with ASPD include neuropeptides. Neuropeptides are compounds that are released by neurons within the brain, where they may act as neurotransmitters. They can also function as hormones, when they are released into the systemic blood supply and act by binding to a variety of receptors expressed by several target organs. Two neuropeptides are of particular relevance to ASPD: oxytocin and vasopressin (Beech et al. 2018). These neuropeptides have similar chemical structures and are produced in the hypothalamic neurons with axons that descend to the pituitary, where they are released into the bloodstream from specialized nerve endings (Beech et al. 2018). They can also be released from dendrites directly into the brain (Beech et al. 2018). Both are released in response to environmental stress and social encounters. As a result, they have both been designated as stress and social compounds (DeLisi and Vaughn 2014). Globally, vasopressin has been shown to enhance social stress, whereas oxytocin promotes social approach behavior (Meyer-Lindenberg et al. 2011).

The effects of vasopressin on antisocial behavior such as aggression have been more established in animal models, with fewer studies conducted in humans (Berends et al. 2019). As for oxytocin, a systematic review by Gedeon and colleagues (2019) found two studies evaluating the effects of oxytocin administration in patients with a diagnosis of ASPD on aggression and the ability to process as well as interpret emotional faces (Alcorn et al. 2015a, 2015b; Timmermann et al. 2017). These studies showed that oxytocin administration fixed their deficits in recognizing fearful and happy faces, but there were no trends between oxytocin administration and aggression. On the other hand, CSF levels of oxytocin have been found to be inversely correlated with lifetime history of aggression (Coccaro et al. 1998; Lee et al. 2009). Thus, literature supports the hypothesis that diminished peripheral and central resting oxytocin levels (reflecting a certain "hypo-oxytocinergic state"; Malik et al. 2012) can predict aggression and antisocial behavior. Yet, more studies are needed before we can draw definitive conclusions. For example, it may seem plausible that individuals high in psychopathic traits would show lower levels of cerebral oxytocin. However, Mitchell et al. (2013) examined the level of urinary oxytocin, used as an index of cerebral oxytocin levels, and found raised oxytocin levels in severe offenders in comparison to nonoffenders. Notably, they found these levels to be correlated with Factor 2 scores on the PCL-R (Mitchell et al. 2013). These findings suggest that direct effects of oxytocin on antisocial behavior are not straightforward and are dependent on several factors, including personality traits (i.e., manipulation, anger) (Alcorn et al. 2015a; Campbell and Hausmann 2013; Ne'eman et al. 2016). With inconsistent evidence concerning the role of oxytocin on social behavior, two distinct premises have been put forward. According to the prosocial hypothesis, oxytocin induces prosocial behavior (Macdonald and Macdonald 2010), whereas according to the social salience hypothesis, oxytocin may have a more general effect of augmenting the salience of social stimuli and may provoke a range of reactions depending on the context (Shamay-Tsoory and Abu-Akel 2016; Shamay-Tsoory et al. 2009). Ne'eman et al. (2016) suggested that the effects of oxytocin are not monolithic and vary depending on social cues (i.e., administration of oxytocin in a hostile environment and friendly environments might increase and decrease aggression, respectively). Furthermore, oxytocin may even interact with cortisol and testosterone. In individuals who have emotion dysregulation, oxytocin has been suggested to have a positive effect on antisocial behavior by attenuating the response of cortisol (Flanagan et al. 2018; Quirin et al. 2011; Simeon et al. 2011). The administration of oxytocin may also alter testosterone levels and, therefore, affect social behavior in a positive manner (Weisman et al. 2014).

Conclusion

Throughout this chapter, stress-regulating and emotion-regulating systems, notably the HPA axis, the ANS, and the HPG axis, have been shown to play a role in the development and maintenance of antisocial behavior. Their relationship with ASPD is not straightforward and fully understood because relatively little literature has examined individuals with an ASPD diagnosis specifically, but several potential biomarkers have been studied in relation to antisociality, including cortisol, heart rate, skin conductance, and testosterone. These associations may be more intricate than initially believed. Because distinct variants of ASPD are likely to exist, it is currently not possible to untangle the specific mechanisms associated with ASPD per se. In this sense, looking into the different concepts may be thought to be more informative in our attempts to understand the mechanisms that may explain specific manifestations and behaviors that are related to ASPD. Indeed, it has been argued that youths and adults with ASPD are heterogeneous, with many presenting distinct comorbidities, symptom severity, and risk factors. Therefore, a specific focus on more homogeneous constructs/conditions might bring us closer to unraveling the biomarkers of the disorder. Moreover, literature has shown that youths with antisocial tendencies have several findings that are similar to those in adults with antisocial personality and psychopathy, which is consistent with a neurodevelopmental perspective of the progression of ASPD.

Divergences in results noted throughout this chapter may be due to differences in samples and other methodological features. First, there is heterogeneity in how antisociality has been operationalized; measures used include delinquency; covert or overt aggressive, oppositional behavior; and psychiatric externalizing disorders such as conduct disorder and psychopathy (Feilhauer et al. 2013). In addition, numerous studies have indeed focused on aggression and psychopathy, but results may not be directly transferable to a full diagnosis of ASPD (Sylvers et al. 2010). Second, research settings have varied widely, with participants drawn from healthy community samples, at-risk community samples, clinic-referred samples with diverse diagnoses, and samples of incarcerated offenders (Feilhauer et al. 2013). Third, studies have differed in their assessment of biomarkers (e.g., basal levels and/or reactivity to experimental stimuli; serum, salivary, or CSF measures) (Feilhauer et al. 2013). Notably, many studies have not controlled for confounding factors in a consistent manner (e.g., substance use, gender, personality traits), and this lack of control may affect findings. Further high-quality studies are consequently necessary to better capture the biomarkers associated with ASPD, while considering the interactions between systems. It is thus unlikely that a single biomarker can fully explicate the pathophysiology of ASPD, and the combination of multiple biomarkers may reflect the development and maintenance of this personality disorder more broadly (Boksa 2013; Ritsner 2009).

Key Points

- Studies on youths who develop antisocial personality disorder (ASPD) suggest that hypoactivity of the hypothalamic-pituitary-adrenal (HPA) axis is associated with low cortisol levels.

- High levels of testosterone, the principal end-product of the hypothalamic-pituitary-gonadal (HPG) axis, may contribute to the development of antisocial behavior.

- Autonomic dysfunctions, evaluated by heart rate and skin conductance, may be linked to antisociality.

- The interaction between the HPA axis and 1) the HPG axis (testosterone-to-cortisol ratio), 2) the monoamine systems (norepinephrine, dopamine, serotonin), and 3) neuropeptides (vasopressin, oxytocin) may better explain the development of ASPD than any single system.

References

Aggarwal I: The role of antisocial personality disorder and antisocial behaviour in crime. Inquiries Journal 5(9):1–2, 2013

Akselrod S, Gordon D, Ubel FA, et al: Power spectrum analysis of heart rate fluctuation: a quantitative probe of beat-to-beat cardiovascular control. Science 213(4504):220–222, 1981 6166045

Alcorn JL 3rd, Green CE, Schmitz J, et al: Effects of oxytocin on aggressive responding in healthy adult men. Behav Pharmacol 26(8 spec no):798–804, 2015a 26241153

Alcorn JL 3rd, Rathnayaka N, Swann AC, et al: Effects of intranasal oxytocin on aggressive responding in antisocial personality disorder. Psychol Rec 65(4):691–703, 2015b 27022201

Alink LR, van Ijzendoorn MH, Bakermans-Kranenburg MJ, et al: Cortisol and externalizing behavior in children and adolescents: mixed meta-analytic evidence for the inverse relation of basal cortisol and cortisol reactivity with externalizing behavior. Dev Psychobiol 50(5):427–450, 2008 18551461

American Psychiatric Association: Diagnostic and Statistical Manual of Mental Disorders, 5th Edition. Arlington, VA, American Psychiatric Association, 2013

Anastassiou-Hadjicharalambous X, Warden D: Physiologically indexed and self-perceived affective empathy in conduct-disordered children high and low on callous-unemotional traits. Child Psychiatry Hum Dev 39(4):503–517, 2008 18792777

Appelhans BM, Luecken LJ: Heart rate variability as an index of regulated emotional responding. Rev Gen Psychol 10(3):229–240, 2006

Archer J, Graham-Kevan N, Davies M: Testosterone and aggression: a reanalysis of Book, Starzyk, and Quinsey's (2001) study. Aggress Violent Behav 10(2):241–261, 2005

Armstrong TA, Keller S, Franklin TW, et al: Low resting heart rate and antisocial behavior: a brief review of evidence and preliminary results from a new test. Criminal Justice Behavior 36(11):1125–1140, 2009

Armstrong TA, Boisvert D, Flores S, et al: Heart rate, serotonin transporter linked polymorphic region (5-HTTLPR) genotype, and violence in an incarcerated sample. J Crim Justice 51:1–8, 2017

Armstrong T, Wells J, Boisvert DL, et al: Skin conductance, heart rate and aggressive behavior type. Biol Psychol 141:44–51, 2019 30584895

Azmitia EC, Segal M: An autoradiographic analysis of the differential ascending projections of the dorsal and median raphe nuclei in the rat. J Comp Neurol 179(3):641–667, 1978 565370

Bagdy G: Role of the hypothalamic paraventricular nucleus in 5-HT1A, 5-HT2A and 5-HT2C receptor-mediated oxytocin, prolactin and ACTH/corticosterone responses. Behav Brain Res 73(1–2):277–280, 1996 8788518

Bandelow B, Wedekind D: Possible role of a dysregulation of the endogenous opioid system in antisocial personality disorder. Hum Psychopharmacol 30(6):393–415, 2015 26250442

Barzman DH, Mossman D, Appel K, et al: The association between salivary hormone levels and children's inpatient aggression: a pilot study. Psychiatr Q 84(4):475–484, 2013 23508357

Bauer AM, Quas JA, Boyce WT: Associations between physiological reactivity and children's behavior: advantages of a multisystem approach. J Dev Behav Pediatr 23(2):102–113, 2002 11943973

Beauchaine TP: Physiological markers of emotional and behavioral dysregulation in externalizing psychopathology. Monogr Soc Res Child Dev 77(2):79–86, 2012 25242827

Beauchaine TP, McNulty T: Comorbidities and continuities as ontogenic processes: toward a developmental spectrum model of externalizing psychopathology. Dev Psychopathol 25(4 pt 2):1505–1528, 2013 24342853

Beauchaine TP, Katkin ES, Strassberg Z, et al: Disinhibitory psychopathology in male adolescents: discriminating conduct disorder from attention-deficit/hyperactivity disorder through concurrent assessment of multiple autonomic states. J Abnorm Psychol 110(4):610–624, 2001 11727950

Beauchaine TP, Klein DN, Crowell SE, et al: Multifinality in the development of personality disorders: a Biology x Sex x Environment interaction model of antisocial and borderline traits. Dev Psychopathol 21(3):735–770, 2009 19583882

Beech AR, Carter AJ, Mann RE, et al (eds): The Wiley Blackwell Handbook of Forensic Neuroscience. New York, Wiley, 2018

Bendezú JJ, Wadsworth ME: Person-centered examination of salivary cortisol and alpha-amylase responses to psychosocial stress: links to preadolescent behavioral functioning and coping. Biol Psychol 132:143–153, 2018 29248565

Benning SD, Patrick CJ, Iacono WG: Psychopathy, startle blink modulation, and electrodermal reactivity in twin men. Psychophysiology 42(6):753–762, 2005 16364071

Berends YR, Tulen JHM, Wierdsma AI, et al: Oxytocin, vasopressin and trust: associations with aggressive behavior in healthy young males. Physiol Behav 204:180–185, 2019 30802507

Boksa P: A way forward for research on biomarkers for psychiatric disorders. J Psychiatry Neurosci 38(2):75–77, 2013 23422052

Booth A, Osgood DW: The influence of testosterone on deviance in adulthood: assessing and explaining the relationship. J Criminol 31(1):93–117, 1993

Booth A, Johnson DR, Granger DA, et al: Testosterone and child and adolescent adjustment: the moderating role of parent-child relationships. Dev Psychol 39(1):85–98, 2003 12518811

Bremne JD, Vermetten E: Stress and development: behavioral and biological consequences. Dev Psychopathol 13(3):473–489, 2001 11523844

Buchanan CM, Eccles JS, Becker JB: Are adolescents the victims of raging hormones: evidence for activational effects of hormones on moods and behavior at adolescence. Psychol Bull 111(1):62–107, 1992 1539089

Burke JD, Loeber R, Lahey BB: Adolescent conduct disorder and interpersonal callousness as predictors of psychopathy in young adults. J Clin Child Adolesc Psychol 36(3):334–346, 2007 17658978

Buss KA, Jaffee S, Wadsworth ME, et al: Impact of psychophysiological stress-response systems on psychological development: moving beyond the single biomarker approach. Dev Psychol 54(9):1601–1605, 2018 30148389

Campbell A, Hausmann M: Effects of oxytocin on women's aggression depend on state anxiety. Aggress Behav 39(4):316–322, 2013 23553462

Carré JM, Mehta PH: Importance of considering testosterone-cortisol interactions in predicting human aggression and dominance. Aggress Behav 37(6):489–491, 2011 21826676

Carré JM, Olmstead NA: Social neuroendocrinology of human aggression: examining the role of competition-induced testosterone dynamics. Neuroscience 286:171–186, 2015 25463514

Carré JM, Campbell JA, Lozoya E, et al: Changes in testosterone mediate the effect of winning on subsequent aggressive behaviour. Psychoneuroendocrinology 38(10):2034–2041, 2013 23587440

Carré JM, Iselin AM, Welker KM, et al: Testosterone reactivity to provocation mediates the effect of early intervention on aggressive behavior. Psychol Sci 25(5):1140–1146, 2014 24681586

Casto KV, Edwards DA: Testosterone, cortisol, and human competition. Horm Behav 82:21–37, 2016 27103058

Cauffman E, Steinberg L, Piquero AR: Psychological, neuropsychological and physiological correlates of serious antisocial behavior in adolescence: the role of self-control. Criminology 43(1):133–176, 2005

Chen FR, Raine A, Granger DA: Tactics for modeling multiple salivary analyte data in relation to behavior problems: additive, ratio, and interaction effects. Psychoneuroendocrinology 51:188–200, 2015a 25462892

Chen FR, Raine A, Rudo-Hutt AS, et al: Harsh discipline and behavior problems: the moderating effects of cortisol and alpha-amylase. Biol Psychol 104:19–27, 2015b 25451383

Chen FR, Raine A, Glenn AL, et al: Hypothalamic pituitary adrenal activity and autonomic nervous system arousal predict developmental trajectories of children's comorbid behavior problems. Dev Psychobiol 58(3):393–405, 2016 26567016

Chen FR, Dariotis JK, Granger DA: Linking testosterone and antisocial behavior in at-risk transitional aged youth: contextual effects of parentification. Psychoneuroendocrinology 91:1–10, 2018 29505951

Chrousos GP, Gold PW: The concepts of stress and stress system disorders: overview of physical and behavioral homeostasis. JAMA 267(9):1244–1252, 1992 1538563

Cima M, Smeets T, Jelicic M: Self-reported trauma, cortisol levels, and aggression in psychopathic and non-psychopathic prison inmates. Biol Psychol 78(1):75–86, 2008 18304719

Coccaro EF: Testosterone and aggression: more than just biology? Biol Psychiatry 82(4):234, 2017 28748784

Coccaro EF, Gabriel S, Siever LJ: Buspirone challenge: preliminary evidence for a role for central 5-HT1a receptor function in impulsive aggressive behavior in humans. Psychopharmacol Bull 26(3):393–405, 1990 2274641

Coccaro EF, Kavoussi RJ, Hauger RL: Physiological responses to d-fenfluramine and ipsapirone challenge correlate with indices of aggression in males with personality disorder. Int Clin Psychopharmacol 10(3):177–179, 1995 8675971

Coccaro EF, Kavoussi RJ, Cooper TB, et al: Central serotonin activity and aggression: inverse relationship with prolactin response to d-fenfluramine, but not CSF 5-HIAA concentration, in human subjects. Am J Psychiatry 154(10):1430–1435, 1997a 9326827

Coccaro EF, Kavoussi RJ, Trestman RL, et al: Serotonin function in human subjects: intercorrelations among central 5-HT indices and aggressiveness. Psychiatry Res 73(1–2):1–14, 1997b 9463834

Coccaro EF, Kavoussi RJ, Hauger RL, et al: Cerebrospinal fluid vasopressin levels: correlates with aggression and serotonin function in personality-disordered subjects. Arch Gen Psychiatry 55(8):708–714, 1998 9707381

Coccaro EF, Beresford B, Minar P, et al: CSF testosterone: relationship to aggression, impulsivity, and venturesomeness in adult males with personality disorder. J Psychiatr Res 41(6):488–492, 2007 16765987

Cohen J: A power primer. Psychol Bull 112(1):155–159, 1992 19565683

Cox J, Edens JF, Magyar MS, et al: Using the Psychopathic Personality Inventory to identify subtypes of antisocial personality disorder. J Crim Justice 41(2):125–134, 2013

Dabbs JM, Dabbs MG: Heroes, Rogues, and Lovers: Testosterone and Behavior. New York, McGraw-Hill, 2000

Dabbs JM Jr, Frady RL, Carr TS, et al: Saliva testosterone and criminal violence in young adult prison inmates. Psychosom Med 49(2):174–182, 1987 3575604

Dabbs JM Jr, Jurkovic GJ, Frady RL: Salivary testosterone and cortisol among late adolescent male offenders. J Abnorm Child Psychol 19(4):469–478, 1991 1757712

Daitzman R, Zuckerman M: Disinhibitory sensation seeking, personality and gonadal hormones. Pers Individ Dif 1(2):103–110, 1980

Darby RR: Neuroimaging abnormalities in neurological patients with criminal behavior. Curr Neurol Neurosci Rep 18(8):47, 2018 29904892

De Deurwaerdère P, Navailles S, Berg KA, et al: Constitutive activity of the serotonin2C receptor inhibits in vivo dopamine release in the rat striatum and nucleus accumbens. J Neurosci 24(13):3235–3241, 2004 15056702 de Kloet ER, Joëls M, Holsboer F: Stress and the brain: from adaptation to disease. Nat Rev Neurosci 6(6):463–475, 2005 15891777

de Wied M, van Boxtel A, Matthys W, et al: Verbal, facial and autonomic responses to empathy-eliciting film clips by disruptive male adolescents with high versus low callous-unemotional traits. J Abnorm Child Psychol 40(2):211–223, 2012 21870040

Dekkers TJ, van Rentergem JAA, Meijer B, et al: A meta-analytical evaluation of the dual-hormone hypothesis: does cortisol moderate the relationship between testosterone and status, dominance, risk taking, aggression, and psychopathy? Neurosci Biobehav Rev 96:250–271, 2019 30529754

Del Giudice M, Hinnant JB, Ellis BJ, et al: Adaptive patterns of stress responsivity: a preliminary investigation. Dev Psychol 48(3):775–790, 2012 22148947

DeLisi M, Vaughn MG (eds): The Routledge International Handbook of Biosocial Criminology. New York, Routledge, 2014

DeLisi M, Drury AJ, Elbert MJ: The etiology of antisocial personality disorder: the differential roles of adverse childhood experiences and childhood psychopathology. Compr Psychiatry 92:1–6, 2019 31079021

Denson TF, Mehta PH, Ho Tan D: Endogenous testosterone and cortisol jointly influence reactive aggression in women. Psychoneuroendocrinology 38(3):416–424, 2013a 22854014

Denson TF, Ronay R, von Hippel W, et al: Endogenous testosterone and cortisol modulate neural responses during induced anger control. Soc Neurosci 8(2):165–177, 2013b 22263640

Deuschle M, Schweiger U, Weber B, et al: Diurnal activity and pulsatility of the hypothalamus-pituitary-adrenal system in male depressed patients and healthy controls. J Clin Endocrinol Metab 82(1):234–238, 1997 8989265

Dinn WM, Harris CL: Neurocognitive function in antisocial personality disorder. Psychiatry Res 97(2–3):173–190, 2000 11166089

Eisenegger C, Haushofer J, Fehr E: The role of testosterone in social interaction. Trends Cogn Sci 15(6):263–271, 2011 21616702

El-Sheikh M, Erath SA, Buckhalt JA, et al: Cortisol and children's adjustment: the moderating role of sympathetic nervous system activity. J Abnorm Child Psychol 36(4):601–611, 2008 18197472

Fairchild G, Van Goozen SH, Stollery SJ, et al: Fear conditioning and affective modulation of the startle reflex in male adolescents with early onset or adolescence-onset conduct disorder and healthy control subjects. Biol Psychiatry 63(3):279–285, 2008 17765205

Fairchild G, Baker E, Eaton S: Hypothalamic-pituitary-adrenal axis function in children and adults with severe antisocial behavior and the impact of early adversity. Curr Psychiatry Rep 20(10):84, 2018 30155579

Fanti KA: Understanding heterogeneity in conduct disorder: a review of psychophysiological studies. Neurosci Biobehav Rev 91:4–20, 2018 27693700

Fanti KA, Henrich CC: Trajectories of pure and co-occurring internalizing and externalizing problems from age 2 to age 12: findings from the National Institute of Child Health and Human Development Study of Early Child Care. Dev Psychol 46(5):1159–1175, 2010 20822230

Fanti KA, Kimonis E: Heterogeneity in externalizing problems at age 3: association with age 15 biological and environmental outcomes. Dev Psychol 53(7):1230–1241, 2017 28406655

Fanti KA, Kyranides MN, Georgiou G, et al: Callous-unemotional, impulsive-irresponsible, and grandiose-manipulative traits: distinct associations with heart rate, skin conductance, and startle responses to violent and erotic scenes. Psychophysiology 54(5):663–672, 2017 28169424

Fanti KA, Eisenbarth H, Goble P, et al: Psychophysiological activity and reactivity in children and adolescents with conduct problems: a systematic review and meta-analysis. Neurosci Biobehav Rev 100:98–107, 2019 30797946

Farrington DP, Coid JW: Early Prevention of Adult Antisocial Behaviour. New York, Cambridge University Press, 2003

Feilhauer J, Cima M, Korebrits A, et al: Salivary cortisol and psychopathy dimensions in detained antisocial adolescents. Psychoneuroendocrinology 38(9):1586–1595, 2013 23466026

Fergusson DM, Horwood LJ, Ridder EM: Show me the child at seven: the consequences of conduct problems in childhood for psychosocial functioning in adulthood. J Child Psychol Psychiatry 46(8):837–849, 2005 16033632

Flanagan JC, Fischer MS, Nietert PJ, et al: Effects of oxytocin on cortisol reactivity and conflict resolution behaviors among couples with substance misuse. Psychiatry Res 260:346–352, 2018 29232576

Fowles DC, Dindo L: A dual-deficit model of psychopathy, in Handbook of Psychopathy, 2nd Edition. Edited by Patrick CJ. New York, Guilford, 2006, pp 14–34

Frick PJ, Morris AS: Temperament and developmental pathways to conduct problems. J Clin Child Adolesc Psychol 33(1):54–68, 2004 16033632

Frick PJ, Ray JV, Thornton LC, et al: Annual research review: a developmental psychopathology approach to understanding callous-unemotional traits in children and adolescents with serious conduct problems. J Child Psychol Psychiatry 55(6):532–548, 2014 24117854

Fuller RW: The involvement of serotonin in regulation of pituitary-adrenocortical function. Front Neuroendocrinol 13(3):250–270, 1992 1334001

Fung MT, Raine A, Loeber R, et al: Reduced electrodermal activity in psychopathy-prone adolescents. J Abnorm Psychol 114(2):187–196, 2005 15869350

Gao Y, Baker LA, Raine A, et al: Brief Report: Interaction between social class and risky decision-making in children with psychopathic tendencies. J Adolesc 32(2):409–414, 2009 18986696

Gao Y, Raine A, Venables PH, et al: Reduced electrodermal fear conditioning from ages 3 to 8 years is associated with aggressive behavior at age 8 years. J Child Psychol Psychiatry 51(5):550–558, 2010 19788551

Gao Y, Raine A, Schug RA: Somatic aphasia: mismatch of body sensations with autonomic stress reactivity in psychopathy. Biol Psychol 90(3):228–233, 2012 22490763

Garralda ME, Connell J, Taylor DC: Psychophysiological anomalies in children with emotional and conduct disorders. Psychol Med 21(4):947–957, 1991 1780407

Gedeon T, Parry J, Völlm B: The role of oxytocin in antisocial personality disorders: a systematic review of the literature. Front Psychiatry 10:76, 2019 30873049

Geniole SN, Carré JM, McCormick CM: State, not trait, neuroendocrine function predicts costly reactive aggression in men after social exclusion and inclusion. Biol Psychol 87(1):137–145, 2011 21382439

Geniole SN, Busseri MA, McCormick CM: Testosterone dynamics and psychopathic personality traits independently predict antagonistic behavior towards the perceived loser of a competitive interaction. Horm Behav 64(5):790–798, 2013 24120551

Geniole SN, Bird BM, Ruddick EL, et al: Effects of competition outcome on testosterone concentrations in humans: an updated meta-analysis. Horm Behav 92:37–50, 2017 27720891

Glenn AL: Cortisol, testosterone, and alpha-amylase in psychopathy. Publicly Accessible Penn Dissertations, May 16, 2011. Available at: www.repository.upenn.edu/cgi/viewcontent.cgi?article=1414&context=edissertations. Accessed April 16, 2021.

Glenn AL, Johnson AK, Raine A: Antisocial personality disorder: a current review. Curr Psychiatry Rep 15(12):427, 2013 24249521

Glenn AL, Remmel RJ, Raine A, et al: Alpha-amylase reactivity in relation to psychopathic traits in adults. Psychoneuroendocrinology 54:14–23, 2015 25662339

Goldstein RB, Grant BF, Ruan WJ, et al: Antisocial personality disorder with childhood- vs. adolescence-onset conduct disorder: results from the National Epidemiologic Survey on Alcohol and Related Conditions. J Nerv Ment Dis 194(9):667–675, 2006 16971818

Gordis EB, Granger DA, Susman EJ, et al: Asymmetry between salivary cortisol and alpha-amylase reactivity to stress: relation to aggressive behavior in adolescents. Psychoneuroendocrinology 31(8):976–987, 2006 16879926

Goulter N, Kimonis ER, Denson TF, et al: Female primary and secondary psychopathic variants show distinct endocrine and psychophysiological profiles. Psychoneuroendocrinology 104:7–17, 2019 30784904

Grebe NM, Del Giudice M, Emery Thompson M, et al: Testosterone, cortisol, and status-striving personality features: a review and empirical evaluation of the dual hormone hypothesis. Horm Behav 109:25–37, 2019 30685468

Grossman P, Taylor EW: Toward understanding respiratory sinus arrhythmia: relations to cardiac vagal tone, evolution and biobehavioral functions. Biol Psychol 74(2):263–285, 2007 17081672

Gunter TD, Vaughn MG, Philibert RA: Behavioral genetics in antisocial spectrum disorders and psychopathy: a review of the recent literature. Behav Sci Law 28(2):148–173, 2010 20422643

Hagenbeek FA, Kluft C, Hankemeier T, et al: Discovery of biochemical biomarkers for aggression: a role for metabolomics in psychiatry. Am J Med Genet B Neuropsychiatr Genet 171(5):719–732, 2016 26913573

Haltigan JD, Roisman GI, Susman EJ, et al: Elevated trajectories of externalizing problems are associated with lower awakening cortisol levels in midadolescence. Dev Psychol 47(2):472–478, 2011 21219067

Hare RD: Psychopathy and electrodermal responses to nonsignal stimulation. Biol Psychol 6(4):237–246, 1978 708810

Hare RD: Manual for the Revised Psychopathy Checklist. Toronto, ON, Canada, Multi-Health Systems, 2003

Hare RD, Neumann CS: Psychopathy: assessment and forensic implications. Can J Psychiatry 54(12):791–802, 2009 20047718

Hawes DJ, Brennan J, Dadds MR: Cortisol, callous-unemotional traits, and pathways to antisocial behavior. Curr Opin Psychiatry 22(4):357–362, 2009 19455037

Herpertz SC, Wenning B, Mueller B, et al: Psychophysiological responses in ADHD boys with and without conduct disorder: implications for adult antisocial behavior. J Am Acad Child Adolesc Psychiatry 40(10):1222–1230, 2001 11589536

Herpertz SC, Mueller B, Wenning B, et al: Autonomic responses in boys with externalizing disorders. J Neural Transm 110(10):1181–1195, 2003

Herpertz SC, Mueller B, Qunaibi M, et al: Response to emotional stimuli in boys with conduct disorder. Am J Psychiatry 162(6):1100–1107, 2005 15930058

Hibbeln JR, Umhau JC, George DT, et al: Plasma total cholesterol concentrations do not predict cerebrospinal fluid neurotransmitter metabolites: implications for the biophysical role of highly unsaturated fatty acids. Am J Clin Nutr 71 (1 suppl):331S–338S, 2000 10617992

Holi M, Auvinen-Lintunen L, Lindberg N, et al: Inverse correlation between severity of psychopathic traits and serum cortisol levels in young adult violent male offenders. Psychopathology 39(2):102–104, 2006 16424682

Horn M, Potvin S, Allaire JF, et al: Male inmate profiles and their biological correlates. Can J Psychiatry 59(8):441–449, 2014 25161069

House TH, Milligan WL: Autonomic responses to modeled distress in prison psychopaths. J Pers Soc Psychol 34(4):556–560, 1976 993975

Insel T, Cuthbert B, Garvey M, et al: Research domain criteria (RDoC): toward a new classification framework for research on mental disorders. Am J Psychiatry 167(7):748–751, 2010 20595427

Jennings WG, Piquero AR, Farrington DP: Does resting heart rate at age 18 distinguish general and violent offending up to age 50? Findings from the Cambridge Study in Delinquent Development. J Crim Justice 41(4):213–219, 2013

Jones EJ, Rohleder N, Schreier HMC: Neuroendocrine coordination and youth behavior problems: a review of studies assessing sympathetic nervous system and hypothalamic-pituitary adrenal axis activity using salivary alpha amylase and salivary cortisol. Horm Behav 122:104750, 2020 32302595

Jones M, Westen D: Diagnosis and subtypes of adolescent antisocial personality disorder. J Pers Disord 24(2):217–243, 2010 20420477

Kimonis ER, Frick PJ, Munoz LC, et al: Callous-unemotional traits and the emotional processing of distress cues in detained boys: testing the moderating role of aggression, exposure to community violence, and histories of abuse. Dev Psychopathol 20(2):569–589, 2008 18423095

Kindlon DJ, Tremblay RE, Mezzacappa E, et al: Longitudinal patterns of heart rate and fighting behavior in 9- through 12-year-old boys. J Am Acad Child Adolesc Psychiatry 34(3):371–377, 1995 7896679

Klinesmith J, Kasser T, McAndrew FT: Guns, testosterone, and aggression: an experimental test of a mediational hypothesis. Psychol Sci 17(7):568–571, 2006 16866740

Koss KJ, George MR, Cummings EM, et al: Asymmetry in children's salivary cortisol and alpha-amylase in the context of marital conflict: links to children's emotional security and adjustment. Dev Psychobiol 56(4):836–849, 2014 24037991

Kreuz LE, Rose RM: Assessment of aggressive behavior and plasma testosterone in a young criminal population. Psychosom Med 34(4):321–332, 1972 5074958

Kudielka BM, Kirschbaum C: Sex differences in HPA axis responses to stress: a review. Biol Psychol 69(1):113–132, 2005 15740829

Kurath J, Mata R: Individual differences in risk taking and endogenous levels of testosterone, estradiol, and cortisol: a systematic literature search and three independent meta-analyses. Neurosci Biobehav Rev 90:428–446, 2018 29730483

Lee R, Ferris C, Van de Kar LD, et al: Cerebrospinal fluid oxytocin, life history of aggression, and personality disorder. Psychoneuroendocrinology 34(10):1567–1573, 2009 19577376

Lidberg L, Tuck JR, Asberg M, et al: Homicide, suicide and CSF 5-HIAA. Acta Psychiatr Scand 71(3):230–236, 1985 2580421

Liening SH, Josephs RA: It is not just about testosterone: physiological mediators and moderators of testosterone's behavioral effects. Social Personality Psychology Compass 4(11):982–994, 2010

Loney BR, Butler MA, Lima EN, et al: The relation between salivary cortisol, callous-unemotional traits, and conduct problems in an adolescent non-referred sample. J Child Psychol Psychiatry 47(1):30–36, 2006 16405638

Loney J, Carlson GA, Salisbury H, et al: Validation of three dimensions of childhood psychopathology in young clinic-referred boys. J Atten Disord 8(4):169–181, 2005 16110047

Lopez-Duran NL, Olson SL, Hajal NJ, et al: Hypothalamic pituitary adrenal axis functioning in reactive and proactive aggression in children. J Abnorm Child Psychol 37(2):169–182, 2009 18696227

Lorber MF: Psychophysiology of aggression, psychopathy, and conduct problems: a meta-analysis. Psychol Bull 130(4):531–552, 2004 15250812

Lynam DR: Early identification of chronic offenders: who is the fledgling psychopath? Psychol Bull 120(2):209–234, 1996 8831297

Macdonald K, Macdonald TM: The peptide that binds: a systematic review of oxytocin and its prosocial effects in humans. Harv Rev Psychiatry 18(1):1–21, 2010 20047458

Malik AI, Zai CC, Abu Z, et al: The role of oxytocin and oxytocin receptor gene variants in childhood-onset aggression. Genes Brain Behav 11(5):545–551, 2012 22372486

Maras A, Laucht M, Gerdes D, et al: Association of testosterone and dihydrotestosterone with externalizing behavior in adolescent boys and girls. Psychoneuroendocrinology 28(7):932–940, 2003 12892659

Marsman R, Swinkels SH, Rosmalen JG, et al: HPA-axis activity and externalizing behavior problems in early adolescents from the general population: the role of comorbidity and gender. The TRAILS study. Psychoneuroendocrinology 33(6):789–798, 2008 18448258

Marsman R, Rosmalen JG, Oldehinkel AJ, et al: Does HPA-axis activity mediate the relationship between obstetric complications and externalizing behavior problems? The TRAILS study. Eur Child Adolesc Psychiatry 18(9):565–573, 2009 19353232

Marsman R, Nederhof E, Rosmalen JG, et al: Family environment is associated with HPA-axis activity in adolescents: the TRAILS study. Biol Psychol 89(2):460–466, 2012 22212280

Matthys W, van Goozen SH, Snoek H, et al: Response perseveration and sensitivity to reward and punishment in boys with oppositional defiant disorder. Eur Child Adolesc Psychiatry 13(6):362–364, 2004 15619048

Mazur A, Booth A: Testosterone and dominance in men. Behav Brain Sci 21(3):353–363, discussion 363–397, 1998 10097017

Mazur A, Booth A: Testosterone is related to deviance in male army veterans, but relationships are not moderated by cortisol. Biol Psychol 96:72–76, 2014 24333104

McBurnett K, Harris SM, Swanson JM, et al: Neuropsychological and psychophysiological differentiation of inattention/overactivity and aggression/defiance symptom groups. J Clin Child Psychol 22(2):165–171, 1993

McBurnett K, Lahey BB, Capasso L, et al: Aggressive symptoms and salivary cortisol in clinic-referred boys with conduct disorder. Ann NY Acad Sci 794:169–178, 1996 8853601

McBurnett K, Lahey BB, Rathouz PJ, et al: Low salivary cortisol and persistent aggression in boys referred for disruptive behavior. Arch Gen Psychiatry 57(1):38–43, 2000 10632231

McKinley S, Patrick C, Verona E: Antisocial personality disorder: neurophysiological mechanisms and distinct subtypes. Curr Behav Neurosci Rep 5(1):72–80, 2018

Mehta PH, Beer J: Neural mechanisms of the testosterone-aggression relation: the role of orbitofrontal cortex. J Cogn Neurosci 22(10):2357–2368, 2010 19925198

Mehta PH, Josephs RA: Testosterone and cortisol jointly regulate dominance: evidence for a dual-hormone hypothesis. Horm Behav 58(5):898–906, 2010 20816841

Mehta PH, Prasad S: The dual-hormone hypothesis: a brief review and future research agenda. Curr Opin Behav Sci 3:163–168, 2015

Mendez MF: The neurobiology of moral behavior: review and neuropsychiatric implications. CNS Spectr 14(11):608–620, 2009 20173686

Meyer-Lindenberg A, Domes G, Kirsch P, et al: Oxytocin and vasopressin in the human brain: social neuropeptides for translational medicine. Nat Rev Neurosci 12(9):524–538, 2011 21852800

Mitchell DGV, Colledge E, Leonard A, et al: Risky decisions and response reversal: is there evidence of orbitofrontal cortex dysfunction in psychopathic individuals? Neuropsychologia 40(12):2013–2022, 2002 12207998

Mitchell IJ, Smid W, Troelstra J, et al: Psychopathic characteristics are related to high basal urinary oxytocin levels in male forensic patients. J Forens Psychiatry Psychol 24(3):309–318, 2013

Moffitt TE, Caspi A: Childhood predictors differentiate life-course persistent and adolescence-limited antisocial pathways among males and females. Dev Psychopathol 13(2):355–375, 2001 11393651

Montoya ER, Terburg D, Bos PA, et al: Testosterone, cortisol, and serotonin as key regulators of social aggression: a review and theoretical perspective. Motiv Emot 36(1):65–73, 2012 22448079

Moore TM, Scarpa A, Raine A: A meta-analysis of serotonin metabolite 5-HIAA and antisocial behavior. Aggress Behav 28(4):299–316, 2002

Muñoz LC, Frick PJ, Kimonis ER, et al: Types of aggression, responsiveness to provocation, and callous-unemotional traits in detained adolescents. J Abnorm Child Psychol 36(1):15–28, 2008 17882544

Murray J, Hallal PC, Mielke GI, et al: Low resting heart rate is associated with violence in late adolescence: a prospective birth cohort study in Brazil. Int J Epidemiol 45(2):491–500, 2016 26822937

Ne'eman R, Perach-Barzilay N, Fischer-Shofty M, et al: Intranasal administration of oxytocin increases human aggressive behavior. Horm Behav 80:125–131, 2016 26862988

Niemelä S, Sourander A, Elonheimo H, et al: What predicts illicit drug use versus police-registered drug offending? Findings from the Finnish "From a Boy to a Man" birth cohort study. Soc Psychiatry Psychiatr Epidemiol 43(9):697–704, 2008 18438733

Northover C, Thapar A, Langley K, et al: Cortisol levels at baseline and under stress in adolescent males with attention-deficit hyperactivity disorder, with or without comorbid conduct disorder. Psychiatry Res 242:130–136, 2016 27280522

O'Brien BS, Frick PJ: Reward dominance: associations with anxiety, conduct problems, and psychopathy in children. J Abnorm Child Psychol 24(2):223–240, 1996 8743246

O'Leary MM, Loney BR, Eckel LA: Gender differences in the association between psychopathic personality traits and cortisol response to induced stress. Psychoneuroendocrinology 32(2):183–191, 2007 17289279

O'Leary MM, Taylor J, Eckel L: Psychopathic personality traits and cortisol response to stress: the role of sex, type of stressor, and menstrual phase. Horm Behav 58(2):250–256, 2010 20302872

Olweus D, Mattsson A, Schalling D, et al: Circulating testosterone levels and aggression in adolescent males: a causal analysis. Psychosom Med 50(3):261–272, 1988 3387509

Oosterlaan J, Geurts HM, Knol DL, et al: Low basal salivary cortisol is associated with teacher-reported symptoms of conduct disorder. Psychiatry Res 134(1):1–10, 2005 15808285

Ortiz J, Raine A: Heart rate level and antisocial behavior in children and adolescents: a meta-analysis. J Am Acad Child Adolesc Psychiatry 43(2):154–162, 2004 14726721

Pajer K, Gardner W, Rubin RT, et al: Decreased cortisol levels in adolescent girls with conduct disorder. Arch Gen Psychiatry 58(3):297–302, 2001 11231837

Pajer K, Tabbah R, Gardner W, et al: Adrenal androgen and gonadal hormone levels in adolescent girls with conduct disorder. Psychoneuroendocrinology 31(10):1245–1256, 2006 17126492

Patrick CJ: Psychophysiological correlates of aggression and violence: an integrative review. Philos Trans R Soc Lond B Biol Sci 363(1503):2543–2555, 2008 18434285

Patrick CJ (ed): Handbook of Psychopathy, 2nd Edition. New York, Guilford, 2018

Patrick CJ, Bernat EM: Neurobiology of psychopathy: a two process theory, in Handbook of Neuroscience for the Behavioral Sciences, Vol 2. Edited by Berntson GG, Cacioppo JT. New York, Wiley, 2009, pp 1110–1131

Paus T, Nawaz-Khan I, Leonard G, et al: Sexual dimorphism in the adolescent brain: role of testosterone and androgen receptor in global and local volumes of grey and white matter. Horm Behav 57(1):63–75, 2010 19703457

Pitts TB: Reduced heart rate levels in aggressive children, in Biosocial Bases of Violence. Edited by Raine A, Brennan P, Farrington DP, et al. New York, Springer, 1997, pp 317–320

Platje E, Jansen LM, Raine A, et al: Longitudinal associations in adolescence between cortisol and persistent aggressive or rule-breaking behavior. Biol Psychol 93(1):132–137, 2013a 23348558

Platje E, Vermeiren RR, Raine A, et al: A longitudinal biosocial study of cortisol and peer influence on the development of adolescent antisocial behavior. Psychoneuroendocrinology 38(11):2770–2779, 2013b 23927935

Popma A, Jansen LM, Vermeiren R, et al: Hypothalamus pituitary adrenal axis and autonomic activity during stress in delinquent male adolescents and controls. Psychoneuroendocrinology 31(8):948–957, 2006 16831519

Portnoy J, Farrington DP: Resting heart rate and antisocial behavior: an updated systematic review and meta-analysis. Aggress Violent Behav 22:33–45, 2015

Portnoy J, Raine A, Chen FR, et al: Heart rate and antisocial behavior: the mediating role of impulsive sensation seeking. Criminology 52(2):292–311, 2014

Posthumus JA, Böcker KB, Raaijmakers MA, et al: Heart rate and skin conductance in four-year-old children with aggressive behavior. Biol Psychol 82(2):164–168, 2009 19596046

Poustka L, Maras A, Hohm E, et al: Negative association between plasma cortisol levels and aggression in a high-risk community sample of adolescents. J Neural Transm (Vienna) 117(5):621–627, 2010 20217435

Quirin M, Kuhl J, Düsing R: Oxytocin buffers cortisol responses to stress in individuals with impaired emotion regulation abilities. Psychoneuroendocrinology 36(6):898–904, 2011 21208748

Raine A: Autonomic nervous system activity and violence, in Aggression and Violence: Genetic, Neurobiological, and Biosocial Perspectives. Edited by Stoff DM, Cairns RB. Hillsdale, NJ, Erlbaum, 1996, pp 145–168

Raine A: The interaction of biological and social measures in the explanation of antisocial and violent behavior, in Developmental Psychobiology of Aggression. Edited by Stoff DM, Susman EJ. New York, Cambridge University Press, 2005, pp 13–42

Raine A: The Psychopathology of Crime: Criminal Behavior as a Clinical Disorder. New York, Elsevier, 2013

Raine A: The neuromoral theory of antisocial, violent, and psychopathic behavior. Psychiatry Res 277:64–69, 2019 30473129

Raine A, Jones F: Attention, autonomic arousal, and personality in behaviorally disordered children. J Abnorm Child Psychol 15(4):583–599, 1987 3437093

Raine A, Venables PH, Williams M: Autonomic orienting responses in 15-year-old male subjects and criminal behavior at age 24. Am J Psychiatry 147(7):933–937, 1990 2356879

Raine A, Venables PH, Williams M: Better autonomic conditioning and faster electrodermal half-recovery time at age 15 years as possible protective factors against crime at age 29 years. Dev Psychol 32(4):624–630, 1996

Raine A, Venables PH, Mednick SA: Low resting heart rate at age 3 years predisposes to aggression at age 11 years: evidence from the Mauritius Child Health Project. J Am Acad Child Adolesc Psychiatry 36(10):1457–1464, 1997 9334560

Raine A, Lencz T, Bihrle S, et al: Reduced prefrontal gray matter volume and reduced autonomic activity in antisocial personality disorder. Arch Gen Psychiatry 57(2):119–127, discussion 128–129, 2000 10665614

Raine A, Fung AL, Portnoy J, et al: Low heart rate as a risk factor for child and adolescent proactive aggressive and impulsive psychopathic behavior. Aggress Behav 40(4):290–299, 2014 24604759

Ritsner MS (ed):The Handbook of Neuropsychiatric Biomarkers, Endophenotypes, and Genes: Volume I: Neuropsychological Endophenotypes and Biomarkers. New York, Springer Science and Business Media, 2009

Ruttle PL, Shirtcliff EA, Serbin LA, et al: Disentangling psychobiological mechanisms underlying internalizing and externalizing behaviors in youth: longitudinal and concurrent associations with cortisol. Horm Behav 59(1):123–132, 2011 21056565

Salis KL, Bernard K, Black SR, et al: Examining the concurrent and longitudinal relationship between diurnal cortisol rhythms and conduct problems during childhood. Psychoneuroendocrinology 71:147–154, 2016 27266968

Sapolsky RM: Behave: The Biology of Humans at Our Best and Worst. New York, Penguin, 2017

Schulkin J: Allostasis: a neural behavioral perspective. Horm Behav 43(1):21–27, discussion 28–30, 2003 12614630

Schulkin J, Gold PW, McEwen BS: Induction of corticotropin-releasing hormone gene expression by glucocorticoids: implication for understanding the states of fear and anxiety and allostatic load. Psychoneuroendocrinology 23(3):219–243, 1998 9695128

Seo D, Patrick CJ, Kennealy PJ: Role of serotonin and dopamine system interactions in the neurobiology of impulsive aggression and its comorbidity with other clinical disorders. Aggress Violent Behav 13(5):383–395, 2008 19802333

Shamay-Tsoory SG, Abu-Akel A: The social salience hypothesis of oxytocin. Biol Psychiatry 79(3):194–202, 2016 26321019

Shamay-Tsoory SG, Fischer M, Dvash J, et al: Intranasal administration of oxytocin increases envy and schadenfreude (gloating). Biol Psychiatry 66(9):864–870, 2009 19640508

Shirtcliff EA, Vitacco MJ, Graf AR, et al: Neurobiology of empathy and callousness: implications for the development of antisocial behavior. Behav Sci Law 27(2):137–171, 2009 19319834

Shoal GD, Giancola PR, Kirillova GP: Salivary cortisol, personality, and aggressive behavior in adolescent boys: a 5-year longitudinal study. J Am Acad Child Adolesc Psychiatry 42(9):1101–1107, 2003 12960710

Siegel A, Douard J: Who's flying the plane: serotonin levels, aggression and free will. Int J Law Psychiatry 34(1):20–29, 2011 21112635

Simeon D, Stanley B, Frances A, et al: Self-mutilation in personality disorders: psychological and biological correlates. Am J Psychiatry 149(2):221–226, 1992 1734743

Simeon D, Bartz J, Hamilton H, et al: Oxytocin administration attenuates stress reactivity in borderline personality disorder: a pilot study. Psychoneuroendocrinology 36(9):1418–1421, 2011 21546164

Sobczak S, Honig A, Nicolson NA, et al: Effects of acute tryptophan depletion on mood and cortisol release in first-degree relatives of type I and type II bipolar patients and healthy matched controls. Neuropsychopharmacology 27(5):834–842, 2002

Soderstrom H, Blennow K, Manhem A, et al: CSF studies in violent offenders, I: 5-HIAA as a negative and HVA as a positive predictor of psychopathy. J Neural Transm 108(7):869–878, 2001

Soderstrom H, Blennow K, Sjodin AK, et al: New evidence for an association between the CSF HVA:5-HIAA ratio and psychopathic traits. J Neurol Neurosurg Psychiatry 74(7):918–921, 2003 12810780

Stålenheim EG, Eriksson E, von Knorring L, et al: Testosterone as a biological marker in psychopathy and alcoholism. Psychiatry Res 77(2):79–88, 1998 9541143

Stoppelbein L, Greening L, Luebbe A, et al: The role of cortisol and psychopathic traits in aggression among at-risk girls: tests of mediating hypotheses. Aggress Behav 40(3):263–272, 2014 24302544

Susman EJ: Psychobiology of persistent antisocial behavior: stress, early vulnerabilities and the attenuation hypothesis. Neurosci Biobehav Rev 30(3):376–389, 2006 16239030

Sylvers P, Brennan PA, Lilienfeld SO, et al: Gender differences in autonomic indicators of antisocial personality disorder features. Pers Disord 1(2):87–96, 2010 22448620

Tarter RE, Kirisci L, Gavaler JS, et al: Prospective study of the association between abandoned dwellings and testosterone level on the development of behaviors leading to cannabis use disorder in boys. Biol Psychiatry 65(2):116–121, 2009 18930183

Terburg D, Morgan B, van Honk J: The testosterone-cortisol ratio: a hormonal marker for proneness to social aggression. Int J Law Psychiatry 32(4):216–223, 2009 19446881

Timmermann M, Jeung H, Schmitt R, et al: Oxytocin improves facial emotion recognition in young adults with antisocial personality disorder. Psychoneuroendocrinology 85:158–164, 2017 28865940

Träskman-Bendz L, Asberg M, Schalling D: Serotonergic function and suicidal behavior in personality disorders. Ann NY Acad Sci 487:168–174, 1986 2436531

Tsigos C, Chrousos GP: Hypothalamic-pituitary-adrenal axis, neuroendocrine factors and stress. J Psychosom Res 53(4):865–871, 2002 12377295

van Bokhoven I, Matthys W, van Goozen SH, et al: Prediction of adolescent outcome in children with disruptive behaviour disorders—a study of neurobiological, psychological and family factors. Eur Child Adolesc Psychiatry 14(3):153–163, 2005a 15959661

van Bokhoven I, Van Goozen SH, van Engeland H, et al: Salivary cortisol and aggression in a population-based longitudinal study of adolescent males. J Neural Transm 112(8):1083–1096, 2005b

van Bokhoven I, van Goozen SH, van Engeland H, et al: Salivary testosterone and aggression, delinquency, and social dominance in a population-based longitudinal study of adolescent males. Horm Behav 50(1):118–125, 2006 16631757

Van de Weijer S, De Jong R, Bijleveld C, et al: The role of heart rate levels in the intergenerational transmission of crime. J Societies 7(3):23, 2017

van de Wiel NM, van Goozen SH, Matthys W, et al: Cortisol and treatment effect in children with disruptive behavior disorders: a preliminary study. J Am Acad Child Adolesc Psychiatry 43(8):1011–1018, 2004 15266196

van der Vegt BJ, Lieuwes N, Cremers TI, et al: Cerebrospinal fluid monoamine and metabolite concentrations and aggression in rats. Horm Behav 44(3):199–208, 2003 14609542

van Goozen SH: The role of early emotion impairments in the development of persistent antisocial behavior. Child Dev Perspect 9(4):206–210, 2015

van Goozen SH, Fairchild G: Neuroendocrine and neurotransmitter correlates in children with antisocial behavior. Horm Behav 50(4):647–654, 2006 16860323

van Goozen SH, Fairchild G: How can the study of biological processes help design new interventions for children with severe antisocial behavior? Dev Psychopathol 20(3):941–973, 2008 18606039

van Goozen SH, Matthys W, Cohen-Kettenis PT, et al: Adrenal androgens and aggression in conduct disorder prepubertal boys and normal controls. Biol Psychiatry 43(2):156–158, 1998 9474448 van Goozen SH, Matthys W, Cohen-Kettenis PT, et al: Hypothalamic-pituitary-adrenal axis and autonomic nervous system activity in disruptive children and matched controls. J Am Acad Child Adolesc Psychiatry 39(11):1438–1445, 2000 11068900

van Goozen SH, Fairchild G, Snoek H, et al: The evidence for a neurobiological model of childhood antisocial behavior. Psychol Bull 133(1):149–182, 2007 17201574

van Honk J, Schutter DJ, Hermans EJ, et al: Low cortisol levels and the balance between punishment sensitivity and reward dependency. Neuroreport 14(15):1993–1996, 2003 14561936

van Honk J, Harmon-Jones E, Morgan BE, et al: Socially explosive minds: the triple imbalance hypothesis of reactive aggression. J Pers 78(1):67–94, 2010 20433613

Virkkunen M: Urinary free cortisol secretion in habitually violent offenders. Acta Psychiatr Scand 72(1):40–44, 1985 2994368

Warner HR, Cox A: A mathematical model of heart rate control by sympathetic and vagus efferent information. J Appl Physiol 17:349–355, 1962 14005012

Weisman O, Zagoory-Sharon O, Feldman R: Oxytocin administration, salivary testosterone, and father-infant social behavior. Prog Neuropsychopharmacol Biol Psychiatry 49:47–52, 2014 24252717

Willner P: The neurobiology of aggression: implications for the pharmacotherapy of aggressive challenging behaviour by people with intellectual disabilities. J Intellect Disabil Res 59(1):82–92, 2015 24467721

Woodman DD, Hinton JW, O'Neill MT: Cortisol secretion and stress in maximum security hospital patients. J Psychosom Res 22(2):133–136, 1978 650613

Yildirim BO, Derksen JJ: A review on the relationship between testosterone and life-course persistent antisocial behavior. Psychiatry Res 200(2–3):984–1010, 2012a 22925371

Yildirim BO, Derksen JJ: A review on the relationship between testosterone and the interpersonal/affective facet of psychopathy. Psychiatry Res 197(3):181–198, 2012b 22342179

Yu YZ, Shi JX: Relationship between levels of testosterone and cortisol in saliva and aggressive behaviors of adolescents. Biomed Environ Sci 22(1):44–49, 2009 19462687

Zahn TP, Kruesi MJP: Autonomic activity in boys with disruptive behavior disorders. Psychophysiology 30(6):605–614, 1993 8248452

Zilioli S, Bird BM: Functional significance of men's testosterone reactivity to social stimuli. Front Neuroendocrinol 47:1–18, 2017 28676436

Zilioli S, Mehta PH, Watson NV: Losing the battle but winning the war: uncertain outcomes reverse the usual effect of winning on testosterone. Biol Psychol 103:54–62, 2014 25148788

Zuckerman M: Sensation Seeking: Beyond the Optimal Level of Arousal. Psychology Revivals. New York, Psychology Press, 2014

CHAPTER 13

Structural MRI Studies of Antisocial Personality Disorder

Olivia Choy, Ph.D.

Our understanding of the biological underpinnings of antisocial personality disorder (ASPD) has been advanced through the contributions of neuroscientific research, which has elucidated the brain's role in antisocial behavior. Brain imaging techniques, such as MRI, allow for the investigation of the neural correlates of this personality disorder. One takeaway point from the past two decades of neuroimaging research on ASPD is that there is empirical evidence of abnormalities in several brain structures in individuals with antisocial behavior.

This chapter focuses on research involving structural MRI. It provides a comprehensive overview of studies that shed light on the anatomical substrates of ASPD. Importantly, these studies investigate brain morphology rather than brain activity. Many of them do so by measuring the volumes of gray and white matter in various brain regions of individuals diagnosed with ASPD and healthy control subjects. Other studies assess the neuroanatomical measures of cortical thickness and cortical surface area separately. Comparisons of these measures of brain structure between ASPD and control groups have yielded significant findings in multiple brain regions.

In this chapter, I review key findings on the prefrontal cortex (PFC), amygdala, hippocampus, striatum, cerebellum, and corpus callosum. A summary of these findings is presented in Table 13–1. Additionally, salient issues relevant to structural neuroimaging studies on ASPD are discussed. These involve disentangling the neural correlates of ASPD from comorbid disorders, interaction effects between biological and psychosocial factors in understanding the etiology of ASPD, and putative sources of structural abnormalities in antisocial individuals. Other pertinent issues include the potential for brain deficits to explain the higher prevalence of ASPD observed in males and the association between early brain structural abnormalities and later ASPD. The chapter concludes with potential areas for future research.

Structural Neuroimaging Findings in Antisocial Personality Disorder

Prefrontal Cortex

A large body of research from the domain of neuropsychology, which involves indirect, behavior-based assessments of brain dysfunction, has identified deficits in executive functioning in antisocial individuals (Ogilvie et al. 2011). The poorer executive functioning observed is thought to represent impairment in frontal lobe functioning. Numerous functional MRI studies that measure regional brain activity in a more direct way have similarly found that increased antisocial behavior is associated with reduced function in the PFC (Yang and Raine 2009), bolstering the neuropsychological findings. By using a different approach that examines brain structure, structural MRI studies can help strengthen our understanding of the role of the frontal cortex on such behavior.

Several structural MRI studies have investigated the PFC in relation to ASPD. In one of the first structural brain imaging studies of antisocial adults, an 11% reduction in gray matter volume was documented in the PFC of 21 men with ASPD compared with 34 healthy control subjects (Raine et al. 2000). Notably, although the ASPD group included individuals with comorbid clinical conditions, such as substance dependence and mood and schizophrenia spectrum disorders, further analyses found that the structural deficits observed in the PFC were not attributable to psychiatric comorbidity. Subsequent studies reported converging evidence of smaller volumes in the PFC in individuals with ASPD (e.g., Laakso et al. 2002; Müller et al. 2008; Raine et al. 2011). This finding was reported in a meta-analysis of 43 structural and functional brain imaging studies of antisocial behavior, which determined that deficits in the structure of the PFC were associated with various forms of antisocial behavior, including the diagnosis of ASPD (Yang and Raine 2009; Figure 13–1). In line with the notion that the PFC is critically involved in executive functions, decision-making, and impulse inhibition (Crews and Boettiger 2009), deficits in the right PFC may be linked to emotional deficits and poor decision-making in antisocial individuals, while reduced volumes in the left dorsolateral PFC may be linked to greater impulsivity and poorer behavioral control, which are in turn associated with increased antisocial behavior (Yang and Raine 2009).

More specifically, studies have identified prefrontal subregions that are particularly implicated in ASPD. One such region is the orbitofrontal cortex (OFC), which occupies the ventral surface of the frontal part of the brain. The OFC is relevant to emotion regulation, behavioral inhibition, and the processing of rewards and punishments (Kringelbach and Rolls 2004).

A technique to examine structural brain differences between groups of subjects from MRI data is voxel-based morphometry. Briefly, it involves spatially normalizing the structural magnetic resonance images to the same stereotactic space, segmenting

TABLE 13–1. Summary of structural neuroimaging findings on antisocial personality disorder (ASPD)

Study	ASPD group (mean age, y, ±SD)	Recruitment of ASPD group	Control group (mean age, y, ±SD)	Magnetic resonance scanner	Main findings
Barkataki et al. 2006	13 males with ASPD (31.62±8.03)	Institutional-based	13 males with schizophrenia and a history of serious violence (34.46±4.94); 15 males with schizophrenia without a history of violence (34.47±7.49); 15 healthy male control subjects (32.13±7.47)	1.5 T	Compared with the healthy control group, males with ASPD had reduced whole brain and temporal lobe volumes and a larger putamen volume. Compared with the group with schizophrenia and a violent history, males with ASPD had smaller temporal lobe and larger hippocampal volumes. Compared with the group with schizophrenia and no history of violence, males with ASPD had smaller temporal lobe volumes and a larger striatum and amygdala.

TABLE 13–1.   Summary of structural neuroimaging findings on antisocial personality disorder (ASPD) *(continued)*

Study	ASPD group (mean age, y, ±SD)	Recruitment of ASPD group	Control group (mean age, y, ±SD)	Magnetic resonance scanner	Main findings
Bertsch et al. 2013	13 male offenders with ASPD and comorbid BPD (28.9±10.1); 12 male offenders with ASPD and high psychopathy scores (27.3±5.4)	Institutional-based	14 healthy male control subjects (26.1±8.3)	1.5 T	Compared with the healthy control group, male offenders with ASPD and comorbid BPD had smaller gray matter volumes in the left frontal pole, left OFC, and right ventromedial PFC, whereas male offenders with ASPD and high levels of psychopathy had reduced gray matter volumes in the left dorsomedial PFC, left postcentral gyrus, right precuneus, and bilateral occipital cortex.
Dolan et al. 2002	18 male patients with personality disorders, of whom 14 had presentations that met diagnostic criteria for ASPD (30.44±7.00)	Institutional-based	19 healthy control subjects (30.52±6.83)	0.5 T	Compared with the healthy control group, patients with personality disorders had reduced temporal volumes. No differences in frontal brain volumes were found.

TABLE 13–1. Summary of structural neuroimaging findings on antisocial personality disorder (ASPD) (*continued*)

Study	ASPD group (mean age, y, ±SD)	Recruitment of ASPD group	Control group (mean age, y, ±SD)	Magnetic resonance scanner	Main findings
Gregory et al. 2012	17 violent male offenders with ASPD and psychopathy (38.9±9.4); 27 violent male offenders with ASPD without psychopathy (36.1±8.2)	Institutional-based	22 healthy male control subjects (32.4±7.7)	1.5 T	Compared with violent male offenders with ASPD but no psychopathy and the healthy control group, violent male offenders with ASPD and high levels of psychopathy had reduced gray matter volumes bilaterally in the anterior rostral medial PFC and temporal poles.
Jiang et al. 2016	27 males with ASPD (20.30±3.01)	Institutional-based	25 healthy male control subjects (21.13±3.16)	3 T	Compared with the healthy control group, males with ASPD showed reduced cortical thickness in the superior frontal gyrus/rostral ACC, precuneus, OFC, pars triangularis, insula cortex, superior temporal sulcus, superior temporal gyrus, and middle frontal gyrus and increased surface area in the medial OFC, precuneus, insula cortex, and superior temporal, superior frontal, middle frontal, precentral, supramarginal, parahippocampal, and postcentral gyri.

TABLE 13–1. Summary of structural neuroimaging findings on antisocial personality disorder (ASPD) *(continued)*

Study	ASPD group (mean age, y, ±SD)	Recruitment of ASPD group	Control group (mean age, y, ±SD)	Magnetic resonance scanner	Main findings
Kolla et al. 2014	9 male offenders with ASPD and high levels of psychopathy (38.7±6.0); 15 male offenders with ASPD and low levels of psychopathy (35.0±9.3)	Institutional-based	13 healthy male control subjects (35.1±8.0)	1.5 T	Compared with male offenders with ASPD and low levels of psychopathy, male offenders with ASPD and high psychopathy scores had smaller gray matter volume in the bilateral temporal poles, right uncus, and posterior cerebellum. No differences in brain structure were reported between ASPD groups and the healthy control group.
Kolla et al. 2017	18 males with ASPD and psychopathy (9 with low-activity *MAOA* [35.7±10.1], 9 with high-activity *MAOA* [36.2±8.7])	Community- and institutional-based	20 healthy male control subjects (9 with low-activity *MAOA* [31.7±6.6], 11 with high-activity *MAOA* [37.1±7.8])	3.0 T	Compared with the healthy control groups, males in the ASPD group had smaller OFC volumes and decreased cortical thickness in the left lateral orbitofrontal gyrus. Compared with the control group with low-activity *MAOA*, males in the ASPD group with low-activity *MAOA* showed decreased surface areas in the right basolateral nucleus and increased surface areas in the right anterior cortical amygdaloid nucleus.

TABLE 13–1. **Summary of structural neuroimaging findings on antisocial personality disorder (ASPD)** *(continued)*

Study	ASPD group (mean age, y, ±SD)	Recruitment of ASPD group	Control group (mean age, y, ±SD)	Magnetic resonance scanner	Main findings
Kumari et al. 2014	14 males with ASPD (34.64±10.96 / 29.33±8.74)[a]	Institutional-based	13 males with schizophrenia and a history of serious violence (32.00±3.79 / 32.13±7.47); 15 males with schizophrenia without a history of violence (39.75±8.06 / 32.55±6.62); 15 healthy male control subjects (32.13±7.47)	1.5 T	Compared with the healthy control group, males with ASPD and those with schizophrenia and a history of violence had significantly lower ACC volumes.
Laakso et al. 2000	19 violent male offenders with ASPD and alcohol dependence (30±8)	Institutional-based	34 healthy control subjects (35±12)	1.0 T / 1.5 T	Compared with the healthy control group, violent male offenders with ASPD and alcohol dependence had smaller right, but not left, hippocampal volume.
Laakso et al. 2002	24 violent male offenders with ASPD and alcohol dependence (31±8)	Institutional-based	33 healthy male control subjects (34±10)	1.0 T / 1.5 T	Compared with the healthy control group, violent male offenders with ASPD and alcohol dependence had smaller volumes in the left dorsolateral PFC, left OFC, and left medial frontal gyrus, but this difference was not significant after controlling for differences in education and duration of alcoholism.

TABLE 13–1. Summary of structural neuroimaging findings on antisocial personality disorder (ASPD) *(continued)*

Study	ASPD group (mean age, y, ±SD)	Recruitment of ASPD group	Control group (mean age, y, ±SD)	Magnetic resonance scanner	Main findings
Müller et al. 2008	17 male patients with ASPD and high levels of psychopathy (33.00±5.81)	Institutional-based	17 healthy male control subjects (30.59±5.92)	1.5 T	Compared with the healthy control group, male patients with ASPD and high psychopathy scores had reduced gray matter in the temporal lobe, PFC, and premotor cortex.
Narayan et al. 2007	14 males with ASPD (33.5±10.4)	Institutional-based	12 males with schizophrenia and a history of violence (34.4±5.2); 15 males with schizophrenia without a history of violence (34.5±7.5); 15 healthy male control subjects (32.1±7.5)	1.5 T	Compared with the healthy control group, males with ASPD showed significant thinning of the medial inferior frontal cortices. The ASPD group and violent males with schizophrenia also showed significant thinning of the frontal pole and the dorsal ACC compared with the healthy control group and nonviolent males with schizophrenia.
Raine et al. 2000	21 males with ASPD (31.9±6.8)	Community-based	34 healthy male control subjects (30.4±6.7); 26 substance-dependent male control subjects (30.2±6.2)	1.5 T	Compared with both the healthy and the substance-dependent control groups, males with ASPD had lower prefrontal gray matter, but not white matter, volumes.

TABLE 13–1. Summary of structural neuroimaging findings on antisocial personality disorder (ASPD) *(continued)*

Study	ASPD group (mean age, y, ±SD)	Recruitment of ASPD group	Control group (mean age, y, ±SD)	Magnetic resonance scanner	Main findings
Raine et al. 2003	15 males with ASPD and high psychopathy scores (31.6±6.6)	Community-based	25 healthy male control subjects (28.8±6.5)	1.5 T	Compared with the healthy control group, males in the ASPD group showed increased white matter volume and length of the corpus callosum and reduced callosal thickness.
Raine et al. 2010	17 males and 1 female with ASPD (32.72±6.54)	Community-based	58 male and 11 female healthy control subjects (31.23±6.83)	1.5 T	Individuals with a CSP had higher ASPD scores compared with individuals without a CSP.
Raine et al. 2011	18 males with ASPD (32.9); 12 females (33.9)[b]	Community-based	30 healthy male control subjects (31.3); 24 substance-dependent male control subjects (30.2)	1.5 T	Compared with both the healthy and the substance-dependent control groups, males with ASPD had lower gray matter, but not white matter, volumes in the OFC and middle frontal gyrus. In males, reduced middle and orbitofrontal volumes were associated with increased ASPD symptoms. In females, reduced orbitofrontal gray matter volume was associated with increased ASPD symptoms.

TABLE 13–1. Summary of structural neuroimaging findings on antisocial personality disorder (ASPD) *(continued)*

Study	ASPD group (mean age, y, ±SD)	Recruitment of ASPD group	Control group (mean age, y, ±SD)	Magnetic resonance scanner	Main findings
Sundram et al. 2012	15 males with ASPD (39±10)	Institutional-based	15 healthy male control subjects (37±11)	1.5 T	Compared with the healthy control group, males with ASPD had reductions in white matter fractional anisotropy bilaterally in the frontal lobe, in the anterior portion of the corpus callosum, and showed increases in mean diffusivity in the right frontal lobe.
Tiihonen et al. 2008	26 male offenders with ASPD and substance dependence (32.5±8.4)	Institutional-based	25 healthy male control subjects (34.6±10.8)	1.0 T	Compared with the healthy control group, male offenders with ASPD and substance dependence had larger white matter volume in the occipital and parietal lobes and left cerebellum; larger gray matter volume in the right cerebellum; smaller gray matter volumes in the postcentral gyri, frontopolar cortex, and OFC; and decreased density of white matter in the right medial frontal gyrus.

Note. ACC=anterior cingulate cortex; BPD=borderline personality disorder; CSP=cavum septum pellucidum; OFC=orbitofrontal cortex; PFC=prefrontal cortex.
[a]The two means and SDs reflect the ages of the ASPD-diagnosed males with and without psychosocial deprivation, respectively.
[b]There was no control group for the female sample as correlational analysis was conducted.

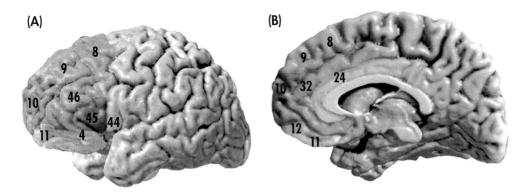

FIGURE 13–1. Lateral (A) and medial (B) illustration of the Brodmann areas (BA) in the orbitofrontal, dorsolateral prefrontal, ventrolateral prefrontal, medial prefrontal, and anterior cingulate cortices.

To view this figure in color, see Plate 6 in Color Gallery.
The orbitofrontal cortex included BA 11, 12, and 47. The dorsolateral prefrontal cortex included BA 8, 9, 10, and 46. The ventrolateral prefrontal cortex included BA 44 and 45. The medial prefrontal cortex included BA 8, 9, 10, 11, and 12. The anterior cingulate cortex included BA 24 and 32.
Source. Reprinted from Yang Y, Raine A: "Prefrontal Structural and Functional Brain Imaging Findings in Antisocial, Violent, and Psychopathic Individuals: A Meta-Analysis." *Psychiatry Research* 174(2):81–88, 2009. Copyright © 2009 Elsevier. Used with permission.

the normalized images into gray and white matter, and smoothing the gray and white matter images in order to perform a statistical comparison of the local composition of brain tissue at the voxel level between the groups (Mechelli et al. 2005). By comparing the voxel-based morphometry of the gray matter of 26 violent male offenders with ASPD and 25 men without ASPD, one study observed lower gray matter volumes of the OFC in the ASPD group compared with the healthy control group (Tiihonen et al. 2008). These results are supported by findings from a recent study in which males with ASPD and high levels of psychopathic traits had reduced OFC volumes relative to volumes of the OFC in healthy control subjects (Kolla et al. 2017).

Structural deficits in other prefrontal subregions have been identified. The ventrolateral PFC also has been implicated in the psychopathology of ASPD. For example, a study comparing 14 males diagnosed with ASPD with 15 healthy control subjects reported significant thinning of the inferior frontal cortex in individuals with ASPD compared with the healthy subjects (Narayan et al. 2007). Another study of 18 ASPD males and 30 healthy control subjects reported that compared with the control group, males with ASPD showed an 8.7%, 17.3%, and 16.1% reduction in orbitofrontal gray volume, middle frontal gray volume, and right rectal gray volume, respectively (Raine et al. 2011). Notably, gray matter volume reductions in these three prefrontal regions were predictive of membership of either ASPD or healthy control groups, with an accuracy of 83.3%.

Neuroimaging research on the frontal lobe of the brain in relation to antisocial behavior has also highlighted the involvement of the anterior cingulate cortex (ACC), which is a medial region in the frontal cortex thought to be involved in the emotional control circuit (Davidson et al. 2000). The ACC also plays an integral role in error detection and in the integration of conflicting inputs (Smith et al. 2016). Thus, it has been suggested that structural impairments in this brain area may lead to dysfunctional emotional conflict evaluation. Empirical evidence shows that structural abnormalities of the ACC may be linked to the violence observed in individuals with ASPD. For instance, a study examining 14 men with ASPD, 13 patients with schizophrenia and a history of violence, and 15 healthy control subjects found that patients with ASPD and those with violent schizophrenia had significantly lower volumes in the ACC compared with healthy control subjects (Kumari et al. 2014).

The prefrontal-ASPD relationship has been evaluated using different brain measures. In addition to smaller gray matter volumes, significant white matter microstructural abnormalities have been found in frontal regions of the brain in adults with ASPD (Sundram et al. 2012). The cortical thickness of the ACC in ASPD patients also has been examined. Findings are consistent with the results obtained from assessing cortical volume. Males with ASPD and violent males with schizophrenia show significant thinning of the dorsal ACC in comparison with healthy control subjects and nonviolent males with schizophrenia (Narayan et al. 2007). Reduced cortical thickness in the OFC, together with reductions in the superior and middle frontal gyri, also have been observed in males with ASPD (e.g., Jiang et al. 2016). In contrast, the study found that compared with healthy control subjects, ASPD patients had increased cortical surface area in these regions. The observed increase in cortical surface areas may be associated with compensatory effects as a result of the reduced cortical thickness in males with ASPD (Jiang et al. 2016). Converging evidence from different measures of brain structure, such as gray matter volume, white matter integrity, and cortical thickness, highlights the important role of the PFC in ASPD.

Amygdala

Structural abnormalities observed in antisocial populations are not restricted to the frontal lobe. Decreased gray matter volumes in temporal brain regions also have been associated with ASPD (Barkataki et al. 2006; Dolan et al. 2002). One brain region that is linked to a neural circuitry involving the orbitofrontal brain regions and the ACC is the amygdala, which is a limbic structure. The limbic system is an aggregation of brain structures that play a major role in activities relating to emotion, memory, and motivation. It is also closely connected to the frontal brain regions where emotional information is modulated and controlled (DeLisi 2011). A body of neuroimaging research has identified the amygdala as a key structure in neurobiological models of antisocial behavior (see, e.g., Fairchild et al. 2011; Raine 2018).

Some indirect evidence indicates that the amygdala may play a role in the pathogenesis of ASPD. For instance, bilateral volume reductions in the amygdala are found in individuals with psychopathy, which is a construct closely associated with ASPD (Yang et al. 2009). Furthermore, in a sample of 191 male adolescents in a youth detention facility, lower amygdala volumes were associated with increased fearlessness, a key characteristic of antisocial individuals (Walters and Kiehl 2015). Given that the amygdala is regarded as the brain locus of fear and plays a major role in fear conditioning (Sah et al. 2003), dysfunction in the amygdala, together with other brain areas of the limbic system, has been linked to greater antisocial and aggressive behavior by impairing the brain's ability to interpret threat cues. In this way, abnormalities of the amygdala have been proposed to be a salient feature of antisocial personalities (Raine 2018).

Hippocampus

Like the amygdala, the hippocampus is part of the limbic system. The hippocampus is involved in cognition and declarative memory, as well as in emotion and the regulation of the stress response (Leclerc et al. 2018). In a forensic sample, Laakso and colleagues (2000) compared 19 violent male offenders with diagnoses of ASPD and alcoholism with a control group of 34 healthy males. Compared with the healthy control group, a reduction in volume of the right hippocampus was observed among the violent offenders with ASPD and alcoholism. Although the study did not tease apart the unique influence of ASPD or alcoholism on volume loss in the hippocampus, some additional support for the notion that smaller hippocampal volumes may be associated with ASPD stems from studies documenting that violent offenders have abnormal hippocampal structure compared with nonviolent control subjects (Boccardi et al. 2010; Yang et al. 2010). These findings implicate the role of the hippocampus in aggressive behavior, which constitutes a feature of ASPD.

Striatum

Despite most empirical findings of reductions in gray matter volume and ASPD, antisocial behavior is not always associated with reduced brain structure. Barkataki and colleagues (2006) conducted a study comparing 13 males with ASPD, 13 violent males with schizophrenia, 15 nonviolent males with schizophrenia, and 15 healthy nonviolent control subjects. They found that males diagnosed with ASPD had larger volumes in the putamen, a subregion of the striatum, compared with the healthy control subjects and nonviolent males with schizophrenia (Barkataki et al. 2006). Although there is a limited number of studies on striatal structure and antisocial behavior, research documenting increased striatal volumes in psychopathy (Glenn et al. 2010), a construct that shares commonalities with ASPD, provides additional support for a role of the striatum in the pathophysiology of ASPD. Both the dorsal and the ventral striatum, of which the putamen can be considered a part, are involved in reward processing, specifically aspects of affective learning (Delgado 2007). The striatum is also linked to decision-making and impulsivity (Kim and Im 2019). Given that the striatum is critically involved in the cognitive processing of reward-related information, these findings are in line with the hypothesis that antisocial individuals are hypersensitive to rewarding stimuli, which in turn promotes their engagement in antisocial behavior.

Cerebellum

In recent years, researchers have begun to consider the possible role of the cerebellum in ASPD. Although the cerebellum is largely regarded as a part of the brain that is responsible for processes related to motor abilities and coordination, there is increasing recognition that this brain region may be involved in other nonmotor functions such as in cognition, emotion, empathy, and moral judgment (Demirtas-Tatlidede and Schmahmann 2013; Van Overwalle et al. 2014). In addition, because impulsivity is a feature of ASPD, empirical findings documenting that the cerebellum is relevant for motor aspects of impulsive acts highlight the value of taking into account the cerebellum in investigations of the brain circuits involved in ASPD (Picazio and Koch 2015).

Studies reporting on the relationship between the cerebellum and ASPD have described mixed findings. One recent study compared the gray matter volumes of 9 male offenders with ASPD and high levels of psychopathy with that of 15 male offenders with ASPD who scored low on psychopathy (Kolla et al. 2014). A reduction in gray matter volume in the cerebellum was found in the ASPD patients with higher levels of psychopathy. However, in another study, persistently violent offenders diagnosed with ASPD and substance dependence showed increased gray matter volume in the right cerebellum (Tiihonen et al. 2008). The differences between the samples in these studies, in addition to the fact that the latter study had the additional confound of substance dependence, make direct comparison between them difficult. Additional research is needed to elucidate the role of the cerebellum in antisocial behavior, but some empirical evidence supports the notion that anomalies of the cerebellum may be associated with disorders characterized by abnormal social behaviors, such as ASPD (Moreno-Rius 2019).

Corpus Callosum

In addition to frontotemporal brain structures often discussed in relation to antisocial behavior, some structural neuroimaging studies have examined whether abnormalities in the corpus callosum, a major white matter bundle that connects the two cerebral hemispheres and supports interhemispheric functional integration, are observed in ASPD patients. In a structural MRI study comparing 15 males who had ASPD and high psychopathy scores with a control group of 25 males without ASPD, the individuals with ASPD showed a 22.6% increase in white matter volume of the corpus callosum (Raine et al. 2003). They also had a 6.9% increase in the length of the corpus callosum and a 15.3% reduction in callosal thickness in comparison with the control group (Raine et al. 2003). These findings suggest that the structural differences in the corpus callosum between antisocial and psychopathic males and healthy individuals reflect atypical neurodevelopmental processes in the former group, involving an arrest of early axonal pruning or an abnormality in the myelination process (Raine et al. 2003). Other neuroimaging studies have found similar structural abnormalities in the corpus callosum. For example, a more recent study conducted voxel-based analyses to assess white matter fractional anisotropy, which is considered to be an index of white matter integrity. The measure is a quantification of the directional dependence of water molecule diffusion in white matter. Fractional anisotropy deficits in the corpus callosum were found in males with ASPD compared with a control group (Sundram et al. 2012). This finding has been suggested to be indicative of information relay impairments between prefrontal and other brain regions in ASPD (Sundram et al. 2012).

Similar to findings in ASPD, abnormalities in the maturation process in the corpus callosum have also been observed in males with conduct disorder (Zhang et al. 2014). Furthermore, it has been noted that abnormalities in the corpus callosum found in individuals who have conduct disorder are present in adulthood even in the absence of an ASPD diagnosis (Lindner et al. 2016). Thus, some researchers suggest that the structural differences in the corpus callosum observed in studies of ASPD may, in fact, reflect a developmental abnormality that is specifically associated with conduct disorder.

Specificity of Structural Brain Abnormalities to Antisocial Personality Disorder

Diagnostic comorbidity presents a challenge to the identification of brain abnormalities specifically associated with ASPD because ASPD has high rates of comorbidity with several psychiatric disorders, such as substance use disorders, schizotypal personality disorder, and borderline personality disorder (Glenn et al. 2013; Sher et al. 2015). A key question pertinent to structural imaging studies of antisocial behavior concerns the specificity of the findings to ASPD.

Some studies have attempted to address this question by comparing a group of ASPD patients with a matched psychiatric control group or by controlling for potential confounding variables. These approaches have resulted in mixed findings. For example, in an effort to disentangle the neural abnormalities associated with substance dependence experienced by ASPD individuals, Raine et al. (2000) compared men with ASPD with a group of individuals who had substance dependence but not antisocial personality. Their finding that the ASPD group had a 13.9% reduction in prefrontal gray matter volume added confidence to the notion that the prefrontal deficits observed in ASPD are not an artifact of comorbid alcohol and substance dependence. The authors took these findings one step further by matching the individuals in the ASPD group with 21 men who were not diagnosed with ASPD to ensure that both groups, on average, had a relatively equal rate of schizophrenia spectrum, affective, and anxiety disorders, as well as other personality disorders, such as borderline, histrionic, narcissistic, avoidant, dependent, and obsessive-compulsive disorders. In line with the previous finding, on average, individuals in the ASPD group had a 14.7% reduction in prefrontal gray matter volumes compared with the psychiatric control group.

A different methodological approach was adopted by Laakso et al. (2002), who assessed prefrontal volumes in 24 nonpsychotic, violent males diagnosed with ASPD and alcoholism and 33 age-matched male control subjects. Males with ASPD were observed to have significantly lower prefrontal volumes. However, this difference in prefrontal volume disappeared after the investigators controlled for duration of alcoholism and education between the ASPD and the control groups. These results suggest that the brain deficits in the ASPD males were associated with substance abuse or education rather than the diagnosis of ASPD. Other studies that used this approach and added variables such as alcohol and substance use, psychosocial deficits, head injury, schizophrenia spectrum disorder, and whole brain volume as covariates in their analysis suggested that structural abnormalities in the corpus callosum could not be attributed to these factors (Raine et al. 2003). Thus, the issue of specificity of structural brain abnormalities to ASPD remains an important one to investigate.

A related issue concerns the association between ASPD and psychopathy. Some neuroimaging studies assess both constructs. Study designs that compare only one group of individuals with ASPD and psychopathic traits with healthy control subjects render it difficult to tease apart the neurobiological mechanisms that may be specific to each condition. However, studies that assess groups that differ on ASPD and on psychopathic traits can help shed light on the underlying neural mechanisms associated with psychopathy distinct from ASPD, and vice versa. For instance, in one study, male offenders with ASPD and high levels of psychopathy were found to have reduced gray matter volumes bilaterally in the anterior rostral medial PFC and temporal poles relative to a matched group of violent offenders who presented with ASPD but scored low on psychopathic features (Gregory et al. 2012). However, individuals with ASPD and low levels of psychopathy did not have significant structural brain differences from healthy, nonoffender control subjects. These results are relevant to our understanding of the etiology of both ASPD and psychopathy. They suggest that certain structural brain deficits are specific to psychopathy but not ASPD. In light of such findings, researchers positing that ASPD is a neurodevelopmental condition have raised the question of whether ASPD with psychopathic features represents a separate clinical manifestation that may be more neurodevelopmental in nature (Raine 2018). Neurobiological evidence in relation to antisocial behavior has also prompted some discussion over the potential for psychopathy to be included as a specifier for the diagnosis of ASPD in DSM (Raine 2018).

Biosocial Interactions Involving Structural Brain Imaging

Research points to the contribution of both biological and psychosocial factors in the development of antisocial behavior (Raine 2013). However, there is a paucity of structural brain imaging studies that also consider the influence of psychosocial factors on antisocial behavior. The issue of whether brain deficits combine with psychosocial deficits to predispose an individual to ASPD has been examined in three studies.

These anatomical MRI studies have tested the accuracy of predicting individuals' group membership into an ASPD group or a healthy control group. One study found that the use of 10 psychosocial variables, such as parental social class, early parental divorce, and physical and sexual abuse, led to the correct classification of individuals with ASPD with an accuracy of 73.9% (Raine et al. 2011). However, including prefrontal gray matter volumes into the statistical model improved the prediction of classification to the ASPD versus control group to 100%. A second structural imaging study on the corpus callosum among individuals with psychopathy documented that the structure of the corpus callosum could add to the prediction of classification of individuals into a group with ASPD and high psychopathic traits or to a control group. It was found that the combination of psychosocial risk factors with measures of corpus callosum structure accounted for 81.5% of the variance in group membership (Raine et al. 2003). A third study found that considering a psychophysiological risk factor for antisocial behavior—namely, low autonomic responsivity—during a social stressor, in combination with reduced prefrontal gray volume and psychosocial deficits, resulted in the correct classification of 88.5% of subjects into an ASPD or control group (compared with 73.0% for psychosocial predictors only and 76.9% for biological predictors only) (Raine et al. 2000). All in all, despite the limited body of extant literature on biosocial interactions involving structural brain measures, some empirical evidence suggests that gray matter volume has the potential to substantially improve the prediction of ASPD versus control group membership over and above psychosocial risk factors for ASPD.

Sources of Structural Brain Abnormalities Associated With Antisocial Personality Disorder

The question of what causes the structural gray matter loss in patients with ASPD is also a critical one that researchers have begun to answer. One proposed mechanism underlying the development of ASPD stems from a biological perspective because ASPD has been documented to have a genetic basis. A recent large-scale, population-based study of 2,794 Norwegian twins reported an estimated heritability of 51% (Rosenström et al. 2017). It has been suggested that genetic influences on ASPD may be expressed, to some extent, through impairments to brain regions (e.g., neural endophenotypes).

Some empirical support for the hypothesis that neural development can be shaped by genetic factors is derived from findings of genotype-related morphological differences in brain regions that are associated with ASPD. In particular, molecular genetic research in relation to antisocial behavior has highlighted the role of the monoamine oxidase A gene (*MAOA*). The monoamine oxidase A enzyme metabolizes monoamine neurotransmitters, including serotonin and norepinephrine (Sabol et al. 1998). The promoter region of *MAOA* on the short arm of the X chromosome contains a 30–base pair variable number of tandem repeats sequence (VNTR) (Ficks and Waldman 2014; Sabol et al. 1998). Variants of the *MAOA*-VNTR polymorphism have been characterized, based on the different number of repeats. Transcription of the 3-repeat (short) allele results in reduced *MAOA* activity, while the 4-repeat (long) allele is associated with increased *MAOA* activity (Ficks and Waldman 2014). Studies have also classified the 2-repeat and 3.5-repeat alleles as low and high activity, respectively. A substantial body of research indicates that low *MAOA* activity is implicated in antisocial behavior (Ficks and Waldman 2014). Additionally, relative to individuals with the high-activity variant of *MAOA*, individuals with low-activity *MAOA* have been documented to have reduced amygdala volumes (Meyer-Lindenberg et al. 2006) and decreased cortical thickness in the bilateral OFC (Cerasa et al. 2010). Although findings need to be replicated, they provide some initial support for the notion that the *MAOA* genotype can have an effect on brain morphology, which may be associated with antisocial outcomes.

Although heritable processes may influence neural development, they are not the only mechanisms. Findings on the influence of adverse environments on brain structure have been obtained from numerous studies. For instance, one study that compared children who were exposed to early life stressors in the form of physical abuse, neglect, and low socioeconomic status with children who were not exposed to early life stress found that individuals who had experienced social adversity early in life had lower amygdala volumes (Hanson et al. 2015). Similar findings have been observed in the hippocampus in child and adult samples. Physically abused and low socioeconomic status children, as well as adults who have suffered from childhood maltreatment, have smaller hippocampal volumes (Bremner et al. 1997; Hanson et al. 2015; Teicher et al. 2012). In the frontal cortex, voxel-based morphometry analysis has indicated an association between early life poverty and reduced gray matter volume in the orbitofrontal cortex at age 25 years (Holz et al. 2015). Moreover, greater childhood psychosocial deprivation, especially physical and sexual abuse, was associated with lower cortical volumes in the ACC in a sample that included patients with ASPD (Kumari et al. 2014). Neuroimaging findings of the association between greater social adversity and impairments in brain structure are also observed when cortical surface areas are measured (Noble et al. 2015) and in children very early in life, at age 5 weeks (Betancourt et al. 2016).

A higher proportion of ASPD patients experience significant psychosocial deprivation early in life (see, e.g., Kumari et al. 2014), and these volumetric brain differences in groups exposed to social adversity are linked to ASPD. Therefore, these findings bring to question whether psychosocial deprivation could predispose individuals to ASPD via structural impairments in frontolimbic regions of the brain. Although not specific to ASPD, some empirical support has arisen from studies on antisocial behavior. In one study consisting of 128 children, left and right hippocampal volumes were found to partially mediate the relationship between early life stress and greater antisocial behavior (Hanson et al. 2015). Another study conducted on a large sample of 1,741 adolescents reported that a combination of lower cortical volumes in the frontomedial and insular cortex and higher volumes in the ventral striatum, hypothalamus, and anterior thalamus partially mediated the association between adverse life events and antisocial behavior (Mackey et al. 2017). These findings are in line with a social neurocriminological theoretical account of antisocial behavior, which posits that the social environment influences biology in a way to predispose to antisocial behavior (Choy et al. 2015). Formal tests of mediation that use ASPD as an outcome variable would extend these findings by testing whether social influences contribute to neural maldevelopment, which, in turn, is associated with ASPD.

Accounting for Sex Differences in Antisocial Personality Disorder

It is well known that ASPD is less prevalent in females than in males. Research suggests that 2%–6% of males and 0.5%–2% of females in the general population meet diagnostic criteria for ASPD (Sher et al. 2015). However, surprisingly little is known about *why* higher rates of ASPD are seen in males.

One viable candidate to account for the sex difference in ASPD is prefrontal volume. Males both with and without ASPD, on average, have been found to have significantly lower gray matter volumes in the orbitofrontal and middle frontal regions of the PFC than do females (Raine et al. 2011). In the only study to date that has tested whether brain differences may underlie the sex difference in ASPD, Raine et al. (2011) found that controlling for gray matter volumes in three regions of the PFC reduced the sex difference in ASPD by 77.3%. Results from the study indicate that the higher rates of ASPD in males can be accounted for, in part, by their smaller prefrontal volumes. These findings are in line with the notion that compared with females, males are more vulnerable over a longer time to stressors in the social environment that have an effect on their brain development (Schore 2017). The negative effects on neurobiological processes particularly in the male brain may place males at greater risk for antisocial behavior (Raine 2019; Schore 2017). At a broader level, these findings suggest that further research on biological characteristics that may help to account for the sex difference in antisocial behavior is warranted.

Early Brain Structure and Prediction of Antisocial Personality Disorder

Brain imaging studies of antisocial behavior are largely correlational in nature. This fact precludes conclusions about whether the structural brain abnormalities observed in individuals diagnosed with ASPD are causes or consequences of antisocial behavior. What remains largely unknown is whether and how early in life brain abnormalities predict later antisocial outcomes.

Longitudinal brain imaging studies on antisocial behavior are scarce. One prospective structural imaging study found that men with lower amygdala volumes measured at age 26 years showed higher levels of aggressive behavior, violence, and psychopathic features 3 years later (Pardini et al. 2014). These results remained after the investigators controlled for earlier levels of these behaviors and a host of other potential confounding variables. The association between brain structure and the development of later ASPD remains to be investigated in longitudinal studies. Nevertheless, because aggressiveness is a feature of ASPD and psychopathy is a closely related construct, these findings provide some initial support for the hypothesis that structural brain abnormalities can help predict ASPD.

Research on the cavum septum pellucidum (CSP) has also helped to shed light on this important research gap. The CSP, which can be evaluated via structural MRI, is a neuroanatomical variant of the septum pellucidum, a thin triangular membrane between the right and the left lateral ventricles in the medial frontal lobe of the brain (Tubbs et al. 2011). During normal human neural development of the septum, a fluid-filled space forms between the two leaves of glia separating the ventricles, but the cavity typically closes between approximately week 20 of gestation and ages 3–6 months (Raine et al. 2010; Sarwar 1989). In some cases, however, the gap does not close. Enlarged CSP and persistence of a CSP beyond infancy thus serve as early indicators of abnormal growth of the limbic structure.

Studies have explored the link between the CSP and antisocial behavior. In a community sample of 87 adults, individuals with a CSP were found to have significantly higher ASPD and psychopathy scores compared with adults without a CSP (Raine et al. 2010). The relation between the CSP and the ASPD could not be attributed to demographic variables, previous trauma exposure, head injury, total brain volume, or comorbid disorders, including alcohol and substance dependence, schizophrenia spectrum, psychotic, and mood disorders. Based on data from their sample, the researchers also identified two subcomponents of ASPD. The presence of a CSP was more strongly associated with the aggressive/life course component of ASPD, which consisted of features such as irritability or aggressiveness, reckless disregard for self or others, and presence of conduct disorder rather than deceptive-irresponsible features such as deceitfulness, consistent irresponsibility, and impulsivity (Raine et al. 2010). In line with these findings, White et al. (2013) documented that adolescents with enlarged CSP showed a higher risk for engaging in aggression, having psychopathic traits, and having a disruptive behavior disorder diagnosis. Although the definition and classification of CSP have differed across studies on antisocial behavior, with some studies defining the CSP as present when it is visible in six or more 1.0 mm–thick coronal slices (e.g., Raine et al. 2010) and others classifying its presence when it is 4 mm or greater in length (e.g., White et al. 2013), conclusions converge to support the hypothesis that very early maldevelopment of the limbic system is associated with increased risk for developing ASPD features. Findings from research on the CSP have supported the proposition of a neurodevelopmental perspective toward understanding ASPD (Raine 2018).

Although further replication of these prospective findings is needed, these studies provide some evidence of temporal order in the link between brain structure and ASPD. It has been suggested that such research that helps to identify observed brain differences before the presence of antisocial behavior can aid in identifying biomarkers to recognize youths who may be at particularly high risk for antisocial behavior compared with other peers (Cope et al. 2014). Brain imaging in prospective longitudinal studies also may prove to be valuable in elucidating the developmental trajectory of ASPD characteristics over time.

Directions for Future Research

The review of the literature on structural brain abnormalities in ASPD highlights that the vast majority of studies of brain morphology and antisocial behavior are collected from samples consisting of males. One limitation of the extant research on brain imaging and ASPD concerns the lack of knowledge about the neural correlates of ASPD in females.

Some preliminary evidence suggests that structural brain abnormalities also characterize females who present with ASPD. For example, in a female sample recruited from the community, reduced orbitofrontal volume was significantly associated with increased antisocial personality scores (Raine et al. 2011). Although these findings were based on a small sample size of 12 females, they are notable in that the association between prefrontal gray matter volume and antisocial behavior found in males was replicated in an independent sample of females. Supporting evidence for the notion that structural brain abnormalities may be present in antisocial females can be derived from neuroimaging research on conduct disorder in female adolescents. Broadly, male and female adolescents with conduct disorder show similar abnormalities in brain structure and function (Fairchild et al. 2011, 2013). While there may indeed be subtle differences in the etiological origins of conduct disorder and ASPD, given that not all youths with conduct disorder will eventually be diagnosed with ASPD, research on the neural correlates of conduct disorder may nevertheless help to provide some insight into the etiology of ASPD in the absence of neuroimaging research on females with ASPD. Future efforts could be directed at examining whether the findings of structural brain abnormalities in ASPD females can be replicated and extended.

Another important area of future research involves disentangling the neural correlates of ASPD from comorbid disorders and other confounding variables. Samples examined in neuroimaging studies of ASPD vary considerably as to whether comorbid disorders, as well as levels of aggressive behavior, criminality, and psychopathic traits, are assessed and controlled for in statistical analyses (Budhiraja et al. 2017; Glenn et al. 2013). Whereas some studies attempt to address the possibility that structural deficits in patients with ASPD may be attributed to comorbid mood and schizophrenia spectrum disorders by comparing individuals diagnosed with ASPD with a psychiatric control group (Raine et al. 2000, 2011), other studies only compare the brain volumes of individuals with ASPD who have comorbid disorders with those of healthy control groups (Bertsch et al. 2013). Future efforts to empirically test whether the observed brain abnormalities are associated with comorbid disorders and social adversity that are common in adults with ASPD can contribute significantly to our understanding of the neural basis of ASPD. A related issue is the small sample size of many neuroimaging studies of ASPD. Larger samples may aid in permitting comparisons between ASPD-only groups and groups of ASPD patients with comorbid disorders.

Conclusion

Numerous structural brain imaging studies have been conducted on individuals with ASPD, examining a wide range of brain regions. Overall, studies have documented that ASPD likely has a neurobiological basis involving structural brain abnormalities, with key impairments commonly found in the prefrontal and temporal cortices. These findings are bolstered not only by results derived from functional imaging studies but also from neuropsychological studies that document executive functioning deficits in populations of individuals with ASPD. Indicators for limbic dysfunction that are associated with ASPD can be observed early in life. Accumulating evidence also suggests that structural brain abnormalities are able to improve the prediction of ASPD when considered alongside psychosocial risk factors for antisocial behavior, are influenced by both genetic and social environmental factors, and can help to account for why males have higher rates of ASPD.

The review of imaging studies presented in this chapter highlights, however, that there is a diversity of findings in individuals with ASPD. Future studies that account for psychiatric comorbidity and other confounding effects may help to reduce some of the observed heterogeneity in these structural imaging findings. More neurobiological testing in prospective longitudinal studies, as well as the inclusion of female subjects and larger samples in structural MRI studies of ASPD, can also help advance our understanding of the neurobiological underpinnings of this personality disorder.

Key Points

- Structural brain differences found between patients with antisocial personality disorder (ASPD) and individuals without ASPD support the notion that ASPD has a neurobiological basis.

- Some of the most consistent neuroimaging findings related to ASPD involve structural deficits in the prefrontal cortex.

- Evidence suggests that very early maldevelopment of the limbic system is linked to a greater risk for developing ASPD features.

- Both genetic and environmental influences likely shape the neural abnormalities associated with ASPD.

- The examination of brain structure can help advance our understanding of key issues such as the prediction of ASPD and the higher rates of ASPD observed in males.

References

Barkataki I, Kumari V, Das M, et al: Volumetric structural brain abnormalities in men with schizophrenia or antisocial personality disorder. Behav Brain Res 169(2):239–247, 2006 16466814

Bertsch K, Grothe M, Prehn K, et al: Brain volumes differ between diagnostic groups of violent criminal offenders. Eur Arch Psychiatry Clin Neurosci 263(7):593–606, 2013 23381548

Betancourt LM, Avants B, Farah MJ, et al: Effect of socioeconomic status (SES) disparity on neural development in female African-American infants at age 1 month. Dev Sci 19(6):947–956, 2016 26489876

Boccardi M, Ganzola R, Rossi R, et al: Abnormal hippocampal shape in offenders with psychopathy. Hum Brain Mapp 31(3):438–447, 2010 19718651

Bremner JD, Randall P, Vermetten E, et al: Magnetic resonance imaging-based measurement of hippocampal volume in posttraumatic stress disorder related to childhood physical and sexual abuse—a preliminary report. Biol Psychiatry 41(1):23–32, 1997 8988792

Budhiraja M, Savic I, Lindner P, et al: Brain structure abnormalities in young women who presented conduct disorder in childhood/adolescence. Cogn Affect Behav Neurosci 17(4):869–885, 2017 28695488

Cerasa A, Cherubini A, Quattrone A, et al: Morphological correlates of MAO A VNTR polymorphism: new evidence from cortical thickness measurement. Behav Brain Res 211(1):118–124, 2010 20303364

Choy O, Raine A, Portnoy J, et al: The mediating role of heart rate on the social adversity-antisocial behavior relationship: a social neurocriminology perspective. Journal of Research Crime and Delinquency 52(3):303–341, 2015

Cope LM, Ermer E, Gaudet LM, et al: Abnormal brain structure in youth who commit homicide. Neuroimage Clin 4:800–807, 2014 24936430

Crews FT, Boettiger CA: Impulsivity, frontal lobes and risk for addiction. Pharmacol Biochem Behav 93(3):237–247, 2009 19410598

Davidson RJ, Putnam KM, Larson CL: Dysfunction in the neural circuitry of emotion regulation—a possible prelude to violence. Science 289(5479):591–594, 2000 10915615

Delgado MR: Reward-related responses in the human striatum. Ann N Y Acad Sci 1104(1):70–88, 2007 17344522

DeLisi M: The limbic system and crime, in The Ashgate Research Companion to Biosocial Theories of Crime. Edited by Walsh A, Beaver KM. New York, Routledge, 2011, pp 167–180

Demirtas-Tatlidede A, Schmahmann JD: Morality: incomplete without the cerebellum? Brain 136(pt 8):e244, 2013 23645927

Dolan MC, Deakin JFW, Roberts N, et al: Quantitative frontal and temporal structural MRI studies in personality-disordered offenders and control subjects. Psychiatry Res 116(3):133–149, 2002 12477598

Fairchild G, Passamonti L, Hurford G, et al: Brain structure abnormalities in early onset and adolescent-onset conduct disorder. Am J Psychiatry 168(6):624–633, 2011 21454920

Fairchild G, Hagan CC, Walsh ND, et al: Brain structure abnormalities in adolescent girls with conduct disorder. J Child Psychol Psychiatry 54(1):86–95, 2013 23082797

Ficks CA, Waldman ID: Candidate genes for aggression and antisocial behavior: a meta-analysis of association studies of the 5HTTLPR and MAOA-uVNTR. Behav Genet 44(5):427–444, 2014 24902785

Glenn AL, Raine A, Yaralian PS, et al: Increased volume of the striatum in psychopathic individuals. Biol Psychiatry 67(1):52–58, 2010 19683706

Glenn AL, Johnson AK, Raine A: Antisocial personality disorder: a current review. Curr Psychiatry Rep 15(12):427, 2013 24249521

Gregory S, ffytche D, Simmons A, et al: The antisocial brain: psychopathy matters. Arch Gen Psychiatry 69(9):962–972, 2012 22566562

Hanson JL, Nacewicz BM, Sutterer MJ, et al: Behavioral problems after early life stress: contributions of the hippocampus and amygdala. Biol Psychiatry 77(4):314–323, 2015 24993057

Holz NE, Boecker R, Hohm E, et al: The long-term impact of early life poverty on orbitofrontal cortex volume in adulthood: results from a prospective study over 25 years. Neuropsychopharmacology 40(4):996–1004, 2015 25315195

Jiang W, Li G, Liu H, et al: Reduced cortical thickness and increased surface area in antisocial personality disorder. Neuroscience 337:143–152, 2016 27600947

Kim B, Im HI: The role of the dorsal striatum in choice impulsivity. Ann N Y Acad Sci 1451(1):92–111, 2019 30277562

Kolla NJ, Gregory S, Attard S, et al: Disentangling possible effects of childhood physical abuse on gray matter changes in violent offenders with psychopathy. Psychiatry Res 221(2):123–126, 2014 24361393

Kolla NJ, Patel R, Meyer JH, et al: Association of monoamine oxidase-A genetic variants and amygdala morphology in violent offenders with antisocial personality disorder and high psychopathic traits. Sci Rep 7(1):9607, 2017 28851912

Kringelbach ML, Rolls ET: The functional neuroanatomy of the human orbitofrontal cortex: evidence from neuroimaging and neuropsychology. Prog Neurobiol 72(5):341–372, 2004 15157726

Kumari V, Uddin S, Premkumar P, et al: Lower anterior cingulate volume in seriously violent men with antisocial personality disorder or schizophrenia and a history of childhood abuse. Aust N Z J Psychiatry 48(2):153–161, 2014 24234836

Laakso MP, Vaurio O, Savolainen L, et al: A volumetric MRI study of the hippocampus in type 1 and 2 alcoholism. Behav Brain Res 109(2):177–186, 2000 10762687

Laakso MP, Gunning-Dixon F, Vaurio O, et al: Prefrontal volumes in habitually violent subjects with antisocial personality disorder and type 2 alcoholism. Psychiatry Res 114(2):95–102, 2002 12036509

Leclerc MP, Regenbogen C, Hamilton RH, et al: Some neuroanatomical insights to impulsive aggression in schizophrenia. Schizophr Res 201:27–34, 2018 29908715

Lindner P, Savic I, Sitnikov R, et al: Conduct disorder in females is associated with reduced corpus callosum structural integrity independent of comorbid disorders and exposure to maltreatment. Transl Psychiatry 6(1):e714, 2016 26784968

Mackey S, Chaarani B, Kan KJ, et al: Brain regions related to impulsivity mediate the effects of early adversity on antisocial behavior. Biol Psychiatry 82(4):275–282, 2017 26971049

Mechelli A, Price CJ, Friston KJ, et al: Voxel-based morphometry of the human brain: methods and applications. Current Medical Imaging 1(2):105–113, 2005

Meyer-Lindenberg A, Buckholtz JW, Kolachana B, et al: Neural mechanisms of genetic risk for impulsivity and violence in humans. Proc Natl Acad Sci U S A 103(16):6269–6274, 2006 16569698

Moreno-Rius J: Is there an "antisocial" cerebellum? Evidence from disorders other than autism characterized by abnormal social behaviours. Prog Neuropsychopharmacol Biol Psychiatry 89:1–8, 2019 30153496

Müller JL, Gänssbauer S, Sommer M, et al: Gray matter changes in right superior temporal gyrus in criminal psychopaths: evidence from voxel-based morphometry. Psychiatry Res 163(3):213–222, 2008 18662867

Narayan VM, Narr KL, Kumari V, et al: Regional cortical thinning in subjects with violent antisocial personality disorder or schizophrenia. Am J Psychiatry 164(9):1418–1427, 2007 17728428

Noble KG, Houston SM, Brito NH, et al: Family income, parental education and brain structure in children and adolescents. Nat Neurosci 18(5):773–778, 2015 25821911

Ogilvie JM, Stewart AL, Chan RC, et al: Neuropsychological measures of executive function and antisocial behavior: a meta-analysis. Criminology 49(4):1063–1107, 2011

Pardini DA, Raine A, Erickson K, et al: Lower amygdala volume in men is associated with childhood aggression, early psychopathic traits, and future violence. Biol Psychiatry 75(1):73–80, 2014 23647988

Picazio S, Koch G: Is motor inhibition mediated by cerebello-cortical interactions? Cerebellum 14(1):47–49, 2015 25283181

Raine A: The Anatomy of Violence: The Biological Roots of Crime. New York, Pantheon Books, 2013

Raine A: Antisocial personality as a neurodevelopmental disorder. Annu Rev Clin Psychol 14:259–289, 2018 29401045

Raine A: A neurodevelopmental perspective on male violence. Infant Ment Health J 40(1):84–97, 2019 30586472

Raine A, Lencz T, Bihrle S, et al: Reduced prefrontal gray matter volume and reduced autonomic activity in antisocial personality disorder. Arch Gen Psychiatry 57(2):119–127, discussion 128–129, 2000 10665614

Raine A, Lencz T, Taylor K, et al: Corpus callosum abnormalities in psychopathic antisocial individuals. Arch Gen Psychiatry 60(11):1134–1142, 2003 14609889

Raine A, Lee L, Yang Y, et al: Neurodevelopmental marker for limbic maldevelopment in antisocial personality disorder and psychopathy. Br J Psychiatry 197(3):186–192, 2010 20807962

Raine A, Yang Y, Narr KL, et al: Sex differences in orbitofrontal gray as a partial explanation for sex differences in antisocial personality. Mol Psychiatry 16(2):227–236, 2011 20029391

Rosenström T, Ystrom E, Torvik FA, et al: Genetic and environmental structure of DSM-IV criteria for antisocial personality disorder: a twin study. Behav Genet 47(3):265–277, 2017 28108863

Sabol SZ, Hu S, Hamer D: A functional polymorphism in the monoamine oxidase A gene promoter. Hum Genet 103(3):273–279, 1998 9799080

Sah P, Faber ES, Lopez De Armentia M, et al: The amygdaloid complex: anatomy and physiology. Physiol Rev 83(3):803–834, 2003 12843409

Sarwar M: The septum pellucidum: normal and abnormal. AJNR Am J Neuroradiol 10(5):989–1005, 1989 2505543

Schore AN: All our sons: the developmental neurobiology and neuroendocrinology of boys at risk. Infant Ment Health J 38(1):15–52, 2017 28042663

Sher L, Siever LJ, Goodman M, et al: Gender differences in the clinical characteristics and psychiatric comorbidity in patients with antisocial personality disorder. Psychiatry Res 229(3):685–689, 2015 26296756

Smith D, Smith R, Misquitta D: Neuroimaging and violence. Psychiatr Clin North Am 39(4):579–597, 2016 27836153

Sundram F, Deeley Q, Sarkar S, et al: White matter microstructural abnormalities in the frontal lobe of adults with antisocial personality disorder. Cortex 48(2):216–229, 2012 21777912

Teicher MH, Anderson CM, Polcari A: Childhood maltreatment is associated with reduced volume in the hippocampal subfields CA3, dentate gyrus, and subiculum. Proc Natl Acad Sci U S A 109(9):E563–E572, 2012 22331913

Tiihonen J, Rossi R, Laakso MP, et al: Brain anatomy of persistent violent offenders: more rather than less. Psychiatry Res 163(3):201–212, 2008 18662866

Tubbs RS, Krishnamurthy S, Verma K, et al: Cavum velum interpositum, cavum septum pellucidum, and cavum vergae: a review. Childs Nerv Syst 27(11):1927–1930, 2011 21687999

Van Overwalle F, Baetens K, Mariën P, et al: Social cognition and the cerebellum: a meta-analysis of over 350 fMRI studies. Neuroimage 86:554–572, 2014 24076206

Walters GD, Kiehl KA: Limbic correlates of fearlessness and disinhibition in incarcerated youth: exploring the brain-behavior relationship with the Hare Psychopathy Checklist: Youth Version. Psychiatry Res 230(2):205–210, 2015 26363777

White SF, Brislin S, Sinclair S, et al: The relationship between large cavum septum pellucidum and antisocial behavior, callous-unemotional traits and psychopathy in adolescents. J Child Psychol Psychiatry 54(5):575–581, 2013 22934662

Yang Y, Raine A: Prefrontal structural and functional brain imaging findings in antisocial, violent, and psychopathic individuals: a meta-analysis. Psychiatry Res 174(2):81–88, 2009 19833485

Yang Y, Raine A, Narr KL, et al: Localization of deformations within the amygdala in individuals with psychopathy. Arch Gen Psychiatry 66(9):986–994, 2009 19736355

Yang Y, Raine A, Han CB, et al: Reduced hippocampal and parahippocampal volumes in murderers with schizophrenia. Psychiatry Res 182(1):9–13, 2010 20227253

Zhang J, Zhu X, Wang X, et al: Increased structural connectivity in corpus callosum in adolescent males with conduct disorder. J Am Acad Child Adolesc Psychiatry 53(4):466.e1–475.e1, 2014 24655656

Functional MRI Studies of Antisocial Personality Disorder

R. James Blair, Ph.D.

Antisocial personality disorder (ASPD) describes an ingrained pattern of behavior in which individuals consistently disregard and violate the rights of others. Symptoms of ASPD include violation of the physical or emotional rights of others, lack of job and home life security, irritability and aggression, lack of remorse, consistent irresponsibility, recklessness and impulsivity, deceitfulness, and symptoms of conduct disorder in childhood. ASPD is typically diagnosed in clinical and research settings using criteria set forth in DSM-5 (American Psychiatric Association 2013).

ASPD is *not* equivalent to psychopathy. Psychopathy characterizes an individual who shows pronounced emotional deficits and is at increased risk for displaying antisocial behavior (Hare 2003). One of the criteria for psychopathy that *could* contribute to a diagnosis of ASPD is a "lack of remorse" (American Psychiatric Association 2013, p. 659). However, whereas a lack of remorse only *contributes* to a diagnosis of ASPD, it is a *core* criterion for the diagnosis of psychopathy, and it is difficult to meet the classification cutoff for psychopathy if this criterion is not met (Hare 2003). This difference in criterion gives rise to very different prevalence rates. Whereas most individuals with psychopathy have presentations that meet criteria for ASPD, only 10%

This research was in part supported by the National Institute of Mental Health under award K22-MH109558. The funders had no role in the design and conduct of the study; collection, management, analysis, and interpretation of the data; preparation, review, or approval of the chapter; and decision to submit the chapter for publication. The author has no conflicts of interest to disclose.

of persons with ASPD present with the core emotional deficit criteria associated with psychopathy and rather have presentations that meet many of the criteria based more on antisocial behavior (Coid and Ullrich 2010). Indeed, the focus on antisocial behavior in the diagnosis of ASPD has given rise to concerns that the disorder pathologizes criminal behavior; nearly 50% of incarcerated individuals in some samples have presentations that meet criteria for the disorder (Fazel and Danesh 2002). Alternatively, the difference in prevalence rates has given rise to suggestions that psychopathy is a more severe form of ASPD (Coid and Ullrich 2010).

The suggestion here is that the veracity of claims that the diagnosis of ASPD pathologizes criminal behavior or that psychopathy is a severe form of ASPD can be fully evaluated only by understanding the neurobiology of ASPD (and psychopathy). If ASPD is associated with neurobiological deficits, then it is unwise to dismiss the diagnosis and consider it simply a pathologizing of criminal behavior. Similarly, if a form of dysfunction is identified that underpins cases of ASPD and is particularly pronounced in cases of psychopathy, then psychopathy could be considered a more severe form of ASPD. Of course, the latter assumes that there is one form of dysfunction that underpins all cases of ASPD and is particularly problematic in cases of psychopathy. A central thesis of this chapter is that this assumption is incorrect.

In this chapter, I consider functional MRI studies of ASPD. Studies using single-photon emission computed tomography and PET studies with patients with ASPD have been well reviewed elsewhere (Kolla and Houle 2019). However, there are relatively few functional MRI studies of ASPD. Importantly, though, given claims that psychopathy is a more severe form of ASPD (Coid and Ullrich 2010), it is possible to consider the rather more extensive literature of functional MRI studies on individuals with psychopathy. In this regard, both dimensional (e.g., correlates of psychopathy severity) and categorical (group difference) studies of psychopathy are considered. However, studies are considered only if they include individuals who show clinical levels of pathology (i.e., individuals who would be likely to receive a *diagnosis* of ASPD). Studies of undergraduates or comparable healthy populations who differ in healthy levels of psychopathic traits are not considered. Although such studies may represent the healthy end of a dimension of pathology, data suggest that they can be misleading. For example, the literature on reward responsiveness and impulsiveness or ADHD has shown that increasing impulsiveness in healthy samples is positively associated with reward responsiveness (Plichta and Scheres 2014). However, increasing impulsiveness in patients with ADHD is *negatively* associated with reward responsiveness (Plichta and Scheres 2014). Clearly, drawing conclusions on the basis of findings in healthy populations would be misleading when attempting to understand the pathology underpinning impulsiveness in patients with ADHD.

In addition to the functional MRI literature on psychopathy, the functional MRI literature on conduct disorder is considered. This is because one of the symptoms of ASPD is the presence of symptoms of conduct disorder in childhood. Given the assumption that there are neurobiological risk factors underpinning the development of at least some cases of ASPD, the assumption is that these same risk factors were leading to the expression of conduct disorder symptoms during the patient's childhood or adolescence.

This chapter is organized around evaluating whether specific forms of dysfunction are seen in patients with ASPD. The functional impairments considered are those in which there are at least some data of impairment in patients with ASPD (i.e., emotional, particularly empathic and threat-based, responsiveness; response control; and reinforcement-based decision-making). Functional impairments seen in psychopathy that are not well documented in cases of ASPD even if likely present (e.g., impairments in moral judgment; see, e.g., Aharoni et al. 2011; Blair 1995; Blair et al. 1995; Harenski et al. 2014) are not considered.

Emotional Responsiveness

The suggestion that antisocial personality might reflect impairment in emotional responsiveness has a long history (Hare 1965, 1970; Lykken 1957). Indeed, the earliest claims predate the ASPD nomenclature. Lykken (1957) characterized individuals with respect to the then DSM description of sociopathic disorder and reported reduced aversive conditioning in this population. This impairment was subsequently also seen in the individuals whom Hare (1965, 1970) was describing as psychopathic.

It is important to remember, though, that not all emotions appear reduced. Anger appears to be intact in individuals with ASPD (Lobbestael et al. 2009) as well as in individuals with psychopathy and in adolescents with conduct disorder (Blair 2018; Marsh 2013; Marsh and Cardinale 2014). Indeed, individuals with ASPD and psychopathy and adolescents with conduct disorder are at increased risk for anger-based reactive aggression (i.e., aggression, underpinned by negative affect, in response to frustration or social provocation) (Cornell et al. 1996; Lobbestael et al. 2013; Thornton et al. 2013).

Emotional functions that do appear profoundly compromised include empathic responding (Bird and Viding 2014; Blair 1995; Brook and Kosson 2013), threat responsiveness (Hare 1965, 1970; Hoppenbrouwers et al. 2016; Lykken 1957; Marsh and Cardinale 2012; Patrick 1994), and, potentially, social affiliation (Viding and McCrory 2019). However, it should be noted that these impairments are more marked in individuals with psychopathy and adolescents with conduct disorder than in participants with ASPD. In fact, a recent review of the literature concluded that threat processing was impaired only in patients with ASPD who also showed psychopathy and that there was no impairment in empathy (Marsden et al. 2019). Although this was likely an overstatement, it reinforces the view that psychopathy is a more severe form of ASPD and/or that different forms of psychopathology can underpin the presentation of ASPD symptoms. The literature on empathy and threat processing are considered in more detail below.

Empathic Responsiveness

Empathic responsiveness is indexed via a variety of paradigms that can involve relatively complicated encoding of social interactions to relatively simple responses to the emotional expressions of others. The difficulty is that not all of these paradigms index the same neurocognitive mechanisms. Worse than this, there is a lack of consistency in the literature regarding nomenclature. A fundamental distinction is often drawn between cognitive and emotional empathy. In my own work, this represents a distinction between tasks that involve coding internal mental states (specifically be-liefs and knowledge; i.e., the classic definition of theory of mind; Baron-Cohen et al. 1985; Leslie 1987) and tasks that involve another individual's emotional states. This distinction is based on neuroimaging data indicating that coding these two different forms of internal states implicates distinct, albeit partially overlapping neurocog-nitive systems (Corradi-Dell'Acqua et al. 2014; Happé and Frith 2014), as discussed below. However, some authors refer to, for example, expression naming or identifica-tion tasks as indexing cognitive empathy and then conclude that cognitive empathy is compromised in ASPD/psychopathy/conduct disorder (Brook and Kosson 2013). This can give rise to suggestions, for example, that the literature with respect to cog-nitive empathy is equivocal—some studies indicate no impairment, whereas others indicate impairment. This is not the case, however. Studies assessing the capacity to represent beliefs and knowledge typically indicate no impairment, whereas studies assessing the capacity to *process* the emotions of others indicate impairment. Studies showing no impairment were assessing a different functional process than those in-dicating impairment—even if both sets of studies used the same name for these dif-ferent functional processes. For this reason, for the rest of this section, I attempt to narrowly specify the functional processes at the neurocognitive levels that are in-cluded within the domain of "empathic processing."

Representing the Intentions and Beliefs of Other Individuals

Representing the intentions and beliefs of other individuals was classically defined as *theory of mind* (Baron-Cohen et al. 1985; Leslie 1987). However, this term is now used far more broadly and so is not used further here. The representation of the intentions, beliefs, and knowledge of other individuals can be indexed through tasks examining whether participants refer to intentions and beliefs when interpreting story vignettes that require reference to such information for their understanding (Baron-Cohen et al. 1985). In the context of functional MRI, the participant might be presented with three image frames telling a story and one final screen with two choices of ending and hav-ing to decide the appropriate ending (Sebastian et al. 2012). A considerable functional MRI literature has indicated that representing the intentions and beliefs of other in-dividuals recruits the temporal pole, superior temporal cortex/temporal-parietal junc-tion, posterior cingulate cortex (PCC), and dorsomedial and rostromedial frontal cortex (Happé and Frith 2014; Molenberghs et al. 2016) (Figure 14–1).

Impairment in representing the intentions and beliefs of other individuals is a characteristic of many individuals with autism (Happé and Frith 2014). Increasing levels of impairment in this function have been associated with increased severity of social and communication symptoms as measured on the Autism Diagnostic Obser-vation Schedule (Tager-Flusberg 2003). However, impairment in this function is not typically seen in adults with ASPD (Bertone et al. 2017), adults with psychopathy (Blair et al. 1996), or children with conduct disorder more generally (Buitelaar et al. 1999). Moreover, the neural regions implicated in representing the intentions and beliefs of other individuals (temporal pole, superior temporal cortex, PCC, and rostro-medial frontal cortex) show appropriate recruitment in youths with conduct problems and elevated callous-unemotional traits when engaged in this functional process (O'Nions et al. 2014; Sebastian et al. 2012).

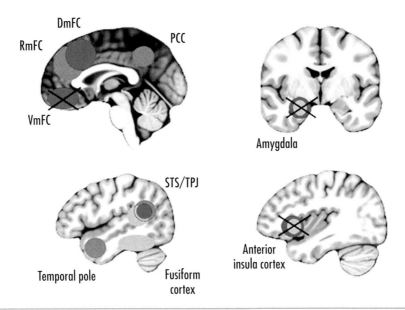

FIGURE 14–1. Core regions implicated in representing the beliefs and knowledge of others (*blue*), the emotional states of others (*red*), and the emotional expressions of others (*orange*).
To view this figure in color, see Plate 7 in Color Gallery.
Size of colored region is not indicative of strength of association. Crosses indicate regions that show significant deficient recruitment in patients with antisocial personality disorder/psychopathy/conduct disorder during relevant tasks.
DmFC=dorsomedial frontal cortex; PCC=posterior cingulate cortex; RmFC=rostromedial frontal cortex; STS/TPJ=superior temporal sulcus/temporal-parietal junction; VmFC=ventromedial frontal cortex.

Responding to the Emotional Expressions of Other Individuals

Face stimuli are processed by a series of neural regions, including those related to emotional processing (e.g., amygdala, anterior insula cortex) as well as temporal cortical regions that are particularly involved in processing faces relative to inanimate objects (e.g., fusiform, superior temporal cortex) (Fusar-Poli et al. 2009) (see Figure 14–1). Many of these regions (e.g., amygdala, anterior insula, fusiform cortex) show stronger responses to emotional than to neutral faces (Fusar-Poli et al. 2009). Moreover, there are indications of regional specification regarding particular emotional expressions; the amygdala appears to be particularly responsive to fearful, sad, and happy expressions but not angry and disgusted expressions, whereas anterior insula cortex is particularly responsive to disgust and anger expressions (Fusar-Poli et al. 2009).

Emotional expressions have a communicatory function: they both modulate ongoing behavior and allow the rapid transmission of valence information about objects and actions (Blair 2003; Fridlund 1992). This is perhaps best documented in the context of social referencing. During social referencing, the observer learns the value of a stimulus based on another individual's emotional reaction to it (e.g., the negative value of a novel threat because the caregiver shows fear toward it). This phenomenon is seen in both humans and monkeys (Klinnert et al. 1987; Mineka and Cook 1993). Functional imaging work and animal studies have stressed the importance of the amygdala in this learning process, at least in response to the fearful expressions of other individuals (Jeon and Shin 2011; Meffert et al. 2015).

Emotional expression recognition has been reported to be impaired in patients with ASPD (Timmermann et al. 2017) as well as in adults with psychopathy and youths with conduct disorder (for a review of this literature, see Blair 2018). This impairment may be particularly marked for fearful, sad, and happy expressions, but this is debated (Blair et al. 2002; Dawel et al. 2012; Marsh and Blair 2008; Muñoz 2009). Moreover, the impaired recognition of fearfulness and sadness is pervasive, applying also to vocal tones and body postures (Blair et al. 2002; Muñoz 2009). The suggestion is that the reduced response to the distress of others should be associated with reduced learning to avoid actions that harm other individuals (the individual finds the "punishment" of the other individual's distress less aversive). This will result in reduced avoidance of the commission of actions that might harm other individuals (Blair 2003).

Adults with ASPD, adults with psychopathy, and adolescents with conduct disorder, particularly those with higher callous-unemotional traits, show reduced neural responses to emotional expression stimuli in emotion or face-processing regions (Decety et al. 2014; Deeley et al. 2006; Ewbank et al. 2018; Jones et al. 2009; Lozier et al. 2014; Marsh et al. 2008; Mier et al. 2014; Passamonti et al. 2010; Shane and Groat 2018; Viding et al. 2012; White et al. 2012). Reduced responsiveness of the amygdala has been reported in the limited work with adults with ASPD (Schiffer et al. 2017) and adolescents with conduct disorder (Jones et al. 2009; Lozier et al. 2014; Marsh et al. 2008; Passamonti et al. 2010; Viding et al. 2012; White et al. 2012). This finding has been less frequently reported in the literature on adults with psychopathy (Decety et al. 2014; Deeley et al. 2006; Mier et al. 2014).

In a particularly interesting study, and consistent with theory (Blair 2003), Lozier and colleagues (2014) reported that the positive relationship between callous-unemotional traits and aggression was mediated by the reduced responsiveness of the amygdala to the distress of other individuals. Work with adults with psychopathy also reports similarly reduced blood oxygenation level–dependent responses in affect or face-processing regions to facial expressions relative to comparison adult groups.

Responding to Pain of Other Individuals

The facial expressions of another individual in pain can also be considered a distress cue. However, many studies examining responsiveness to the pain of another individual in persons with psychopathic or callous-unemotional traits have used visual stimuli depicting painful *events* (e.g., a hand caught in a slamming door) rather than facial *expressions* of pain. These are depictions of events associated with another individual's pain and require either interpretation or some association with the aversiveness of such events in the viewer's past.

A series of studies have identified a "pain matrix"—a network of brain regions that respond to the sight of another individual in pain. These regions include the neural regions related to emotional processing listed earlier as well as supplementary motor area (for a meta-analytic review of this literature, see Lamm et al. 2011). The activation of the supplementary motor area is interesting because it probably reflects activity relating to the association of the visual image with comparable events in the observer's past.

Although responsiveness to other individuals' pain has not received much attention in studies focused on participants specifically with ASPD, it has been known for some time that individuals with psychopathy show reduced emotional (autonomic) responses to the sight of other individuals in apparent pain (House and Milligan 1976). Moreover, functional MRI studies with both adults with psychopathy and adolescents with conduct disorder have reported that observing others in pain is associated with *reduced* activity within rostral medial/anterior cingulate cortex, amygdala, and insula cortex (Decety et al. 2013a, 2013b; Lockwood et al. 2013; Marsh et al. 2013; Meffert et al. 2013; Michalska et al. 2016).

Representing the Emotional States of Other Individuals

Representing the emotional states of other individuals has been referred to as *affective perspective taking*. Tasks assessing the representation of the emotional states of other individuals often involve participants being asked to identify an individual's emotional state on the basis of complex socioaffective pictorial stimuli or from verbal narratives describing a protagonist's emotional state. Such tasks recruit regions also recruited by tasks assessing the representation of intentions, beliefs, and knowledge (specifically anterior dorsomedial frontal cortex and bilateral temporal-parietal junction; for a meta-analytic review of this literature, see Molenberghs et al. 2016). In addition, they recruit greater activation in areas including the amygdala and ventromedial frontal cortex (vmFC) (Gonzalez-Liencres et al. 2013; Molenberghs et al. 2016), regions implicated in emotional responding (see Figure 14–1).

There has been little work with participants with ASPD specifically focusing on representing the emotional states of other individuals beyond expression processing studies. However, impairments in tasks requiring the representational capacity of affective perspective taking have been found both in studies with adults with psychopathy (Brook and Kosson 2013; Shamay-Tsoory et al. 2010) and in studies with adolescents with conduct disorder (Anastassiou-Hadjicharalambous and Warden 2008). Moreover, functional MRI studies with both adults with psychopathy and adolescents with conduct problems have reported reduced recruitment of amygdala and anterior insula cortex in the context of tasks requiring the representation of the emotional states of other individuals (Decety et al. 2013a, 2013b; Sebastian et al. 2012).

Threat Responsiveness

Neural systems that mediate the acute response to threat are the amygdala, hypothalamus, and periaqueductal gray (Gregg and Siegel 2001; Panksepp 1998). Core neural systems that allow learning from emotional information include the amygdala, anterior insula cortex, and striatum (the last-mentioned region is more implicated with respect to reward information and will be considered later) (LeDoux 2007). Neural regions involved in emotional decision-making include not only the amygdala, anterior insula cortex, and striatum but also the vmFC and PCC (Clithero and Rangel 2014). Visual and temporal cortices are critical for the representation of emotional information, and reciprocal connections between these regions and the amygdala mean that representations associated with emotional responses (amygdala responses) can be primed and their representation strengthened (i.e., they will be attended to; see Desimone and Duncan 1995; Pessoa et al. 2002). Finally, there have been suggestions that the intensity of an emotional experience is due in part to the role of these cortical midline structures in affect-based self-referential processing (De Pisapia et al. 2019; Waugh et al. 2010) with rostromedial prefrontal cortex being particularly implicated in the maintenance of this emotional response (Waugh et al. 2014).

There are indications of dysfunctional threat processing, or at least dysfunctional aversive conditioning, in patients with ASPD. The aversive conditioning paradigm involves learning to associate a threat (e.g., an electric shock) with a previously neutral cue. Impairment in aversive conditioning was first documented with respect to "sociopathic disorder," a DSM diagnostic precursor to ASPD (Lykken 1957). Since then, deficits in aversive conditioning have been reported in adults with psychopathy (Birbaumer et al. 2005; Hare 1965; Hare and Quinn 1971; Rothemund et al. 2012) and adolescents with conduct disorder (Fairchild et al. 2010). Indeed, in a seminal work, Raine and colleagues have shown that reduced aversive conditioning at age 3 years is a risk factor for increased antisocial behavior at 8 years and in adulthood (Gao et al. 2010a, 2010b). A related paradigm is the anticipated fear paradigm, in which a participant is told that a particular stimulus anticipates shock (Phelps and LeDoux 2005). Work has found that patients with ASPD show reduced anticipation responses to impending threat (Kumari et al. 2009). At the neutral level, this has been associated with reduced amygdala responses during aversive conditioning in adults with psychopathy and youths with conduct disorder (Birbaumer et al. 2005; van Lith et al. 2018). It should be noted that one study reported *increased* amygdala responses in patients with ASPD during aversive conditioning (Schneider et al. 2000). However, some caution must be taken with the result because the sample size was relatively small, and, inconsistent with considerable previous literature (LeDoux 2007; Phelps and LeDoux 2005), the healthy comparison adults in this study showed decreased amygdala responding during aversive conditioning.

Increased Threat Responsiveness

Mammalian species show a gradated response to threat, from freezing to flight to reactive aggression (aggression in response to threat or frustration) as the threat grows more proximal (Blanchard et al. 1977). Considerable animal work has shown that this response is mediated by the amygdala and its connections through the hypothalamus to the periaqueductal gray (Gregg and Siegel 2001; Panksepp 1998). More recent, functional MRI work with humans has largely confirmed this (Coker-Appiah et al. 2013; Mobbs et al. 2007, 2009, 2010). The more proximal the threat, the greater the activity within this system and the more likely that reactive aggression will be shown in response to this threat. Notably, the suggestion that these systems mediate reactive aggression to frustrating stimuli (Blair 2004) has also received empirical support (Yu et al. 2014). In short, the probability of reactive aggression is increased if the threat is sufficiently intense (or is at least processed as if it were sufficiently intense) and/or systems responsible for the regulation of the basic threat response are dysfunctional.

There have been suggestions that some individuals showing significant antisocial behavior but no callous-unemotional traits or high levels of psychopathy may show heightened, rather than reduced, threat responsiveness (Blair 2004, 2012). Such indi-

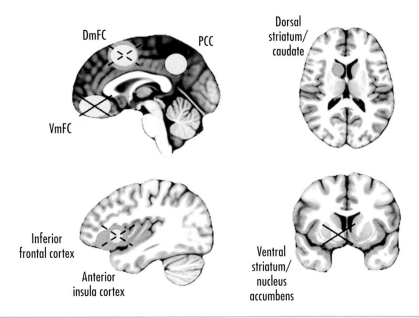

FIGURE 14–2.   Core regions implicated in response control (*green*) and reinforcement-based decision-making (*yellow*).

To view this figure in color, see Plate 8 in Color Gallery.

Crosses indicate regions that show significant deficient recruitment in patients with antisocial personality disorder/psychopathy/conduct disorder during relevant tasks (hashed crosses indicate less consistent data).

DmFC=dorsomedial frontal cortex; PCC=posterior cingulate cortex; VmFC=ventromedial frontal cortex.

viduals would be at increased risk for reactive aggression; they would respond with aggression rather than freezing or taking flight to provocations (threat, frustration, or social) (Blair 2004, 2012). Data indicate that heightened threat sensitivity may be seen in antisocial adolescents with low psychopathic (callous-unemotional) traits (see, e.g., Hwang et al. 2016; Viding et al. 2012). Increased responses to social threat are also associated with a heightened risk for reactive aggression (Choe et al. 2015). Moreover, heightened threat sensitivity likely underpins the development of hostile attribution biases (Dodge et al. 1995, 1997; Lopez-Duran et al. 2009). It should be noted, however, that this has not been systematically examined in adults with ASPD.

Response Control

Response control refers to the control of actions that interfere with goal-driven behavior. Classic response control tasks are the Go/No-Go, Stop, and Stroop tasks (Aron et al. 2016). Response control typically requires the recruitment of dorsomedial and inferior frontal/anterior insula cortices and the striatum (Aron et al. 2016) (Figure 14–2).

There are indications of response control impairments in adults with ASPD (Dolan 2012; Turner et al. 2017) in which they respond impulsively to stimuli that they are instructed not to respond to. This complements a rather more extensive literature indicating that many adolescents with conduct disorder (Hwang et al. 2016; McDonald et al. 2021) and a less extensive literature indicating that at least some adults with psychopathy show response inhibition impairments (Krakowski et al. 2015; Weidacker et al. 2017), although these impairments are seen in nonpsychopathic offenders also (Morgan and Lilienfeld 2000). Indeed, response control problems have long been linked to externalizing problems generally (Miyake and Friedman 2012; Young et al. 2009).

Relatively few data have indicated that recruitment of these regions during response control is compromised, at least as a function of severity of ASPD or psychopathy. A series of event-related potential studies have indicated that individuals with psychopathy show compromised responses to rare target and novel stimuli on odd-ball tasks (for a review, see Gao and Raine 2009). However, a recent functional MRI study with 168 incarcerated adult men reported that Factor 1 (emotion-related) scores on the Psychopathy Checklist—Revised (Hare 2003) were inversely related to responsiveness within a broad array of frontal, parietal, temporal, limbic, occipital, subcortical, and cerebellar regions to the common nontarget stimuli rather than the novel stimuli (Anderson et al. 2018). But both of these results, even in their inconsistency, would suggest compromised attentional responses to salient stimuli rather than problems in response control (Meffert et al. 2016).

Given the neuropsychological data and the data from adolescents with conduct disorder, it seems likely that at least some individuals with ASPD show impairment in the recruitment of neural systems necessary for response control. However, this impairment is likely not a major component of the pathology of ASPD per se. Instead, dysfunction in response control is a core component of the pathophysiology of ADHD (Dalley and Robbins 2017), which is highly comorbid with ASPD (Lenzenweger et al. 2007; Storebø and Simonsen 2016).

Reinforcement-Based Decision-Making

Reinforcement-based decision-making is a global term covering a variety of computations involved when choosing one response or object over another on the basis of the likelihood that the choice will result in reward or avoid punishment. Core regions implicated in reinforcement-based decision-making include the striatum, vmFC, dorsomedial prefrontal cortex, anterior insula cortex, and PCC (Clithero and Rangel 2014; Knutson and Bossaerts 2007) (see Figure 14–2).

Individuals with ASPD show significant impairment on a variety of reinforcement-based decision-making tasks. For example, they show poorer learning to avoid stimuli associated with punishment on the passive avoidance task, poorer reversal learning, and poorer decision-making in tasks requiring an evaluation of reward versus risk (De Brito et al. 2013). These forms of impairment are seen in adults with psychopathy (Blair et al. 2004; Budhani et al. 2006) and adolescents with conduct problems (Budhani and Blair 2005).

There is debate regarding what form of reinforcement-based dysfunction might be a risk factor for antisocial behavior. One view is that *hyperresponsiveness to reward* is a risk factor for conduct disorder and/or psychopathic traits (Murray et al. 2018). In this view, hyperresponsiveness to potential rewards results in insensitivity to potential negative consequences of any action. An alternative view is that the risk factor is hyporesponsiveness to reward (Blair et al. 2018). The suggestion here is that reduced reward sensitivity/responsiveness, particularly within regions critical for the representation of long-term goals, should result in an individual who makes poorer decisions (response choices will be less well guided by goal-modifiable reward expectations) and is thus more likely to be impulsive or become frustrated and aggressive as a function of his or her frustration (Blair et al. 2018). The situation is already complex because existing data with respect to "healthy" impulsiveness indicate that increased reward sensitivity is related to impulsiveness in healthy participants, probably reflecting increased reward seeking, but that severity of clinical levels of impulsiveness, as seen in patients with ADHD, is related to decreased reward sensitivity, potentially reflecting consequent impaired decision-making (Plichta and Scheres 2014).

There has been little functional MRI work with patients with ASPD examining neural responding during decision-making. There have been studies reporting atypical striatal morphology (Payer et al. 2015) and atypical striatal–medial prefrontal cortex connectivity (in interaction with the *MAOA* genotype; Kolla et al. 2018) in participants with ASPD. There has also been a report that individuals with ASPD show *increased* responses in right orbitofrontal and subgenual cingulate cortices to the receipt of reward (Völlm et al. 2010), consistent with the first of the views described earlier. However, a second study failed to report any indications of heightened reward responsiveness in participants with ASPD (Gregory et al. 2015), although this study did report a relative lack of the suppression of PCC responding to *punishment* when reward had been expected in patients with ASPD who also showed high levels of psychopathic traits (Gregory et al. 2015). PCC and vmFC both encode expected value (Clithero and Rangel 2014) and show suppression in activity when punishment is received following a change in reinforcement contingencies (Budhani et al. 2007). Notably, adolescents with conduct disorder with psychopathic traits show suppression of the vmFC while responding to punishment when reward had been expected on the same task (Finger et al. 2008).

Several studies have examined reinforcement processing in adolescents with conduct disorder. Most of this work supports the suggestion of decreased reward responsiveness in adolescents who have clinically concerning levels of conduct problems, conduct disorder, or callous-unemotional traits. It is true that one study did report increased striatal responsiveness to reward in youths with externalizing difficulties relative to comparison youths, but the sample size was very small ($n = 12$ in each group) (Bjork et al. 2010). A second study found that within a group of adolescents with conduct disorder, increasing callous-unemotional traits were associated with increased striatal responses to watching *another* win reward—although callous-unemotional traits did not relate to reward responding when *they themselves* won reward (i.e., there were no indications of heightened responsiveness for reward for the self) (Schwenck et al. 2017). In contrast, a series of studies have reported that youths with conduct problems or conduct disorder show reduced neural responsiveness to reward and reward omissions within the striatum and vmFC (Cohn et al. 2015; Crowley et al. 2010; Finger et al. 2011; Rubia et al. 2009; Veroude et al. 2016; White et al. 2013). However, it should be noted that at least one study reported no indications of heightened reward responsiveness but reported, instead, reduced responsiveness to punishment within the amygdala (Byrd et al. 2018).

The literature focusing on adults with psychopathy is less clear cut but has indicated either no impairment or increased reward responsiveness. Thus, one study reported that psychopathy was associated with stronger subjective value-related activity within the nucleus accumbens during intertemporal choice (Hosking et al. 2017). A second study indicated that individuals with psychopathy show increased nucleus accumbens responses during reward anticipation (Geurts et al. 2016). However, it is notable that this last result held only if the individuals with psychopathy were compared with healthy participants who scored below the healthy participant sample median for impulsivity on a personality measure. There were no group differences between the individuals with psychopathy and the healthy participants matched for impulsiveness. Two further studies reported no group differences in reward responsiveness (Gregory et al. 2015; Pujara et al. 2014). Pujara and colleagues (2014) found no significant relation between psychopathy and nucleus accumbens response to reward relative to neutral reinforcement, but they did report a significant inverse relation between psychopathy and loss relative to neutral reinforcement. As noted earlier, Gregory and colleagues (2015) observed a failure in adults with psychopathy to suppress responding within the PCC and insula cortex to unexpected punishment. Finally, an additional study reported diminished responding within the rostral anterior cingulate cortex during high-uncertainty, relative to low-uncertainty, choice conditions in a decision-making task (Prehn et al. 2013).

Conclusion

The goal of this chapter was to review functional MRI studies of ASPD (and related studies with conduct disorder and psychopathy). Several functional capacities were considered. Some showed no significant evidence of dysfunction (the representation of the intentions and beliefs of other individuals). However, data indicate that systems implicated in emotional responsiveness show reduced responding in at least some patients with ASPD in response to emotional expressions or pain cues and when representing the emotional states of other individuals. There are also data indicating reduced threat responsiveness, at least during aversive conditioning. Neural systems engaged in response control are likely disrupted in at least some individuals with ASPD, even if the disruption in these systems appears to relate principally to the expression of ADHD symptoms rather than ASPD symptoms (although these, of course, may be exacerbated by this pathology). Behaviorally, there are indications of impairment in reinforcement-based decision-making even if the neural underpinnings of these impairments remain unclear. Both neutrally increased and decreased reinforcement sensitivity have been documented in adults with ASPD (and for that matter, adults with psychopathy). It is only in the literature with adolescents with conduct disorder that there are more consistent indications of reduced reward sensitivity, and it is then notable that these indications are shared by patients with ADHD.

An aim of this chapter was to reconsider the suggestion that psychopathy might be considered a more severe form of ASPD (Coid and Ullrich 2010) on the basis of the functional MRI data. The crucial studies to address this suggestion have not been conducted. No supportive data have been provided showing that a group of individuals with ASPD but without psychopathy show a specific form of impairment and that this impairment is much more severe in a group of individuals with ASPD and psychopathy. Indeed, the very limited data available indicate that the individuals with ASPD but without psychopathy do not show reinforcement-based decision-making impairment, whereas those with ASPD and psychopathy show impairment (Gregory et al. 2015). However, data are insufficient to draw any conclusions with confidence.

The core functional impairment seen in ASPD, psychopathy, and conduct disorder is the deficit in emotional responding. This impairment is unique to psychopathy and likely some cases of ASPD and conduct disorder. The impairment in response control and reduced reward sensitivity are shared with patients with ADHD (Dalley and Robbins 2017; Plichta and Scheres 2014). Moreover, patients with substance use disorders show impairments in response control (Feldstein Ewing et al. 2014; Silveri et al. 2016) and reinforcement-based decision-making (Claus et al. 2018; Feldstein Ewing et al. 2014; Silveri et al. 2016), and it is likely that these impairments are exaggerated by the neurotoxic effect of the substances used (Aloi et al. 2018, 2020). If several patients have ASPD/psychopathy/conduct disorder with heightened reward sensitivity, then these individuals share this proclivity with healthy individuals showing heightened levels of presumably healthy impulsiveness (Plichta and Scheres 2014). Assuming that the core functional impairment is the deficit in emotional responding, it can then be considered whether those with psychopathy have a more severe form of this impairment than individuals meeting diagnostic criteria only for ASPD. Currently, the relevant studies in patients with ASPD/psychopathy have not been conducted (cf. Marsden et al. 2019). However, data indicate that among participants with conduct problems or conduct disorder, increasing callous-unemotional traits (the emotional component of psychopathy) are associated with progressively reduced emotional responsiveness (Hwang et al. 2016; Viding et al. 2012).

Another aim of this chapter was to reconsider the concern that because so many criminals have presentations that meet criteria for ASPD (see, e.g., Fazel and Danesh 2002), ASPD might be considered an attempt to pathologize criminal behavior. The consideration was that if a significant number of patients with ASPD show atypical neurobiological functioning, as appears to be the case, the diagnosis should not be considered to be a pathologizing of criminal behavior. Of course, the data reviewed here did not show that *all* patients with ASPD have the same neurobiological deficits or even that all patients with ASPD show some level of deficit. In other words, the literature cannot currently answer the question whether the behavior of all cases of ASPD is underpinned by a neurobiological deficit or perhaps overlapping deficits. It is quite possible—and, given reported diagnostic rates (e.g., Fazel and Danesh 2002), perhaps probable—that in some cases of apparent ASPD, the behavior will be present but will have arisen through totally nonbiological developmental routes. This reinforces the importance of having neurobiologically informed diagnoses in the future. If we are not correctly characterizing the causal underpinnings of the symptoms of individual cases of ASPD, then the treatment in at least some cases is likely to be nonoptimal.

Key Points

- Antisocial personality disorder (ASPD) is not equivalent to psychopathy. But individuals with psychopathy are a subset of those individuals with ASPD.

- Psychopathy is not a more severe form of ASPD. Rather, different forms of dysfunction are associated with ASPD; some, but not all, are particularly severe in patients with psychopathy.

- Most patients with psychopathy and many patients with ASPD show impairment in processing the distress of other individuals and reduced recruitment of the amygdala and associated regions to these expressions.

- Some patients with ASPD (and psychopathy) show dysfunctional response control.

- Patients who have ASPD show impairment in reinforcement-based decision-making that may relate to dysfunction within the striatum and medial frontal cortex and the interaction of these systems.

References

Aharoni E, Antonenko O, Kiehl KA: Disparities in the moral intuitions of criminal offenders: the role of psychopathy. J Res Pers 45(3):322–327, 2011 21647247

Aloi J, Blair KS, Crum KI, et al: Adolescents show differential dysfunctions related to alcohol and cannabis use disorder severity in emotion and executive attention neuro-circuitries. Neuroimage Clin 19:782–792, 2018 29988822

Aloi J, Blair KS, Crum KI, et al: Alcohol use disorder, but not cannabis use disorder, symptomatology in adolescents is associated with reduced differential responsiveness to reward versus punishment feedback during instrumental learning. Biol Psychiatry Cogn Neurosci Neuroimaging 5(6):610–618, 2020 32299790

American Psychiatric Association: Diagnostic and Statistical Manual of Mental Disorders, 5th Edition. Arlington, VA, American Psychiatric Association, 2013

Anastassiou-Hadjicharalambous X, Warden D: Cognitive and affective perspective-taking in conduct-disordered children high and low on callous-unemotional traits. Child Adolesc Psychiatry Ment Health 2(1):16, 2008 18601753

Anderson NE, Maurer JM, Steele VR, et al: Psychopathic traits associated with abnormal hemodynamic activity in salience and default mode networks during auditory oddball task. Cogn Affect Behav Neurosci 18(3):564–580, 2018 29633199

Aron AR, Herz DM, Brown P, et al: Frontosubthalamic circuits for control of action and cognition. J Neurosci 36(45):11489–11495, 2016 27911752

Baron-Cohen S, Leslie AM, Frith U: Does the autistic child have a "theory of mind"? Cognition 21(1):37–46, 1985 2934210

Bertone MS, Diaz-Granados EA, Vallejos M, et al: Differences in social cognition between male prisoners with antisocial personality or psychotic disorder. Int J Psychol Res (Medellin) 10(2):16–25, 2017 32612761

Birbaumer N, Veit R, Lotze M, et al: Deficient fear conditioning in psychopathy: a functional magnetic resonance imaging study. Arch Gen Psychiatry 62(7):799–805, 2005 15997022

Bird G, Viding E: The self to other model of empathy: providing a new framework for understanding empathy impairments in psychopathy, autism, and alexithymia. Neurosci Biobehav Rev 47:520–532, 2014 25454356

Bjork JM, Chen G, Smith AR, et al: Incentive-elicited mesolimbic activation and externalizing symptomatology in adolescents. J Child Psychol Psychiatry 51(7):827–837, 2010 20025620

Blair RJR: A cognitive developmental approach to mortality: investigating the psychopath. Cognition 57(1):1–29, 1995 7587017

Blair RJR: Facial expressions, their communicatory functions and neuro-cognitive substrates. Philos Trans R Soc Lond B Biol Sci 358(1431):561–572, 2003 12689381

Blair RJR: The roles of orbital frontal cortex in the modulation of antisocial behavior. Brain Cogn 55(1):198–208, 2004 15134853

Blair RJR: Considering anger from a cognitive neuroscience perspective. Wiley Interdiscip Rev Cogn Sci 3(1):65–74, 2012 22267973

Blair RJR: Traits of empathy and anger: implications for psychopathy and other disorders associated with aggression. Philos Trans R Soc Lond B Biol Sci 373(1744):20170155, 2018 29483341

Blair RJR, Jones L, Clark F, et al: Is the psychopath "morally insane"? Pers Individ Dif 19(5):741–752, 1995

Blair RJR, Sellars C, Strickland I, et al: Theory of mind in the psychopath. Journal of Forensic Psychiatry 7:15–25, 1996

Blair RJR, Mitchell DG, Richell RA, et al: Turning a deaf ear to fear: impaired recognition of vocal affect in psychopathic individuals. J Abnorm Psychol 111(4):682–686, 2002 12428783

Blair RJR, Mitchell DGV, Leonard A, et al: Passive avoidance learning in individuals with psychopathy: modulation by reward but not by punishment. Pers Individ Dif 37(6):1179–1192, 2004

Blair RJR, Veroude K, Buitelaar JK: Neuro-cognitive system dysfunction and symptom sets: a review of fMRI studies in youth with conduct problems. Neurosci Biobehav Rev 91:69–90, 2018 27794436

Blanchard RJ, Blanchard DC, Takahashi T, et al: Attack and defensive behaviour in the albino rat. Anim Behav 25(3):622–634, 1977 562631

Brook M, Kosson DS: Impaired cognitive empathy in criminal psychopathy: evidence from a laboratory measure of empathic accuracy. J Abnorm Psychol 122(1):156–166, 2013 23067260

Budhani S, Blair RJR: Response reversal and children with psychopathic tendencies: success is a function of salience of contingency change. J Child Psychol Psychiatry 46(9):972–981, 2005 16109000

Budhani S, Richell RA, Blair RJ: Impaired reversal but intact acquisition: probabilistic response reversal deficits in adult individuals with psychopathy. J Abnorm Psychol 115(3):552–558, 2006 16866595

Budhani S, Marsh AA, Pine DS, et al: Neural correlates of response reversal: considering acquisition. Neuroimage 34(4):1754–1765, 2007 17188518

Buitelaar JK, van der Wees M, Swaab-Barneveld H, et al: Theory of mind and emotion-recognition functioning in autistic spectrum disorders and in psychiatric control and normal children. Dev Psychopathol 11(1):39–58, 1999 10208355

Byrd AL, Hawes SW, Burke JD, et al: Boys with conduct problems and callous-unemotional traits: neural response to reward and punishment and associations with treatment response. Dev Cogn Neurosci 30:51–59, 2018 29324299

Choe DE, Shaw DS, Forbes EE: Maladaptive social information processing in childhood predicts young men's atypical amygdala reactivity to threat. J Child Psychol Psychiatry 56(5):549–557, 2015 25142952

Claus ED, Feldstein Ewing SW, Magnan RE, et al: Neural mechanisms of risky decision making in adolescents reporting frequent alcohol and/or marijuana use. Brain Imaging Behav 12(2):564–576, 2018 28429160

Clithero JA, Rangel A: Informatic parcellation of the network involved in the computation of subjective value. Soc Cogn Affect Neurosci 9(9):1289–1302, 2014 23887811

Cohn MD, Veltman DJ, Pape LE, et al: Incentive processing in persistent disruptive behavior and psychopathic traits: a functional magnetic resonance imaging study in adolescents. Biol Psychiatry 78(9):615–624, 2015 25497690

Coid J, Ullrich S: Antisocial personality disorder is on a continuum with psychopathy. Compr Psychiatry 51(4):426–433, 2010 20579518

Coker-Appiah DS, White SF, Clanton R, et al: Looming animate and inanimate threats: the response of the amygdala and periaqueductal gray. Soc Neurosci 8(6):621–630, 2013 24066700

Cornell DG, Warren J, Hawk G, et al: Psychopathy in instrumental and reactive violent offenders. J Consult Clin Psychol 64(4):783–790, 1996 8803369

Corradi-Dell'Acqua C, Hofstetter C, Vuilleumier P: Cognitive and affective theory of mind share the same local patterns of activity in posterior temporal but not medial prefrontal cortex. Soc Cogn Affect Neurosci 9(8):1175–1184, 2014 23770622

Crowley TJ, Dalwani MS, Mikulich-Gilbertson SK, et al: Risky decisions and their conse-quences: neural processing by boys with antisocial substance disorder. PLoS One 5(9):e12835, 2010 20877644

Dalley JW, Robbins TW: Fractionating impulsivity: neuropsychiatric implications. Nat Rev Neurosci 18(3):158–171, 2017 28209979

Dawel A, O'Kearney R, McKone E, et al: Not just fear and sadness: meta-analytic evidence of pervasive emotion recognition deficits for facial and vocal expressions in psychopathy. Neurosci Biobehav Rev 36(10):2288–2304, 2012 22944264

De Brito SA, Viding E, Kumari V, et al: Cool and hot executive function impairments in violent offenders with antisocial personality disorder with and without psychopathy. PLoS One 8(6):e65566, 2013 23840340

De Pisapia N, Barchiesi G, Jovicich J, et al: The role of medial prefrontal cortex in processing emotional self-referential information: a combined TMS/fMRI study. Brain Imaging Be-hav 13(3):603–614, 2019 29744797

Decety J, Chen C, Harenski C, et al: An fMRI study of affective perspective taking in individu-als with psychopathy: imagining another in pain does not evoke empathy. Front Hum Neurosci 7:489, 2013a 24093010

Decety J, Skelly LR, Kiehl KA: Brain response to empathy-eliciting scenarios involving pain in incarcerated individuals with psychopathy. JAMA Psychiatry 70(6):638–645, 2013b 23615636

Decety J, Skelly L, Yoder KJ, et al: Neural processing of dynamic emotional facial expressions in psychopaths. Soc Neurosci 9(1):36–49, 2014 24359488

Deeley Q, Daly E, Surguladze S, et al: Facial emotion processing in criminal psychopathy: pre-liminary functional magnetic resonance imaging study. Br J Psychiatry 189:533–539, 2006 17139038

Desimone R, Duncan J: Neural mechanisms of selective visual attention. Annu Rev Neurosci 18:193–222, 1995 7605061

Dodge KA, Pettit GS, Bates JE, et al: Social information-processing patterns partially mediate the effect of early physical abuse on later conduct problems. J Abnorm Psychol 104(4):632–643, 1995 8530766

Dodge KA, Lochman JE, Harnish JD, et al: Reactive and proactive aggression in school children and psychiatrically impaired chronically assaultive youth. J Abnorm Psychol 106(1):37–51, 1997 9103716

Dolan M: The neuropsychology of prefrontal function in antisocial personality disordered offend-ers with varying degrees of psychopathy. Psychol Med 42(8):1715–1725, 2012 22142550

Ewbank MP, Passamonti L, Hagan CC, et al: Psychopathic traits influence amygdala-anterior cingulate cortex connectivity during facial emotion processing. Soc Cogn Affect Neurosci 13(5):525–534, 2018 29660102

Fairchild G, Stobbe Y, van Goozen SH, et al: Facial expression recognition, fear conditioning, and startle modulation in female subjects with conduct disorder. Biol Psychiatry 68(3):272–279, 2010 20447616

Fazel S, Danesh J: Serious mental disorder in 23000 prisoners: a systematic review of 62 sur-veys. Lancet 359(9306):545–550, 2002 11867106

Feldstein Ewing SW, Sakhardande A, Blakemore SJ: The effect of alcohol consumption on the adolescent brain: a systematic review of MRI and fMRI studies of alcohol-using youth. Neuroimage Clin 5:420–437, 2014 26958467

Finger EC, Marsh AA, Mitchell DGV, et al: Abnormal ventromedial prefrontal cortex function in children with psychopathic traits during reversal learning. Arch Gen Psychiatry 65(5):586–594, 2008 18458210

Finger EC, Marsh AA, Blair KS, et al: Disrupted reinforcement signaling in the orbitofrontal cortex and caudate in youths with conduct disorder or oppositional defiant disorder and a high level of psychopathic traits. Am J Psychiatry 168(2):152–162, 2011 21078707

Fridlund A: Darwin's anti-Darwinism in the "Expression of the Emotions in Man and Ani-mals," in International Review of Studies on Emotion, Volume 2. Edited by Strongman KT. New York, Wiley, 1992, pp 117–137

Fusar-Poli P, Placentino A, Carletti F, et al: Functional atlas of emotional faces processing: a voxel-based meta-analysis of 105 functional magnetic resonance imaging studies. J Psychiatry Neurosci 34(6):418–432, 2009 19949718

Gao Y, Raine A: P3 event-related potential impairments in antisocial and psychopathic individuals: a meta-analysis. Biol Psychol 82(3):199–210, 2009 19576948

Gao Y, Raine A, Venables PH, et al: Association of poor childhood fear conditioning and adult crime. Am J Psychiatry 167(1):56–60, 2010a 19917592

Gao Y, Raine A, Venables PH, et al: Reduced electrodermal fear conditioning from ages 3 to 8 years is associated with aggressive behavior at age 8 years. J Child Psychol Psychiatry 51(5):550–558, 2010b 19788551

Geurts DE, von Borries K, Volman I, et al: Neural connectivity during reward expectation dissociates psychopathic criminals from non-criminal individuals with high impulsive/antisocial psychopathic traits. Soc Cogn Affect Neurosci 11(8):1326–1334, 2016 27217111

Gonzalez-Liencres C, Shamay-Tsoory SG, Brüne M: Towards a neuroscience of empathy: ontogeny, phylogeny, brain mechanisms, context and psychopathology. Neurosci Biobehav Rev 37(8):1537–1548, 2013 23680700

Gregg TR, Siegel A: Brain structures and neurotransmitters regulating aggression in cats: implications for human aggression. Prog Neuropsychopharmacol Biol Psychiatry 25(1):91–140, 2001 11263761

Gregory S, Blair RJ, Ffytche D, et al: Punishment and psychopathy: a case-control functional MRI investigation of reinforcement learning in violent antisocial personality disordered men. Lancet Psychiatry 2(2):153–160, 2015 26359751

Happé F, Frith U: Annual research review: towards a developmental neuroscience of atypical social cognition. J Child Psychol Psychiatry 55(6):553–557, 2014 24963529

Hare RD: Temporal gradient of fear arousal in psychopaths. J Abnorm Psychol 70(6):442–445, 1965 5846428

Hare RD: Psychopathy: Theory and Research. New York, Wiley, 1970

Hare RD: Manual for the Revised Psychopathy Checklist, 2nd Edition. Toronto, ON, Canada, Multi-Health Systems, 2003

Hare RD, Quinn MJ: Psychopathy and autonomic conditioning. J Abnorm Psychol 77(3):223–235, 1971 5556930

Harenski CL, Edwards BG, Harenski KA, et al: Neural correlates of moral and non-moral emotion in female psychopathy. Front Hum Neurosci 8:741, 2014 25309400

Hoppenbrouwers SS, Bulten BH, Brazil IA: Parsing fear: a reassessment of the evidence for fear deficits in psychopathy. Psychol Bull 142(6):573–600, 2016 26854867

Hosking JG, Kastman EK, Dorfman HM, et al: Disrupted prefrontal regulation of striatal subjective value signals in psychopathy. Neuron 95(1):221.e4–231.e4, 2017 28683266

House TH, Milligan WL: Autonomic responses to modeled distress in prison psychopaths. J Pers Soc Psychol 34(4):556–560, 1976 993975

Hwang S, Nolan ZT, White SF, et al: Dual neurocircuitry dysfunctions in disruptive behavior disorders: emotional responding and response inhibition. Psychol Med 46(7):1485–1496, 2016 26875722

Jeon D, Shin HS: A mouse model for observational fear learning and the empathetic response. Curr Protoc Neurosci Chapter 8:Unit 8.27, 2011 21971850

Jones AP, Laurens KR, Herba CM, et al: Amygdala hypoactivity to fearful faces in boys with conduct problems and callous-unemotional traits. Am J Psychiatry 166(1):95–102, 2009 18923070

Klinnert MD, Emde RN, Butterfield P, et al: Social referencing: the infant's use of emotional signals from a friendly adult with mother present. Annual Progress in Child Psychiatry and Child Development 22:427–432, 1987

Knutson B, Bossaerts P: Neural antecedents of financial decisions. J Neurosci 27(31):8174–8177, 2007 17670962

Kolla NJ, Houle S: Single-photon emission computed tomography and positron emission tomography studies of antisocial personality disorder and aggression: a targeted review. Curr Psychiatry Rep 21(4):24, 2019 30852703

Kolla NJ, Dunlop K, Meyer JH, et al: Corticostriatal connectivity in antisocial personality disorder by MAO-A genotype and its relationship to aggressive behavior. Int J Neuropsychopharmacol 21(8):725–733, 2018 29746646

Krakowski MI, Foxe J, de Sanctis P, et al: Aberrant response inhibition and task switching in psychopathic individuals. Psychiatry Res 229(3):1017–1023, 2015 26257091

Kumari V, Das M, Taylor PJ, et al: Neural and behavioural responses to threat in men with a history of serious violence and schizophrenia or antisocial personality disorder. Schizophr Res 110(1–3):47–58, 2009 19230621

Lamm C, Decety J, Singer T: Meta-analytic evidence for common and distinct neural networks associated with directly experienced pain and empathy for pain. Neuroimage 54(3):2492–2502, 2011 20946964

LeDoux J: The amygdala. Curr Biol 17(20):R868–R874, 2007 17956742

Lenzenweger MF, Lane MC, Loranger AW, et al: DSM-IV personality disorders in the National Comorbidity Survey Replication. Biol Psychiatry 62(6):553–564, 2007 17217923

Leslie AM: Pretense and representation: the origins of "theory of mind." Psychol Rev 94(4):412–426, 1987

Lobbestael J, Arntz A, Cima M, et al: Effects of induced anger in patients with antisocial personality disorder. Psychol Med 39(4):557–568, 2009 19171078

Lobbestael J, Cima M, Arntz A: The relationship between adult reactive and proactive aggression, hostile interpretation bias, and antisocial personality disorder. J Pers Disord 27(1):53–66, 2013 23342957

Lockwood PL, Sebastian CL, McCrory EJ, et al: Association of callous traits with reduced neural response to others' pain in children with conduct problems. Curr Biol 23(10):901–905, 2013 23643836

Lopez-Duran NL, Olson SL, Hajal NJ, et al: Hypothalamic pituitary adrenal axis functioning in reactive and proactive aggression in children. J Abnorm Child Psychol 37(2):169–182, 2009 18696227

Lozier LM, Cardinale EM, VanMeter JW, et al: Mediation of the relationship between callous-unemotional traits and proactive aggression by amygdala response to fear among children with conduct problems. JAMA Psychiatry 71(6):627–636, 2014 24671141

Lykken DT: A study of anxiety in the sociopathic personality. J Abnorm Psychol 55(1):6–10, 1957 13462652

Marsden J, Glazebrook C, Tully R, et al: Do adult males with antisocial personality disorder (with and without co-morbid psychopathy) have deficits in emotion processing and empathy? A systematic review. Aggress Violent Behav 48:197–217, 2019

Marsh AA: What can we learn about emotion by studying psychopathy? Front Hum Neurosci 7:181, 2013 23675335

Marsh AA, Blair RJ: Deficits in facial affect recognition among antisocial populations: a meta-analysis. Neurosci Biobehav Rev 32(3):454–465, 2008 17915324

Marsh AA, Cardinale EM: Psychopathy and fear: specific impairments in judging behaviors that frighten others. Emotion 12(5):892–898, 2012 22309726

Marsh AA, Cardinale EM: When psychopathy impairs moral judgments: neural responses during judgments about causing fear. Soc Cogn Affect Neurosci 9(1):3–11, 2014 22956667

Marsh AA, Finger EC, Fowler KA, et al: Reduced amygdala response to fearful expressions in children and adolescents with callous-unemotional traits and disruptive behavior disorders. Am J Psychiatry 165(6):712–720, 2008 18281412

Marsh AA, Finger EC, Fowler KA, et al: Empathic responsiveness in amygdala and anterior cingulate cortex in youths with psychopathic traits. J Child Psychol Psychiatry 54(8):900–910, 2013 23488588

McDonald JB, Bozzay ML, Bresin K, Verona E: Facets of externalizing psychopathology in relation to inhibitory control and error processing. Int J Psychophysiol 163:79–91, 2021 31634490

Meffert H, Gazzola V, den Boer JA, et al: Reduced spontaneous but relatively normal deliberate vicarious representations in psychopathy. Brain 136(pt 8):2550–2562, 2013 23884812

Meffert H, Brislin SJ, White SF, et al: Prediction errors to emotional expressions: the roles of the amygdala in social referencing. Soc Cogn Affect Neurosci 10(4):537–544, 2015 24939872

Meffert H, Hwang S, Nolan ZT, et al: Segregating attention from response control when performing a motor inhibition task: segregating attention from response control. Neuroimage 126:27–38, 2016 26584863

Michalska KJ, Zeffiro TA, Decety J: Brain response to viewing others being harmed in children with conduct disorder symptoms. J Child Psychol Psychiatry 57(4):510–519, 2016 26472591

Mier D, Haddad L, Diers K, et al: Reduced embodied simulation in psychopathy. World J Biol Psychiatry 15(6):479–487, 2014 24802075

Mineka S, Cook M: Mechanisms involved in the observational conditioning of fear. J Exp Psychol Gen 122(1):23–38, 1993 8440976

Miyake A, Friedman NP: The nature and organization of individual differences in executive functions: four general conclusions. Curr Dir Psychol Sci 21(1):8–14, 2012 22773897

Mobbs D, Petrovic P, Marchant JL, et al: When fear is near: threat imminence elicits prefrontal-periaqueductal gray shifts in humans. Science 317(5841):1079–1083, 2007 17717184

Mobbs D, Marchant JL, Hassabis D, et al: From threat to fear: the neural organization of defensive fear systems in humans. J Neurosci 29(39):12236–12243, 2009 19793982

Mobbs D, Yu R, Rowe JB, et al: Neural activity associated with monitoring the oscillating threat value of a tarantula. Proc Natl Acad Sci USA 107(47):20582–20586, 2010 21059963

Molenberghs P, Johnson H, Henry JD, et al: Understanding the minds of others: a neuroimaging meta-analysis. Neurosci Biobehav Rev 65:276–291, 2016 27073047

Morgan AB, Lilienfeld SO: A meta-analytic review of the relation between antisocial behavior and neuropsychological measures of executive function. Clin Psychol Rev 20(1):113–136, 2000 10660831

Muñoz LC: Callous-unemotional traits are related to combined deficits in recognizing afraid faces and body poses. J Am Acad Child Adolesc Psychiatry 48(5):554–562, 2009 19318989

Murray L, Waller R, Hyde LW: A systematic review examining the link between psychopathic personality traits, antisocial behavior, and neural reactivity during reward and loss processing. Pers Disord 9(6):497–509, 2018 30080060

O'Nions E, Sebastian CL, McCrory E, et al: Neural bases of theory of mind in children with autism spectrum disorders and children with conduct problems and callous-unemotional traits. Dev Sci 17(5):786–796, 2014 24636205

Panksepp J: Affective Neuroscience: The Foundations of Human and Animal Emotions. New York, Oxford University Press, 1998

Passamonti L, Fairchild G, Goodyer IM, et al: Neural abnormalities in early onset and adolescence-onset conduct disorder. Arch Gen Psychiatry 67(7):729–738, 2010 20603454

Patrick CJ: Emotion and psychopathy: startling new insights. Psychophysiology 31(4):319–330, 1994 10690912

Payer DE, Park MT, Kish SJ, et al: Personality disorder symptomatology is associated with anomalies in striatal and prefrontal morphology. Front Hum Neurosci 9:472, 2015 26379535

Pessoa L, Kastner S, Ungerleider LG: Attentional control of the processing of neural and emotional stimuli. Brain Res Cogn Brain Res 15(1):31–45, 2002 12433381

Phelps EA, LeDoux JE: Contributions of the amygdala to emotion processing: from animal models to human behavior. Neuron 48(2):175–187, 2005 16242399

Plichta MM, Scheres A: Ventral-striatal responsiveness during reward anticipation in ADHD and its relation to trait impulsivity in the healthy population: a meta-analytic review of the fMRI literature. Neurosci Biobehav Rev 38:125–134, 2014 23928090

Prehn K, Schlagenhauf F, Schulze L, et al: Neural correlates of risk taking in violent criminal offenders characterized by emotional hypo- and hyper-reactivity. Soc Neurosci 8(2):136–147, 2013 22747189

Pujara M, Motzkin JC, Newman JP, et al: Neural correlates of reward and loss sensitivity in psychopathy. Soc Cogn Affect Neurosci 9(6):794–801, 2014 23552079

Rothemund Y, Ziegler S, Hermann C, et al: Fear conditioning in psychopaths: event-related potentials and peripheral measures. Biol Psychol 90(1):50–59, 2012 22387928

Rubia K, Smith AB, Halari R, et al: Disorder-specific dissociation of orbitofrontal dysfunction in boys with pure conduct disorder during reward and ventrolateral prefrontal dysfunction in boys with pure ADHD during sustained attention. Am J Psychiatry 166(1):83–94, 2009 18829871

Schiffer B, Pawliczek C, Müller BW, et al: Neural mechanisms underlying affective theory of mind in violent antisocial personality disorder and/or schizophrenia. Schizophr Bull 43(6):1229–1239, 2017 28199713

Schneider F, Habel U, Kessler C, et al: Functional imaging of conditioned aversive emotional responses in antisocial personality disorder. Neuropsychobiology 42(4):192–201, 2000 11096335

Schwenck C, Ciaramidaro A, Selivanova M, et al: Neural correlates of affective empathy and reinforcement learning in boys with conduct problems: fMRI evidence from a gambling task. Behav Brain Res 320:75–84, 2017 27888020

Sebastian CL, McCrory EJ, Cecil CA, et al: Neural responses to affective and cognitive theory of mind in children with conduct problems and varying levels of callous-unemotional traits. Arch Gen Psychiatry 69(8):814–822, 2012 22868935

Shamay-Tsoory SG, Harari H, Aharon-Peretz J, et al: The role of the orbitofrontal cortex in affective theory of mind deficits in criminal offenders with psychopathic tendencies. Cortex 46(5):668–677, 2010 19501818

Shane MS, Groat LL: Capacity for upregulation of emotional processing in psychopathy: all you have to do is ask. Soc Cogn Affect Neurosci 13(11):1163–1176, 2018 30257006

Silveri MM, Dager AD, Cohen-Gilbert JE, et al: Neurobiological signatures associated with alcohol and drug use in the human adolescent brain. Neurosci Biobehav Rev 70:244–259, 2016 27377691

Storebø OJ, Simonsen E: The association between ADHD and antisocial personality disorder (ASPD): a review. J Atten Disord 20(10):815–824, 2016 24284138

Tager-Flusberg H: Exploring the relationships between theory of mind and social-communicative functioning in children with autism, in Individual Differences in Theory of Mind: Implications for Typical and Atypical Development. Edited by Repacholi B, Slaughter V. London, Psychology Press, 2003, pp 197–212

Thornton LC, Frick PJ, Crapanzano AM, et al: The incremental utility of callous-unemotional traits and conduct problems in predicting aggression and bullying in a community sample of boys and girls. Psychol Assess 25(2):366–378, 2013 23244642

Timmermann M, Jeung H, Schmitt R, et al: Oxytocin improves facial emotion recognition in young adults with antisocial personality disorder. Psychoneuroendocrinology 85:158–164, 2017 28865940

Turner D, Sebastian A, Tüscher O: Impulsivity and Cluster B personality disorders. Curr Psychiatry Rep 19(3):15, 2017 28251591

van Lith K, Veltman DJ, Cohn MD, et al: Effects of methylphenidate during fear learning in antisocial adolescents: a randomized controlled fMRI trial. J Am Acad Child Adolesc Psychiatry 57(12):934–943, 2018 30522739

Veroude K, von Rhein D, Chauvin RJ, et al: The link between callous-unemotional traits and neural mechanisms of reward processing: an fMRI study. Psychiatry Res Neuroimaging 255:75–80, 2016 27564545

Viding E, McCrory E: Towards understanding atypical social affiliation in psychopathy. Lancet Psychiatry 6(5):437–444, 2019 31006435

Viding E, Sebastian CL, Dadds MR, et al: Amygdala response to preattentive masked fear in children with conduct problems: the role of callous-unemotional traits. Am J Psychiatry 169(10):1109–1116, 2012 23032389

Völlm B, Richardson P, McKie S, et al: Neuronal correlates and serotonergic modulation of behavioural inhibition and reward in healthy and antisocial individuals. J Psychiatr Res 44(3):123–131, 2010 19683258

Waugh CE, Hamilton JP, Gotlib IH: The neural temporal dynamics of the intensity of emotional experience. Neuroimage 49(2):1699–1707, 2010 19833213

Waugh CE, Lemus MG, Gotlib IH: The role of the medial frontal cortex in the maintenance of emotional states. Soc Cogn Affect Neurosci 9(12):2001–2009, 2014 24493835

Weidacker K, Snowden RJ, Boy F, et al: Response inhibition in the parametric Go/No-Go task in psychopathic offenders. Psychiatry Res 250:256–263, 2017 28171793

White SF, Marsh AA, Fowler KA, et al: Reduced amygdala response in youths with disruptive behavior disorders and psychopathic traits: decreased emotional response versus increased top-down attention to nonemotional features. Am J Psychiatry 169(7):750–758, 2012 22456823

White SF, Pope K, Sinclair S, et al: Disrupted expected value and prediction error signaling in youths with disruptive behavior disorders during a passive avoidance task. Am J Psychiatry 170(3):315–323, 2013 23450288

Young SE, Friedman NP, Miyake A, et al: Behavioral disinhibition: liability for externalizing spectrum disorders and its genetic and environmental relation to response inhibition across adolescence. J Abnorm Psychol 118(1):117–130, 2009 19222319

Yu R, Mobbs D, Seymour B, et al: The neural signature of escalating frustration in humans. Cortex 54:165–178, 2014 24699035

CHAPTER 15

SPECT and PET Studies of Antisocial Personality Disorder and Aggression

Nathan J. Kolla, M.D., Ph.D., FRCPC

Sylvain Houle, M.D., Ph.D., FRCPC

Most violent crime is perpetrated by a small group of males who have conduct-disordered behavior in childhood and meet diagnostic criteria for antisocial personality disorder (ASPD) as adults. Although ASPD is not as prevalent as other psychiatric conditions in the community (some estimates indicate that ASPD affects 1% of American adults; Lenzenweger et al. 2007), nearly 50% of incarcerated individuals meet criteria for the disorder (Fazel and Danesh 2002). Furthermore, 85% of individuals with ASPD have acted violently toward others (Robins and Regier 1991; Samuels et al. 2004). Hence, these statistics underscore the importance of a research framework that takes into account multiple levels of information to understand the pathology, including neurochemistry, of ASPD.

A common mistake made by clinicians and researchers is the interchangeable use of the terms *ASPD* and *psychopathy*. ASPD and psychopathy share some features in common (e.g., impulsivity and involvement in criminal activity), but prototypical psychopathy also includes the personality characteristics of deficient affective experience, lack of empathy, and callousness, which are not necessarily observed in ASPD. Most individuals with psychopathy meet criteria for ASPD, whereas only 10% of per-

This chapter was adapted from Kolla NJ, Houle S: "Single-Photon Emission Computed Tomography and Positron Emission Tomography Studies of Antisocial Personality Disorder and Aggression: A Targeted Review." *Current Psychiatry Reports* 21(4):24, 2019. Used with permission of Springer Nature.

sons with ASPD present with psychopathy (National Collaborating Centre for Mental Health 2010). Some evidence also indicates that psychopathy is a more severe form of ASPD (Coid and Ullrich 2010).

ASPD is typically diagnosed in clinical and research settings using criteria set forth in DSM-5 (American Psychiatric Association 2013). By contrast, the most common instrument used to classify individuals with psychopathy is the Hare Psychopathy Checklist–Revised (PCL-R; Hare 2003). The PCL-R contains 20 items that are each rated as 0 (not present), 1 (partially present), or 2 (fully present), ideally based on file review and clinical interview. Scores between 0 and 40 are thus generated. In North America, a score of 30 or more denotes the presence of psychopathy. Important to note is that psychopathy is not universally viewed as a taxon (e.g., presence or absence of a disorder) but, instead, is often conceptualized as a dimensional construct (Blackburn and Coid 1998). The same is true of ASPD (Marcus et al. 2006).

Aggressive behavior is a common feature of ASPD, psychopathy, and other psychiatric disorders. Healthy individuals without psychiatric illness also engage in aggressive behavior under certain circumstances. As such, trait aggression is thought to occur along a continuum (Anderson and Huesmann 2003), where some people rarely, if ever, act aggressively, but others (usually when psychiatric disorder is present) have lower thresholds for becoming aggressive. Aggression that is impulsive and typically manifests in response to a threat or anger is known as *reactive aggression*. By contrast, aggression that is premeditated or used to achieve an aim or increase dominance is labeled *proactive* or *instrumental aggression* (Raine et al. 2006). A lack of differentiation of these two main types of aggression often leads to conflicting results in the literature. Research investigating the neural mechanisms of aggressive behavior has also been plagued by this issue, although some PET studies, as discussed later in this chapter, have differentiated reactive from proactive aggression and report on the neurochemical indexes of each. The distinction between reactive and proactive aggression is important because these entities likely have different neural underpinnings.

The purpose of this chapter is to critically examine single-photon emission computed tomography (SPECT) and PET brain imaging studies of ASPD and aggression in nonclinical populations. We discuss each in turn. Studies that included at least one patient with ASPD were included in the analysis on ASPD.

SPECT

SPECT is a three-dimensional nuclear imaging technique. Following the intravenous injection of a radiopharmaceutical, a molecule tagged with a gamma-emitting radionuclide—most commonly, technetium-99m (^{99m}Tc), a radiation detector rotates around the subject's body acquiring multiple two-dimensional images. These images are then fed to a tomographic reconstruction program that produces three-dimensional maps of the radiopharmaceutical concentration within the body. The most widely used SPECT radiopharmaceutical for brain imaging is ^{99m}Tc-hexamethylpropylene-amine oxide (^{99m}Tc-HMPAO) (Neirinckx et al. 1987), which provides an index of regional cerebral blood flow (rCBF). Because blood flow in the brain is closely linked to local brain metabolism and energy use, ^{99m}Tc-HMPAO can offer an indirect measure of brain metabolism.

SPECT Studies of Antisocial Personality Disorder

In the five SPECT studies that follow, 37 individuals with ASPD were scanned out of a total of 198 participants. One report that examined rCBF using ^{99m}Tc-HMPAO SPECT sampled 40 patients hospitalized on an alcoholism inpatient ward (Kuruoglu et al. 1996). Of these patients, 15 met criteria for ASPD, 21 had primarily dependent personality disorder, and 4 had other personality disorders. Axis I comorbidity (besides alcohol misuse) was exclusionary. All individuals were scanned at the termination of alcohol withdrawal symptoms. Ten males who did not drink and had no relatives with alcohol misuse served as the comparison group. The main finding to emerge was that the ASPD group had anterior frontal hypoperfusion relative to the other personality groups. A reduction in cerebral lobe rCBF ratio was also reported in 87.5% of the ASPD group. This study is notable for the fact that ASPD participants were tested as a single group rather than as part of a heterogeneous sample of aggressive or antisocial individuals.

Another ^{99m}Tc-HMPAO investigation (Gerra et al. 1998) that studied healthy participants and detoxified opiate misusers with either depression, ASPD (7 men and 2 women), or no comorbid Axis I or II psychopathology found that the ASPD group had lower rCBF in the right frontal lobes compared with healthy control subjects and opiate misusers without comorbid psychiatric conditions. On the other hand, the study reported no differences between the ASPD and the depression samples, even though other SPECT studies of depression have reported alterations in several brain regions (Ito et al. 1996; Mayberg et al. 1994).

A subsequent ^{99m}Tc-HMPAO study (Soderstrom et al. 2002) investigated 32 violent offenders without severe and persistent mental illness; only 2 subjects had ASPD. There was no comparison group, and statistical tests were limited to correlational analyses. The authors reported significant negative correlations between the interpersonal features of psychopathy (e.g., callousness, lack of empathy, deficient affective experience) and frontal and temporal perfusion. Given the small number of ASPD participants, it would seem that these results have less relevance for understanding CBF alterations in ASPD.

A ^{99m}Tc-HMPAO protocol (Goethals et al. 2005) scanned 37 participants with either borderline personality disorder (BPD) or ASPD ($n=10$) and 34 healthy control subjects. Axis I psychopathology was exclusionary for all groups. Compared with the healthy group, reduced rCBF in the right lateral temporal cortex, right frontopolar cortex, and right ventrolateral prefrontal cortex was reported among the participants with personality disorders. Importantly, no difference in rCBF between ASPD and BPD was seen, suggesting that these conditions might share similar pathologies, although subsequent PET studies of ASPD and BPD have reported important differences in other neural substrates studied (Kolla et al. 2015, 2016a).

An innovative study that used ^{99m}Tc-HMPAO (Anckarsäter et al. 2007) scanned nine pretrial violent offenders and then rescanned them on average 4 years later in what was essentially a test-retest design. Only one participant was diagnosed with ASPD, and the study had no healthy control subjects. Notably, all subjects had improved clinically from the first scan, which included the absence of any psychotic symptoms, drug abuse, or treatment with psychoactive medication. Group results from the first scans were compared with amalgamated data from the second set of SPECT scans. No quantitative differences between groups were detected. Violent offenders showed unchanged frontotemporal hypoactivity from the initial SPECT scan. Moreover, the mean changes in all of the regions sampled were less than 5%. These results raise the important question of whether frontotemporal hypoactivity is a state or trait phenomenon in violent offenders and what role, if any, the presence of psychoactive substances contributes to these findings. Of course, because this study included only one ASPD participant, it is difficult to generalize to this population.

Early SPECT studies tended to focus on violent offenders or substance misusers as groups that failed to include large numbers of ASPD participants. As a result, findings may be less relevant to ASPD. These investigations also were likely underpowered to detect differences between patient groups, such as ASPD versus depression or BPD. Some evidence supports decreased frontotemporal rCBF in ASPD, but, again, this pattern was observed in offender groups with very little representation from ASPD subjects. However, the phenomenon of frontotemporal hypoperfusion is bolstered by structural MRI findings in ASPD that document reduced volumes of gray matter in these regions (Dolan et al. 2002; Kolla et al. 2014; Raine et al. 2000). Because the frontal lobes exert control over neural threat response systems, structural or functional alterations of this complex could weaken threat-response regulation (Pemment 2013), ultimately leading to increased reactive or impulsive aggression. Finally, some evidence indicates that structural alteration of temporal lobes in ASPD relates to impairment in aggression control, heightened impulsivity, and deficits in emotion processing (Barkataki et al. 2006).

PET

PET is another three-dimensional nuclear imaging technique. It differs from SPECT by using positron-emitting radiopharmaceuticals rather than single gamma photon-emitting radionuclides. Given the size of the technetium atom and the fact that it must be chelated to the target molecule, the number of useful SPECT radiopharmaceuticals for brain imaging is severely limited. Carbon-11 and fluorine-18 are the most widely used radionuclides for PET. Because the nuclides are nearly identical to the nonradioactive carbon-12 and fluorine-19 atoms, they can radiolabel a much wider range of natural molecules or drugs to probe specific biochemical processes, enzymes, transporter substrates, ligands for receptor systems, hormones, antibodies, peptides, drugs, and oligonucleotides (Phelps 2000). When positron emitters decay, two annihilation photons are produced, and the PET scanner detects these photons. After intravenous injection into the subject, the PET scanner records the three-dimensional concentration of the positron-emitting radiopharmaceutical over time. Although PET imaging offers several technical and biological advantages over SPECT, its widespread use is limited by the short half-lives of carbon-11 (20.4 minutes) and fluorine-18 (110 minutes), requiring their production by cyclotrons located close to the PET scanners.

Depending on the positron-emitting radiopharmaceutical used, different biological indexes, such as metabolic rate, binding potential, neuroreceptor occupancy, or distribution volume, can be obtained from the PET data by a mathematical technique known as kinetic modeling. In some instances, simpler measures are used, such as standardized uptake values.

The glucose analog 2-deoxy-2-[fluorine-18]-fluoro-D-glucose ([^{18}F]FDG) is the most commonly used PET radiopharmaceutical (Scam et al. 2007). On injection, [^{18}F]FDG is transported into cells and phosphorylated much like glucose to FDG-6-phosphate. However, because FDG-6-phosphate is not a substrate for glucose-6-phosphate isomerase, it remains trapped in the cell, reaching near equilibrium approximately 1 hour after injection. For brain scans, the regional cerebral metabolic rate of glucose (rCMRglu) is then measured for individual brain regions.

FDG-PET Studies in Antisocial Personality Disorder

Among the eight investigations in which it was possible to discern the number of ASPD participants who received an FDG-PET scan, 36 subjects with ASPD out of 310 participants were scanned. An initial FDG-PET study (Volkow et al. 1995) analyzing brain metabolism examined eight patients admitted to a state psychiatric hospital who endorsed repetitive violence and who had either intermittent explosive disorder (IED), a behavioral condition marked by volatile outbursts of explosion and anger, or ASPD. However, only one individual in the sample met criteria for ASPD. Patients with chronic psychotic conditions were also included in the analysis. Eight healthy control subjects were also tested. Results showed that violent patients had significantly lower metabolism in the left and right prefrontal regions, left frontal regions, and left and right temporal medial areas. Given the paucity of ASPD participants, it was not possible to test the individual effects of ASPD on the results obtained.

Another FDG-PET investigation (Goyer et al. 1994) compared patients with personality disorder (6 with ASPD out of 17 total participants) with 43 healthy control subjects who had no psychiatric history. The experimental group comprised military personnel admitted to an inpatient ward. No differences in rCMRglu were detected between the ASPD patients and the healthy control subjects. Moreover, there was no interaction between ASPD subjects and the image plane. The authors suggested that a history of alcohol abuse (four of six subjects) may have produced sufficient variability in the data to lead to a false-negative finding. Insufficient power was also cited as a possibility. On the other hand, for the six BPD participants, an interaction emerged between diagnosis and image plane. For example, BPD patients showed significant differences between normalized rCMRglu in two planes of the frontal lobes, one showing an increase and the other a decrease. These results tentatively suggest a dissection of neural correlates in ASPD and BPD that further supports the notion of these disorders as distinct conditions.

One FDG-PET scan examined seven extremely violent offenders (Seidenwurm et al. 1997) (murder was the index offense for all subjects—in all cases unprovoked—and some individuals had multiple victims), one of whom was diagnosed with ASPD. Nine control subjects without organic brain damage were also included. Quantitative PET data were evaluated as standardized uptake values that compared the greatest occipital region with the lowest temporal region. The mean percentage of decreased activity in the violent group was 39%, which was statistically greater than the mean decrease in the control group (27%). The authors suggested that, similar to other studies, glucose metabolism abnormalities in the temporal lobe were related to violent behavior. Because all episodes of violence exclusively involved proactive or instrumental aggression, these results could shed some light on the neural correlates of this form of aggression.

A two-scan FDG-PET protocol (New et al. 2002) examined 13 subjects with impulsive aggression (4 with comorbid ASPD) and 13 healthy control subjects. Meta-chlorophenylpiperazine (m-CPP), a serotonergic probe, was administered prior to one scan, and the other scan had no stimulus. m-CPP is a partial agonist at serotonin type 2A (5-HT$_{2A}$) and 2C (5-HT$_{2C}$) receptors and also targets presynaptic 5-HT sites (Baumann et al. 1995). PET images were standardized as mean relative glucose metabolic rate (rGMR). The authors reported that, unlike healthy control subjects, impulsive patients showed no activation in the left anteromedial orbital cortex in response to m-CPP and that the left anterior cingulate cortex (ACC), which is typically activated by m-CPP, was deactivated in the experimental group. On the other hand, the posterior cingulate gyrus was activated in impulsive patients and deactivated in healthy control subjects. No group differences were detected in the baseline scans. The authors interpreted their results to mean that activation of the anterior cingulate gyrus and posterior orbital cortex in concert with serotonergic input may act to constrain aggressive behavior.

Another investigation that used fenfluramine (FEN), an indirect agonist of 5-HT receptors (Rothman and Baumann 2002), and FDG-PET sampled a cohort of 22 BPD patients, one of whom had comorbid ASPD, and 24 control subjects (Soloff et al. 2005). Study participants received placebo on day 1 and FEN on day 2 before the PET scans. Gender differences in FDG uptake emerged between BPD participants in terms of response to placebo by diagnosis, within-group comparisons in response to FEN, and between-group comparisons in response to FEN. Importantly, when measures of trait impulsivity and aggression were included as covariates in each of the models, all group comparisons and differences between BPD and control groups in response to placebo were rendered insignificant. These results suggest that impulsive and aggressive personality traits may have been driving the observed associations. Given the small number of individuals with comorbid ASPD, it is not unexpected that none of the analyses controlled for this covariate.

A double-blind, placebo-controlled study of fluoxetine, a selective serotonin reuptake inhibitor (SSRI), was conducted with FDG-PET (New et al. 2004). Subjects received a PET scan before and after 12 weeks of SSRI treatment. Initially, 22 nondepressed, impulsive-aggressive patients with BPD (4 patients had ASPD) were enrolled. However, only 10 of the 15 participants receiving active treatment and 3 of the 5 taking placebo completed the investigation. The authors did not report how many patients with concomitant ASPD had completed the trial. Results indicated that rGMR was increased in the orbitofrontal cortex (OFC) and medial anterior temporal regions relative to baseline in the SSRI-treated group at the conclusion of the study. The study authors proposed a relationship between increased OFC rGMR and improvement in aggressive symptomatology.

An additional FDG-PET study by New et al. (2009) evaluated 38 patients with BPD (10 patients had comorbid ASPD) and impulsive aggression (met criteria for IED-

Revised [IED-R]; Coccaro et al. 1998) and 36 healthy control subjects in a two-scan protocol employing the Point Subtraction Aggression Paradigm (PSAP). The PSAP is a psychometric task that assesses provoked aggression in a laboratory setting with a computer protocol (Cherek et al. 1997). Participants' aggressive responding to the loss of "points" worth money over the 35 minutes of testing is evaluated. In the study, each participant underwent two PET scans with a provocation and nonprovocation version. Patients increased mean (provoked responses on the task–nonprovoked responses on the task) rGMR in the OFC and amygdala when provoked, whereas healthy control subjects showed a decrease in mean rGMR in these same regions. Subgroups involving participants with comorbid major depressive disorder and PTSD were analyzed (no differences were appreciated), although ASPD as a subgroup was not considered.

A reanalysis of the same data set (Perez-Rodriguez et al. 2012) found that male patients had lower mean striatal rGMR in both provoked and nonprovoked groups compared with all other groups. Interestingly, the investigators found no relation between striatal activity and behavioral aggression among the patients. Also, an ASPD diagnosis was not treated as a covariate. Based on their findings, the study authors opined that the striatum could contribute to social aggression as exemplified by BPD subjects with comorbid IED-R.

In a more recent investigation (Park et al. 2016), 72 adults received an FDG-PET scan and also completed Cloninger's Temperament and Character Inventory (Cloninger 1987). Based on these results, 13 subjects (18%) were designated as having antisocial personality. None of the participants were administered structured instruments typically used to diagnose ASPD. Among the antisocial personality group, elevated rCMRglu was detected in the left hemisphere, including the inferior frontal gyrus, whereas decreased metabolism was present bilaterally in the right OFC gyrus and hippocampus. Although the investigators suggested that differences in the level of rCMRglu between cortical and subcortical structures could be central to the pathology of antisocial personality, many of these subjects may not have met the diagnostic criteria for ASPD, and, as such, results cannot generalize to the wider group of individuals with rigorously diagnosed ASPD.

A major limitation of the FDG-PET studies described in this section is the narrow representation of ASPD in the study samples. Most studies intentionally recruited BPD participants with IED-R, some of whom happened to have comorbid ASPD. Thus, it is unclear how these results relate to ASPD, because very few studies examined an ASPD diagnosis as a covariate. Furthermore, at least one study whose aim it was to report on findings of antisocial individuals did not use structured assessments to diagnose ASPD but instead relied on self-report psychometric data. FDG-PET results of BPD cannot be assumed to translate to ASPD, because some data have shown differing neural correlates between the two disorders.

PET Studies With Serotonergic Probes

Among the following seven studies that reported the number of ASPD participants scanned, one-quarter (67 of 268) sampled ASPD participants. When serotonergic positron-emitting radiopharmaceuticals became available, many researchers started investigating 5-HT transporter (SERT) and 5-HT receptor occupancies in personality disorder populations. The advent of these serotonergic probes provided a new avenue to study the neurochemistry of ASPD.

The radiopharmaceutical [^{11}C]McN 5652 was first used to quantify SERT distribution in the brains of 10 individuals with impulsive aggression (2 patients had comorbid ASPD) and 10 healthy control subjects (Frankle et al. 2005). Outcome measures included binding potential (BP$_{ND}$: ratio at equilibrium of specifically bound radioligand to nondisplaceable radioligand in tissue) of the SERT and the specific-to-nonspecific partition coefficient (V$_3$″). The authors reported that both indexes of SERT in the ACC were lower in the IED group. Along with the OFC, the ACC provides top-down control of subcortical structures to inhibit impulsive, reactive responding (Rosell and Siever 2015). In addition to the small sample size, an important limitation of this study was that [^{11}C]McN 5652 has been linked to high levels of nonspecific binding, which limits the ability to measure SERT in regions of low SERT density (Parsey et al. 2000).

Another study (Rosell et al. 2010) that sampled IED-R used the radiopharmaceutical [^{11}C]MDL100907 to quantify 5-HT$_{2A}$ receptor availability in 25 healthy control subjects and two groups of patients with IED-R and personality disorders: 14 with current physical aggression and 15 without current physical aggression. The former group had four ASPD patients, and the latter group had six ASPD participants. When comparing group differences, OFC 5-HT$_{2A}$ receptor BP$_p$ (ratio at equilibrium of specifically bound radioligand to amount of total parent radioligand) and BP$_{ND}$ were higher among IED-R patients with current physical aggression compared with IED-R subjects without current physical aggression or healthy control subjects. No other differences were detected between groups or brain regions. Strengths of the study included a medication-free sample, the absence of concurrent major depressive episodes, and no active alcohol or substance abuse. These results imply that increased OFC 5-HT$_{2A}$ receptor availability may be specifically related to IED-R with current physical aggression.

A notable investigation (Meyer et al. 2008) that measured 5-HT$_{2A}$ receptor density using an alternative radioligand ([^{18}F]setoperone) sampled 16 individuals with ASPD with violent behavior and 16 healthy control subjects. One of the principal findings was decreased dorsolateral prefrontal cortex (DLPFC) 5-HT$_{2A}$ receptor availability among the ASPD group. DLPFC 5-HT$_{2A}$ receptor density was reduced among participants ages 19–24 years compared with healthy control subjects, but no differences were detected in ASPD subjects ages 25–33 years. Similar to the study by Rosell et al. (2010), an increase in PFC 5-HT$_{2A}$ receptor availability was present in the participants ages 34–39 years. One criticism of the investigation is that it did not measure aggression with an operationalized construct. However, this study is one of very few to retain a clinical sample composed entirely of ASPD participants. Thus, these findings should be regarded as especially relevant to the neurochemistry of ASPD with current violence.

Twenty-nine patients with IED-R, including a substantial contingent of ASPD patients (n=17), were compared with 30 healthy control subjects using [^{11}C]DASP PET to measure SERT density in the pregenual ACC, amygdala, and other subcortical structures (van de Giessen et al. 2014). As noted earlier, this research group had previously found lower ACC SERT density in the experimental group using a different radiopharmaceutical sensitive to SERT. In the current study, contrary to the authors' hypothesis, there was no difference in ACC SERT binding between IED-R participants and healthy subjects. Interestingly, a significant positive correlation between ACC SERT availability and trait callousness, measured with the Dimensional Assessment of Personality Pathology (Pukrop et al. 2009), was detected in the IED-R group. The researchers conjectured that the previously demonstrated association between low presynaptic 5-HT and aggression was mainly applicable to reactive aggression and that proactive aggression, including callousness as one component, could be related to high presynaptic 5-HT. van de Giessen et al. (2014) believe that this finding has not been replicated in subsequent PET studies.

A dual-tracer PET investigation that sampled males with high impulsive aggression and excluded those with callous-unemotional traits evaluated SERT binding using [^{11}C]DASP and 5-HT$_{2A}$ receptor availability with [^{11}C]MDL100907 (Rylands et al. 2012). As noted, individuals (all male) had no callous-unemotional traits and were grouped into two categories: high impulsivity and low impulsivity. All of the high-impulsivity participants met diagnostic criteria for either ASPD ($n=11$), BPD ($n=7$), or both ($n=4$). Impulsivity was measured with the Psychopathic Personality Inventory-Revised (Lillenfield and Widows 2005) and the Impulsiveness, Venturesomeness, and Empathy Scale (Eysenck and Eysenck 1991). It was not clear how many ASPD participants were actually scanned. However, 22 high- and low-impulsivity participants completed a [^{11}C]DASP scan, and 24 high- and low-impulsivity subjects underwent [^{11}C]MDL100907 scanning. The authors reported a group difference among eight brain regions testing 5-HT$_{2A}$ receptor BP$_{ND}$ between the high-impulsivity and the low-impulsivity groups, with lower BP$_{ND}$ in the high-impulsivity group. Conversely, SERT BP$_{ND}$ was significantly higher in the high-impulsivity group among all of the regions sampled, although results were driven primarily by differences in the brain stem. Among the entire sample, brain-stem SERT BP$_{ND}$ was positively correlated with impulsivity, aggression, and ratings of childhood trauma. Furthermore, in the high-impulsivity group, a positive correlation emerged between brain-stem SERT BP$_{ND}$ and a measure of childhood trauma. The authors posited that childhood adverse experiences could have affected serotonergic gene function to give rise to neurodevelopmental alterations of 5-HT function, ultimately resulting in high impulsivity. Whether these results were due to neurochemical differences present in ASPD or an altered neural substrate underlying high impulsivity could not be determined. Studies involving ASPD participants with varying levels of impulsivity could help parse these results.

A study targeting 5-HT$_{2A}$ receptor binding that used [^{18}F]altanserin sampled 33 BPD patients (8 with comorbid ASPD) and 27 healthy control subjects (Soloff et al. 2014). The authors reported that BPD participants with comorbid ASPD, compared with those without ASPD, had lower BP$_{ND}$ in the basal ganglia, left thalamus, medial temporal cortex, pregenual cingulate, and ACC. Conversely, depression, current substance use disorder, and suicide attempter status did not relate to 5-HT$_{2A}$ receptor binding in any brain region. These results suggest that BPD with comorbid ASPD may represent a different phenotype than either disorder alone, with corresponding alterations in 5-HT$_{2A}$ receptor binding.

One novel study to examine serotonergic targets beyond the SERT and 5-HT$_{2A}$ receptor used [^{11}C]AZ10419360 to measure 5-HT$_{1B}$ receptor BP$_{ND}$ in 19 incarcerated violent offenders (14 individuals with ASPD) and 24 healthy control subjects (da Cunha-Bang et al. 2017b). 5-HT$_{1B}$ receptor functions as an autoreceptor presynaptically and a heteroreceptor postsynaptically, and basic science research suggests that 5-HT$_{1B}$ heteroreceptors may mediate aggression and impulsivity (Nautiyal et al. 2015). Although no group differences in 5-HT$_{1B}$ receptor BP$_{ND}$ were discerned (OFC, ACC, and striatum were examined), post-hoc analyses examined the relation between the brain regions and the clinical characteristics of violent offenders. For example, striatal 5-HT$_{1B}$ receptor BP$_{ND}$ was associated with trait aggression; trait psychopathy, which was primarily related to self-centered impulsivity; and PCL-R score. Trait anger also showed a relationship with ACC and OFC BP$_{ND}$. Moreover, caudate 5-HT$_{1B}$ receptor BP$_{ND}$ showed a strong association with trait anger, trait psychopathy, and PCL-R score. Whole-brain voxelwise analysis in the violent offender group replicated the positive correlation of trait anger with caudate/OFC 5-HT$_{1B}$ receptor BP$_{ND}$. Importantly, none of these associations were present in the healthy control group, although it was noted that the low range of trait anger within the comparison group could have been responsible for the group interaction effect. The high proportion of ASPD participants in this study group helps generalize these findings to the larger population of male ASPD patients who engage in violent behavior.

Using the same PET scan data as in the study described in the previous paragraph, the investigators tested whether 5-HT$_{1B}$ receptor BP$_{ND}$ showed a relationship with performance on a computerized version of an emotional Go/No-go task (da Cunha-Bang et al. 2017a). The results of the violent offenders and healthy control subjects were pooled for the analyses. The authors hypothesized that 5-HT$_{1B}$ receptor binding would be positively correlated with proportion of false alarms in response to threat-related facial expressions (angry and fearful). Primary outcome measures were false alarms for neutral Go trials, in which angry and fearful faces functioned as No-go trials, and false alarms for angry and fearful Go trials, in which neutral faces acted as No-go trials. Post-hoc analyses found that false alarms in blocks where angry faces were Go stimuli showed a significant positive correlation with ACC 5-HT$_{1B}$ receptor binding. The authors concluded that men (whose level of aggression varied tremendously given that it was a sample of violent offenders and healthy subjects) with high 5-HT$_{1B}$ receptor binding had relative difficulty withholding responses to neutral No-go stimuli when Go stimuli were angry faces. They suggested that ACC 5-HT$_{1B}$ receptors could be implicated in the neural underpinnings of response inhibition when presented with socially threatening cues.

Earlier 5-HT PET studies focused on examining IED-R subjects with comorbid BPD. In most instances, the proportion of ASPD subjects was minimal. It is, therefore, doubtful whether these findings contribute substantially to our knowledge about the neurochemistry of ASPD. Additionally, some of these studies produced contrary results—one study reported that ACC SERT binding was lower in IED-R, but another study, by the same research group, noted that ACC SERT binding was higher. Limitations of the radiopharmaceuticals used may have contributed to divergent results. One investigation that studied ASPD exclusively found that lower 5-HT$_{2A}$ receptor density was present in the DLPFC (Meyer et al. 2008). However, results were significant only in younger populations. An interesting hypothesis advanced by van de Giessen et al. (2014) suggested that increased ACC SERT availability could be related to proactive aggression. However, to date, little evidence supports this conclusion.

On the other hand, a dual-radiopharmaceutical PET study whose intent was to examine measures of serotonergic function in highly impulsive ASPD groups found that brain-stem SERT BP_{ND} was related to both impulsivity and aggression. Finally, more studies of ASPD participants that use radiopharmaceuticals to probe previously uncharted serotonergic receptors, such as $5\text{-}HT_{1B}$ receptor, are necessary to advance the field.

PET Studies With Alternative Probes

To the best of our knowledge, only two PET studies that used a nonserotonergic ligand to study ASPD have been published (Kolla et al. 2015, 2021). [^{11}C]Harmine was the radiopharmaceutical used in one study to measure monoamine oxidase A (MAO A) distribution volume (V_T) in 18 male violent offenders with ASPD and 18 male control participants (Kolla et al. 2015). MAO A is a brain enzyme located on outer mitochondrial membranes that degrades 5-HT, dopamine, and norepinephrine (Youdim et al. 2006). In each study group, nine of the subjects had alcohol dependence. The authors chose the OFC and ventral striatum as the primary brain regions given their biological abnormalities in ASPD and aggression (Blair 2004; Glenn and Yang 2012). A global reduction in MAO A V_T was observed in ASPD, including the a priori regions. Several self-report, clinician-administered, and behavioral measures of impulsivity also showed an inverse correlation with ventral striatum V_T. Results supported previous findings of MAO A knockout models in rodents exhibiting aggressive behavior (Cases et al. 1995; Godar et al. 2011) and a rare MAO A missense mutation in human males leading to extreme aggression and impulsivity (Brunner et al. 1993). The extent to which comorbid alcohol dependence may have altered results is unknown. A subsequent multimodal PET–functional MRI study based on the same sample reported that functional coupling of ventral striatum seeds to frontal regions and hippocampus was positively and negatively associated with ventral striatum MAO A V_T, respectively, and that ventral striatum resting state networks were negatively correlated with impulsivity (Kolla et al. 2016b). These results suggest that brain MAO A phenotypic markers may have relevance to understanding functional connectivity and impulsivity. The disadvantage of this study is that it did not include a healthy control group.

A more recent PET study examined the role of the endocannabinoid system in ASPD (Kolla et al. 2021). The endocannabinoid system is composed of receptors, endogenous ligands, and enzymes that regulate cognitive functions and social behaviors, including aggression (Zanettini et al. 2011). Fatty acid amide hydrolase (FAAH), an enzyme, is a particular molecule of interest as it degrades anandamide, an endocannabinoid that binds to cannabinoid 1 receptors to stimulate neurotransmission (Zanettini et al. 2011). Because reactive aggression in humans has been associated with increased amygdala responsiveness (Siep et al. 2019), Kolla and colleagues hypothesized that decreased FAAH levels in the amygdala using [^{11}C]CURB PET could be related to heightened anandamide–cannabinoid 1 receptor signaling. Sixteen male participants with ASPD (some with comorbid schizophrenia) and 16 male control subjects completed the experiment. Results showed that amygdala FAAH binding was lower in the amygdala and that cerebellar and striatal FAAH binding were inversely related with impulsivity. Cerebellar FAAH binding was also negatively associated with assaultive aggression. The investigation of novel therapeutics to target the endocannabinoid system was proposed as a potential remedy for ASPD.

PET Studies of Aggression

A [^{99m}Tc]HMPAO SPECT study examined 20 patients with schizophrenia spectrum disorders and a history of severe violence and 9 patients with schizophrenia spectrum disorders without a history of violence as a comparison group (Jacobsen et al. 2017). Violent patients who had Historical Clinical Risk Management–20 (Webster et al. 1997) scores higher than 20 showed reduced accrual of [^{99m}Tc]HMPAO in left temporal lobes. Furthermore, 12 violent patients manifested bilateral reduced perfusion, and 11 subjects had frontally hypoperfused areas. In the control group, only 2 patients had frontal and temporal lobe hypoperfusion. The results of the violent schizophrenia spectrum disorder subjects largely parallel those seen in ASPD as discussed earlier (see section "SPECT Studies of Antisocial Personality Disorder"), which may imply that frontal and temporal hypoperfusion is not as specific a marker of ASPD because it is a more general correlate of aggressive behavior. Some of the violent schizophrenia spectrum disorder participants also may have had comorbid ASPD that was not measured.

An elegant investigation using FDG-PET analyzed brain metabolic activity and physiological measures in participants at rest, during exposure to violent media, and during exposure to emotional, nonviolent media (Alia-Klein et al. 2014). Study groups were relatively small, albeit carefully designed. Participants included males who had a history of physical fights in the last year and scored above the seventy-fifth percentile on the Physical Aggression scale of the Buss Perry Aggression Questionnaire (BPAQ; Buss and Perry 1992) ($n=12$) and another group of males who did not get into fights and scored at or below the fiftieth percentile on the same aggression questionnaire ($n=13$). The most consistent neuroimaging finding to emerge was hyperactivity of the default mode network (e.g., medial PFC, posterior cingulate cortex, precuneus, inferior parietal lobules, and medial temporal regions) in the aggressive versus nonaggressive group as well as hypoactivity of the OFC and cerebellum at rest. These findings were largely replicated during exposure to violent media and suggested a dissection of brain metabolism as a function of trait aggression.

A series of PET studies have examined dopamine receptor binding in relation to trait aggression. Plavén-Sigray and colleagues (2014) used [^{11}C]SCH23390, a dopamine D_1 receptor ligand, to analyze the association between scores on the Verbal Trait Aggression and Physical Trait Aggression scales of the Swedish universities Scales of Personality (Gustavsson et al. 2000) and D_1 receptor availability. Although the striatum was identified as the main target region, the study was highly exploratory and tested numerous extrastriatal areas, presumably because D_1 receptors are prevalent outside of the striatum (Hall et al. 1994). Among the 23 healthy participants (13 males, 10 females) who participated, D_1 receptor BP_{ND} in the limbic striatum showed an inverse correlation with physical trait aggression. Because D_1 receptor binding was also associated with social desirability, the authors concluded that increased D_1 receptor availability was related to high affiliation and low dominance. However, in a follow-up study by the same authors who aimed to replicate this result (Plavén-Sigray et al. 2018), no relationship emerged between limbic striatum D_1 receptor binding and physical trait aggression. Lack of a diverse sample (the second study recruited only males) and relatively small sample sizes may have led to decreased sensitivity to detect associations. The authors also acknowledged that their first result could have occurred as a result of a type I error.

A carefully conceived investigation (Schlüter et al. 2016) that aimed to measure dopamine release following observation of a violent movie used [^{18}F]desmethoxy-fallypride ([^{18}F]DFMP), a radiotracer that is comparable to raclopride in terms of its binding affinity to D_2 and D_3 receptors (Gründer et al. 2003) but has the advantage of slower kinetics and a longer half-life. The investigators separated male participants into two groups based on high ($n=11$) or low ($n=12$) MAO A promoter variable nucleotide tandem repeats (VNTRs). The main study objective was to examine the effect of the MAO A VNTR on stimulus-related dopamine release and emergence of aggressive behavior. To achieve this aim, subjects were scanned twice under differing conditions: once while watching a violent movie and on another occasion while viewing a neutral movie. Afterward, the participants completed the PSAP. The two groups did not differ on measures of aggression or psychopathic traits at baseline. Results showed that the high-activity MAO A group had greater dopamine release in the ventral caudate nucleus and putamen (calculated as the change in dopamine release while viewing the violent movie compared with the emotionally neutral movie) and increased aggression, according to results from the PSAP, after viewing the violent movie. Like many of the other studies reviewed in this chapter, the sample size was very small. Thus, results should be viewed as tentative. Yet, the data showed that simplified mechanisms linking lower in vitro MAO A genotypes to greater dopamine release and subsequent aggression in humans may be less relevant to understanding the influence of the MAO A VNTR polymorphism on aggression. Moreover, this study supports findings of a previous PET investigation that used [^{18}F]fluorodopa to investigate the relationship between dopamine synthesis capacity and aggression, in which lower aggression was associated with greater dopamine storage capacity in striatum and midbrain (Schlüter et al. 2013). One of the main advantages of the study by Schlüter et al. (2016) is that they investigated aspects of both reactive and proactive forms of aggression.

A final [^{11}C]SB207145 PET investigation tested the relationship between 5-HT$_4$ receptor binding and results from the BPAQ (da Cunha-Bang et al. 2016). An inverse relationship between 5-HT$_4$ receptor binding and extracellular levels of 5-HT had been previously demonstrated. The authors assembled 18 brain regions to calculate a global volume-weighted 5-HT$_4$ receptor BP_{ND} as a biomarker of central 5-HT tone. They also performed post-hoc voxel-based analyses. Sixty-one individuals participated in the experiment (47 males and 14 females); analyses were subsequently adjusted for age, sex, SERT polymorphism, and type of PET scanner (subjects were scanned between 2006 and 2013 on two different scanners). A positive correlation was discerned between BPAQ total score and global 5-HT$_4$ receptor as well as BPAQ physical aggression and global 5-HT$_4$ receptor but only in males. No main effect was seen in the mixed-sex sample. Sex interaction effects were present in the association of 5-HT$_4$ receptor binding and BPAQ physical aggression. Whole brain voxel-based analysis, conducted in males who were younger than 50 years, identified two clusters in which

BPAQ total score showed a significant positive correlation with 5-HT$_4$ receptor binding: left ACC and left middle cingulate gyrus and right anterior insula and inferior frontal gyrus. The authors concluded that low cerebral levels of 5-HT were correlated with high trait aggression in males but not in females. However, the sample may have been underpowered to observe an effect in females, or there may have been too little variance to detect an association.

Conclusion

A common theme throughout this chapter is the lack of SPECT and PET studies that have examined large samples of ASPD participants or have conducted subgroup analyses of ASPD groups. However, the following are exceptions: da Cunha-Bang et al. 2017b; Gerra et al. 1998; Goethals et al. 2005; Goyer et al. 1994; Kolla et al. 2015, 2021; Kuruoğlu et al. 1996; Meyer et al. 2008; and Soloff et al. 2014. Most of the reviewed investigations evaluated criminals, psychiatric inmates, and individuals with BPD and IED-R, which included some individuals with ASPD. Therefore, it is unclear how relevant these studies are to understanding the neurochemistry of ASPD. Hypoperfusion of frontotemporal regions, alterations in cortical and subcortical 5-HT receptor or transporter function, and reduced MAO A V$_T$ in the OFC and ventral striatum are the principal PET and SPECT findings of ASPD. However, results are not uniform, and some studies with similar paradigms yielded conflicting results.

Yet, it is encouraging to note that the use of PET ligands to investigate ASPD has largely paralleled the evolution of radiopharmaceutical development. Still, many more molecular targets could be pursued with existing positron-emitting radiopharmaceuticals, and the hope is that these probes will be used to further investigate ASPD. Importantly, some studies clearly differentiated state versus trait aggression in their subjects by scanning them when they were aggressive or nonaggressive. This distinction is important because neurotransmitter systems likely to be active during aggression may not be responsive when aggression is absent and vice versa.

The trend in psychiatric research is to investigate basic dimensions of functioning ranging from genomics to neural circuitry, as exemplified by the Research Domain Criteria of the National Institute of Mental Health (2021). We have seen this focus in some of the reviewed studies that measured impulsivity, aggression, and psychopathic traits in relation to a molecular target. Ultimately, mapping the symptoms, especially aggression, that characterize ASPD in nonclinical populations may prove to be just as beneficial as studying categorical diagnoses.

In summary, relatively few SPECT or PET studies of ASPD have been done. Investigating ASPD and its symptom clusters is highly relevant given the burden that this diagnosis poses to society. To date, no pharmacological interventions are specifically targeted for ASPD. Examining alternative neuroreceptor systems could be particularly beneficial in this regard to help yield novel pharmacological treatments.

Key Points

- Most PET studies of personality disorder populations include very few individuals with antisocial personality disorder (ASPD); as such, it is difficult to generalize findings of these investigations to ASPD.

- Radiopharmaceuticals that target the serotonergic system have been used in ASPD. These studies have advanced the field by investigating different subtypes of aggression. However, results are inconsistent.

- To the best of our knowledge, two PET studies have exclusively targeted ASPD participants with novel radioligands. One study found reduced monoamine oxidase A distribution volume in the orbitofrontal cortex and ventral striatum of ASPD, and the other reported reduced fatty acid amide hydrolase binding in the amygdala of ASPD.

- PET studies that have examined the dopaminergic systems have uncovered links between dopaminergic neurotransmission and aggression, independent of ASPD.

References

Alia-Klein N, Wang GJ, Preston-Campbell RN, et al: Reactions to media violence: it's in the brain of the beholder. PLoS One 9(9):e107260, 2014 25208327

American Psychiatric Association: Diagnostic and Statistical Manual of Mental Disorders, 5th Edition. Arlington, VA, American Psychiatric Association, 2013

Anckarsäter H, Piechnik S, Tullberg M, et al: Persistent regional frontotemporal hypoactivity in violent offenders at follow-up. Psychiatry Res 156(1):87–90, 2007 17689934

Anderson CA, Huesmann LR: Human aggression: a social-cognitive view, in The Sage Handbook of Social Psychology. Edited by Hogg MA, Cooper J. Thousand Oaks, CA, Sage, 2003, pp 296–323

Barkataki I, Kumari V, Das M, et al: Volumetric structural brain abnormalities in men with schizophrenia or antisocial personality disorder. Behav Brain Res 169(2):239–247, 2006 16466814

Baumann MH, Mash DC, Staley JK: The serotonin agonist m-chlorophenylpiperazine (mCPP) binds to serotonin transporter sites in human brain. Neuroreport 6(16):2150–2152, 1995 8595191

Blackburn R, Coid JW: Psychopathy and the dimensions of personality disorder in violent offenders. Pers Individ Dif 25(1):129–145, 1998

Blair RJ: The roles of orbital frontal cortex in the modulation of antisocial behavior. Brain Cogn 55(1):198–208, 2004 15134853

Brunner HG, Nelen M, Breakefield XO, et al: Abnormal behavior associated with a point mutation in the structural gene for monoamine oxidase A. Science 262(5133):578–580, 1993 8211186

Buss AH, Perry M: The aggression questionnaire. J Pers Soc Psychol 63(3):452–459, 1992 1403624

Cases O, Seif I, Grimsby J, et al: Aggressive behavior and altered amounts of brain serotonin and norepinephrine in mice lacking MAOA. Science 268(5218):1763–1766, 1995 7792602

Cherek DR, Moeller FG, Dougherty DM, et al: Studies of violent and nonviolent male parolees, II: laboratory and psychometric measurements of impulsivity. Biol Psychiatry 41(5):523–529, 1997 9046984

Cloninger CR: A systematic method for clinical description and classification of personality variants: a proposal. Arch Gen Psychiatry 44(6):573–588, 1987 3579504

Coccaro EF, Kavoussi R, Berman M, Lish J: Intermittent explosive disorder-revised: development, reliability, and validity of research criteria. Compr Psychiatry 39:368–376, 1998 9829145

Coid J, Ullrich S: Antisocial personality disorder is on a continuum with psychopathy. Compr Psychiatry 51(4):426–433, 2010 20579518

da Cunha-Bang S, Mc Mahon B, Fisher PM, et al: High trait aggression in men is associated with low 5-HT levels, as indexed by 5-HT4 receptor binding. Soc Cogn Affect Neurosci 11(4):548–555, 2016 26772668

da Cunha-Bang S, Hjordt LV, Dam VH, et al: Anterior cingulate serotonin 1B receptor binding is associated with emotional response inhibition. J Psychiatr Res 92:199–204, 2017a 28502766

da Cunha-Bang S, Hjordt LV, Perfalk E, et al: Serotonin 1B receptor binding is associated with trait anger and level of psychopathy in violent offenders. Biol Psychiatry 82(4):267–274, 2017b 27108021

Dolan MC, Deakin JFW, Roberts N, et al: Quantitative frontal and temporal structural MRI studies in personality-disordered offenders and control subjects. Psychiatry Res 116(3):133–149, 2002 12477598

Eysenck HJ, Eysenck SBG: Adult Impulsiveness, Venturesomeness, and Empathy Scale. London, Hodder & Stoughton, 1991

Fazel S, Danesh J: Serious mental disorder in 23000 prisoners: a systematic review of 62 surveys. Lancet 359(9306):545–550, 2002 11867106

Frankle WG, Lombardo I, New AS, et al: Brain serotonin transporter distribution in subjects with impulsive aggressivity: a positron emission study with [11C]McN 5652. Am J Psychiatry 162(5):915–923, 2005 15863793

Gerra G, Calbiani B, Zaimovic A, et al: Regional cerebral blood flow and comorbid diagnosis in abstinent opioid addicts. Psychiatry Res 83(2):117–126, 1998 9818737

Glenn AL, Yang Y: The potential role of the striatum in antisocial behavior and psychopathy. Biol Psychiatry 72(10):817–822, 2012 22672927

Godar SC, Bortolato M, Frau R, et al: Maladaptive defensive behaviours in monoamine oxidase A-deficient mice. Int J Neuropsychopharmacol 14(9):1195–1207, 2011 21156093

Goethals I, Audenaert K, Jacobs F, et al: Brain perfusion SPECT in impulsivity-related personality disorders. Behav Brain Res 157(1):187–192, 2005 15617785

Goyer PF, Andreason PJ, Semple WE, et al: Positron-emission tomography and personality disorders. Neuropsychopharmacology 10(1):21–28, 1994 8179791

Gründer G, Siessmeier T, Piel M, et al: Quantification of D2-like dopamine receptors in the human brain with 18F-desmethoxyfallypride. J Nucl Med 44(1):109–116, 2003 12515884

Gustavsson JP, Bergman H, Edman G, et al: Swedish universities Scales of Personality (SSP): construction, internal consistency and normative data. Acta Psychiatr Scand 102(3):217–225, 2000 11008858

Hall H, Sedvall G, Magnusson O, et al: Distribution of D1- and D2-dopamine receptors, and dopamine and its metabolites in the human brain. Neuropsychopharmacology 11(4):245–256, 1994 7531978

Hare RD: Manual for the Revised Psychopathy Checklist, 2nd Edition. Toronto, ON, Canada, Multi-Health Systems, 2003

Ito H, Kawashima R, Awata S, et al: Hypoperfusion in the limbic system and prefrontal cortex in depression: SPECT with anatomic standardization technique. J Nucl Med 37(3):410–414, 1996 8772633

Jacobsen M, Jensen A, Storvestre GB, et al: Experiences with 99mTc-HMPAO in a diagnostic pathway for violent patients with schizophrenic spectrum disorders. Curr Radiopharm 10(2):115–122, 2017 28637403

Kolla NJ, Gregory S, Attard S, et al: Disentangling possible effects of childhood physical abuse on gray matter changes in violent offenders with psychopathy. Psychiatry Res 221(2):123–126, 2014 24361393

Kolla NJ, Matthews B, Wilson AA, et al: Lower monoamine oxidase-A total distribution volume in impulsive and violent male offenders with antisocial personality disorder and high psychopathic traits: an [(11)C] harmine positron emission tomography study. Neuropsychopharmacology 40(11):2596–2603, 2015 26081301

Kolla NJ, Chiuccariello L, Wilson AA, et al: Elevated monoamine oxidase-A distribution volume in borderline personality disorder is associated with severity across mood symptoms, suicidality, and cognition. Biol Psychiatry 79(2):117–126, 2016a 25698585

Kolla NJ, Dunlop K, Downar J, et al: Association of ventral striatum monoamine oxidase-A binding and functional connectivity in antisocial personality disorder with high impulsivity: a positron emission tomography and functional magnetic resonance imaging study. Eur Neuropsychopharmacol 26(4):777–786, 2016b 26908392

Kolla NJ, Boileau I, Karas K, et al: Lower amygdala fatty acid amide hydrolase in violent offenders with antisocial personality disorder: an [^{11}C]CURB positron emission tomography study. Transl Psychiatry 11(1):57, 2021 33462180

Kuruoğlu AC, Arikan Z, Vural G, et al: Single photon emission computerised tomography in chronic alcoholism: antisocial personality disorder may be associated with decreased frontal perfusion. Br J Psychiatry 169(3):348–354, 1996 8879722

Lenzenweger MF, Lane MC, Loranger AW, et al: DSM-IV personality disorders in the National Comorbidity Survey Replication. Biol Psychiatry 62(6):553–564, 2007 17217923

Lillenfield SO, Widows MR: Psychopathic Personality Inventory-Revised. Lutz, FL, Psychological Assessment Resources, 2005

Marcus DK, Lilienfeld SO, Edens JF, et al: Is antisocial personality disorder continuous or categorical? A taxometric analysis. Psychol Med 36(11):1571–1581, 2006 16836795

Mayberg HS, Lewis PJ, Regenold W, et al: Paralimbic hypoperfusion in unipolar depression. J Nucl Med 35(6):929–934, 1994 8195877

Meyer JH, Wilson AA, Rusjan P, et al: Serotonin2A receptor binding potential in people with aggressive and violent behaviour. J Psychiatry Neurosci 33(6):499–508, 2008 18982172

National Collaborating Centre for Mental Health: Antisocial Personality Disorder: The NICE Guideline on Treatment, Management and Prevention. National Clinical Practice Guideline, No 77. London, British Psychological Society and Royal College of Psychiatrists, 2010

National Institute of Mental Health: Research Domain Criteria (RDoC). Available at: www.nimh.nih.gov/research-priorities/rdoc/index.shtml. Accessed April 19, 2021.

Nautiyal KM, Tanaka KF, Barr MM, et al: Distinct circuits underlie the effects of 5-HT1B receptors on aggression and impulsivity. Neuron 86(3):813–826, 2015 25892302

Neirinckx RD, Canning LR, Piper IM, et al: Technetium-99m d,l-HM-PAO: a new radiopharmaceutical for SPECT imaging of regional cerebral blood perfusion. J Nucl Med 28(2):191–202, 1987 3492596

New AS, Hazlett EA, Buchsbaum MS, et al: Blunted prefrontal cortical 18fluorodeoxyglucose positron emission tomography response to meta-chlorophenylpiperazine in impulsive aggression. Arch Gen Psychiatry 59(7):621–629, 2002 12090815

New AS, Buchsbaum MS, Hazlett EA, et al: Fluoxetine increases relative metabolic rate in prefrontal cortex in impulsive aggression. Psychopharmacology (Berl) 176(3–4):451–458, 2004 15160265

New AS, Hazlett EA, Newmark RE, et al: Laboratory induced aggression: a positron emission tomography study of aggressive individuals with borderline personality disorder. Biol Psychiatry 66(12):1107–1114, 2009 19748078

Park SH, Park HS, Kim SE: Regional cerebral glucose metabolism in novelty seeking and antisocial personality: a positron emission tomography study. Exp Neurobiol 25(4):185–190, 2016 27574485

Parsey RV, Kegeles LS, Hwang DR, et al: In vivo quantification of brain serotonin transporters in humans using [11C]McN 5652. J Nucl Med 41(9):1465–1477, 2000 10994724

Pemment J: The neurobiology of antisocial personality disorder: the quest for rehabilitation and treatment. Aggress Violent Behav 18(1):79–82, 2013

Perez-Rodriguez MM, Hazlett EA, Rich EL, et al: Striatal activity in borderline personality dis-
    order with comorbid intermittent explosive disorder: sex differences. J Psychiatr Res
    46(6):797–804, 2012 22464337

Phelps ME: Positron emission tomography provides molecular imaging of biological processes.
    Proc Natl Acad Sci USA 97(16):9226–9233, 2000 10922074

Plavén-Sigray P, Gustavsson P, Farde L, et al: Dopamine D1 receptor availability is related to
    social behavior: a positron emission tomography study. Neuroimage 102(pt 2):590–595,
    2014 25134976

Plavén-Sigray P, Matheson GJ, Gustavsson P, et al: Is dopamine D1 receptor availability related
    to social behavior? A positron emission tomography replication study. PLoS One
    13(3):e0193770, 2018 29543812

Pukrop R, Steinbring I, Gentil I, et al: Clinical validity of the "Dimensional Assessment of Per-
    sonality Pathology (DAPP)" for psychiatric patients with and without a personality disor-
    der diagnosis. J Pers Disord 23(6):572–586, 2009 20001176

Raine A, Lencz T, Bihrle S, et al: Reduced prefrontal gray matter volume and reduced auto-
    nomic activity in antisocial personality disorder. Arch Gen Psychiatry 57(2):119–127, dis-
    cussion 128–129, 2000 10665614

Raine A, Dodge K, Loeber R, et al: The reactive-proactive aggression questionnaire: differential
    correlates of reactive and proactive aggression in adolescent boys. Aggress Behav
    32(2):159–171, 2006 20798781

Robins LN, Regier DA: Psychiatric Disorders in America. New York, Free Press, 1991

Rosell DR, Siever LJ: The neurobiology of aggression and violence. CNS Spectr 20(3):254–279,
    2015 25936249

Rosell DR, Thompson JL, Slifstein M, et al: Increased serotonin 2A receptor availability in the
    orbitofrontal cortex of physically aggressive personality disordered patients. Biol Psychi-
    atry 67(12):1154–1162, 2010 20434136

Rothman RB, Baumann MH: Therapeutic and adverse actions of serotonin transporter sub-
    strates. Pharmacol Ther 95(1):73–88, 2002 12163129

Rylands AJ, Hinz R, Jones M, et al: Pre- and postsynaptic serotonergic differences in males with
    extreme levels of impulsive aggression without callous unemotional traits: a positron
    emission tomography study using (11)C-DASB and (11)C-MDL100907. Biol Psychiatry
    72(12):1004–1011, 2012 22835812

Samuels J, Bienvenu OJ, Cullen B, et al: Personality dimensions and criminal arrest. Compr
    Psychiatry 45(4):275–280, 2004 15224270

Schlüter T, Winz O, Henkel K, et al: The impact of dopamine on aggression: an [18F]-FDOPA
    PET study in healthy males. J Neurosci 33(43):16889–16896, 2013 24155295

Schlüter T, Winz O, Henkel K, et al: MAOA-VNTR polymorphism modulates context-
    dependent dopamine release and aggressive behavior in males. Neuroimage 125:378–385,
    2016 26481676

Seam P, Juweid ME, Cheson BD: The role of FDG-PET scans in patients with lymphoma. Blood
    110(10):3507–3516, 2007 17709603

Seidenwurm D, Pounds TR, Globus A, et al: Abnormal temporal lobe metabolism in violent
    subjects: correlation of imaging and neuropsychiatric findings. AJNR Am J Neuroradiol
    18(4):625–631, 1997 9127022

Siep N, Tonnaer F, van de Ven V, et al: Anger provocation increases limbic and decreases me-
    dial prefrontal cortex connectivity with the left amygdala in reactive aggressive violent of-
    fenders. Brain Imaging Behav 13(5):1311–1323, 2019 30145716

Soderstrom H, Hultin L, Tullberg M, et al: Reduced frontotemporal perfusion in psychopathic
    personality. Psychiatry Res 114(2):81–94, 2002 12036508

Soloff PH, Meltzer CC, Becker C, et al: Gender differences in a fenfluramine-activated FDG PET
    study of borderline personality disorder. Psychiatry Res 138(3):183–195, 2005 15854787

Soloff PH, Chiappetta L, Mason NS, et al: Effects of serotonin-2A receptor binding and gender
    on personality traits and suicidal behavior in borderline personality disorder. Psychiatry
    Res 222(3):140–148, 2014 24751216

van de Giessen E, Rosell DR, Thompson JL, et al: Serotonin transporter availability in impulsive aggressive personality disordered patients: a PET study with [11C]DASB. J Psychiatr Res 58:147–154, 2014 25145808

Volkow ND, Tancredi LR, Grant C, et al: Brain glucose metabolism in violent psychiatric patients: a preliminary study. Psychiatry Res 61(4):243–253, 1995 8748468

Webster C, Douglas KS, Eaves D, et al: HCR-20: Assessing Risk for Violence, Version 2. Vancouver, BC, Canada, Mental Health, Law, and Policy Institute, 1997

Youdim MB, Edmondson D, Tipton KF: The therapeutic potential of monoamine oxidase inhibitors. Nat Rev Neurosci 7(4):295–309, 2006 16552415

Zanettini C, Panlilio LV, Alicki M, et al: Effects of endocannabinoid system modulation on cognitive and emotional behavior. Front Behav Neurosci 5:57, 2011 21949506

CHAPTER 16

New Insights Into the Causes of and Potential for Prevention of Psychopathy—A Syndrome Distinct From Antisocial Personality Disorder

Sheilagh Hodgins, Ph.D., FRSC

Psychopathy is a profound disorder of personality that negatively affects the life of the afflicted and those around them. Individuals with psychopathy wreak havoc on society by committing serious violence, some of which leads to criminal prosecution, and much that does not. Adults presenting with the syndrome show multiple stable characteristics including grandiosity, pathological lying, manipulation, callousness, a lack of empathy and guilt, shallow affect, failure to take responsibility for their own actions, stimulation seeking, a parasitic orientation, a lack of goals, impulsivity, irresponsibility, and poor anger control. The adult syndrome denoting an array of symptoms indicative of severe personality pathology is rare. By contrast, the traits of psychopathy vary dimensionally in the population and are associated with negative outcomes even at low levels. To prevent the development of the syndrome of psychopathy (hereafter, syndrome of psychopathy will be referred to as psychopathy for brevity), and of psychopathic traits, it is critical to acknowledge that psychopathy differs in presentation, etiology, and treatment response from other forms of antisocial personality disturbance.

There is a population of individuals, more males than females, who display early-onset antisocial and aggressive behavior that remains stable across the life span (ESAAB). These individuals score high on behavior ratings of conduct problems and meet criteria for conduct disorder (CD) and oppositional defiant disorder in childhood and for antisocial personality disorder (ASPD) in adulthood. Much evidence from prospective, longitudinal studies conducted in countries with different cultures and health, social, and criminal justice systems has confirmed the existence of this population, the early onset, and the stability (Moffitt 2018). For example, one prospective investigation of a New Zealand birth cohort showed that ESAAB individuals were distinguished at age 3 years by neurological soft signs and slower motor development; in childhood by lower IQ and reading scores; and among the boys by lower heart rate, uncontrolled temperament, and poor memory. The boys also were found to be impulsive, hostile, alienated, suspicious, cynical, and callous and cold toward others (Moffitt 2018). From age 7 to 15 years, ESAAB females and males differed from same-sex healthy peers as to three individual factors—low IQ, poor reading achievement, and ADHD symptoms—and seven parent characteristics—low socioeconomic status, maltreatment, inconsistent parenting, family conflict, poor maternal mental health, low maternal IQ, and parents' criminality (Moffitt and Caspi 2001). At age 32, the men and women characterized by ESAAB were engaging in serious violence and experiencing significant mental health, physical health, and economic problems. A greater proportion of the men (33%) than the women (3%) had been convicted of violent crimes, but 42% of the women and 10% of the men reported hitting a child. Although 11.1% of the women reported engaging in violence toward others, informants reported that 47.1% of them had, in fact, engaged in violence. Among the men, 30.6% self-reported engaging in violence, and informants reported that 26.7% had engaged in violence (Odgers et al. 2008). As shown in Figure 16–1, the ESAAB population includes individuals who will develop psychopathy and those who will have ASPD accompanied by various levels of psychopathic traits.

I begin this chapter with descriptions of the subgroups within the population of ESAAB, the prevalence of these disorders, and criminality. I then focus on adults presenting with psychopathy. I review evidence of abnormalities of brain structure and function and of cognition, highlighting the differences from healthy adults and from those with ASPD. Next, neural abnormalities associated with psychopathic traits in community samples are reviewed, as are those identified in clinical samples with low levels of psychopathic traits. Subsequently, I discuss the limits of studies of adults and the reasons for focusing the remaining sections of the chapter on children who have conduct problems and callous-unemotional traits, the predictive power of conduct problems plus callous-unemotional traits, the age at onset and stability, neural correlates, intergenerational transfer, and parenting. Before closing, the emerging evidence on the key role of anxiety in psychopathy is discussed. Finally, I briefly address clinical and scientific implications of the reviewed literature.

Subgroups Within the Population of Early-Onset Stable Antisocial and Aggressive Behavior

Psychopathy

Using Cleckley's vivid and detailed descriptions (Cleckley 1976), Robert Hare constructed a scale to identify criminal offenders presenting with psychopathy. The scale

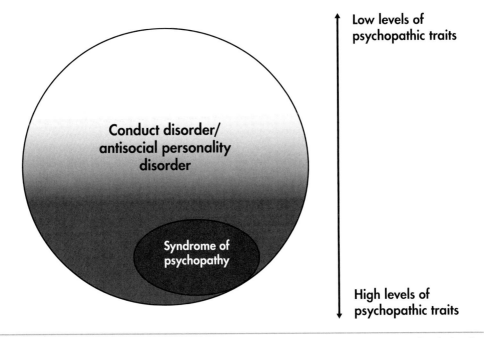

FIGURE 16–1. Population of persons with early-onset antisocial and aggressive behavior that remains stable across the life span.

was subsequently revised and became the Psychopathy Checklist–Revised (PCL-R; Hare 2003; Hare and Neumann 2006). Psychopathy comprises four facets of personality and behavior:

1. Interpersonal—impression management, grandiose sense of self-worth, pathological lying, and manipulation
2. Affective—callousness, lack of empathy and guilt, shallow affect, and failure to take responsibility for one's own actions
3. Lifestyle—stimulation seeking, parasitic orientation, lacking goals, impulsivity, and irresponsibility
4. Antisocial behavior—poor anger control, early behavior problems, and juvenile delinquency

The PCL-R is administered by clinicians trained to use the instrument and involves coding information from institutional files, conducting the PCL interview, and then rating 20 items. Studies of offenders in Canada and the United States indicated that scores of 30 or higher identified psychopathy (Hare 2003; Hare and Neumann 2006). These individuals obtain high scores on all four facets of the PCL-R. Interestingly, in Europe the cutoff score to identify the syndrome was set at 25 (Hare 2003). Most research on psychopathy has used this definition, although other measures are available (Patrick and Drislane 2015). Evidence has accumulated showing that these traits, or facets of psychopathy, vary dimensionally in the general population (Guay et al. 2007) and that they can be measured by clinical assessment or self-report (Sellbom et al. 2018).

Syndrome of Psychopathy

Eddie was raised with his older brother and sister by his biological parents. His mother had worked at the post office for years and also cared for the children and the family home. His father worked in the warehouse of a plumbing company. Eddie was an easy child and did not care about much of anything. His mother noticed that even as a toddler, he showed little sympathy when, for example, she squeezed her fingers in the kitchen drawer or his sister fell from the top bunk and hurt herself. He seemed somewhat perplexed by their crying. In the years before attending school, Eddie liked to be outside with the neighborhood children, organizing games. He was somewhat of a leader among the preschoolers. Few noticed that he took new baseballs, hockey pucks, and other small items from the other children. Even if other children noticed, they were frightened to mention it as Eddie's revenge would be to exclude them from all future games. He was less fearful than the other children, often succeeding at physical feats that they wouldn't even attempt. When a tricycle race down a big hill ended in an accident, he didn't try to help his injured friend or get help from an adult. Again, he was bewildered by all the screaming and crying.

Once Eddie started school, he found it boring. The work was not difficult. The other kids were stupid and seemed to waste so much energy being afraid and upset. He wondered why he had to put up with them. When teachers would organize the children into workgroups, they noticed that he quickly finished his work—never perfect but simply acceptable—and never helped the children who were having difficulty even when encouraged to do so. He quickly realized how easy it was to intimidate some of the other children and to take their lunch money. When one boy finally stood up to him, he simply gave him back his money. Later that afternoon, on the way home, he severely beat the boy. No one at that school ever stood up to him again. He used the lunch money that he collected to buy himself a mobile phone. He told his parents that he had earned some money doing odd jobs for an elderly neighbor. By late childhood, he realized that pictures taken of the girls when they were changing clothes for gym class could be sent online to all the boys at school and that the girls would pay him to take them down. When a group of teachers confronted him about his bullying, he denied it all, blaming other kids who were jealous of him for spreading lies. When the teachers called his parents to a meeting and told them what was suspected, the parents talked to Eddie who again successfully lied about his activities. He was so charming, a nice boy, even if a bit frightening.

High school was more fun than primary school because there were more students and more opportunities. Again, he found his peers rather dumb and failed to understand their enthusiasm for sports and for girls. He was so much smarter. Eddie had seen a guy who regularly showed up outside the schoolyard to sell cannabis and Ecstasy pills. He finally approached this guy to ask if he could help and said that he had better contacts with more potential buyers. A deal was made about prices, and it became known around the high school that Eddie sold drugs. He kept his end of the deal and always paid up-front for the drugs. One day, his drug supplier asked if he would be interested in working at another school. Eddie was ambitious and agreed. By chance, a teacher saw him give a package of weed to a student. When the teacher confronted him, again he made up a story about the package and convinced the teacher that he was not selling drugs. He started a rumor that the teacher was having sex with one of his pupils.

Eddie's schoolwork was mediocre, and he often handed in assignments late or not at all. He didn't care much, and his parents were unable to motivate him to do better. The guy who sold Eddie drugs asked him if he wanted to meet some men who were planning to extend their drug sales downtown. At the meeting, Eddie agreed to recruit girls his age to work in strip clubs and massage parlors. As his drug sales increased, the police closed in, and he was sent to a juvenile detention facility. Here, he quickly became a leader, using force when necessary to keep other boys in line, and set up visits by boys who would bring in drugs and mobile phones, which he sold.

Once back outside, Eddie no longer went to school but joined the gang downtown who sold drugs and girls. Life was good—lots of money, girls, and parties. He had developed strategies to recruit young girls who recently arrived in the city to find work. Seduction, intimidation, money, and drugs were his primary tools. He found girls at the bus station or nearby rooming houses and even liked some of them. But he established no relationships as he made money, selling the girls to clubs once they were drug dependent. However, one girl died. A police investigation began when a rival gang identified him as having recruited the girl. He was arrested and convicted of manslaughter for injecting her with too much heroin.

Within the prison, his charm and verbal skills set him apart from the other inmates and guaranteed him jobs in the library or hospital office. Relatively quickly, he understood the hierarchy of inmates and found his way into the top-ranking clan. In the first few years, when ordered by the clan bosses to steal or assault, he followed orders. He quickly rose in the ranks and consolidated his place by sometimes severely beating a rival but more often by setting a trap so that an enemy was thought to have committed an infraction of the prison rules and sent to segregation. Just as he had lied to his parents, teachers, and police investigators, Eddie convincingly lied to psychiatrists and psychologists who assessed him. Most of his past antisocial and aggressive behavior, and his juvenile conviction, were therefore unknown. With only one conviction, and a good record of employment within the prison, he was considered to be at low risk for future offending. After a few years, Eddie was released from detention. As required by his parole conditions, he got a job, but it was in a strip club previously known to him and owned by his former associates. Life was good—girls, money, and parties.

Antisocial Personality Disorder

Psychopathy differs from ASPD by definition, but some criteria overlap. Almost all, if not all, individuals who present with psychopathy will meet the criteria for ASPD, but only a minority of those presenting with ASPD will meet the criteria for psychopathy, and others will have lower levels of psychopathic traits (Hare 1996; Warren and South 2006). Importantly, the two behavioral facets of psychopathy—lifestyle and antisocial behavior—assess the same behavior patterns indexing ASPD as defined by DSM-5 (American Psychiatric Association 2013). Furthermore, the key personality trait of deficient affective experience reflecting lack of empathy overlaps with one of the pathological traits of ASPD.

Antisocial Personality Disorder With Low Levels of Psychopathic Traits

Frank was the third of four children raised in a blended family by his biological parents in a poor neighborhood of a medium-sized city. His mother cared for the children and the house but often took part-time jobs outside the home in retail outlets to supplement the family income. His father worked on-and-off, usually driving small delivery trucks. He drank a lot and sometimes disappeared for a few days. When drunk at home, he would become excessively angry and hit his wife and on occasion some of the children. Money was limited, but the family had enough food, a warm house, and a large television. In the years before he went to school, Frank's parents were often frustrated by his persistent disobedience. His older brother was in trouble for fighting at school, and social services had threatened to send him to a juvenile facility. Frank's parents did not want to have to deal with similar problems with him. When he misbehaved, his parents sometimes scolded or hit him, other times yelled, or failed to notice what he had done. Frank often grabbed things and broke them. Sometimes this led to a slap, other times his parents simply yelled, and when he could hide what he had done, he got no reaction from his parents. When he grabbed and broke the joystick of his older brother's video game, he was promptly beaten. At age 3 years, his mother stopped taking him to the grocery store, because he was constantly grabbing items off the shelf. As he got older, the minute his mother arrived home from the grocery store, Frank would grab the cookies and run and hide. Frank often got into fights with the neighborhood children, usually as a result of them calling him names or refusing to play with him when he had broken or stolen their toys. A few times, the parents of neighborhood children knocked on the door of the family home to complain to his parents about his behavior. Following these visits, he would sometimes get slapped or whacked on his bottom, other times be sent to the room he shared with his brother, or receive no consequences, but he would hear his parents muttering that "boys will be boys."

Shortly after starting school, Frank's failure to follow rules and difficulty with schoolwork became apparent. The teacher's attempts to talk with his parents were rebuffed. Frank's frustration at not being able to complete his schoolwork, as the other children did, grew. He often flew into a rage and attempted to punch his peers who made fun of his difficulties. In the schoolyard, he was not popular. He would not follow the rules of various games and consequently was often not allowed to join in. When other children accidentally banged into him, or made a remark about him, he punched them. Fighting led to detentions, extra homework, and calls to his parents. The family home was somewhat chaotic, with little structure to support Frank's need to complete schoolwork. His parents provided little encouragement to succeed as they saw no good coming from educational success. Frank often hit his sister when she would not wait on him as he ordered and regularly stole money from his mother's purse. By late childhood, Frank had fallen behind his peers in school and no longer tried to complete school assignments.

As Frank transitioned to a high school with hundreds of pupils, he quickly found other boys who shared his negative attitude toward school. Together, they flaunted the rules, began stealing, and sometimes bought beer or other forms of alcohol. His quick temper that typically led to him beating someone up became well known throughout the school. Frank soon realized that he liked to drink. It made him feel good and powerful. Some days, he and his friends skipped school and went downtown, always managing to jump the turnstiles in the subway. Buoyed by their success at stealing food and alcohol from convenience stores, they tried but were unsuccessful in stealing mobile phones. They met older boys who paid them to deliver small bags of marijuana, and with these funds Frank was able to buy a mobile phone. This allowed the older boys to contact Frank and his friends to deliver drugs and also to steal from local stores and businesses. He attended school less and less frequently and was drinking and experimenting with all kinds of drugs. On the weekends, alcohol- and drug-fueled parties occupied his time. The police had picked him up several times for shoplifting. He was arrested for a robbery of batteries and other small items from a convenience store. The store was situated on one corner of a park diagonally opposite another convenience store. When Frank robbed the store, there was a police car out front. An investigator asked Frank, "Why did you rob the store with a police car in front?" "I dunno," he replied.

Frank was eventually convicted in juvenile court and sent to a correctional facility. Inside the juvenile facility, his education in how to steal and buy and use drugs began in earnest. Although he had no access to alcohol, drugs were easy to get on the inside. To pay for the drugs, he used the money his parents gave him for "treats" when they visited. Sometimes he was paid by other juveniles to steal cigarettes and phones, and this money also was used to buy drugs. When he left the institution, he had a wide circle of friends who were just like him. He supported himself by stealing and selling drugs. Often, when flush, he would take small amounts of money to his mother. He lived with his friends, and several times he found a girl who would let him stay with her. These arrangements never lasted long as he would end up beating her up when she repeatedly demanded that he get a job and help pay for the household expenses. He typically got on well in his job of selling drugs, but occasionally he annoyed his bosses when he would fly off the handle in response to a negative remark and occasionally hurt a client or member of a rival drug empire. His first sentence to adult prison resulted from driving the getaway car for a bank robbery. And life went on for several decades following a similar pattern.

Conduct Disorder or Conduct Problems and Callous-Unemotional Traits

Evidence has accumulated to suggest that in childhood a similar distinction may be evident, with a subgroup of children with conduct problems presenting elevated levels of the antecedents of psychopathic traits. Initially, research aimed at extending the concept of psychopathy to children showed that callous-unemotional, narcissistic, and impulsive dimensions could be observed among boys and girls. Among children with conduct problems, callous-unemotional traits identified those with the most serious conduct problems (Christian et al. 1997). Children with conduct problems plus callous-unemotional traits do obtain high scores for the interpersonal and impulsive dimensions of psychopathy (Christian et al. 1997), but research has focused on callous-unemotional traits defined as lack of empathy and guilt, failure to put forth effort on important tasks, and shallow and deficient emotions. To identify this subgroup of children, DSM-5 (American Psychiatric Association 2013) includes a specifier to the CD diagnosis—"with limited prosocial emotions"—that is applied when children with CD show two or more of the following characteristics persistently over 12 months in more than one relationship or setting: lack of remorse or guilt; callous—lack of empathy; unconcerned about performance at school, at work, or in other important activities; and shallow or deficient affect. A study of a randomly selected population sample in the United Kingdom estimated that close to half of both the girls and the boys with CD presented elevated levels of callous-unemotional traits (Rowe et al. 2010). These children were five times more likely than others with CD to show serious conduct problems 3 years later. Another study reported that children with CD who met criteria for the specifier with limited prosocial emotions presented more aggressive and cruel behavior than did other children with CD (Kahn et al. 2012). As is discussed in subsequent sections of this chapter, children presenting elevated levels of callous-unemotional traits plus conduct problems display several of the behavior patterns, impairments in emotion processing, and neural abnormalities that are characteristic of adults with psychopathy, albeit to a lesser degree.

Summary

As illustrated in Figure 16–1, within the population of people who present ESAAB, all would meet criteria for CD or oppositional defiant disorder before age 15 years and ASPD in adulthood. Within this population is a subgroup with psychopathy that is distinguished most clearly from CD or ASPD by higher scores for the two personality facets of psychopathy: interpersonal and deficient affective experience and predatory or proactive aggressive behaviors. Importantly, those with CD or ASPD obtain higher psychopathy scores than healthy individuals (Frick et al. 2014b; Hemphälä et al. 2015).

Prevalence

Psychopathy is estimated to affect approximately 1% of males and few females (Hare 2003). Among offenders in Canada sentenced to 2 years or more of incarceration, approximately 20% met criteria for psychopathy (Hare 2003). Most estimates of lifetime prevalence of ASPD vary among men from 4.5% to 6.5% and among women from 0.8% to 2.5% (Compton et al. 2005; Robins et al. 1991; Samuels et al. 2002; J. Samuels, personal communication, June 4, 2007; Swanson et al. 1994). Not all children who have elevated levels of conduct problems or CD will develop ASPD. Findings from large community samples in the United States and Great Britain have reported prevalence rates of CD as high as 12.0% in boys and 7.1% in girls (Green et al. 2005; Maughan et al. 2004; Nock et al. 2006). The prevalence of the subgroup with conduct problems plus callous-unemotional traits is difficult to establish because the definition of "high" callous-unemotional traits varies across studies, as do the items used to rate callous-unemotional traits and the rater—parent, teacher, or participant. In a large sample of twins representative of U.K. children, teacher reports of callous-unemotional traits at ages 7, 9, and 12 years were used to compute trajectories. The stable high trajectory included 3.4% of the children, 81% of whom were male (Fontaine et al. 2010). In a U.K. population sample, mother reports indicated that among the 3,367 boys, 8.5% presented conduct problems, 6.9% had callous-unemotional traits, and 5.5% had callous-unemotional traits plus conduct problems and that among the 3,306 girls, 7.3% presented with conduct problems, 7.5% had callous-unemotional traits, and 5.7% had callous-unemotional traits plus conduct problems (Barker et al. 2011).

Criminality and Aggressive Behavior

Most research on psychopathy has been conducted with incarcerated offenders. Among male offenders, those with ASPD and psychopathy begin offending earlier, acquire more convictions for both nonviolent and violent crimes, and show more versatility than do those with only ASPD (Frick and White 2008; Wong 1985). Furthermore, psychopathy is associated with premeditated, instrumental, or proactive aggression aimed at obtaining something or at maintaining dominance (Cornell et al. 1996). By contrast, only one-half of adults with CD or ASPD are convicted of crimes (Robins et al. 1991; J. Samuels, personal communication, June 1, 2007), even though large proportions of incarcerated offenders present with ASPD (Fazel and Danesh 2002). The degree to which CD or ASPD is associated with violent offending is unclear, with estimates in community samples ranging from 50% to 85% (Coid et al. 2006; Robins et al. 1991).

Attempting to Identify Neural Abnormalities

Studies using MRI to identify neural correlates of psychopathy compare groups, such as offenders with psychopathy and offenders without the syndrome or healthy adults. However, the participants in each group present many other characteristics that are reflected in brain structure and function. Consequently, the challenge is to determine which characteristic is associated with which neural abnormality (Schiffer et al. 2011). The first major confound is substance misuse. Most adults with psychopathy and ASPD have a history of substance misuse going back to at least mid-adolescence (Compton et al. 2005). Depending on the type of substance, dose, duration of use, age at use, and structural and functional abnormalities differ (Bagga et al. 2014; Harris et al. 2008; Luciana et al. 2013; Niciu and Mason 2014). Yet eliciting such information from adult participants with psychopathy or ASPD is almost impossible because they have used so many substances, for so long, that they cannot provide an accurate history. A second major confound not taken into account in past studies is childhood maltreatment, which also leads to structural and functional neural abnormalities (Teicher and Samson 2016). A third major confound is comorbid mental disorders, such as anxiety, that are common and that are discussed later in the chapter. Other confounds such as poverty (Holz et al. 2015) and toxic prenatal factors (e.g., maternal substance misuse; Haghighi et al. 2013) are no doubt also involved. The effects of all these factors on the brain are conditioned by genes that have not yet been taken into account.

Structural Abnormalities

Men with psychopathy exhibit reduced gray matter volume in prefrontal and orbital-frontal cortices and in limbic/paralimbic regions including the amygdala, insula, and anterior cingulate cortex (Anderson and Kiehl 2012). Some of the challenges in identifying such abnormalities are illustrated by a study we conducted. We compared two groups of violent offenders with ASPD who were on probation: one group had psychopathy and one group did not, and a group of nonoffenders recruited at unemployment offices in a deprived neighborhood. Over a period of 4 days at the university, participants completed interviews, questionnaires, neuropsychological tests, and an MRI brain scan. They were paid minimum hourly wage for their time. PCL-R scores were determined based on criminal justice files, the PCL-R interview, and all other available information. Diagnostic interviews confirmed that no participant had a major mental disorder. Despite the request to refrain from substance use, urine and saliva samples on the day of the scan indicated that some participants had recently used. These participants were interviewed to ensure that they were not intoxicated and would be safe within the scanner. The two groups of offenders had similar IQ and levels of education that were lower than those of the nonoffenders. Lifetime diagnoses of abuse and dependence were similar for the two offender groups and significantly more common than among the nonoffenders. The group with ASPD and psychopathy was significantly younger at first conviction for a violent offense than the offenders with ASPD only, and there was a trend suggesting that they had accumulated more convictions for violent crimes. The three groups differed on measures of total aggression, reactive aggression, and proactive aggression, with offenders who had ASPD and psychopathy obtaining significantly higher scores for proactive aggression than the offenders with ASPD only.

In all comparisons, age and IQ were entered as covariates. Violent offenders who had ASPD and psychopathy, as compared with the nonoffenders, showed reduced gray matter volume in the bilateral anterior rostral medial prefrontal cortex, bilateral anterior temporal areas, and bilateral anterior insula. Violent offenders who had ASPD and psychopathy, as compared with the ASPD-only violent offenders, showed significantly reduced gray matter volume bilaterally in the anterior rostral medial prefrontal and temporal pole regions. Results changed somewhat when we took account of confounders. Unlike most studies, we had objectively assessed recent substance use on the day of the scan. Excluding participants who tested positive did not alter the highly significant differences between the violent offenders with ASPD and psychopathy and those with ASPD only in the bilateral anterior temporal cortex but weakened differences in the bilateral anterior rostral medial prefrontal cortex (Gregory et al. 2012).

In subsequent studies with the same sample (Kolla et al. 2013, 2014), we found that the offenders with ASPD and psychopathy reported significantly more childhood physical abuse than did the ASPD-only offenders and the nonoffenders. When taking account of childhood physical abuse, offenders with ASPD and psychopathy, relative to ASPD-only offenders, displayed less volume only in the right temporal pole and right uncus. Our finding was consistent with previous evidence from children and adolescents who had experienced maltreatment (De Brito et al. 2013). Thus, our study detected differences in gray matter volume between violent offenders with ASPD who differed only with regard to psychopathy and were similar in terms of age, IQ, histories of substance use disorders, and absence of major mental disorders in brain areas central to the development of self-conscious emotions, such as guilt or embarrassment, which promote prosocial behaviors and form the basis of moral learning. In addition, reductions in the volume of the insula may underlie difficulties in experiencing emotions, emotion processing, decision-making, and empathy. We ruled out some possible confounds by matching groups (e.g., IQ, education, lifetime substance use disorders, no major mental disorders) and showed that others such as recent drug use prior to the scan and childhood maltreatment affected group comparisons. Yet, even though most current studies of structural correlates of psychopathy covary for history of substance misuse, they do not use objective measures of substance misuse at the scan or consider childhood maltreatment or other traumas.

In a recent study of 716 adult male inmates that controlled for age, IQ, and substance dependence, PCL-R scores were negatively associated with measures of gyrification within the right hemisphere in the mid-cingulate cortex and adjacent regions of the superior frontal gyrus and the lateral superior parietal cortex. The total of the interpersonal and affective facet scores were associated with decreased gyrification within the right mid-cingulate cortex and adjacent dorsomedial frontal cortex and greater gyrification in the bilateral occipital cortex. By contrast, scores for the lifestyle and antisocial facets were not associated with gyrification (Miskovich et al. 2018). The authors noted that these gyrification findings were consistent with previous evidence of dysfunction in paralimbic regions and abnormalities in regions supporting attention and control processes. As noted, gyrification abnormalities may reflect structural connectivity and cortical organization that takes place in utero or during adolescence when gyrification decreases.

Consistent with the gyrification findings, alterations to white matter structures have been identified in individuals with psychopathy. But, as in studies of gray matter volume, there are problems disentangling psychopathy and confounds from white matter structure abnormalities. A study of a large sample of incarcerated offenders showed that psychopathy was associated with reduced fractional anisotropy[1] in the right uncinate fasciculus, the primary tract connecting the ventral frontal and anterior temporal cortices, when controlling for age, race, and substance use disorders. This finding was almost entirely a result of the association with the PCL-R interpersonal facet (Wolf et al. 2015). The authors noted that the uncinate fasciculus connects two brain regions, the amygdala and ventromedial prefrontal cortex, believed to be involved in moral judgment, empathy, aggression, value representation, and stimulus reinforcement learning.

Neural Dysfunction

Offenders with psychopathy, as compared with those without, show less activity in the anterior insula, amygdala, and prefrontal cortex in response to emotional words, negative odors, pain, and negative mood induction. In response to emotions in faces, the reduced activity has been detected principally in the fusiform gyrus, frontal gyrus, and orbitofrontal cortex, with increased activity in the insula to negative faces (Seara-Cardoso and Viding 2015). Low autonomic and neural reactivity to fearful or unpleasant stimuli was thought to underlie the reported deficit in fear conditioning and passive avoidance learning (Newman and Kosson 1986). However, this evidence belies the multiple examples of learning through fear conditioning, and of passive avoidance learning, that are shown by individuals with psychopathy as they go about their daily lives. In childhood, for example, they use passive avoidance learning to not put their hands on hot stoves to avoid being burned and to avoid walking in front of cars that could injure or kill them. In summary, although individuals with psychopathy display reduced biological indexes of fear, they also continually show instances when they appropriately use fear to learn to protect themselves.

Neural activity in response to pictures of injured people depends on instructions given to offenders with psychopathy. When instructed to imagine themselves in the pictures, they showed increased activity in the anterior insula, dorsal anterior cingulate, and inferior frontal gyrus as compared with nonpsychopathic offenders. However, when instructed to imagine another person in the pictures, they showed reduced response and connectivity in the anterior insula and orbitofrontal cortex as well as in the amygdala. In tasks of moral reasoning and decision-making, psychopathic persons show less activity in brain regions associated with emotions and more activity in regions associated with cognitive processing (for a systematic review, see Seara-Cardoso and Viding 2015).

Amygdala activity may depend on attention. One study reported that offenders with psychopathy showed decreased amygdala activity in response to threat only when attention was already engaged in another task. During this experimental condition, the psychopathic offenders also showed greater activation in selective attention regions of the lateral prefrontal cortex than did nonpsychopathic offenders. When

---

[1] The integrity of white matter structures was measured with diffusion-weighted MRI. Fractional anisotropy is a scalar value between zero and one that describes the degree of anisotropy of a diffusion process. Fractional anisotropy is thought to reflect fiber density, axonal diameter, and myelination in white matter.

explicitly attending to threat, amygdala activation did not differ in those with and without psychopathy (Larson et al. 2013). Thus, the poor decision-making consistently shown by individuals with psychopathy may reflect this difficulty in taking account of the possibility of future punishment when engaged in goal-directed behavior. Consistent with these findings, in our study of violent offenders that was described earlier, we found that the offenders who had ASPD and psychopathy, as compared with those who had ASPD only, showed atypical punishment prediction error signaling indicating altered organization of the information processing system responsible for reinforcement learning and appropriate decision-making (Gregory et al. 2015).

Thus, male offenders with psychopathy use information about emotions when it is consistent with their focus on a rewarding goal but fail to take account of such information, typically about the likelihood of punishment, when it is not essential for attaining their immediate goal. In real life, for example, when an individual who has psychopathy is focused on maintaining dominance within a group, he or she may fail to notice an impending attack by a rival gang. In one study, male prisoners performed a gaze detection task involving affective faces. As predicted, high PCL-R scores, but not high scores for externalizing behaviors, were associated with better performance on the gaze detection task when the necessity of using contextual affect to regulate goal-directed behavior was minimized. Conversely, high externalizing, not psychopathy, was associated with increased errors on trials that required prisoners to use affective face expressions, specifically fear, as a cue to inhibit dominant responses (Baskin-Sommers and Newman 2014). Another study also indicated that higher-order cognitive processes moderated the fear deficits of offenders with high PCL-R scores. In this study, the high scorers showed the expected deficit in fear-potentiated startle response consistent with them being labeled as fearless but displayed fear-potentiated startle response typical of individuals without psychopathy when instructed to focus on threat. Similar findings were obtained when using only scores for the interpersonal and affective PCL-R facets to categorize offenders (Newman et al. 2010). The authors suggested that the diminished reactivity to fear stimuli, and emotion-related cues more generally, shown by the offenders with psychopathy reflect idiosyncrasies in attention that limit their processing of peripheral information. Another study compared brain activity of psychopathic offenders and healthy individuals while viewing videos of emotional hand interactions and while experiencing similar interactions. Brain regions involved in experiencing these interactions were not spontaneously activated as strongly among the offenders as in the comparison group participants while viewing the videos. The group difference was markedly reduced when the offenders were instructed to feel like the actors in the videos (Meffert et al. 2013).

This evidence is the basis of the Impaired Integration Theory (Hamilton et al. 2015; Newman and Baskin-Sommers 2016). The theory proposes that individuals with psychopathy are impaired in processing stimuli that are presented simultaneously and show enhanced performance when information is presented in series. The affective and disinhibitory symptoms of psychopathy may be a consequence of difficulty in rapidly integrating components of multidimensional sensory stimuli. In other words, inefficient processing may limit psychopathic individuals' use of affective and inhibitory cues (Hamilton and Newman 2018).

> This attention style may also explain how psychopathic individuals can use information that is directly relevant to their goal to effectively regulate behavior (for example, modulate behavior to con someone), but display impulsive behavior (for example, quitting one's job in the absence of an alternative one) and egregious decision making (for example, seeking publicity for a con while wanted by police) when information escapes their awareness (Baskin-Sommers and Newman 2014, p. 375)

While presenting with this atypical attentional style, persons with psychopathy do not have impairments in executive functions (Rodman et al. 2016) as do those with externalizing-only problems and those with ASPD only, who show multiple deficits in executive functions, including selective attention, interference suppression, and response inhibition associated with reduced activity in the dorsolateral prefrontal cortex during response inhibition. These latter findings among externalizing-only offenders are consistent with results of structural imaging studies showing reductions in dorsolateral prefrontal cortex gray matter volume and cortical thickness. However, studies have shown that the dysfunction in the prefrontal cortex associated with impulsive antisocial behaviors actually reflects a dysfunction in the striatum (Buckholtz 2015; Buckholtz and Faigman 2014; Rodman et al. 2016).

One study of incarcerated offenders reported that those with high psychopathy scores showed increased activity in the striatum in response to reward (Pujara et al. 2014), consistent with increased striatum gray matter volume (Buckholtz et al. 2010) and increased activity in response to reward in the nucleus accumbens (Schiffer et al. 2011). In a subsequent study, striatal subjective value signaling during decision-making was found to be dysregulated among inmates with psychopathy resulting from weakened corticostriatal connectivity that led to heightened striatal value encoding during decision-making. This pattern of dysfunction was positively associated with the number of criminal convictions (Hosking et al. 2017).

In summary, adult men with psychopathy show abnormalities of gray matter volume and white matter structures in frontal, limbic, and paralimbic regions, as do the few females with psychopathy who have been studied (Edwards et al. 2019). They also show reduced activity in limbic structures in response to stimuli that typically elicit an emotional response that is altered by cognitive processes—specifically, a failure to take account of information that is peripheral to their primary focus.

Neural Correlates of Psychopathic Traits Self-Reported by General Population Samples

Psychopathic traits not severe enough to denote the syndrome of psychopathy have been associated with multiple negative outcomes, including antisocial behavior, aggressive behavior, nonviolent and violent crime (Leistico et al. 2008), substance use disorders (Asscher et al. 2011; Hemphälä and Hodgins 2014; Leistico et al. 2008), and nonoptimal parenting (Beaver et al. 2014). By mid-adolescence, scores for psychopathic traits that are not high enough to denote psychopathy predict multiple adverse psychosocial and mental health outcomes and criminal offending over and above conduct problems (Hemphälä and Hodgins 2014; Leistico et al. 2008). Evidence now shows that the primary neural abnormalities characterizing adults with psychopathy also characterize adults with psychopathic traits (Seara-Cardoso and Viding 2015). Individuals self-reporting high levels of psychopathic traits show many characteristics similar to those who have psychopathy, including reduced startle potentiation, reduced autonomic responses to aversive images, reduced affective responses to others' emotions, atypical moral processing, and poor decision-making during gambling tasks (Seara-Cardoso and Viding 2015). For example, in a sample of young adult men from low-income families in the United States, self-reported antisocial behaviors accompanied by high levels of callous-unemotional traits were associated with widespread abnormalities of white matter structures, including the uncinate fasciculus, cingulum, inferior fronto-occipital fasciculus, superior longitudinal fasciculus, inferior longitudinal fasciculus, and anterior thalamic radiation (Dotterer et al. 2019). In a large community sample of adolescents, amygdala reactivity to fearful faces was negatively associated with self-reports of the interpersonal trait of psychopathy and positively associated with lifestyle trait (Carré et al. 2013). A systematic review of functional MRI studies with general population samples concluded that psychopathic traits are negatively associated with activity in brain regions associated with affect processing during tasks that involve affective stimuli, including emotion recognition and social interactions, and positively associated with activity in the ventral striatum typically engaged during reward processing (Seara-Cardoso and Viding 2015).

Studies of neural correlates of self-reported psychopathic traits in community samples have not fully characterized the participants. Consequently, little is known about the antisocial and aggressive behaviors of those reporting high levels of traits. Are they part of the population with ESAAB? Do they have CD or ASPD? Furthermore, studies vary in defining "high" levels of traits. Many questions remain to be answered.

Neural Correlates of Low Levels of Psychopathic Traits

We studied a sample of 99 females and 81 males who had consulted a clinic for substance misuse in adolescence. We assessed them at an average age of 16.8 years using the Psychopathy Checklist: Youth Version (PCL:YV; Forth et al. 2003) and 5 years later using the PCL-R. Consistent with much evidence (Verona and Vitale 2018), the female scores were lower than the male scores. PCL scores were slightly higher than those reported in community samples and lower than those identified among offenders. Among both females and males, moderate to high rank-order stability was observed for total PCL and facet scores. The principal predictor of PCL-R scores in early adulthood were mid-adolescent PCL:YV scores, even when taking into account family and individual characteristics (Hemphälä et al. 2015). In another study of this same sample, we showed that PCL-YV scores measured in mid-adolescence predicted mental disorders, psychosocial functioning, substance misuse, ASPD symptoms, aggressive behaviors, and criminality during the subsequent 5 years (Hemphälä and Hodgins 2014).

We studied the association of Psychopathy Checklist: Screening Version (PCL:SV; Hart et al. 1995) scores with white matter structures in 44 of these women, 31 of their sisters, and 24 healthy women (Lindner et al. 2017). Diffusion tensor imaging, tractography, and tract-based spatial statistics indicated that right uncinate fasciculus microstructure was negatively associated with the interpersonal facet. Whole-brain analyses found that both affective and lifestyle facets were negatively correlated with white matter structures adjacent to the fusiform gyrus, and the interpersonal facet correlated negatively with the integrity of the fornix. Findings survived adjustment for the other facet scores and age, verbal IQ, and performance IQ (Lindner et al. 2017). A similar negative association between the interpersonal facet and uncinate fasciculus integrity was previously observed in male offenders (Wolf et al. 2015). Thus, in a sample of women, few of whom met criteria for ASPD, who obtained low total PCL:SV scores (mean=3.32; SD=3.87; range=0–18) and low scores on the interpersonal trait of psychopathy (mean=0.57; SD=0.86; range=0–4), the associated abnormality of white matter structures in the tract connecting the amygdala and orbital frontal cortex was similar to that observed in male offenders with psychopathy. In another study of the same sample, we found that neural circuits also varied with low levels of psychopathic traits (Lindner et al. 2018). These initial findings associating low levels of psychopathic traits with abnormalities of white matter structures and neural circuits are preliminary but dramatic.

In summary, studies have reported that self-reported psychopathic traits in community samples and low levels of clinically assessed psychopathic traits in young adults with histories of externalizing problems are associated with neural abnormalities similar to those associated with psychopathy. Further research is needed to determine what "dose" of each trait is associated with what level of neural abnormality, antisocial and aggressive behaviors, and other negative outcomes.

Limits of Studying Adults

Studies of adults, such as those reviewed earlier, do not provide objective evidence about causal factors or how psychopathy develops. Two sets of findings indicate the necessity of refocusing research on psychopathy and ASPD away from studies of adults to prospective, longitudinal investigations of genetically informed cohorts recruited in utero.

The first set of findings indicating the necessity for reorienting studies of psychopathy away from adults to investigations of development relate to the abundant evidence that has accumulated to suggest that conduct problems plus callous-unemotional traits are the antecedents of psychopathy and that callous-unemotional traits are observed among toddlers. Although prospective, longitudinal studies are needed to confirm this proposition, current findings indicate similarity between aggressive behaviors, neurocognition, emotion processing, and brain structure and functioning in children and adolescents with conduct problems plus callous-unemotional traits and psychopathy in adults (Viding and Kimonis 2018).

The second set of findings indicating the need to reorient research on psychopathy confirms high heritability for psychopathy (Forsman et al. 2008; Larsson et al. 2006) and conduct problems plus callous-unemotional traits (Tuvblad et al. 2017; Viding et al. 2008) and medium heritability for CD or ASPD (Krueger et al. 2002; Waldman et al. 2018) and associations with specific genetic variants and with epigenetic changes to specific genes. Single nucleotide polymorphisms of the oxytocin receptor gene are associated with callous-unemotional traits (Dadds et al. 2014b; Ezpeleta et al. 2019) and with reduced gray matter volume in the hypothalamus, reduced amygdala activation, increased coupling of the amygdala and hypothalamus when processing social information (Tost et al. 2010), and low levels of peripheral oxytocin (Dadds et al. 2014b; Levy et al. 2015). Callous-unemotional traits also have been associated with functional polymorphisms of the serotonin 2A and 1B receptor genes and with lower serum levels of serotonin (Moul et al. 2018). Furthermore, callous-unemotional traits have been associated with a variant of a dopamine gene that confers vulnerability to nonoptimal parenting (Moul et al. 2018). Candidate genes associated with callous-unemotional traits differ from those found to be associated with CD or ASPD (e.g., see Byrd and Manuck 2014; Nilsson et al. 2018).

The genetic variants associated with callous-unemotional traits likely modify the risk of callous-unemotional traits in the presence of negative environmental factors and decrease the risk in the presence of positive environmental factors. For example, callous-unemotional traits have been associated with one variant of the serotonin transporter gene among individuals who were raised in families with low socioeconomic status (Sadeh et al. 2010). In order to understand the role played by individual genetic variants, it is necessary to take account of not only negative and positive environmental factors but also epistasis, the interactions of genetic variants with one another (e.g., see Nilsson et al. 2014). Furthermore, current evidence suggests that genotypes that increase sensitivity to environmental factors also may increase the likelihood of epigenetic changes (Checknita et al. 2021).

Callous-unemotional traits also have been associated with epigenetic changes. In a clinical sample of boys, those who were diagnosed with conduct problems plus callous-unemotional traits showed altered methylation of a serotonin receptor gene (*HTR1B*) (Moul et al. 2015) and of an oxytocin receptor gene that was correlated with lower circulating oxytocin levels (Dadds et al. 2014a). Furthermore, high oxytocin receptor gene methylation and callous-unemotional traits among youths with CD were associated with frontoparietal hyperactivity and amygdala-frontoparietal disconnection when recognizing or resonating angry and fearful faces (Aghajani et al. 2018). Epigenetic changes may result from stress experienced by parents before the pregnancy, maternal stress and behaviors such as smoking during pregnancy, and adverse events after birth (Barker et al. 2018). Notably, stress is associated with epigenetic alterations in several candidate genes (Booij et al. 2015) and in genomewide studies (Szyf et al. 2016). Childhood maltreatment has been associated with epigenetic alterations in the promoters of several genes in hippocampal neurons (Labonté et al. 2013). Some experts in the field have suggested that in addition to gene-by-environment interactions, epistasis, and epigenetics, rare variants contribute to the high heritability of conduct problems plus callous-unemotional traits (Viding and Kimonis 2018).

Taken together, these two sets of findings indicate that in order to elucidate the etiology of psychopathy, investigations are needed that study the early emergence of callous-unemotional traits, high heritability that can be modified by environmental factors, genetic variants conferring sensitivity to environmental factors, epistasis, and epigenetic changes to gene activity by pre- and postnatal adversity. Furthermore, future studies need to begin in utero. Although such studies are not yet available, consistent evidence about conduct problems plus callous-unemotional traits and callous-unemotional traits is accumulating. These findings are the focus of subsequent sections of the chapter.

Predictive Power of Conduct Problems Plus Callous-Unemotional Traits

As noted earlier, among adults with ESAAB, those with psychopathy commit more violent offenses than the others. Similarly, among children with conduct problems, those with callous-unemotional traits show more serious conduct problems and more frequent and more serious aggressive behavior than those with conduct problems only (Frick et al. 2014b). Furthermore, they engage in proactive aggression. Among children who have CD, those with callous-unemotional traits show the earliest onset and persistence of delinquency (Frick et al. 2014a). We studied a sample of 1,593 males and 1,423 females from age 6 to 24 years when we obtained their official criminal records (Hodgins et al. 2013). At ages 6 and 10 years, their classroom teachers rated their behaviors, allowing us to classify them into four groups: 1) neither conduct problems nor callous-unemotional traits; 2) conduct problems but no callous-unemotional traits; 3) callous-unemotional traits but no conduct problems; and 4) conduct problems plus callous-unemotional traits. Table 16–1 presents ORs for convictions for violent and nonviolent crimes from ages 12 to 24 years comparing each risk group with those who had neither conduct problems nor callous-unemotional traits. Among both males and females, those who had presented with conduct problems plus callous-unemotional traits at age 6 years were more likely than those with neither conduct problems nor callous-unemotional traits at this age to be convicted of a criminal offense by age 24, as were those who presented this combination at age 10 years. Among boys who had presented with conduct problems plus callous-unemotional traits at age 6 years, as compared with those who had neither conduct problems nor callous-unemotional traits, the risk of conviction for violent crimes was three times higher and the risk of conviction for nonviolent crimes was five times higher. Among girls, conduct problems plus callous-unemotional traits at age 6 years were associated with a sixfold increase in the risk of a conviction for a nonviolent crime. Age 10 risk groups showed similar elevations in risk for criminal convictions. Thus, consistent with other prospective, longitudinal investigations conducted in countries with different health, social, and justice systems (Fergusson et al. 2009; Odgers et al. 2008; Sourander et al. 2007), children with conduct problems showed an increased risk for criminal convictions in adolescence and adulthood. Extending this evidence, our findings showed that children with conduct problems plus callous-unemotional traits had even higher risks for criminality than did children who had conduct problems without callous-unemotional traits. In a U.S. study, conduct problems plus callous-unemotional traits in seventh-grade children were highly predictive of juvenile and adult arrests and ASPD (McMahon et al. 2010). These findings contribute to the accumulating evidence that childhood conduct problems plus callous-unemotional traits have lifelong negative consequences.

As can be seen in Table 16–1, among females, conduct problems without callous-unemotional traits were not associated with future criminality. Our findings on fe-

TABLE 16–1.   ORs for criminal convictions at age 24 of males and females who had conduct problems (CP) without callous-unemotional (CU) traits, CU traits without CP, and both CP and CU traits at ages 6 and 10 years as compared with children without CP or CU traits

	No. of participants	Criminal convictions up to age 24	
		Violent crimes, OR (95% CI)	Nonviolent crimes, OR (95% CI)
Males (N=1,593)			
Age 6			
No CP; no CU	1,354		
CP; no CU	86	2.49* (1.23–5.03)	1.48 (0.86–2.53)
CU; no CP	71	0.83 (0.26–2.75)	1.89 (1.09–3.30)
CP+CU	82	2.93* (1.48–5.79)	4.58* (2.89–7.26)
Age 10			
No CP; no CU	1,071		
CP; no CU	89	4.32* (2.31–8.08)	2.91* (1.80–4.70)
CU; no CP	50	2.37 (0.90–6.24)	2.46* (1.30–4.68)
CP+CU	64	2.62* (1.13–6.04)	3.32* (1.93–5.72)
Females (N=1,423)			
Age 6			
No CP; no CU	1,241		
CP; no CU	64		2.17 (0.75–6.28)
CU; no CP	55		1.88 (0.56–6.29)
CP+CU	82		6.38* (3.01–13.54)
Age 10			
No CP; no CU	1,028		
CP; no CU	54		1.37 (0.32–5.92)
CU; no CP	57		4.17* (1.75–9.93)
CP+CU	64		4.37* (1.73–11.05)

*Significant.

males are consistent with the results from the New Zealand cohort described earlier, showing that females who had conduct problems in childhood were rarely convicted for violence despite the fact that they assaulted others at high rates. Finally, the results presented in Table 16–1 show that among males, callous-unemotional traits without conduct problems at ages 6 and 10 were associated with elevations in risk for nonviolent convictions, as was the age 10 measure among females.

Age at Onset of Psychopathic Traits and Stability

Much evidence shows that aggressive behavior is most frequent in toddlerhood and declines by age 4 years, except among those children who will develop ESAAB

(Broidy et al. 2003). Their aggressive behavior emerges at an early age and remains stable. Results are accumulating to suggest that callous-unemotional traits, and perhaps the other traits of psychopathy, also emerge very early in life and remain relatively stable. Parents have used various instruments to identify children presenting high levels of callous-unemotional traits as early as ages 2 and 3 years. At even younger ages, precursors of callous-unemotional traits are observed (Dadds et al. 2012a; Fanti and Kimonis 2017; Hyde et al. 2013; Waller et al. 2012). For example, at age 6 months, infants' reactions to their mother's unresponsive face (typically a stressor), and duration of time the infant focused on the mother's face, were measured. Among infants with scores for mother-directed gaze at or below the mean of the sample, reduced reactivity to her unresponsive face predicted callous-unemotional traits at 24, 30, and 36 months (Wagner et al. 2016). (Older children and adolescents presenting callous-unemotional traits show deficient eye contact with caregivers during dyadic interactions; Frick et al. 2014b.) A study of 7-month-old infants reported that increased attention to faces (regardless of facial expression) was related to more frequent helping responses at 24 months and reduced callous-unemotional traits at age 48 months (Peltola et al. 2018). Another study showed that fearlessness at 24 months predicted callous-unemotional traits at age 13 years (Barker et al. 2011).

Callous-unemotional traits show moderate to strong stability across childhood (Frick et al. 2003; Obradović et al. 2007). In a regression model that included 27-month-old children, ADHD and oppositional behavior, gender, relationship between biological and adoptive parents, perinatal complications, and age 27-month callous-unemotional traits predicted teacher-rated externalizing problems at age 7 years (Waller et al. 2017). As previously noted (Viding and Kimonis 2018), however, correlations of scores for callous-unemotional traits across time mask individual change, even when relatively high. For example, in one study, intraclass correlations for psychopathic trait scores rated by parents were 0.93 and for self-reports were 0.79. Yet only 30% of the children who were rated high in the first assessment remained high in the 3 subsequent years (Frick et al. 2003). In another study of a large U.K. population sample of 9,462 twins, trajectory analyses of callous-unemotional traits rated by teachers at ages 7, 9, and 12 years identified a subgroup of 3.4%, mostly boys, who had high stable callous-unemotional traits. This subgroup showed the highest level of conduct problems prior to school entry and in early adolescence, and these children were raised in chaotic family environments in which parents used negative discipline (Fontaine et al. 2010). A study of a U.S. sample of children showed stability of callous-unemotional traits and conduct problems from ages 3 to 15 (Fanti and Kimonis 2017).

In our study described earlier (Hodgins et al. 2013), conduct problems plus callous-unemotional traits identified by classroom teachers in the spring of the first year of school predicted criminal convictions to age 24. In a follow-up of a small sample of these males, we found that 28% of the variance in total PCL-R scores at age 33 was explained by three parent characteristics—father's violent criminality, mother's criminality, and mother's age at participant's birth; three teacher-rated childhood behaviors—anxiety at age 6 years, hurtful behavior at age 10 years, and reactive aggression at age 12 years; and mathematics grades at age 12 years (Bamvita et al. 2017). One study of boys showed moderate stability in psychopathic traits from ages 7 to 17 (Lynam et al. 2009), whereas another showed stability from ages 13 to 24 (Lynam et al. 2008). In one study of a clinical sample of boys with disruptive behavior disorders, callous-unemotional traits at ages 7–12 years predicted PCL-R scores at ages 18–19 (Burke et al. 2007). In a clinical sample of Swedish adolescents with substance misuse, we found that PCL:YV scores were the strongest predictor of PCL-R scores 5 years later (Hemphälä et al. 2015). In a prospective, longitudinal study of males from the United Kingdom, PCL:SV scores at age 48 were associated with childhood neighborhood socioeconomic status, family structure, inconsistent discipline, participants' behavioral impulsivity, and age 13 psychopathy ratings (Piquero et al. 2012). Studies of young children provide evidence of change in levels of callous-unemotional traits, with few presenting high stable levels, but studies of older children and adolescents suggest that the trait levels consolidate before adulthood. For example, a study of boys that showed moderate stability of psychopathic traits from ages 7 to 17 examined multiple individual and family factors to determine whether they modified stability of the traits. Eight of 65 tests identified moderation of stability but only among boys with low, not high, psychopathy scores at age 13 (Lynam et al. 2009).

In summary, callous-unemotional traits are observed by age 2 or 3 years, and predictors of callous-unemotional traits are observed by age 6 or 7 months. Callous-unemotional traits show change during childhood but stability in a small group. By adolescence, levels of psychopathic traits appear to be relatively consolidated.

Neural Structures and Functioning

Several studies have indicated that autonomic system abnormalities (Fanti 2018) and brain structure and function are specifically associated with conduct problems plus callous-unemotional traits. In one of the first studies, 11-year-old boys with conduct problems plus callous-unemotional traits, as compared with typically developing boys, presented increased gray matter concentration in the medial orbitofrontal and anterior cingulate cortices, as well as increased gray matter volume and concentration in the temporal lobes, bilaterally, controlling for cognitive ability and hyperactivity-inattention symptoms (De Brito et al. 2009). Additionally, they showed decreased white matter concentration in some of these brain regions, including the right superior frontal lobe (subgyral), right dorsal anterior cingulate (limbic lobe), right superior temporal gyrus, and left precuneus, and increased white matter concentration, bilaterally, in the middle frontal gyrus. A preliminary exploratory analysis indicated that boys with conduct problems plus callous-unemotional traits showed decreasing white matter concentration with age, a pattern opposite to that detected among the typically developing boys (De Brito et al. 2011). A meta-analysis focusing on youths with conduct problems (Rogers and De Brito 2016) reported that higher levels of callous-unemotional traits were associated with less reduction of gray matter volume of the left putamen. A subsequent study showed that callous-unemotional traits mediated the association between externalizing behaviors and reduced gray matter volume of the amygdala (Cardinale et al. 2019). Another study of adolescent boys with conduct problems indicated that white matter structure abnormalities distinguished those with conduct problems plus callous-unemotional traits and those with callous-unemotional traits only (Puzzo et al. 2018).

A recent study of a population cohort of 2,146 children ages 8–11 years from the Netherlands reported that callous-unemotional traits were negatively associated with total cortical gray matter volume, right amygdala volume (but this association did not survive false discovery rate correction), cortical surface area bilaterally in the frontal and temporal lobes, and superior frontal gyrus gyrification. Results were robust to corrections for comorbid disorders and nonverbal IQ. No sex differences were found. By contrast, in females only, callous-unemotional traits were negatively associated with total white matter volume and global mean diffusivity, notably in the superior longitudinal fasciculus, corticospinal tract, uncinate, and cingulum (Bolhuis et al. 2019).

Emotion recognition, especially fear and sadness, is impaired among adolescents who have high levels of conduct problems plus callous-unemotional traits as in adults with psychopathy (Marsh and Blair 2008). Conduct problems plus callous-unemotional traits are also associated with reduced startle potentiation by aversive stimuli (Kimonis et al. 2017). Functional MRI studies have consistently shown that amygdala and insula activity when processing fearful faces is inversely associated with levels of callous-unemotional traits (Seara-Cardoso and Viding 2015; Viding et al. 2012). Furthermore, activity in the amygdala when processing fearful faces has been shown to mediate the association between callous-unemotional traits and instrumental aggression (Lozier et al. 2014). A review of functional MRI studies concluded that boys with conduct problems plus callous-unemotional traits showed reduced ventromedial prefrontal-hypothalamic-limbic activation and hyperactivation in cognitive control mediating dorsolateral prefrontal-dorsal and striatal regions (Alegria et al. 2016).

In summary, evidence is accumulating to suggest that abnormalities of brain structure and functioning similar to those observed among adults with psychopathy characterize youths with conduct problems plus callous-unemotional traits. Maturation rate may affect findings and be related to some identified sex differences. What causes these abnormalities?

Intergenerational Transfer of Psychopathic Traits

Parents contribute to their offspring's conduct problems plus callous-unemotional traits by transmitting genes, by creating chaotic family environments, and by engaging in harsh parenting. Nonoptimal parenting practices (e.g., harsh punishments, sanctions that do not immediately follow inappropriate behavior and that are not systematically applied, and few rewards for appropriate behavior; Jaffee et al. 2006) are associated with offspring conduct problems (Shaw and Gross 2008; Shaw and Shelleby 2014) and callous-unemotional traits (Frick et al. 2003; Pardini et al. 2007). Some studies suggest that parents' lack of warmth toward their child is associated with callous-unemotional traits (Pasalich et al. 2011), as are a chaotic family environment (Fontaine et al. 2011), low socioeconomic status of the family (Barker et al. 2011), and exposure to violence (Waller et al. 2018a).

Parents' characteristics are associated with their parenting style. For example, in a study of a U.K. population sample of approximately 7,000 infants, mothers' psychopathology at 8–32 weeks of gestation was positively associated with offspring's fearless temperament at age 2 years in boys, not girls, and with conduct problems and callous-unemotional traits at age 13 years (Barker et al. 2011). Parents who show antisocial behavior are more likely than other parents to have children with conduct problems to whom they provide a chaotic family environment and nonoptimal parenting (Jaffee et al. 2006) and to mate with antisocial partners (Krueger et al. 1998).

Several studies have examined the links between parent and child psychopathic traits. One study showed that parent callous-unemotional traits influenced adolescent callous-unemotional traits indirectly through hostile parenting practices for those dyads in chaotic homes (Kahn et al. 2016). In another study, fathers' interpersonal and affective facet scores predicted similarly high scores in their young adult offspring (Auty et al. 2015). Another study showed that the association between mothers' interpersonal and affective facet scores and offspring callous-unemotional traits depended on mothers' parenting style (Loney et al. 2007). In a study of a clinical sample of young children with conduct problems, fathers' interpersonal and affective facet scores predicted callous-unemotional traits in their children, even after taking into account parents' psychopathology, warmth, and harsh parenting. The association of a mother's lifestyle and affective facet scores and her offspring's callous-unemotional traits depended on her level of warmth (Mendoza Diaz et al. 2018).

One study of 561 children adopted in the days following birth has provided more evidence of the factors determining the association of parent and offspring psychopathic traits. Among the children, higher fearlessness and lower affiliative behavior at age 18 months were associated with callous-unemotional traits at age 27 months (punishment does not change behavior, does not feel guilty after misbehaving, shows too little fear, does not show affection, and is unresponsive to affection), after controlling for ADHD and oppositional behavior, gender, perinatal factors, and relationships of biological and adoptive parents. Children's callous-unemotional traits at age 27 months were also predicted by their biological mothers' fearlessness and affiliative behaviors. This association differed depending on the adoptive mother's positive parenting, such that child fearlessness predicted higher callous-unemotional traits at low and mean scores for adoptive mother positive parenting but not at high levels of positive parenting. The adoptive father's positive parenting did not influence child callous-unemotional traits (Waller et al. 2016). In another study with the same sample, child callous-unemotional traits at age 27 months were found to be related to the biological mother's antisocial behavior. Among the children whose biological mother had antisocial behavior, the adoptive mothers' positive parenting was associated with reduced levels of callous-unemotional traits (Hyde et al. 2016). Another study of this same sample reported that among children at higher inherited risk (biological mother's high fearlessness and low interpersonal affiliation), callous-unemotional traits at age 27 months were associated with the adoptive mother's harsh parenting at 54 months, and the adoptive father's harsh parenting at age 27 months was predictive of callous-unemotional behaviors at 54 months (Trentacosta et al. 2019).

A study of monozygotic twins showed the effect of parenting while holding heritable factors constant. The twin who received harsher parenting showed more aggressive behavior and higher callous-unemotional traits than the co-twin. The twin who received warmer parenting showed lower callous-unemotional traits. The relationship between parental harshness and child aggression was stronger among low-income families (Waller et al. 2018b). Older findings that focused on children with conduct problems without distinguishing those with and without callous-unemotional traits showed that maltreatment increases the risk for conduct problems among children at high, not

low, genetic risk (Jaffee et al. 2005) and that both mothers' and fathers' antisocial behavior increased the likelihood of maltreatment approximately threefold. Parents'
history of antisocial behavior accounted for nearly 50% of the effect of physical maltreatment on conduct problems at age 7 years (Jaffee et al. 2004). Importantly, the consequences of childhood maltreatment are determined, at least in part, by genotypes.

Thus, early emerging callous-unemotional traits are associated with similar traits
in parents, as well as their antisocial behaviors, and with the type of parenting provided to their offspring. Callous-unemotional traits and their precursor, fearless temperament, appear to promote harsh parenting.

Parenting

Much research has confirmed that nonoptimal parenting, principally inconsistent
and harsh discipline and a failure to consistently reward appropriate behavior, is a
key factor in promoting conduct problems. For example, in a large U.K. population
sample, among the boys, two pathways to conduct problems plus callous-unemotional
traits were identified: 1) prenatal stress predicted fearless temperament at age 2 years,
which was associated with elevated levels of harsh parenting at age 4 years that further resulted in increased conduct problems and callous-unemotional traits at age
13 years; and 2) fearless temperament at age 2 years was associated with an increase
in levels of harsh parenting at age 4 years, which resulted in increased conduct problems and callous-unemotional traits at age 13 years (Barker et al. 2011). Another study
found that the combination of mothers' low sensitivity to distress and low positive
regard elevated the risk for callous-unemotional traits among their preschool-age
offspring (Wright et al. 2018). In a sample of U.S. males recruited in low-income neighborhoods, maternal aggression, low empathic awareness, and difficult infant temperament predicted maternal warmth at age 2 years, which predicted limited prosocial
emotions at ages 10–12 years. Additionally, there were indirect effects of parental
warmth on limited prosocial emotions at age 20, via limited prosocial emotions at ages
10–12 years (Waller et al. 2015). In another study, less sensitive parenting at 24, 36, and
58 months predicted higher levels of conduct problems plus callous-unemotional
traits in first grade after controlling for earlier measures of conduct problems plus
callous-unemotional behaviors. The children's drawings showing family dysfunction
were associated with callous-unemotional traits, not conduct problems (Wagner et al.
2015). Another study showed that maternal prenatal substance use and socioeconomic adversity in infancy were prospectively associated with lower levels of maternal sensitivity, which was associated with decreases in children's conscience in early
childhood, and, in turn, lower conscience predicted increases in teacher-reported conduct problems in middle childhood (Ettekal et al. 2020). Many studies have shown a
link between various forms of childhood maltreatment (physical, sexual, emotional,
emotional and physical neglect) and psychopathy scores (Kimonis et al. 2013; Saukkonen et al. 2016).

Parenting appears to be key to reducing conduct problems plus callous-unemotional
traits, even among children at high genetic risk. Nonoptimal and harsh parenting are
associated with parents' antisocial behaviors and psychopathic traits and appear to
be promoted by child conduct problems plus callous-unemotional traits.

Comorbid Anxiety

As illustrated in Figure 16–2, the population of individuals with ESAAB is heterogeneous with respect not only to levels of psychopathic traits but also to anxiety in childhood (Dadds et al. 2018; Kimonis et al. 2016), adolescence (Fanti et al. 2013; Kimonis et al. 2012; Salihovic et al. 2014), and adulthood (Newman et al. 1992; Vassileva et al. 2005). Many studies have shown that approximately one-half of individuals with ASPD in community samples, and one-half of offenders with ASPD, present anxiety disorders (Hodgins et al. 2018). In 1941, Karpman identified a subgroup of individuals with psychopathy who also had high levels of anxiety. He labeled these individuals *secondary psychopaths* and proposed that they had experienced maltreatment (Karpman 1941). Some children with conduct problems plus callous-unemotional traits also have high levels of anxiety. For example, a study of a large sample of U.S. children at age 3 years identified one group without conduct problems or callous-unemotional traits or internalizing problems and three groups with conduct problems: 1) high callous-unemotional traits and high internalizing problems, 2) high callous-unemotional traits and no internalizing problems, and 3) low callous-unemotional traits and internalizing problems. Importantly, these groups and their defining characteristics remained stable up to age 15 years (Fanti and Kimonis 2017).

A recent study suggested that the attentional dysfunction described by the Impaired Integration Theory characterizes only children with conduct problems plus callous-unemotional traits who have not experienced maltreatment or who do not also have anxiety (Dadds et al. 2018), those designated as having the antecedents of primary psychopathy. Among children and adolescents, those with conduct problems plus callous-unemotional traits and anxiety have the antecedents of secondary psychopathy. This latter subtype is more prevalent than the first subtype and includes a greater proportion of females. Individuals with conduct problems plus callous-unemotional traits plus anxiety show heightened threat perception and greater autonomic and central nervous system reactivity that triggers reactive aggression (Dackis et al. 2015). This subtype with conduct problems plus callous-unemotional traits plus anxiety includes greater proportions of children who have experienced maltreatment compared with those with conduct problems plus callous-unemotional traits (Dackis et al. 2015; Fanti 2018; Kimonis et al. 2013), and changes in autonomic nervous system reactivity following maltreatment have been found to vary as a function of callous-unemotional traits (Dackis et al. 2015). Children with conduct problems plus callous-unemotional traits plus anxiety show lower than average intelligence, poor academic achievement, and weak self-regulation (Fanti and Kimonis 2017). Adolescents and adults with conduct problems plus callous-unemotional traits plus anxiety, unlike those with conduct problems plus callous-unemotional traits and no anxiety, do not have deficits in recognizing or responding to emotional expressions (Bagley et al. 2009; Kimonis et al. 2012), but they are more behaviorally and emotionally dysregulated (Kimonis et al. 2012). In childhood, those who have conduct problems plus callous-unemotional traits plus anxiety are fearful and hypersensitive to threat. Despite the presence of callous-unemotional traits, it is hypothesized that internalizing problems are associated with physiological hyperreactivity (Fanti 2018).

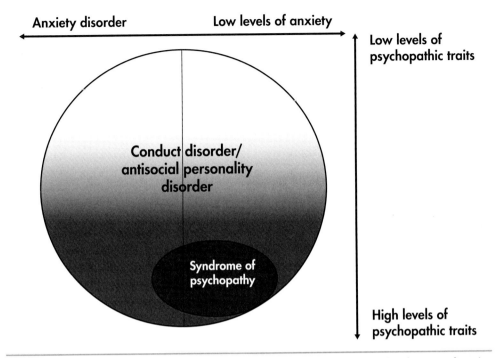

FIGURE 16–2.   Population of persons with early-onset antisocial behavior that remains stable across the life span.

In summary, as Karpman noted in 1941, some individuals with psychopathy experience anxiety probably as a result of childhood maltreatment. Despite this clinical observation, research on psychopathy, and on children with conduct problems plus callous-unemotional traits, has largely ignored the distinction between primary and secondary psychopathy. Emerging evidence indicates, however, that furthering understanding of psychopathy will require distinguishing the two subtypes. Although some of the biopsychosocial mechanisms may be common to those with conduct problems plus callous-unemotional traits with and without anxiety, the accumulated evidence suggests that emotion processing, attention, intelligence, and abnormalities of the autonomic nervous system and brain differ. Could it be that children with conduct problems plus callous-unemotional traits plus anxiety present as adults with ASPD and levels of psychopathic traits higher than in community samples but that are not high enough to denote the syndrome of psychopathy? If the mechanisms underlying conduct problems plus callous-unemotional traits differ depending on anxiety, such research is essential for informing early childhood intervention programs.

Clinical and Scientific Implications of the Extant Literature

The early emergence and stability of conduct problems plus callous-unemotional traits indicate that prevention, treatment, and research need to focus on early childhood. Furthermore, taking account of comorbid anxiety is critical to success. Given observations of callous-unemotional trait–like behaviors or callous-unemotional trait precursors in infants, the stability of callous-unemotional traits, and the multiple negative outcomes throughout life, interventions with parents are warranted. Teaching optimal parenting skills, emphasizing warmth, and discouraging maltreatment and harshness would benefit all children. Encouraging high-risk parents (i.e., those with antisocial behavior and/or psychopathic traits) to complete parent management training has the potential to reduce conduct problems plus callous-unemotional traits in their offspring. Consistent with the evidence on the role of warm, positive parenting in reducing callous-unemotional traits, even among genetically high-risk children (Hyde et al. 2016), parent management training programs that teach parent monitoring and how to establish positive, warm relationships with children have been shown to reduce both conduct problems and callous-unemotional traits (Kimonis et al. 2019; Kjøbli et al. 2018). Interventions to improve emotion recognition are also indicated (Dadds et al. 2012b). It is critical that such interventions are undertaken when children with conduct problems and callous-unemotional traits are young in order to prevent a cascade of negative outcomes, including rejection by parents, teachers, and peers; falling behind in school because of conduct problems; and bullying and assaulting other children. As is evident from the studies reviewed in this chapter, teachers and daycare educators are precious resources who can identify children with conduct problems plus callous-unemotional traits.

It is currently unknown at what age the dysfunction in attention and the correlated neural abnormalities that are observed in adults with psychopathy emerge. However, such a deficit would have to be modified in childhood in order to alter behavioral and neural development toward healthy outcomes. In adults with psychopathy, a cognitive program was shown to remedy this deficit (Baskin-Sommers et al. 2015). A similar intervention is needed for children.

Adolescents with conduct problems plus callous-unemotional traits who have begun to use alcohol and drugs and to engage in delinquency present a huge challenge. Programs such as Reasoning and Rehabilitation (Antonowicz and Parker 2014) use cognitive-behavioral strategies to curb antisocial behavior, attitudes, and ways of thinking. Adolescents may benefit from programs designed to increase their emotion recognition abilities and emotion sensitivity and to reduce the attentional dysfunction. Given the stability of conduct problems plus callous-unemotional traits, and the seeming consolidation of psychopathic traits in adolescence, trials are urgently needed to identify what works with this population.

Learning changes the brain. The effectiveness of treatment and prevention trials should be measured not only by changes in behaviors, emotion recognition, and so forth but also in the neural correlates of the original deficits. If the neural correlates are not modified to resemble those of healthy children and adolescents, it is unlikely that changes in behaviors or symptoms will be maintained. Additionally, taking account of genes, and epigenetic changes to gene activity, may enhance treatment outcomes. Importantly, changes in children's behaviors when their parents complete parent management training programs have been shown to differ depending on the variant of the glucocorticoid gene (NR3C1) (Albert et al. 2015) or of the serotonin transporter gene (5HTTLPR) (Brody et al. 2009) that they carry.

The prevention of psychopathy depends on understanding the etiology. To achieve this goal, prospective, longitudinal investigations that begin in utero, are genetically informed, and include repeated brain imaging are needed.

Key Points

- The syndrome of psychopathy is a rare neurodevelopmental disorder that is characterized by manipulation of others, pathological lying, callousness, and predatory violent behavior that afflicts more males than females.

- Males with psychopathy have distinctive features of neural gray and white matter structures in frontal, limbic, and paralimbic regions and reduced activity in limbic structures resulting from limiting attention to a primary task.

- Males with psychopathy have a history of childhood-onset callousness, conduct problems, and aggressive behavior.

- The combination of childhood callousness and conduct problems is highly heritable; callousness among toddlers is also highly heritable and can be reduced by warm, positive parenting.

- Psychopathic traits are observed in general population samples and are associated with antisocial behavior and neural abnormalities.

References

Aghajani M, Klapwijk ET, Colins OF, et al: Interactions between oxytocin receptor gene methylation and callous-unemotional traits impact socioaffective brain systems in conduct-disordered offenders. Biol Psychiatry Cogn Neurosci Neuroimaging 3(4):379–391, 2018 29628070

Albert D, Belsky DW, Crowley DM, et al: Can genetics predict response to complex behavioral interventions? Evidence from a genetic analysis of the fast track randomized control trial. J Policy Anal Manage 34(3):497–518, 2015 26106668

Alegria AA, Radua J, Rubia K: Meta-analysis of fMRI studies of disruptive behavior disorders. Am J Psychiatry 173(11):1119–1130, 2016 27523497

American Psychiatric Association: Diagnostic and Statistical Manual of Mental Disorders, 5th Edition. Arlington, VA, American Psychiatric Association, 2013

Anderson NE, Kiehl KA: The psychopath magnetized: insights from brain imaging. Trends Cogn Sci 16(1):52–60, 2012 22177031

Antonowicz DH, Parker J: Reducing recidivism: evidence from 26 years of international evaluations of reasoning and rehabilitation programs. 2014. Available at: www.academia.edu/6939168/Reducing_Recidivism_Evidence_from_26_Years_of_International_Evaluations_of_Reasoning_and_Rehabilitation_Programs. Accessed April 20, 2021.

Asscher JJ, van Vugt ES, Stams GJJM, et al: The relationship between juvenile psychopathic traits, delinquency and (violent) recidivism: a meta-analysis. J Child Psychol Psychiatry 52(11):1134–1143, 2011 21599664

Auty KM, Farrington DP, Coid JW: Intergenerational transmission of psychopathy and mediation via psychosocial risk factors. Br J Psychiatry 206(1):26–31, 2015 25395688

Bagga D, Sharma A, Kumari A, et al: Decreased white matter integrity in fronto-occipital fasciculus bundles: relation to visual information processing in alcohol-dependent subjects. Alcohol 48(1):43–53, 2014 24388377

Bagley AD, Abramowitz CS, Kosson DS: Vocal affect recognition and psychopathy: converging findings across traditional and cluster analytic approaches to assessing the construct. J Abnorm Psychol 118(2):388–398, 2009 19413412

Bamvita J-M, Larm P, Checknita D, et al: Childhood predictors of adult psychopathy scores among males followed from age 6 to 33. J Crim Justice 53(11):55–65, 2017

Barker ED, Oliver BR, Viding E, et al: The impact of prenatal maternal risk, fearless temperament and early parenting on adolescent callous-unemotional traits: a 14-year longitudinal investigation. J Child Psychol Psychiatry 52(8):878–888, 2011 21410472

Barker ED, Walton E, Cecil CAM: Annual Research Review: DNA methylation as a mediator in the association between risk exposure and child and adolescent psychopathology. J Child Psychol Psychiatry 59(4):303–322, 2018 28736860

Baskin-Sommers AR, Newman JP: Psychopathic and externalizing offenders display dissociable dysfunctions when responding to facial affect. Pers Disord 5(4):369–379, 2014 24932762

Baskin-Sommers AR, Curtin JJ, Newman JP: Altering the cognitive-affective dysfunctions of psychopathic and externalizing offender subtypes with cognitive remediation. Clin Psychol Sci 3(1):45–57, 2015 25977843

Beaver KM, da Silva Costa C, Poersch AP, et al: Psychopathic personality traits and their influence on parenting quality: results from a nationally representative sample of Americans. Psychiatr Q 85(4):497–511, 2014 25092358

Bolhuis K, Viding E, Muetzel RL, et al: Neural profile of callous traits in children: a population-based neuroimaging study. Biol Psychiatry 85(5):399–407, 2019 30554676

Booij L, Tremblay RE, Szyf M, et al: Genetic and early environmental influences on the serotonin system: consequences for brain development and risk for psychopathology. J Psychiatry Neurosci 40(1):5–18, 2015 25285876

Brody GH, Beach SRH, Philibert RA, et al: Prevention effects moderate the association of 5-HTTLPR and youth risk behavior initiation: gene x environment hypotheses tested via a randomized prevention design. Child Dev 80(3):645–661, 2009 19489894

Broidy LM, Nagin DS, Tremblay RE, et al: Developmental trajectories of childhood disruptive behaviors and adolescent delinquency: a six-site, cross-national study. Dev Psychol 39(2):222–245, 2003 12661883

Buckholtz JW: Social norms, self-control, and the value of antisocial behavior. Curr Opin Behav Sci 3:122–129, 2015

Buckholtz JW, Faigman DL: Promises, promises for neuroscience and law. Curr Biol 24(18):R861–R867, 2014 25247363

Buckholtz JW, Treadway MT, Cowan RL, et al: Mesolimbic dopamine reward system hypersensitivity in individuals with psychopathic traits. Nat Neurosci 13(4):419–421, 2010 20228805

Burke JD, Loeber R, Lahey BB: Adolescent conduct disorder and interpersonal callousness as predictors of psychopathy in young adults. J Clin Child Adolesc Psychol 36(3):334–346, 2007 17658978

Byrd AL, Manuck SB: MAOA, childhood maltreatment, and antisocial behavior: meta-analysis of a gene-environment interaction. Biol Psychiatry 75(1):9–17, 2014 23786983

Cardinale EM, O'Connell K, Robertson EL, et al: Callous and uncaring traits are associated with reductions in amygdala volume among youths with varying levels of conduct problems. Psychol Med 49(9):1449–1458, 2019 30139402

Carré JM, Hyde LW, Neumann CS, et al: The neural signatures of distinct psychopathic traits. Soc Neurosci 8(2):122–135, 2013 22775289

Checknita D, Tiihonen J, Hodgins S, Nilsson KW: Associations of age, sex, sexual abuse, and genotype with monoamine oxidase a gene methylation. J Neural Transm (Vienna) 128(11):1721–1739, 2021 34424394

Christian RE, Frick PJ, Hill NL, et al: Psychopathy and conduct problems in children, II: implications for subtyping children with conduct problems. J Am Acad Child Adolesc Psychiatry 36(2):233–241, 1997 9031576

Cleckley HM: The Mask of Sanity: An Attempt to Clarify Some Issues About the So-Called Psychopathic Personality, 5th Edition. St. Louis, MO, Mosby, 1976

Coid J, Yang M, Roberts A, et al: Violence and psychiatric morbidity in the national household population of Britain: public health implications. Br J Psychiatry 189:12–19, 2006 16816300

Compton WM, Conway KP, Stinson FS, et al: Prevalence, correlates, and comorbidity of DSM-IV antisocial personality syndromes and alcohol and specific drug use disorders in the United States: results from the National Epidemiologic Survey on Alcohol and Related Conditions. J Clin Psychiatry 66(6):677–685, 2005 15960559

Cornell DG, Warren J, Hawk G, et al: Psychopathy in instrumental and reactive violent offenders. J Consult Clin Psychol 64(4):783–790, 1996 8803369

Dackis MN, Rogosch FA, Cicchetti D: Child maltreatment, callous-unemotional traits, and defensive responding in high-risk children: an investigation of emotion-modulated startle response. Dev Psychopathol 27(4 pt 2):1527–1545, 2015 26535942

Dadds MR, Allen JL, Oliver BR, et al: Love, eye contact and the developmental origins of empathy v. psychopathy. Br J Psychiatry 200(3):191–196, 2012a 21852303

Dadds MR, Cauchi AJ, Wimalaweera S, et al: Outcomes, moderators, and mediators of empathic-emotion recognition training for complex conduct problems in childhood. Psychiatry Res 199(3):201–207, 2012b 22703720

Dadds MR, Moul C, Cauchi A, et al: Methylation of the oxytocin receptor gene and oxytocin blood levels in the development of psychopathy. Dev Psychopathol 26(1):33–40, 2014a 24059811

Dadds MR, Moul C, Cauchi A, et al: Polymorphisms in the oxytocin receptor gene are associated with the development of psychopathy. Dev Psychopathol 26(1):21–31, 2014b 24059750

Dadds MR, Kimonis ER, Schollar-Root O, et al: Are impairments in emotion recognition a core feature of callous-unemotional traits? Testing the primary versus secondary variants model in children. Dev Psychopathol 30(1):67–77, 2018 28420457

De Brito SA, Mechelli A, Wilke M, et al: Size matters: increased grey matter in boys with conduct problems and callous-unemotional traits. Brain 132(pt 4):843–852, 2009 19293245

De Brito SA, McCrory EJP, Mechelli A, et al: Small, but not perfectly formed: decreased white matter concentration in boys with psychopathic tendencies. Mol Psychiatry 16(5):476–477, 2011 20548295

De Brito SA, Viding E, Sebastian CL, et al: Reduced orbitofrontal and temporal grey matter in a community sample of maltreated children. J Child Psychol Psychiatry 54(1):105–112, 2013 22880630

Dotterer HL, Waller R, Shaw DS, et al: Antisocial behavior with callous-unemotional traits is associated with widespread disruptions to white matter structural connectivity among low-income, urban males. Neuroimage Clin 23:101836, 2019 31077985

Edwards BG, Carre JR, Kiehl KA: A review of psychopathy and Cluster B personality traits and their neural correlates in female offenders. Biol Psychol 148:107740, 2019 31415792

Ettekal I, Eiden RD, Nickerson AB, et al: Developmental cascades to children's conduct problems: the role of prenatal substance use, socioeconomic adversity, maternal depression and sensitivity, and children's conscience. Dev Psychopathol 32(1):85–103, 2020 30704548

Ezpeleta L, Penelo E, de la Osa N, et al: Association of OXTR rs53576 with the developmental trajectories of callous-unemotional traits and stressful life events in 3- to 9-year-old community children. J Abnorm Child Psychol 47(10):1651–1662, 2019 31030321

Fanti KA: Understanding heterogeneity in conduct disorder: a review of psychophysiological studies. Neurosci Biobehav Rev 91:4–20, 2018 27693700

Fanti KA, Kimonis E: Heterogeneity in externalizing problems at age 3: association with age 15 biological and environmental outcomes. Dev Psychol 53(7):1230–1241, 2017 28406655

Fanti KA, Demetriou CA, Kimonis ER: Variants of callous-unemotional conduct problems in a community sample of adolescents. J Youth Adolesc 42(7):964–979, 2013 23644815

Fazel S, Danesh J: Serious mental disorder in 23000 prisoners: a systematic review of 62 surveys. Lancet 359(9306):545–550, 2002 11867106

Fergusson DM, Boden JM, Horwood LJ: Situational and generalised conduct problems and later life outcomes: evidence from a New Zealand birth cohort. J Child Psychol Psychiatry 50(9):1084–1092, 2009 19298467

Fontaine NMG, Rijsdijk FV, McCrory EJP, et al: Etiology of different developmental trajectories of callous-unemotional traits. J Am Acad Child Adolesc Psychiatry 49(7):656–664, 2010 20610135

Fontaine NMG, McCrory EJP, Boivin M, et al: Predictors and outcomes of joint trajectories of callous-unemotional traits and conduct problems in childhood. J Abnorm Psychol 120(3):730–742, 2011 21341879

Forsman M, Lichtenstein P, Andershed H, et al: Genetic effects explain the stability of psychopathic personality from mid- to late adolescence. J Abnorm Psychol 117(3):606–617, 2008 18729612

Forth AE, Kosson DS, Hare RD: Hare Psychopathy Checklist: Youth Version (PCL:YV). Toronto, ON, Canada, Multi-Health Systems, 2003

Frick PJ, White SF: Research review: the importance of callous-unemotional traits for developmental models of aggressive and antisocial behavior. J Child Psychol Psychiatry 49(4):359–375, 2008 18221345

Frick PJ, Kimonis ER, Dandreaux DM, et al: The 4 year stability of psychopathic traits in non-referred youth. Behav Sci Law 21(6):713–736, 2003 14696028

Frick PJ, Ray JV, Thornton LC, et al: Annual research review: a developmental psychopathology approach to understanding callous-unemotional traits in children and adolescents with serious conduct problems. J Child Psychol Psychiatry 55(6):532–548, 2014a 24117854

Frick PJ, Ray JV, Thornton LC, et al: Can callous-unemotional traits enhance the understanding, diagnosis, and treatment of serious conduct problems in children and adolescents? A comprehensive review. Psychol Bull 140(1):1–57, 2014b 23796269

Green H, McGinnity A, Meltzer H, et al: Mental Health of Children and Young People in Great Britain, 2004. New York, Palgrave Macmillan, 2005

Gregory S, ffytche D, Simmons A, et al: The antisocial brain: psychopathy matters. Arch Gen Psychiatry 69(9):962–972, 2012 22566562

Gregory S, Blair RJ, Ffytche D, et al: Punishment and psychopathy: a case-control functional MRI investigation of reinforcement learning in violent antisocial personality disordered men. Lancet Psychiatry 2(2):153–160, 2015 26359751

Guay J-P, Ruscio J, Knight RA, Hare RD: A taxometric analysis of the latent structure of psychopathy: evidence for dimensionality. J Abnorm Psychol 116(4):701–716, 2007 18020717

Haghighi A, Schwartz DH, Abrahamowicz M, et al: Prenatal exposure to maternal cigarette smoking, amygdala volume, and fat intake in adolescence. JAMA Psychiatry 70(1):98–105, 2013 22945562

Hamilton RKB, Newman JP: Information processing capacity in psychopathy: effects of anomalous attention. Pers Disord 9(2):182–187, 2018 27775411

Hamilton RKB, Hiatt Racer K, Newman JP: Impaired integration in psychopathy: a unified theory of psychopathic dysfunction. Psychol Rev 122(4):770–791, 2015 26437150

Hare RD: Psychopathy and antisocial personality disorder: a case of diagnostic confusion. Psychiatr Times (13):39–40, 1996

Hare RD: Manual for the Revised Psychopathy Checklist, 2nd Edition. Toronto, ON, Canada, Multi-Health Systems, 2003

Hare RD, Neumann CS: The PCL-R assessment of psychopathy: development, structural properties and new directions, in Handbook of Psychopathy. Edited by Patrick CJ. New York, Guilford, 2006, pp 58–88

Harris GJ, Jaffin SK, Hodge SM, et al: Frontal white matter and cingulum diffusion tensor imaging deficits in alcoholism. Alcohol Clin Exp Res 32(6):1001–1013, 2008 18422840

Hart SD, Cox DN, Hare RD: Manual for the Hare Psychopathy Checklist: Screening Version (PCL:SV). Toronto, ON, Canada, Multi-Health Systems, 1995

Hemphälä M, Hodgins S: Do psychopathic traits assessed in mid-adolescence predict mental health, psychosocial, and antisocial, including criminal outcomes, over the subsequent 5 years? Can J Psychiatry 59(1):40–49, 2014 24444323

Hemphälä M, Kosson D, Westerman J, et al: Stability and predictors of psychopathic traits from mid-adolescence through early adulthood. Scand J Psychol 56(6):649–658, 2015 26565733

Hodgins S, Larm P, Ellenbogen M, et al: Teachers' ratings of childhood behaviours predict adolescent and adult crime among 3016 males and females. Can J Psychiatry 58(3):143–150, 2013 23461885

Hodgins S, Checknita D, Lindner P, et al: Antisocial personality disorder, in The Wiley Blackwell Handbook of Forensic Neuroscience, Volume 33. Edited by Beech AR, Carter AJ, Mann RE, et al. Hoboken, NJ, Chichester, UK, Wiley Blackwell, 2018, pp 229–271

Holz NE, Boecker R, Hohm E, et al: The long-term impact of early life poverty on orbitofrontal cortex volume in adulthood: results from a prospective study over 25 years. Neuropsychopharmacology 40(4):996–1004, 2015 25315195

Hosking JG, Kastman EK, Dorfman HM, et al: Disrupted prefrontal regulation of striatal subjective value signals in psychopathy. Neuron 95(1):221.e4–231.e4, 2017 28683266

Hyde LW, Shaw DS, Gardner F, et al: Dimensions of callousness in early childhood: links to problem behavior and family intervention effectiveness. Dev Psychopathol 25(2):347–363, 2013 23627949

Hyde LW, Waller R, Trentacosta CJ, et al: Heritable and nonheritable pathways to early callous-unemotional behaviors. Am J Psychiatry 173(9):903–910, 2016 27056607

Jaffee SR, Caspi A, Moffitt TE, et al: Physical maltreatment victim to antisocial child: evidence of an environmentally mediated process. J Abnorm Psychol 113(1):44–55, 2004 14992656

Jaffee SR, Caspi A, Moffitt TE, et al: Nature X nurture: genetic vulnerabilities interact with physical maltreatment to promote conduct problems. Dev Psychopathol 17(1):67–84, 2005 15971760

Jaffee SR, Belsky J, Harrington H, et al: When parents have a history of conduct disorder: how is the caregiving environment affected? J Abnorm Psychol 115(2):309–319, 2006 16737395

Kahn RE, Frick PJ, Youngstrom E, et al: The effects of including a callous-unemotional specifier for the diagnosis of conduct disorder. J Child Psychol Psychiatry 53(3):271–282, 2012 21950481

Kahn RE, Deater-Deckard K, King-Casas B, et al: Intergenerational similarity in callous-unemotional traits: contributions of hostile parenting and household chaos during adolescence. Psychiatry Res 246:815–820, 2016 28029442

Karpman B: On the need of separating psychopathy into two distinct clinical types: the symptomatic and the idiopathic. J Crim Psychopathol 3:112–137, 1941

Kimonis ER, Frick PJ, Cauffman E, et al: Primary and secondary variants of juvenile psychopathy differ in emotional processing. Dev Psychopathol 24(3):1091–1103, 2012 22781873

Kimonis ER, Fanti KA, Isoma Z, et al: Maltreatment profiles among incarcerated boys with callous-unemotional traits. Child Maltreat 18(2):108–121, 2013 23553263

Kimonis ER, Fanti KA, Anastassiou-Hadjicharalambous X, et al: Can callous-unemotional traits be reliably measured in preschoolers? J Abnorm Child Psychol 44(4):625–638, 2016 26344015

Kimonis ER, Fanti KA, Goulter N, et al: Affective startle potentiation differentiates primary and secondary variants of juvenile psychopathy. Dev Psychopathol 29(4):1149–1160, 2017 28031056

Kimonis ER, Fleming G, Briggs N, et al: Parent-child interaction therapy adapted for preschoolers with callous-unemotional traits: an open trial pilot study. J Clin Child Adolesc Psychol 48 (suppl 1):S347–S361, 2019 29979887

Kjøbli J, Zachrisson HD, Bjørnebekk G: Three randomized effectiveness trials—one question: can callous-unemotional traits in children be altered? J Clin Child Adolesc Psychol 47(3):436–443, 2018 27359164

Kolla NJ, Malcolm C, Attard S, et al: Childhood maltreatment and aggressive behaviour in violent offenders with psychopathy. Can J Psychiatry 58(8):487–494, 2013 23972111

Kolla NJ, Gregory S, Attard S, et al: Disentangling possible effects of childhood physical abuse on gray matter changes in violent offenders with psychopathy. Psychiatry Res 221(2):123–126, 2014 24361393

Krueger RF, Moffitt TE, Caspi A, et al: Assortative mating for antisocial behavior: developmental and methodological implications. Behav Genet 28(3):173–186, 1998 9670593

Krueger RF, Hicks BM, Patrick CJ, et al: Etiologic connections among substance dependence, antisocial behavior, and personality: modeling the externalizing spectrum. J Abnorm Psychol 111(3):411–424, 2002 12150417

Labonté B, Suderman M, Maussion G, et al: Genome-wide methylation changes in the brains of suicide completers. Am J Psychiatry 170(5):511–520, 2013 23511308

Larson CL, Baskin-Sommers AR, Stout DM, et al: The interplay of attention and emotion: top-down attention modulates amygdala activation in psychopathy. Cogn Affect Behav Neurosci 13(4):757–770, 2013 23712665

Larsson H, Andershed H, Lichtenstein P: A genetic factor explains most of the variation in the psychopathic personality. J Abnorm Psychol 115(2):221–230, 2006 16737387

Leistico A-MR, Salekin RT, DeCoster J, et al: A large-scale meta-analysis relating the Hare measures of psychopathy to antisocial conduct. Law Hum Behav 32(1):28–45, 2008 17629778

Levy T, Bloch Y, Bar-Maisels M, et al: Salivary oxytocin in adolescents with conduct problems and callous-unemotional traits. Eur Child Adolesc Psychiatry 24(12):1543–1551, 2015 26433370

Lindner P, Budhiraja M, Westerman J, et al: White matter correlates of psychopathic traits in a female community sample. Soc Cogn Affect Neurosci 12(9):1500–1510, 2017 28992269

Lindner P, Flodin P, Budhiraja M, et al: Associations of psychopathic traits with local and global brain network topology in young adult women. Biol Psychiatry Cogn Neurosci Neuroimaging 3(12):1003–1012, 2018 29945829

Loney BR, Huntenburg A, Counts-Allan C, et al: A preliminary examination of the intergenerational continuity of maternal psychopathic features. Aggress Behav 33(1):14–25, 2007 17441002

Lozier LM, Cardinale EM, VanMeter JW, et al: Mediation of the relationship between callous-unemotional traits and proactive aggression by amygdala response to fear among children with conduct problems. JAMA Psychiatry 71(6):627–636, 2014 24671141

Luciana M, Collins PF, Muetzel RL, et al: Effects of alcohol use initiation on brain structure in typically developing adolescents. Am J Drug Alcohol Abuse 39(6):345–355, 2013 24200204

Lynam DR, Loeber R, Stouthamer-Loeber M: The stability of psychopathy from adolescence into adulthood: the search for moderators. Crim Justice Behav 35(2):228–243, 2008 20593007

Lynam DR, Charnigo R, Moffitt TE, et al: The stability of psychopathy across adolescence. Dev Psychopathol 21(4):1133–1153, 2009 19825261

Marsh AA, Blair RJ: Deficits in facial affect recognition among antisocial populations: a meta-analysis. Neurosci Biobehav Rev 32(3):454–465, 2008 17915324

Maughan B, Rowe R, Messer J, et al: Conduct disorder and oppositional defiant disorder in a national sample: developmental epidemiology. J Child Psychol Psychiatry 45(3):609–621, 2004 15055379

McMahon RJ, Witkiewitz K, Kotler JS, et al: Predictive validity of callous-unemotional traits measured in early adolescence with respect to multiple antisocial outcomes. J Abnorm Psychol 119(4):752–763, 2010 20939651

Meffert H, Gazzola V, den Boer JA, et al: Reduced spontaneous but relatively normal deliberate vicarious representations in psychopathy. Brain 136(pt 8):2550–2562, 2013 23884812

Mendoza Diaz A, Overgaauw S, Hawes DJ, et al: Intergenerational stability of callous-unemotional traits. Child Psychiatry Hum Dev 49(3):480–491, 2018 29119362

Miskovich TA, Anderson NE, Harenski CL, et al: Abnormal cortical gyrification in criminal psychopathy. Neuroimage Clin 19:876–882, 2018 29946511

Moffitt TE: Male antisocial behaviour in adolescence and beyond. Nat Hum Behav 2(3):177–186, 2018 30271880

Moffitt TE, Caspi A: Childhood predictors differentiate life-course persistent and adolescence-limited antisocial pathways among males and females. Dev Psychopathol 13(2):355–375, 2001 11393651

Moul C, Dobson-Stone C, Brennan J, et al: Serotonin 1B receptor gene (HTR1B) methylation as a risk factor for callous-unemotional traits in antisocial boys. PLoS One 10(5):e0126903, 2015 25993020

Moul C, Hawes DJ, Dadds MR: Mapping the developmental pathways of child conduct problems through the neurobiology of empathy. Neurosci Biobehav Rev 91:34–50, 2018 28377098

Newman JP, Baskin-Sommers AR: Smith and Lilienfeld's meta-analysis of the response modulation hypothesis: important theoretical and quantitative clarifications. Psychol Bull 142(12):1384–1393, 2016 27869458

Newman JP, Kosson DS: Passive avoidance learning in psychopathic and nonpsychopathic offenders. J Abnorm Psychol 95(3):252–256, 1986 3745647

Newman JP, Kosson DS, Patterson CM: Delay of gratification in psychopathic and nonpsychopathic offenders. J Abnorm Psychol 101(4):630–636, 1992 1430601

Newman JP, Curtin JJ, Bertsch JD, et al: Attention moderates the fearlessness of psychopathic offenders. Biol Psychiatry 67(1):66–70, 2010 19793581

Niciu MJ, Mason GF: Neuroimaging in alcohol and drug dependence. Curr Behav Neurosci Rep 1(1):45–54, 2014 24678450

Nilsson KW, Comasco E, Hodgins S, et al: Genotypes do not confer risk for delinquency but rather alter susceptibility to positive and negative environmental factors: gene-environment interactions of BDNF Val66Met, 5-HTTLPR, and MAOA-uVNTR [corrected]. Int J Neuropsychopharmacol 18(5):pyu107, 2014 25522433

Nilsson KW, Åslund C, Comasco E, et al: Gene-environment interaction of monoamine oxidase A in relation to antisocial behaviour: current and future directions. J Neural Transm (Vienna) 125(11):1601–1626, 2018 29881923

Nock MK, Kazdin AE, Hiripi E, et al: Prevalence, subtypes, and correlates of DSM-IV conduct disorder in the National Comorbidity Survey Replication. Psychol Med 36(5):699–710, 2006 16438742

Obradović J, Pardini DA, Long JD, et al: Measuring interpersonal callousness in boys from childhood to adolescence: an examination of longitudinal invariance and temporal stability. J Clin Child Adolesc Psychol 36(3):276–292, 2007 17658974

Odgers CL, Moffitt TE, Broadbent JM, et al: Female and male antisocial trajectories: from childhood origins to adult outcomes. Dev Psychopathol 20(2):673–716, 2008 18423100

Pardini DA, Lochman JE, Powell N: The development of callous-unemotional traits and antisocial behavior in children: are there shared and/or unique predictors? J Clin Child Adolesc Psychol 36(3):319–333, 2007 17658977

Pasalich DS, Dadds MR, Hawes DJ, et al: Do callous-unemotional traits moderate the relative importance of parental coercion versus warmth in child conduct problems? An observational study. J Child Psychol Psychiatry 52(12):1308–1315, 2011 21726225

Patrick CJ, Drislane LE: Triarchic model of psychopathy: origins, operationalizations, and observed linkages with personality and general psychopathology. J Pers 83(6):627–643, 2015 25109906

Peltola MJ, Yrttiaho S, Leppänen JM: Infants' attention bias to faces as an early marker of social development. Dev Sci 21(6):e12687, 2018 29971869

Piquero AR, Farrington DP, Fontaine NMG, et al: Childhood risk, offending trajectories, and psychopathy at age 48 years in the Cambridge Study in delinquent development. Psychol Public Policy Law 18(4):577–598, 2012

Pujara M, Motzkin JC, Newman JP, et al: Neural correlates of reward and loss sensitivity in psychopathy. Soc Cogn Affect Neurosci 9(6):794–801, 2014 23552079

Puzzo I, Seunarine K, Sully K, et al: Altered white-matter microstructure in conduct disorder is specifically associated with elevated callous-unemotional traits. J Abnorm Child Psychol 46(7):1451–1466, 2018 29273881

Robins LN, Tipp J, Przybeck T: Antisocial personality, in Psychiatric Disorders in America: The Epidemiologic Catchment Area Study. Edited by Robins LN, Regier DA. New York, Free Press, 1991, pp 258–290

Rodman AM, Kastman E, Dorfman HM, et al: Selective mapping of psychopathy and externalizing to dissociable circuits for inhibitory self-control. Clin Psychol Sci 4(3):559–571, 2016 27453803

Rogers JC, De Brito SA: Cortical and subcortical gray matter volume in youths with conduct problems: a meta-analysis. JAMA Psychiatry 73(1):64–72, 2016 26650724

Rowe R, Maughan B, Moran P, et al: The role of callous and unemotional traits in the diagnosis of conduct disorder. J Child Psychol Psychiatry 51(6):688–695, 2010 20039995

Sadeh N, Javdani S, Jackson JJ, et al: Serotonin transporter gene associations with psychopathic traits in youth vary as a function of socioeconomic resources. J Abnorm Psychol 119(3):604–609, 2010 20677849

Salihovic S, Kerr M, Stattin H: Under the surface of adolescent psychopathic traits: high-anxious and low-anxious subgroups in a community sample of youths. J Adolesc 37(5):681–689, 2014 24680581

Samuels J, Eaton WW, Bienvenu OJ 3rd, et al: Prevalence and correlates of personality disorders in a community sample. Br J Psychiatry 180(6):536–542, 2002 12042233

Saukkonen S, Aronen ET, Laajasalo T, et al: Victimization and psychopathic features in a population-based sample of Finnish adolescents. Child Abuse Negl 60:58–66, 2016 27690216

Schiffer B, Müller BW, Scherbaum N, et al: Disentangling structural brain alterations associated with violent behavior from those associated with substance use disorders. Arch Gen Psychiatry 68(10):1039–1049, 2011 21646569

Seara-Cardoso A, Viding E: Functional neuroscience of psychopathic personality in adults. J Pers 83(6):723–737, 2015 25041571

Sellbom M, Lilienfeld SO, Fowler KA, et al: The self-report assessment of psychopathy: challenges, pitfalls, and promises, in Handbook of Psychopathy, 2nd Edition. Edited by Patrick CJ. New York, Guilford, 2018, pp 211–258

Shaw DS, Gross HE: What we have learned about early childhood and the development of delinquency, in The Long View of Crime: A Synthesis of Longitudinal Research, Volume 12. Edited by Liberman AM. New York, Springer, 2008, pp 79–127

Shaw DS, Shelleby EC: Early starting conduct problems: intersection of conduct problems and poverty. Annu Rev Clin Psychol 10:503–528, 2014 24471370

Sourander A, Jensen P, Davies M, et al: Who is at greatest risk of adverse long-term outcomes? The Finnish From a Boy to a Man study. J Am Acad Child Adolesc Psychiatry 46(9):1148–1161, 2007 17712238

Swanson MC, Bland RC, Newman SC: Epidemiology of psychiatric disorders in Edmonton: antisocial personality disorders. Acta Psychiatr Scand Suppl 376(suppl):63–70, 1994 8178687

Szyf M, Tang Y-Y, Hill KG, et al: The dynamic epigenome and its implications for behavioral interventions: a role for epigenetics to inform disorder prevention and health promotion. Transl Behav Med 6(1):55–62, 2016 27012253

Teicher MH, Samson JA: Annual Research Review: Enduring neurobiological effects of childhood abuse and neglect. J Child Psychol Psychiatry 57(3):241–266, 2016 26831814

Tost H, Kolachana B, Hakimi S, et al: A common allele in the oxytocin receptor gene (OXTR) impacts prosocial temperament and human hypothalamic-limbic structure and function. Proc Natl Acad Sci USA 107(31):13936–13941, 2010 20647384

Trentacosta CJ, Waller R, Neiderhiser JM, et al: Callous-unemotional behaviors and harsh parenting: reciprocal associations across early childhood and moderation by inherited risk. J Abnorm Child Psychol 47(5):811–823, 2019 30306411

Tuvblad C, Fanti KA, Andershed H, et al: Psychopathic personality traits in 5 year old twins: the importance of genetic and shared environmental influences. Eur Child Adolesc Psychiatry 26(4):469–479, 2017 27683227

Vassileva J, Kosson DS, Abramowitz CS, et al: Psychopathy versus psychopathies in classifying criminal offenders. Legal Criminol Psychol 10(1):27–43, 2005

Verona E, Vitale J: Psychopathy in women: assessment, manifestations, and etiology, in Handbook of Psychopathy, 2nd Edition. Edited by Patrick CJ. New York, Guilford, 2018, pp 508–528

Viding E, Kimonis ER: Callous-unemotional traits, in Handbook of Psychopathy, 2nd Edition. Edited by Patrick CJ. New York, Guilford, 2018, pp 144–164

Viding E, Jones AP, Frick PJ, et al: Heritability of antisocial behaviour at 9: do callous-unemotional traits matter? Dev Sci 11(1):17–22, 2008 18171362

Viding E, Sebastian CL, Dadds MR, et al: Amygdala response to preattentive masked fear in children with conduct problems: the role of callous-unemotional traits. Am J Psychiatry 169(10):1109–1116, 2012 23032389

Wagner NJ, Mills-Koonce WR, Willoughby MT, et al: Parenting and children's representations of family predict disruptive and callous-unemotional behaviors. Dev Psychol 51(7):935–948, 2015 26010385

Wagner NJ, Mills-Koonce WR, Propper CB, et al: Associations between infant behaviors during the face-to-face still-face paradigm and oppositional defiant and callous-unemotional behaviors in early childhood. J Abnorm Child Psychol 44(8):1439–1453, 2016 26936036

Waldman ID, Rhee SH, LoParo D, Park Y: Genetic and environmental influences on psychopathy and antisocial behavior, in Handbook of Psychopathy, 2nd Edition. Edited by Patrick CJ. New York, Guilford, 2018, pp 335–353

Waller R, Gardner F, Hyde LW, et al: Do harsh and positive parenting predict parent reports of deceitful-callous behavior in early childhood? J Child Psychol Psychiatry 53(9):946–953, 2012 22490064

Waller R, Shaw DS, Forbes EE, et al: Understanding early contextual and parental risk factors for the development of limited prosocial emotions. J Abnorm Child Psychol 43(6):1025–1039, 2015 25510355

Waller R, Trentacosta CJ, Shaw DS, et al: Heritable temperament pathways to early callous-unemotional behaviour. Br J Psychiatry 209(6):475–482, 2016 27765772

Waller R, Shaw DS, Neiderhiser JM, et al: Toward an understanding of the role of the environment in the development of early callous behavior. J Pers 85(1):90–103, 2017 26291075

Waller R, Baskin-Sommers AR, Hyde LW: Examining predictors of callous unemotional traits trajectories across adolescence among high-risk males. J Clin Child Adolesc Psychol 47(3):444–457, 2018a 26799585

Waller R, Hyde LW, Klump KL, et al: Parenting is an environmental predictor of callous-unemotional traits and aggression: a monozygotic twin differences study. J Am Acad Child Adolesc Psychiatry 57(12):955–963, 2018b 30522741

Warren JI, South SC: Comparing the constructs of antisocial personality disorder and psychopathy in a sample of incarcerated women. Behav Sci Law 24(1):1–20, 2006 16491474

Wolf RC, Pujara MS, Motzkin JC, et al: Interpersonal traits of psychopathy linked to reduced integrity of the uncinate fasciculus. Hum Brain Mapp 36(10):4202–4209, 2015 26219745

Wong S: Criminal and Institutional Behaviors of Psychopaths. Ottawa, ON, Ministry of the Solicitor General of Canada, 1985

Wright N, Hill J, Sharp H, et al: Maternal sensitivity to distress, attachment and the development of callous-unemotional traits in young children. J Child Psychol Psychiatry 59(7):790–800, 2018 29380375

PART IV

Clinical Management

CHAPTER 17

Psychosocial Treatment of Antisocial Personality Disorder

James McGuire, Ph.D.

A pivotal question facing mental health services is whether antisocial personality disorder (ASPD) can be ameliorated by planned intervention, or whether any form of individual or group psychotherapy or system of case management or service provision can make a positive difference to its progress. In this chapter, I focus on that area of concern and on a series of issues that arise within it.

The question of whether antisocial individuals can change, particularly whether they may do so in response to planned therapeutic effort, has been a matter of debate. Traditionally, there has been a widespread belief that individuals diagnosed with ASPD—at least with a serious form of it—are "untreatable." More concerning, there has been a belief in some quarters that treatment makes them worse. Over about the past two decades, however, professional and scientific opinions have become more nuanced and have shifted in a more optimistic direction.

The objective in this chapter is to provide an overview of the main interrelated issues within this debate. First, the prospects of working successfully with this group are addressed: is there evidence that any kind of interventions "work" to reduce the features of ASPD? To answer this question, I collate the findings from previous reviews of the subject and from a collection of primary studies in which the efficacy of treatment has been directly investigated. Second, I review the role of the *therapeutic alliance* in provision of psychosocial interventions. Third, given that the volume of relevant research remains low and there is not enough of it to provide definitive practical guidance, I review other recommendations for the clinical management of antisocial individuals.

Effectiveness of Psychosocial Treatment

The "Untreatability" Myth

For most of the time since the definition of ASPD was formulated, the prevalent view was that ASPD is not amenable to change. In common with other forms of personality disorder, ASPD generally has been considered chronic and lifelong (Black 2015; Black et al. 1995). However, it is with specific reference to ASPD, and the related concept of psychopathy, that the term *untreatable* came into circulation. Although these terms are often used interchangeably, psychopathy appears to represent the severe end of the antisociality spectrum (Black 2013; Coid and Ullrich 2010).

Although ASPD's presumed untreatability is regarded as having held some sort of dominant or mainstream position, it is not clear that a preponderance of clinicians ever actually endorsed this concept. In a survey of practitioners working in mental health and criminal justice services in the United Kingdom, Tennet et al. (1993) found that 62% of psychiatrists, 95% of psychologists, and 82% of probation officers considered that the disorder was either "always" or "sometimes" remediable. Only a small minority of these three professional groups (1%, 2%, and 8%, respectively) considered that it was "never" remediable. If that was the perception of what is regarded as the most severe end of the continuum of ASPD, beliefs about the disorder more generally may never have been as outright dismissive as was thought. A more recent Delphi study of 61 experts from a range of professional backgrounds in different countries reported that regarding ASPD, "the experts unanimously argued against the judgment that treatment is not possible" (van den Bosch et al. 2018, p. 75).

In the past two decades, several conclusions have emerged that bring the untreatability standpoint into doubt. Reporting on an extensive review of the evaluation studies available at the time, Lösel (1998) noted the methodological problems that bedevil research in this area and the lack of well-controlled studies. In this survey of a wide variety of approaches to intervention, outcome evidence was mixed. Rather than comparing types of treatment and attempting to discern any that had consistently superior outcomes, Lösel (1998) found that "research in the treatment of antisociality suggests differentiated pathways that may lead to more successful interventions with at least some groups of psychopaths under particular conditions" (p. 330). This suggested the potential value of developing a broad set of principles as a guide to intervention and service delivery. Lösel made a series of 14 proposals concerning such principles. They include, for example, carrying out thorough dynamic assessments of individual patients and developing and sustaining a prosocial institutional climate and regime within organizations delivering treatment.

Subsequently, in putting to test the "therapeutic pessimism" of conclusions drawn elsewhere, Salekin (2002, p. 79) drew together tentative signs of positive results from a series of 42 studies. These studies used a variety of research designs, and only 8 involved comparisons between treated and untreated samples. The dependent variables were intermediate measures rather than mental health or recidivism outcomes. Of these studies, 5 reported use of behavioral, cognitive, personal construct, or interpersonal therapies, with a combined sample of 246 participants. Results showed high effect sizes on mediating variables. Salekin (2002) concluded that these therapies "addressed patients' thoughts about themselves, others and society…[and] they tended to treat some psychopathic traits" (p. 93). Although somewhat tenuous as an evidence base, this set of findings nevertheless contradicted the view that therapeutic change was out of reach for this patient population.

In a critique of Salekin's review, Harris and Rice (2006) discounted the results as being of little value on the grounds of the weak methodology of almost all the studies. Their own overview of the field went beyond skepticism to a position that led them to dismiss the prospects of being able to modify core traits of psychopathic personality. This conclusion was based on an evolutionary model of the advantages of antisocial traits in securing reproductive success. Harris and Rice not only reinforced the long-standing position of virtual intractability but also proposed an explanation for it. High levels of antisocial traits were purportedly of significant value in enabling individuals to ensure that their genes are passed on to the next generation. The researchers described this as an evolution-based, nonpathological approach to understanding psychopathy. They did not exclude the possibility of a treatment solution being found at some stage, although they thought that it most likely would come from neuroscience and molecular genetics.

Can Treatment Make Antisocial Individuals Worse?

In a review with a different emphasis, D'Silva et al. (2004) examined whether there were real grounds for the belief that treatment makes antisocial individuals worse. They located 24 studies that had used some version of Hare's Psychopathy Checklist–Revised (PCL-R) as a method of defining psychopathy (Hare 1991). The studies had numerous methodological weaknesses, and only 3 of the studies included an untreated control sample. Although some of the studies showed poorer outcomes for individuals who had high PCL-R scores, others showed the reverse. The authors concluded that evidence was insufficient to permit the conclusion that treatment made the participants worse.

It is interesting to explore the provenance of the "making people worse" notion. The most striking example of such an effect comes from an evaluation by Rice et al. (1992) of the Social Therapy Unit based in what was then known as Oak Ridge, the maximum-security division of Penetanguishene Mental Health Centre (later renamed Waypoint) in Ontario, Canada. The study compared rates of violent recidivism for "psychopaths" and "nonpsychopaths" over a period of 10.5 years following discharge. There was a significant difference among nonpsychopaths in percentage reoffending between treated and untreated groups for both general recidivism (44% vs. 58%) and violent recidivism (22% vs. 39%). Thus, there was evidence of a treatment effect. For the psychopathic group, on the other hand, there was no significant difference between treated and untreated groups for general recidivism (87% vs. 90%), although the treated group had a far higher rate of new violent offenses (77% vs. 55%). These findings of course relate to individuals who were assessed as being at the upper end of the scale of antisociality, so the study could shed only limited light on what we can infer about ASPD as a broader concept.

It could be that the damaging effect of treatment has an explanation other than the inability of those designated as psychopathic to change. The explanation might reside instead in the inappropriateness of the treatment regimen, one described by D'Silva et al. (2004) as "insidious and extreme," for this population. The Social Therapy Unit at Oak Ridge was conceptualized as a therapeutic community, but the basic model was modified in selected ways to an extent that it departed sharply from the meaning of the concept of therapeutic. Allocation to the unit was not on a voluntary basis; selected prisoners were mandated to go there. Whereas interaction with staff is often a key engine of change in such circumstances, at Oak Ridge it was kept to a minimal level. Prisoners spent periods of up to 2 weeks in small groups in a windowless room, in a state of nudity, in what was called the "Total Encounter Capsule" (Barker and McLaughlin 1977; Bazar 2015; Weisman 1995). The evaluation team themselves later expressed reservations about the project (Harris et al. 1994), and the methods used in Oak Ridge were later ruled by a Canadian judge as amounting to torture (Power 2017).

Against the background of the Oak Ridge findings, and given the evolving nature of psychosocial interventions, Hatchett (2015) reviewed other studies that included initial reports of treatment having had deleterious effects on participants assessed as psychopathic. Closer analysis indicated that any such outcomes had been insubstantial or were interim or short-term results, and Hatchett concluded that "there is little if any evidence that modern treatment interventions are iatrogenic for individuals classed as psychopathic" (p. 19).

Systematic Reviews of the Evidence

During the same time that researchers were reviewing treatment for antisociality, systematic reviews appeared that were concerned with interventions for personality disorders in general (Budge et al. 2013, 2014; Duggan et al. 2007), with some of the studies focusing on ASPD. Gibbon et al. (2010) reported a systematic review of randomized controlled trials (RCTs) of psychological interventions for ASPD or dissocial personality disorder, a closely corresponding category in the International Classification of Diseases. A search of 26 databases produced 48 studies (11 of which met specified inclusion criteria), containing a total of 14 comparisons between an intervention and a waiting list, treatment as usual, or no-treatment control. Several forms of intervention were reviewed, including contingency management, cognitive-behavioral therapy (CBT), supportive-expressive psychotherapy, schema therapy, relapse prevention, social problem-solving, strengths-based case management, a driving while intoxicated program, and judicial supervision. As found in all reviews to date, there was wide variation in the outcome measures used, making comparisons difficult. However, some positive, statistically significant, and practically meaningful results were found for several of these approaches, including various combinations of contingency management, maintenance therapy, and CBT, plus the driving while intoxicated program. Positive outcomes were confined to the area of clinical change, levels of substance abuse, or family functioning; no positive results emerged for variables associated with antisocial behavior. Collectively, therefore, the evidence up to that point must be regarded as rather thin. The authors' overall conclusion was that there was "insufficient trial evidence to justify using any psychological intervention for those with a diagnosis" of ASPD (Gibbon et al. 2010, p. 28). Reviewing the field not long afterward, Felthous (2011) also found no conclusive evidence to confirm or disconfirm the usefulness of psychological treatment.

Salekin et al. (2010) located and reviewed eight studies of treatment with adults assessed as psychopathic on the basis of their PCL-R scores. In most of the studies, there was no evidence that participants benefited from treatment; they often had high rates of dropout or poor postintervention results. However, three studies showed evidence of either treatment effects or no association between PCL-R scores and records or measures of aggression; that is, no evidence that high antisociality had a differential effect on responsiveness. Describing the effects across studies as ranging from "low-moderate to poor," Salekin et al. (2010) questioned whether this outcome reflected "no treatment response at all, or simply less gain than the non-psychopathic individuals, for some of these studies" (p. 248). Although none of the studies examined was a controlled trial, in some practical trials in clinical settings, there were significant relationships between level of participation in treatment and effects on later functioning, including lower rates of violent recidivism.

For example, Skeem et al. (2002) analyzed the progress of 871 patients from the MacArthur Violence Risk Assessment Study, who were supervised in a community setting. Within the study population, 72 patients were classified as psychopathic and 195 as potentially psychopathic. Members of the first group who had attended seven or more treatment sessions were 3.5 times less likely to commit violent offenses than were those who attended fewer sessions, and those designated as potentially psychopathic were 2.5 times less likely. These findings held with several other hypothetically influential variables controlled.

Olver and Wong (2009, 2013) and Wong et al. (2012) have reported evidence from evaluation of the Clearwater program, a group-based intervention for high-risk sexual offenders lasting approximately 8 months that was delivered in a secure psychiatric center. Of the participants classified as psychopathic, 73% completed treatment, and following release they had a reoffending rate one-third lower than that of those who did not complete treatment (61% vs. 92%).

Emmelkamp and Vedel (2010) acknowledged that it is difficult to conduct controlled trials in the settings where those diagnosed with ASPD receive treatment and recommended instead using high-quality quasi-experimental designs analyzed with propensity score matching or other forms of statistical adjustment. However, they disputed the status of evidence concerning outcomes from criminal justice research on the grounds that unless ASPD had been specifically assessed, it could not be known what fraction of a sample would have met diagnostic criteria, indeed even whether any individuals did. Although other evidence points to the existence of sizable proportions of persons with ASPD in most prison samples (Black et al. 2010; Fazel and Danesh 2002), no valid conclusion can be drawn unless ASPD is explicitly assessed. Thus, although there is now considerable evidence of the possibility of reducing violence by adult offenders (McGuire 2020; Papalia et al. 2019; Ross et al. 2013), such evidence cannot be presumed to be evidence of successful intervention with individuals with ASPD. Emmelkamp and Vedel (2010) also voiced concern that the group-based interventions thought suitable for delivery in correctional settings, which are widely used in some jurisdictions, might be undermined by highly manipulative individuals.

In a later review, Wilson (2014) collated results from six studies of treatments for ASPD. In most of the studies, participants had other concomitant psychiatric diagnoses. There were three RCTs, one of which was included in the review by Gibbon et al. (2010), and three uncontrolled studies. Two of the RCTs also yielded uncontrolled comparisons between groups with and without ASPD. All the resultant ORs were in a direction that favored treatment, but because of CIs, only one study was statistically significant: a study of an institution-based therapeutic community in which the key outcome variable was rates of reincarceration 12 months after release (McKendrick et al. 2006) (see Table 17–1 in the section "Controlled Trials of Antisocial Personality Disorder Treatment"). Among the experimental sample, none of the participants was reincarcerated. When individuals with ASPD diagnoses were compared with those without a diagnosis, no significant difference in outcome was seen between the groups. That is, treatment was "equally effective for individuals, regardless of ASPD status" (Wilson 2014, p. 43).

Other reviewers have responded in a similar vein. Polaschek and colleagues contested the untreatability stance and identified a growing consensus that an effective intervention can be devised (Polaschek 2014; Polaschek and Daly 2013). On the basis of a review of 17 studies of the association between psychopathy and violence, Reidy et al. (2013) noted that "there is good preliminary evidence to suggest that although they are more treatment resistant likely requiring more resources and dosage, a specifically and carefully crafted intervention may be effective in reducing violence by psychopathic individuals" (p. 536). Similarly, Wilson and Tamatea (2013, p. 493) depicted the expectation of untreatability as an "urban myth" and suggested that the fundamental problem is rather that we just have not yet found what effective treatment involves.

Reviewing studies of both psychological and pharmacological therapy, Black (2017) noted that there is a dearth of research in both areas and that treatment of ASPD is widely deemed "unsatisfactory and vexing" (p. 296) but found a mixture of outcomes from several sources. There have been positive reports of some individual progress in case series studies. In research on persons with ASPD and concomitant substance abuse disorders, no differences were found between those allocated to different treatments, but there were indicators of responsiveness in all groups. There was further evidence, albeit limited, from some other forms of intervention. These studies are discussed more fully in the next section.

Olver (2018; see also Wong 2016) adopted a novel approach with the objective of identifying what might be likely elements of successful intervention or service provision. He placed them in two main categories to form a dual-component model of treatment, corresponding to Factor 1 and Factor 2 of the PCL-R as originally conceived by Hare (Hare and Neumann 2008). Evidence suggested that Factor 1 (interpersonal and affective facets of psychopathy) changes relatively little over time; therefore, it may need to be managed rather than treated. By contrast, Factor 2 (lifestyle and antisocial behavior facets) alters over time and can be placed alongside other aspects of antisociality that are targeted in criminal justice rehabilitation programs. In some respects, this conceptualization accords well with the idea of treatment or service guidelines that are discussed later in this chapter. Although the reviews by Olver (2018) and Wong (2016) differ in their perspectives, they both add weight to the objection that the untreatability standpoint has no sound clinical backing.

Controlled Trials of
Antisocial Personality Disorder Treatment

On the basis of their review discussed in the subsection "The 'Untreatability' Myth," Harris and Rice (2006) maintained that "only controlled studies can be informative regarding treatment efficacy, and no conclusions can be drawn from uncontrolled studies" (p. 558). Some people would consider this a narrow interpretation; Polaschek and Skeem (2018) described it as "unduly conservative." Valid conclusions can be drawn from other kinds of studies. Arguably, quasi-experimental designs in natural or everyday practice settings can achieve higher *external* validity than specially designed experiments, which, in trying to attain high *internal* validity, often impose requirements that are so far removed from the constraints of routine practice that they are almost artificial. Nevertheless, the controlled trial is widely accepted as the most consistent strategy for hypothesis testing. In this section, we review such controlled studies of interventions for ASPD and psychopathy.

Table 17–1 provides details extracted from 18 articles or sets of articles pertaining to 17 independent studies of the effects of psychosocial interventions on features of ASPD, evaluated using RCT designs. In these studies, either 1) participants diagnosed with ASPD were randomly allocated to the different conditions being compared, or 2) a group containing individuals with and without ASPD was randomly divided and allotted to different conditions, with subsequent separate analyses of the subgroups, to test whether one showed better, similar, or poorer outcomes than the other. In some cases, the comparison was between an experimental condition (intervention to be tested) and no treatment or treatment as usual, the nature of which was also described. In other cases, the comparison was between two separate kinds of treatment. Studies that contained parallel samples of individuals with and without ASPD are included here only if the ASPD subgroup was analyzed separately. In other words, studies that consisted solely of a comparison between an ASPD group and a non-ASPD group were not retained for this summary. Only studies of adult participants were included.

This exercise was not formally designed following customary systematic review procedures of treatment effects but was undertaken to test a general hypothesis that we can express in crude terms as whether individuals with ASPD benefit from a psychosocial intervention. Among these studies, 14 were conducted in the United States, 3 in the United Kingdom, and 1 in Denmark, and all were published between 1985 and 2016. The entries were assembled from reviews by Gibbon et al. (2010) and Wilson and Tamatea (2013), although some of the studies they retained were excluded from the table for reasons given below.

In addition, reference lists were scrutinized in meta-analyses or systematic reviews by Hesse and Pederson (2006), Carr (2014), and Newton-Howes et al. (2017), with a briefer literature review by Hatchett (2015). These authors addressed the question of differential responsiveness to treatment between participants with and without ASPD, with particular reference to alcohol or other substance abuse treatment. Three of the studies cited in these reviews were randomized trials and are included in Table 17–1. The 10 other studies these authors cited used less rigorous types of design, and

TABLE 17–1.   Randomized controlled trials of psychosocial interventions for ASPD

Study	Participants	Interventions and comparators	Monitoring and outcome measures	Main findings
Bateman et al. 2016	*N*=40 outpatients (75% male) with diagnoses of both ASPD and BPD seen in a community mental health setting	Mentalization-based treatment (MBT): 18 months of weekly sessions vs. structured clinical management by nonspecialist practitioners	Wide range of clinical assessments and self-report measures: anger, aggression, hostility, anxiety, depression, impulsivity, relationships, paranoid symptoms and ideation, suicide attempts, self-harm	At 18-month end of treatment, equivalent beneficial changes were found in both groups on most outcome variables, but there was significantly greater improvement for the MBT group in relation to anger, paranoid symptoms and ideation, suicide attempts, and self-harm.
Brooner et al. 1998	*N*=40 drug-abusing adults (81% male, 50% African American) in methadone treatment who met DSM-III-R ASPD criteria (American Psychiatric Association 1987), randomly assigned to two conditions	Contingency management (CM; positive consequences for abstinence plus counseling) vs. no-treatment control	Retention in treatment, self-reported drug abuse, ASI scores, urinalysis test results, reported psychosocial problems	At 90-day follow-up, no significant between-group differences were found; both groups showed reductions in substance misuse (i.e., there was no evidence of greater effectiveness for the CM condition), which was taken to indicate a better than expected response to treatment by individuals diagnosed with ASPD.
Cullen et al. 2012a, 2012b	*N*=84 male inpatients (30%–34% white, 47%–52% Black) in medium-security psychiatric units with a psychotic disorder and history of violence, of whom 45% met criteria for ASPD	Structured 36×2-hour sessions of a cognitive-skills program, Reasoning and Rehabilitation, vs. TAU	Program completion, scores on social and cognitive skills measures (SPSI), anger (NAS), antisocial attitudes, perspective-taking (IRI), substance use, and rates of verbal and physical violence	At 12-month posttreatment follow-up, program completers showed gains in cognitive and social skills relative to control subjects, showed significant gains in perspective taking, were less likely to have antisocial attitudes, and showed lower levels of verbal aggression. However, level of attrition was high (≈50%).

TABLE 17–1. Randomized controlled trials of psychosocial interventions for ASPD *(continued)*

Study	Participants	Interventions and comparators	Monitoring and outcome measures	Main findings
Davidson et al. 2009	$N=52$ males (67% white) with an ASPD diagnosis and recent violence in two community settings in different parts of the United Kingdom	Cognitive-behavioral therapy (CBT): either 15 or 30 1-hour sessions over 6 or 12 months, allocated randomly plus TAU vs. TAU alone	Occurrence of acts of verbal or physical aggression (MCVSI), drug and alcohol use (AUDIT), levels of self-reported anger (NAS), core schemas, and social functioning	At 12-month follow-up (79% contact rate), both groups showed reductions in physical and verbal aggression and there were no significant between-group differences on any measure; however, some trends favored the CBT group with respect to less harmful drinking and improved social functioning.
Easton et al. 2012	$N=136$ marijuana-dependent young adults ages 18–25 with probation, parole, or court involvement, 44% of whom met criteria for ASPD	Four conditions: motivational enhancement with skills training vs. drug counseling, each or without CM	Numbers or rates of treatment sessions attended, marijuana-abstinent days, positive urine screens, and arrest + a range of secondary clinical outcomes; ASPD subgroups were matched at baseline	At end of treatment + 6-month follow-up, no evidence was found to indicate that participants with ASPD had poorer attendance levels, fewer abstinent days, or more positive urine screens; CM groups had higher rates of treatment attendance regardless of ASPD diagnosis.
Festinger et al. 2002	$N=181$ individuals (77% male) admitted to a 14-week drug court treatment program over a 15-month period; 33% were diagnosed with ASPD on the basis of a brief (30-minute) interview only	Comparison of two reporting conditions: biweekly attendance vs. "as-needed" attendance	Rates of program completion and of drug abstinence tested by urinalysis	The study found an interaction effect between attendance condition and ASPD diagnosis: the ASPD subgroup had a higher abstinence rate than the non-ASPD subgroup with reporting biweekly, but the reverse was found with "as-needed" reporting. The ASPD group had a lower completion rate than the non-ASPD group in the "as-needed" condition but was equal to it in the biweekly condition.

TABLE 17–1. Randomized controlled trials of psychosocial interventions for ASPD (continued)

Study	Participants	Interventions and comparators	Monitoring and outcome measures	Main findings
Frisman et al. 2009	Subsample from $N=198$ individuals with co-occurring psychoses and SUDs; a secondary analysis compared $n=36$ individuals with ASPD and $n=88$ without ASPD; all in community mental health centers	Study of integrated dual disorder treatment, comparing assertive community treatment (ACT) vs. standard clinical case management (SCCM)	Substance use (ASI), self-report and official records of housing history and stays in hospital or jail; self-report and laboratory measures of alcohol and drug use	The study found no between-condition differences in outcomes for the non-ASPD group. For individuals with ASPD, those receiving ACT showed significantly lower rates of both alcohol consumption and incarceration than did those receiving SCCM.
Havens et al. 2007	$N=162$ injection drug users (75.9% Black), of whom 22.8% were diagnosed with ASPD, enrolled in evaluation of Treatment Retention Intervention (TRI) in the Baltimore Needle Exchange Program	Random assignment to strengths-based case management intervention with several proactive elements vs. no active case management	Principal outcome: level of participation in treatment at 1-month follow-up visit after initial assessment; other variables (ASPD diagnosis, assigned group, site of treatment) were entered in regression	Individuals with ASPD who received ≥25 minutes of case management time were more likely to enter treatment than were those with <5 minutes or no exposure (OR=3.51; CI=1.03–11.90).
Longabaugh et al. 1994	$N=31$ persons with severe alcohol problems diagnosed with ASPD and $n=118$ non-ASPD problem drinkers attending an outpatient treatment setting	Individual CBT vs. joint relationship enhancement (RE) sessions with partner, both totaling 20 sessions	Alcohol consumption using TLFB procedure, days abstinent, and number of drinks per drinking day	At 13- to 18-month follow-up, differential outcome effects were observed; in both treatment conditions, ASPD groups had more days abstinent, with larger effect from individual CBT sessions. ASPD groups showed significantly lower drinking rate following CBT than RE; rates for non-ASPD groups were same in both.

TABLE 17–1. Randomized controlled trials of psychosocial interventions for ASPD *(continued)*

Study	Participants	Interventions and comparators	Monitoring and outcome measures	Main findings
McKay et al. 2000	*N*=127 male veteran cocaine-dependent hospital patients (84% African American), of whom 46 (36.2%) met criteria for diagnosis of ASPD	Individualized relapse prevention for 20 weeks vs. standard care (some addictions counseling and 12-step recovery practices)	ASI administered at 3-, 6-, and 12-month follow-up; self-report of cocaine and alcohol use (employing TLFB) at 12 months→days of substance use or abstinence; urine toxicology measures; rate of continuation in care	Follow-up rates were very high for main outcome variables (86.4%–96.2%). No differences were found between ASPD and non-ASPD groups in continuation of care or substance use from self-report or urine toxicology data. This was despite the finding that ASPD patients had more severe ASI indicators at initial assessment and therefore improved significantly more than did non-ASPD patients over time.
McKendrick et al. 2006	*N*=139 male prisoners with mental illness and chemical abuse disorders, of whom 49% were also classified as having a current diagnosis of ASPD	Modified therapeutic community (MTC) vs. standard mental health services (MH), all prison-based	Two outcome domains: self-reported involvement in crime and substance use (alcohol, illicit drugs) and official information on rates of reincarceration	Follow-up ("retrieval") rates at 12 months postrelease were 82% with MTC and 69% with MH; the rate for ASPD was 76%, and the rate without ASPD was 74%. Significant gains were made with MTC relative to MH regardless of ASPD status, ASPD reincarceration rate was zero, and outcome domains both showed significant effects.
Messina et al. 1999, 2002	*N*=275 adults (72% male, 98% Black) meeting ASPD criteria who had histories of substance abuse and criminality	Comparison of two therapeutic communities with different periods of inpatient and outpatient time (10+2 vs. 6+6 months)	Treatment completion rates, urinalysis, postdischarge criminal arrest records	No association was found between ASPD diagnosis and treatment outcomes; people diagnosed did as well as those who were not. Messina et al. (2002) concluded that individuals diagnosed with ASPD can benefit from therapeutic communities treatment and "do as well as those with no" ASPD (p. 209).

TABLE 17–1. Randomized controlled trials of psychosocial interventions for ASPD (*continued*)

Study	Participants	Interventions and comparators	Monitoring and outcome measures	Main findings
Messina et al. 2003	N=120 diagnosed cocaine-dependent clinic attendees (56% male, 38% white, 31% African American, 28% Hispanic), 44% of whom met criteria for ASPD, randomly assigned to one of four conditions, each lasting 16 weeks	Four conditions: CBT, CM, CBT+CM, and methadone maintenance	Level of treatment retention; substance use monitored by urinalysis 3 × a week during treatment and at 17-, 26-, and 52-week follow-up	No significant differences were found in treatment retention between ASPD and non-ASPD attendees. The ASPD group had a significantly higher rate of cocaine-negative samples during treatment and at 17 and 26 weeks. At 52 weeks, the rate of negative samples was still higher but was nonsignificant. Analysis showed effects were mainly related to the CM condition, although CBT results were also positive.
Neufeld et al. 2008	N=100 patients (77% male, 60% African American) diagnosed with ASPD and opioid dependence	CM of abstinence vs. standard methadone treatment	Attendance and retention rates, self-reported drug abuse, urinalysis test results, levels of psychosocial problems	At 6-month follow-up, the experimental group had significantly higher attendance in counseling sessions and significantly lower levels of psychosocial impairment. There were no differences in urinalysis results.
Swogger et al. 2016	N=105 substance-using adults (68 men, 37 women; 52% minority, 48% white) in a pretrial jail diversion program assessed for psychopathy using PCL-R	Brief motivational intervention+standard care vs. standard care alone	Daily substance use using TLFB; breathalyzer and urine screening; consequences of substance use (self-report); up to 6-month follow-up	Follow-up rates were similar in both arms (36/53 and 37/52), with overall 74.3% retention. Regression analysis found an interaction effect with the study condition: for high PCL-R Factor 1 and Factor 2 scores, more frequent substance abuse was indicated in both self-report and toxicology data.
Thylstrup and Hesse 2016; Thylstrup et al. 2015, 2017	N=175 (156 males) with comorbid ASPD and SUDs in community-based substance abuse treatment centers in Denmark	Impulsive Lifestyle Counseling psychoeducation program (6 sessions) vs. TAU (opioid substitution)	Reports of receiving help with ASPD recorded on Likert scales, days drug-abstinent (ASI), self-reported aggression (BPAQ)	At final follow-up (15 months, 61% contact), those assigned to experimental treatment perceived themselves as having had more help with both ASPD and SUDs; this was associated with having more days abstinent and a lower rate of dropout.

TABLE 17–1.　Randomized controlled trials of psychosocial interventions for ASPD *(continued)*

Study	Participants	Interventions and comparators	Monitoring and outcome measures	Main findings
Woodall et al. 2007	$N=52$ first-time driving while intoxicated (DWI) offenders diagnosed with ASPD, primarily male (86.5%) and indigenous American (71.2%), compared with a larger sample of DWI offenders	Incarceration (28 days)+a treatment program with 10 components and a motivational interviewing emphasis vs. incarceration alone	Self-reported measures of the frequency of drinking and driving; official records of DWI arrests 6, 12, and 24 months after discharge	ASPD participants had higher levels of drinking than others prior to intake; however, the ASPD group showed a larger improvement over time than did the non-ASPD cohort in self-reported DWI. ASPD participants in the treatment condition were considerably (but nonsignificantly) less likely to be rearrested for DWI than were those in the control group.
Woody et al. 1985	$N=110$ male patients referred for psychotherapy, including $n=16$ with opioid dependence (OP) alone; $n=16$ with OP and depression; $n=13$ with OP and ASPD; and $n=17$ with OP, ASPD, and depression	Three conditions: drug counseling alone, supportive-expressive psychotherapy+ counseling, and CBT+counseling	A range of clinical measures, ASI, and levels of drug use comparing four groups, two with ASPD and two without, at 7-month evaluation	Although the OP+ASPD group had the poorest outcome and the OP+depression group had the best results, the OP+ASPD+depression group fared almost as well as the latter subgroup (respective Cohen's *d* effect sizes of 0.50 and 0.53). The authors suggested that ASPD alone led to problems in forming relationships; and the experience of depression may have made participants more amenable to psychotherapy.

Note.　ASI=Addiction Severity Index; ASPD=antisocial personality disorder; AUDIT=Alcohol Use Disorders Identification Test; BPAQ=Buss-Perry Aggression Questionnaire; BPD=borderline personality disorder; IRI=Interpersonal Reactivity Index; MCVSI=MacArthur Community Violence Screening Instrument; NAS=Novaco Anger Scale; PCL-R=Psychopathy Checklist–Revised; SPSI=Social Problem-Solving Inventory; SUDs=substance use disorders; TAU=treatment as usual; TLFB=Timeline Followback.

8 of them found no evidence of differences with respect to retention in treatment or in recorded treatment effects.

Finally, the process of compiling reviews for the table was supplemented by a separate literature search of the PsycINFO and MEDLINE electronic databases from January 2012 to March 2020 using the terms *antisocial personality disorder or ASPD or dissocial personality disorder, intervention or treatment or therapy,* and *randomized (or randomised) controlled trial or RCT* and inspecting the reference lists of the located research reports. Studies are listed in Table 17–1 in alphabetical order by the first author's surname.

Potentially, many outcome variables could be evaluated in this field, and the listed studies contain an assortment of them. They include aspects of clinical symptoms that constitute the diagnostic criteria for ASPD: social functioning; psychological well-being; and behavioral indicators, principally relating to aggression or violence, and recorded criminality. No single criterion can be used to measure whether an intervention "works," but the concept of being untreatable does not specify precisely in what sense that term applies. In principle, presumably almost any clinical or behavioral indicator used in mental health or criminal justice research could be of interest.

A controlled trial of an intervention combining psychoeducation and a group problem-solving training program was omitted because it included participants with a range of types of personality disorder (Huband et al. 2007; McMurran et al. 2016). Only a small proportion (15%) of the treatment sample met criteria for ASPD, and data for that group were not analyzed separately. It was also unclear what proportion of the sample met criteria for more than one type of personality disorder. For similar reasons, an evaluation of the structured group program Systems Training for Emotional Predictability and Problem Solving (Black et al. 2016) was excluded because it focused primarily on participants diagnosed with borderline personality disorder (BPD), comparing those with and without a concomitant diagnosis of ASPD. However, it is noteworthy that participants with comorbid BPD and ASPD did as well as, and on some measures marginally better than, those with BPD alone. A study by Tyrer et al. (2004) was eliminated because no separate data were given for the 15 participants diagnosed with dissocial personality disorder, who, in any event, constituted only a small fraction (3%) of the sample. A study by Marlowe et al. (2007) was excluded because it did not allocate participants with ASPD to different conditions or provide separate data on the ASPD group relative to others. Instead, ASPD was used as part of a high-risk selection strategy in group assignment. Again, however, it is of note that during the study, participants with ASPD and a history of drug treatment attended drug court more frequently than did their lower-risk counterparts.

Although the studies listed in Table 17–1 all used randomized designs and most subgroups were of approximately similar size, there are interpretative difficulties in some instances. For example, the studies by Brooner et al. (1998) and Neufeld et al. (2008) were conducted at the same clinic and contained overlapping rather than independent samples, but because the latter report involved many more participants after a 10-year gap, the two studies have been listed separately in the table. In the studies of Cullen et al. (2012a, 2012b), the process of social-cognitive skills assessment was not conducted blind, and there was a rather high level of treatment attrition. Thus, despite the initial randomization, it was not possible to conclude that observed changes were treatment effects. Equally, however, Table 17–1 presents only key outcomes.

There are many discrete findings within the studies. For example, in the study by Swogger et al. (2016), data were analyzed for associations with specific PCL-R traits. Analysis of their results showed that the affective but not the interpersonal facets of psychopathy Factor 1 had a moderating effect on the percentage of days on which study participants attended substance abuse treatment. This provides partial support for the proposals of Olver (2018) and Wong (2016), as outlined earlier.

As can be seen in the second column of Table 17–1, the sample sizes in most studies were not large, and in most cases follow-up periods were short as compared with treatment outcome research in some other fields. None of the studies entailed a comparison with a non-ASPD group equivalent to the experimental participants in other key respects, although any such design would give rise to other methodological objections.

Drawing all this together, what can we conclude? A small number of studies evaluating psychosocial interventions have used RCT designs. In these studies, sample sizes were relatively modest, follow-up periods were short, and the results were mixed in that the designated experimental intervention did not always outperform the comparison condition. On the contrary, in most of the studies, positive changes were observed in ASPD groups, and some of them were statistically significant and clinically meaningful. In addition, reviews of other research that used quasi-experimental, nonequivalent, or simply before-and-after designs have found a variety of positive outcomes. To this can be added other reviews of intervention studies concerned with reducing violence, with study samples highly likely to contain a proportion, if not a majority, of participants with features of ASPD. The overall picture as it stands is far from amounting to one that can identify a treatment of choice. Equally, however, the evidence is incompatible with the long-held view that this clinical group is not susceptible to change or amenable to intervention.

Therapeutic Relationship

Psychosocial therapy is an interactive process and necessarily requires the formation and management of a collaborative relationship between the therapist (however the role is designated) and the patient or service user. The extent to which the *working alliance* is perceived as central or as the vehicle of change and the importance accorded to it differ greatly between therapeutic orientations. It is commonly anticipated that establishing a therapeutic liaison presents additional demands when attempting engagement with someone with ASPD. This may be a broader expectation about working with people who have broken the law. However, in comparison to the volume of mental health research on the therapeutic relationship, there have been few studies focused on working with offenders. Hence, the issues at stake are less well understood (Blasko et al. 2018).

However, within the available studies, it is possible to distinguish different treatment approaches. In clinical therapies informed by psychodynamic models, a concern is that engaging persons with a diagnosis of ASPD in therapy is problematic because of a likely negative countertransference on the part of the therapist. A productive therapeutic alliance cannot then be established, and therapy probably will not succeed. Describing one variant of psychodynamically based practice, transference focused therapy, Kernberg (2016) contended that the approach has had success in treating "personality disordered patients with significant antisocial traits and behavior, but not antisocial personality disorder proper" (p. 386). There are, however, no evaluative data supporting these points. In contrast, Evans (2011) reported several case studies of psychoanalytic work with detained patients diagnosed with ASPD. He described the mental states associated with the disorder as "infectious" (p. 146), which can leave clinicians "feeling either helpless and ineffective or intimidated and frightened" (p. 153). To protect the professional's mental health, it is vital when undertaking work of this kind to have available both clinical supervision and opportunities for reflective practice. These support mechanisms can help "to decontaminate unhealthy aspects of the clinical situation that get lodged inside staff in an unhelpful way" (p. 155).

From other directions, a small quantity of research findings indicate that it is feasible to establish and maintain effective therapeutic relationships with individuals diagnosed with ASPD. Ross et al. (2008) proposed a model of how the working alliance concept can be applied in the field of offender rehabilitation. Several studies have investigated levels of therapeutic collaboration with high-risk offenders convicted of sexual or violent offenses. In some research, a similar problem arises as found elsewhere: although it is likely that some of the participants met ASPD diagnostic criteria, this cannot be ascertained because it was not reported.

Other studies, however, have undertaken assessments of the therapeutic relationship with individuals who have ASPD. Polaschek and Ross (2010) described a study of 50 men convicted of violent offenses who took part in a prison-based treatment program in New Zealand. The authors used the Working Alliance Inventory (WAI; Horvath and Greenberg 1989), a measure well attested for this purpose, to explore the client-therapist relationship at different stages of the 93-session program. More than half of the participants scored in the psychopathic range on the PCL-R. These men completed the WAI at different stages of treatment, as did a total of 10 therapists who worked with them in different treatment groups over 3.5 years. In the opening phase of the program, therapists' ratings on the WAI showed low expectations of prisoners' levels of motivation. However, the men's scores on the WAI were in a similar range to those found in populations without ASPD. Moreover, as the program progressed, there was a significant correlation between change scores on several risk measures and increases over time in scores on the WAI.

In a study of 89 convicted sex offenders in a U.S. maximum security prison, Walton et al. (2018) found low, nonsignificant correlations between PCL-R scores and scores on the WAI. There were no indications that individuals scoring in the upper range of antisocial personality variables were incapable of forming a therapeutic alliance. Working with 111 incarcerated male federal sex offenders in Canada who participated in the Clearwater treatment program mentioned earlier, DeSorcy et al. (2020) found that "even high PCL-R scoring men demonstrated the capacity to establish working alliances with their primary therapist within the context of sex offender treatment" (p. 1753). These findings call into question the expectation that individuals who have committed serious crimes and who are assessed as showing high levels of antisociality are not amenable to forming and benefiting from a therapeutic alliance.

Treatment and Service Guidelines

In the absence of a reasonable quantity or a consolidated array of clinical research findings, which could form an unambiguous basis for making treatment decisions, the next best option is often believed to be the development of a set of principles or guidelines that can inform clinical decision-making and service planning. As noted in the subsection "The 'Untreatability' Myth," such a suggestion was made by Lösel (1998) with reference to psychopathy, and since then the possibility has also been pursued in relation to the broader category of ASPD.

Probably the most extensive and elaborate set of proposals was devised by the National Institute for Health and Care Excellence (NICE) in the United Kingdom. Since the introduction of NICE in 1999, the organization's appointed role has been to compile and publish evidence-based guidance for the delivery of health and social care. To prepare such a document in relation to ASPD, a multiprofessional development group was formed and then embarked on a detailed review of research and patterns of practice and service delivery pertaining to ASPD (National Collaborating Centre for Mental Health 2010). The relative sparsity of well-validated evidence—previous systematic reviews at that point had identified only five controlled trials—led to the decision to adopt a "pragmatic, practical, threefold strategy" (Duggan and Kane 2010, p. 5) drawing on related areas of relevance. In the first part, the researchers examined the possibility of preventing ASPD, collating research on whether the treatment of childhood conduct disorder could avert its continuation into personality disorder in adulthood. In the second part, they considered findings from criminology and applied psychology on the reduction of offending behavior and criminal recidivism. Third, the group examined clinical research on conditions that are frequently comorbid with ASPD.

The ASPD guideline was developed against a background of increasing awareness that people with any type of personality disorder often have problems accessing health care services and that efforts had been made to change relevant policy (National Institute for Mental Health in England 2003). The resultant guideline contained a series of proposals with the principal objective of rectifying this detrimental position. The document was intended to "promote the implementation of best clinical practice" (National Collaborating Centre for Mental Health 2010, p. 13) and therefore provided a series of recommendations focused on the organization and delivery of services for the management of ASPD. These recommendations included the following:

- Assessment of both clinical problems and antisocial behavior as far as possible using structured methods
- Providing equality of access to services and minimizing disruption while doing so
- Ensuring proper coordination of services and collaboration between care providers through interagency networks of referral systems and specialized facilities
- Training and ongoing supervision of staff at all levels of service in developing awareness of ASPD and in acquiring the necessary competences for providing the most constructive responses to need and risk

The last point was thought to apply not only to clinicians or therapists working in mental health but also to general medical practitioners, who, as the first port of call for persons seeking medical help, are the gateway to secondary services such as general hospitals and tertiary services such as secure psychiatric units or specialized community services for individuals with personality disorders (National Collaborating Centre for Mental Health 2010). Numerous other detailed proposals were made in the NICE document concerning quality assurance and maintenance of standards, access to services by members of ethnic minorities, and transparency in the communication of information. It was recommended that care providers discuss with service users the implications of an ASPD diagnosis to build trusting relationships with the health care staff. Overall, given the sparse amount of knowledge on effective treatment, the NICE guidance was concerned primarily with management.

There continues to be wide recognition that when individuals likely to meet criteria for an ASPD diagnosis seek help, it is typically for other problems they are experiencing, such as depression, anxiety, substance misuse, or relationship discord. Given the complexity of presentation, the presence of ASPD can sometimes detract from efforts to ameliorate those problems, with some individuals resisting or even refusing treatment. For a proportion of these individuals, resistance is likely to occur in the context of criminal justice or secure mental health services, where they may show what are construed as treatment-interfering behaviors, although these behaviors remain poorly understood (Klein Haneveld et al. 2018), and the research reviewed earlier suggests that their frequency may be overestimated.

Nevertheless, safety issues must be considered, and necessary precautionary procedures must be introduced. For example, attempts to provide treatment on a solitary clinical basis are inadvisable. In routine services in hospitals or in community clinical settings, solitary treatment is unlikely to occur because the modal pattern of service delivery is reliant on multidisciplinary teams, usually comprising a minimum of a psychiatrist, a clinical or forensic psychologist, nursing or residential care staff, and a range of other professionals such as occupational therapists, probation officers, and social workers. However, for therapists working in private practice who become aware of serious personality dysfunction in their patients, it is wise for them to make interagency contacts or seek other forms of peer support. Doing so is important in order to have a mechanism for monitoring of progress, to guard against the possibility of boundary violations, and, in some circumstances, also to ensure personal safety. Risk management is further discussed in Chapter 19, "Treatment Issues With Antisocial Personality Disorder."

The ASPD guideline was the subject of generally welcoming and positive comments from a range of experienced clinicians and researchers (Black and Blum 2020; Emmelkamp and Vedel 2010; Evans 2010; Polaschek 2010; Trestman and Lazrove 2010). However, there were also some reservations and criticisms. Evans (2010) expressed disappointment at the exclusion of studies that included patients who had comorbid ASPD and serious psychoses such as schizophrenia. Polaschek (2010) considered that the guideline took insufficient account of the "poorly defined nature" (p. 20) of ASPD, drawing attention to some of the conceptual and empirical implications of this lack of definition and illustrating how it affected the interpretation of some areas of research covered in the review. Other authors had raised such definitional issues even while the work of the NICE group was in progress (Pickersgill 2009). Polaschek (2010) also described some of the guideline recommendations as "disappointingly generic" (p. 27), potentially applying to service users with other types of mental health problems.

According to the NICE website, the guideline was revised in 2013 and audited again in 2018 to check whether further revisions were required. In 2018, a "surveillance decision" was made, to the effect that no new evidence had been found that required altering the advice given in the guideline (National Institute of Health and Care Excellence 2018). This took account of changes to the classification of personality disorder in the (then pending) eleventh revision of the International Classification of Diseases (ICD-11). NICE planned to perform an exceptional surveillance review in 2021 in order to gauge the reaction of the community to ICD-11 and to consider any potential effect on the recommendations made. At the time of writing, that work was still under way, but the National Institute for Health and Care Excellence (2021) published an online interactive flowchart facilitating access to all its published material.

Ensuing service developments followed similar lines in operationalizing procedures for the provision of services that can meet the needs of individuals with ASPD within a context of risk management, where appropriate (Joseph and Benefield 2012). In England and Wales, this included the development of the Offender Personality Disorder Pathway program (Campbell and Craissati 2018; Minoudis and Kane 2017). This program was set up to provide nearly 1,000 new places in prisons and probation hostels for the treatment of offenders with personality disorder between 2012 and 2017. Drawing on examples from other countries, notably the Netherlands and Canada, the strategy involved introducing new and more thorough screening and assessment methods, creating a specialized model of care, and training staff in their implementation. This also entailed developing processes for interagency commissioning of services according to the levels and types of need identified in the target population (Burns et al. 2018). A central feature of this development has been the use of case formulation as a means of understanding the interconnections of different needs at an individual level (Minoudis and Shaw 2018), a point amplified more broadly by Franke et al. (2019).

For many individuals with ASPD, the route to health care is often through the criminal courts, to imprisonment or detention in secure psychiatric units. The Offender Personality Disorder Pathway is designed to enhance the joint working of these parallel but in some ways markedly different systems. An evaluation framework has been developed for the program (Craissati and Campbell 2018), but information on outcomes was not yet available at the time of writing. However, some preliminary studies of components of the project have yielded promising results (Bruce et al. 2017; Jolliffe et al. 2017). At the same time, this departure has also been the target of some trenchant criticism because it was the successor to an earlier initiative, the Dangerous and Severe Personality Disorder program, which was very widely deemed to have been a failure (O'Loughlin 2014; Tyrer et al. 2010). The public profile of any innovation in this area is such that it becomes very difficult to evaluate it without also considering its context in wider public-political debates.

Conclusion

Given what is known, if precise treatment recommendations for ASPD cannot be made, the likeliest explanation is that we have not yet succeeded in inventing them.

Until we do, the disparaging "untreatable" label should be dispensed with. This is not to deny that some individuals are extremely unresponsive or resistant to change. Most mental health practitioners can probably think of examples of antisocial individuals with whom they made very little or even no progress. But that difficulty is not confined to working with people who have received an ASPD diagnosis. It could arise with many types of mental health problems or because of personal history, abusive or traumatic experience, extreme circumstances, the perceived threats or costs of change, or previous treatment failures due to other factors, including poor service. Difficult-to-treat patients or clients can be found who have received varied kinds of diagnoses. Such difficulty is not an inherent characteristic of just one type of mental health problem. It is more likely a function of the severity of the problem, of the complexity of factors influencing it, or of the time that lapsed before the individual was able to seek help. Overall, further refinement of the concept of ASPD may be warranted if significant improvements are to be achieved in the nature and range of clinical interventions.

Key Points

- Although there is a long-standing debate about the "treatability" of antisocial personality disorder (ASPD), there is no evidence that treatment makes people with ASPD worse.

- Surveys of mental health professionals do not support the view that the likelihood of treatment success is universally believed to be low.

- Reviews have reported mixed results for psychosocial treatments, but most studies reviewed here found equivalent outcomes for participants with and without ASPD. This calls into question the untreatability of ASPD.

- Therapeutic alliance and involvement of multidisciplinary mental health teams are important considerations in treating this patient population.

References

American Psychiatric Association: Diagnostic and Statistical Manual of Mental Disorders, 3rd Edition, Revised. Washington, DC, American Psychiatric Association, 1987
Barker ET, McLaughlin AJ: The total encounter capsule. Can Psychiatr Assoc J 22(7):355–360, 1977 589550
Bateman A, O'Connell J, Lorenzini N, et al: A randomised controlled trial of mentalization-based treatment versus structured clinical management for patients with comorbid borderline personality disorder and antisocial personality disorder. BMC Psychiatry 16:304, 2016 27577562
Bazar JL: The Oak Ridge program. Remembering Oak Ridge: Digital Archive and Exhibit. Toronto, ON, Canada, Waypoint Centre for Health Care. 2015. Available at: https://historyexhibit.waypointcentre.ca/exhibits/show/treatment/or-program. Accessed April 20, 2021.
Black DW: Bad Boys, Bad Men: Confronting Antisocial Personality Disorder (Sociopathy). New York, Oxford University Press, 2013

Black DW: The natural history of antisocial personality disorder. Can J Psychiatry 60(7):309–314, 2015 26175389

Black DW: The treatment of antisocial personality disorder. Curr Treat Options Psychiatry 4(4):295–302, 2017

Black DW, Blum N: Commentary: Response to NICE: guidelines for the treatment of antisocial personality disorder. Personal Ment Health 4(2):9–11, 2020

Black DW, Baumgard CH, Bell SE: A 16- to 45-year follow-up of 71 men with antisocial personality disorder. Compr Psychiatry 36(2):130–140, 1995 7758299

Black DW, Gunter T, Loveless P, et al: Antisocial personality disorder in incarcerated offenders: psychiatric comorbidity and quality of life. Ann Clin Psychiatry 22(2):113–120, 2010 20445838

Black DW, Simsek-Duran F, Blum N, et al: Do people with borderline personality disorder complicated by antisocial personality disorder benefit from the STEPPS treatment program? Personal Ment Health 10(3):205–215, 2016 26671625

Blasko BL, Serran G, Abracen J: The role of the therapeutic alliance in offender therapy, in New Frontiers in Offender Treatment. Edited by Jeglic EL, Calkins C. Cham, Switzerland, Springer Nature, 2018, pp 87–108

Brooner RK, Kidorf M, King VL, et al: Preliminary evidence of good treatment response in antisocial drug abusers. Drug Alcohol Depend 49(3):249–260, 1998 9571389

Bruce M, Horgan H, Kerr R, et al: Psychologically informed practice (PIP) for staff working with offenders with personality disorder: a pragmatic exploratory trial in approved premises. Crim Behav Ment Health 27(4):290–302, 2017 26864888

Budge SL, Moore JT, Del Re AC, et al: The effectiveness of evidence-based treatments for personality disorders when comparing treatment-as-usual and bona fide treatments. Clin Psychol Rev 33(8):1057–1066, 2013 24060812

Budge SL, Moore JT, Del Re AC, et al: Corrigendum to "The effectiveness of evidence-based treatments for personality disorders when comparing treatment-as-usual and bona fide treatments." Clin Psychol Rev 34:451–452, 2014

Burns M, Campbell C, Craissati J: The offender personality disorder pathway: modelling collaborative commissioning in the NHS and criminal justice system, in Managing Personality Disordered Offenders: A Pathways Approach. Edited by Campbell C, Craissati J. Oxford, UK, Oxford University Press, 2018, pp 175–202

Campbell C, Craissati J: Introduction, in Managing Personality Disordered Offenders: A Pathways Approach. Edited by Campbell C, Craissati J. Oxford, UK, Oxford University Press, 2018, pp 1–25

Carr WA: The impact of personality disorders on legally supervised community treatment: a systematic literature review. Community Ment Health J 50(6):664–672, 2014 24068584

Coid J, Ullrich S: Antisocial personality disorder is on a continuum with psychopathy. Compr Psychiatry 51(4):426–433, 2010 20579518

Craissati J, Campbell C: Making an impact: have we got it right yet? in Managing Personality Disordered Offenders: A Pathways Approach. Edited by Campbell C, Craissati J. Oxford, UK, Oxford University Press, 2018, pp 203–215

Cullen AE, Clarke AY, Kuipers E, et al: A multi-site randomized controlled trial of a cognitive skills programme for male mentally disordered offenders: social-cognitive outcomes. Psychol Med 42(3):557–569, 2012a 21846425

Cullen AE, Clarke AY, Kuipers E, et al: A multisite randomized trial of a cognitive skills program for male mentally disordered offenders: violence and antisocial behavior outcomes. J Consult Clin Psychol 80(6):1114–1120, 2012b 23025249

Davidson KM, Tyrer P, Tata P, et al: Cognitive behaviour therapy for violent men with antisocial personality disorder in the community: an exploratory randomized controlled trial. Psychol Med 39(4):569–577, 2009 18667099

DeSorcy DR, Olver ME, Wormith JS: Working alliance and psychopathy: linkages to treatment outcome in a sample of treated sexual offenders. J Interpers Violence 35(7–8):1739–1760, 2020 29294686

D'Silva K, Duggan C, McCarthy L: Does treatment really make psychopaths worse? A review of the evidence. J Pers Disord 18(2):163–177, 2004 15176755

Duggan C, Kane E: Commentary: Developing a national institute of clinical excellence and health guideline for antisocial personality disorder. Personal Ment Health 4(1):3–8, 2010

Duggan C, Huband N, Smailagic N, et al: The use of psychological treatments for people with personality disorder: a systematic review of randomized controlled trials. Personal Ment Health 1(2):95–125, 2007

Easton CJ, Oberleitner LM, Scott MC, et al: Differences in treatment outcome among marijuana-dependent young adults with and without antisocial personality disorder. Am J Drug Alcohol Abuse 38(4):305–313, 2012 22242558

Emmelkamp PMG, Vedel E: Commentary: Psychological treatments for antisocial personality disorder: where is the evidence that group treatment and therapeutic community should be recommended? Personal Ment Health 4(1):30–33, 2010

Evans C: Commentary: The NICE ASPD guidelines: a clinical perspective. Personal Ment Health 4:16–19, 2010

Evans M: Pinned against the ropes: understanding antisocial personality-disordered patients through use of the countertransference. Psychoanal Psychother 25:143–156, 2011

Fazel S, Danesh J: Serious mental disorder in 23000 prisoners: a systematic review of 62 surveys. Lancet 359(9306):545–550, 2002 11867106

Felthous AR: The "untreatability" of psychopathy and hospital commitment in the USA. Int J Law Psychiatry 34(6):400–405, 2011 22079085

Festinger DS, Marlowe DB, Lee PA, et al: Status hearings in drug court: when more is less and less is more. Drug Alcohol Depend 68(2):151–157, 2002 12234644

Franke I, Nigel S, Dudeck M: What might work when nothing seems to work: case formulation in the treatment of antisocial personality disorder in a forensic mental health setting, in Case Formulation for Personality Disorders: Tailoring Psychotherapy to the Individual Client. Edited by Kramer U, Zanarini MC. London, Academic Press, 2019, pp 161–180

Frisman LK, Mueser KT, Covell NH, et al: Use of integrated dual disorder treatment via assertive community treatment versus clinical case management for persons with co-occurring disorders and antisocial personality disorder. J Nerv Ment Dis 197(11):822–828, 2009 19996720

Gibbon S, Duggan C, Stoffers J, et al: Psychological interventions for antisocial personality disorder. Cochrane Database Syst Rev (6):CD007668, 2010 20556783

Hare RD: The Hare Psychopathy Checklist—Revised. North Tonawanda, NY, Multi-Health Systems, 1991

Hare RD, Neumann CS: Psychopathy as a clinical and empirical construct. Annu Rev Clin Psychol 4:217–246, 2008 18370617

Harris GT, Rice ME: Treatment of psychopathy: a review of empirical findings, in Handbook of Psychopathy. Edited by Patrick CJ. New York, Guilford, 2006, pp 555–572

Harris GT, Rice ME, Cormier CA: Psychopaths: is a therapeutic community therapeutic? Ther Commun 15(4):283–299, 1994

Hatchett GT: Treatment guidelines for clients with antisocial personality disorder. J Ment Health Couns 37(1):15–27, 2015

Havens JR, Cornelius LJ, Ricketts EP, et al: The effect of a case management intervention on drug treatment entry among treatment-seeking injection drug users with and without comorbid antisocial personality disorder. J Urban Health 84(2):267–271, 2007 17334939

Hesse M, Pedersen MU: Antisocial personality disorder and retention: a systematic review. Ther Commun 27:495–504, 2006

Horvath AO, Greenberg LS: Development and validation of the Working Alliance Inventory. J Couns Psychol 36(2):223–233, 1989

Huband N, McMurran M, Evans C, et al: Social problem-solving plus psychoeducation for adults with personality disorder: pragmatic randomised controlled trial. Br J Psychiatry 190:307–313, 2007 17401036

Jolliffe D, Cattell J, Raza A, et al: Evaluating the impact of the London Pathway Project. Crim Behav Ment Health 27(3):238–253, 2017 28677902

Joseph N, Benefield N: A joint offender personality disorder pathway strategy: an outline summary. Crim Behav Ment Health 22(3):210–217, 2012 22711617

Kernberg OF: New developments in transference focused psychotherapy. Int J Psychoanal 97(2):385–407, 2016 27112823

Klein Haneveld E, Neumann CS, Smid W, et al: Treatment responsiveness of replicated psychopathy profiles. Law Hum Behav 42(5):484–495, 2018 30272468

Longabaugh R, Rubin A, Malloy P, et al: Drinking outcomes of alcohol abusers diagnosed as antisocial personality disorder. Alcohol Clin Exp Res 18(4):778–785, 1994 7978086

Lösel F: Treatment and management of psychopaths, in Psychopathy: Theory, Research, and Implications for Society. Edited by Cooke D, Forth AE, Hare RA. Dordrecht, The Netherlands, Springer Science and Business Media, 1998, pp 303–354

Marlowe DB, Festinger DS, Dugosh KL, et al: Adapting judicial supervision to the risk level of drug offenders: discharge and 6-month outcomes from a prospective matching study. Drug Alcohol Depend 88 (suppl 2):S4–S13, 2007 17071020

McGuire J: What works with violent offenders? A response to "nothing works," in The Wiley Handbook of What Works in Violence Risk Management: Theory, Research, and Practice. Edited by Wormith JS, Craig LA, Hogue TE. Chichester, UK, Wiley, 2020, pp 53–78

McKay JR, Alterman AI, Cacciola JS, et al: Prognostic significance of antisocial personality disorder in cocaine-dependent patients entering continuing care. J Nerv Ment Dis 188(5):287–296, 2000 10830566

McKendrick K, Sullivan C, Banks S, et al: Modified therapeutic community treatment for offenders with MICA disorders: antisocial personality disorder and treatment outcomes. J Offender Rehabil 44(2):133–159, 2006

McMurran M, Crawford MJ, Reilly J, et al: Psychoeducation with problem-solving (PEPS) therapy for adults with personality disorder: a pragmatic randomised controlled trial to determine the clinical effectiveness and cost-effectiveness of a manualised intervention to improve social functioning. Health Technol Assess 20(52):1–250, 2016 27431341

Messina NP, Wish ED, Nemes S: Therapeutic community treatment for substance abusers with antisocial personality disorder. J Subst Abuse Treat 17(1–2):121–128, 1999 10435260

Messina NP, Wish ED, Hoffman JA, et al: Antisocial personality disorder and TC treatment outcomes. Am J Drug Alcohol Abuse 28(2):197–212, 2002 12014812

Messina N, Farabee D, Rawson R: Treatment responsivity of cocaine-dependent patients with antisocial personality disorder to cognitive-behavioral and contingency management interventions. J Consult Clin Psychol 71(2):320–329, 2003 12699026

Minoudis P, Kane E: It's a journey, not a destination—from dangerous and severe personality disorder (DSPD) to the offender personality disorder (OPD) pathway. Crim Behav Ment Health 27(3):207–213, 2017 28677904

Minoudis P, Shaw J: Case identification and formulation, in Managing Personality Disordered Offenders: A Pathways Approach. Edited by Campbell C, Craissati J. Oxford, UK, Oxford University Press, 2018, pp 55–81

National Collaborating Centre for Mental Health: Antisocial Personality Disorder: The NICE Guideline on Treatment, Management and Prevention. National Clinical Practice Guideline No 77. London, British Psychological Society and the Royal College of Psychiatrists, 2010

National Institute of Health and Care Excellence: 2018 surveillance of personality disorders. 2018. Available at: www.nice.org.uk/guidance/cg77/resources/2018-surveillance-of-personality-disorders-nice-guidelines-cg77-and-cg78-4906490080/chapter/Surveillance-decision?tab=evidence. Accessed April 20, 2021.

National Institute of Health and Care Excellence: Personality disorders overview: antisocial personality disorder. 2021. Available at: https://pathways.nice.org.uk/pathways/personality-disorders#path=view%3A/pathways/personality-disorders/antisocial-personality-disorder.xml&content=view-index. Accessed October 4, 2021.

National Institute for Mental Health in England: Personality Disorder: No Longer a Diagnosis of Exclusion. Policy Implementation Guidance for the Development of Services for People With Personality Disorder. London, National Institute for Mental Health in England, 2003

Neufeld KJ, Kidorf MS, Kolodner K, et al: A behavioral treatment for opioid-dependent pa-
     tients with antisocial personality. J Subst Abuse Treat 34(1):101–111, 2008 17574801
Newton-Howes GM, Foulds JA, Guy NH, et al: Personality disorder and alcohol treatment out-
     come: systematic review and meta-analysis. Br J Psychiatry 211(1):22–30, 2017 28385703
O'Loughlin A: The offender personality disorder pathway: expansion in the face of failure?
     Howard Journal of Crime and Justice 53(2):173–192, 2014
Olver ME: Can psychopathy be treated? What the research tells us, in New Frontiers in Of-
     fender Treatment: The Translation of Evidence-Based Practices to Correctional Settings.
     Edited by Jeglic EL, Calkins C. Cham, Switzerland, Springer Nature, 2018, pp 287–306
Olver ME, Wong SC: Therapeutic responses of psychopathic sexual offenders: treatment attri-
     tion, therapeutic change, and long-term recidivism. J Consult Clin Psychol 77(2):328–336,
     2009 19309191
Olver ME, Wong SCP: A description and research review of the Clearwater Sex Offender Treat-
     ment Programme. Psychol Crime Law 19(5–6):477–492, 2013
Papalia N, Spivak B, Daffern M, et al: A meta-analytic review of the efficacy of psychological
     treatments for violent offenders in correctional and forensic mental health settings. Clin
     Psychol Sci Pract 26(1):e12282, 2019
Pickersgill MD: NICE guidelines, clinical practice and antisocial personality disorder: the eth-
     ical implications of ontological uncertainty. J Med Ethics 35(11):668–671, 2009 19880702
Polaschek DLL: Commentary: What do mental health services offer to people with antisocial
     personality disorder? A commentary on the NICE clinical guideline. Personal Ment Health
     4(1):20–29, 2010
Polaschek DLL: Adult criminals with psychopathy: common beliefs about treatability and
     change have little empirical support. Current Directions in Psychological Science
     23(4):296–301, 2014
Polaschek DLL, Daly TE: Treatment and psychopathy in forensic settings. Aggress Violent Be-
     hav 18:592–603, 2013
Polaschek DLL, Ross EC: Do early therapeutic alliance, motivation, and stages of change pre-
     dict therapy change for high-risk, psychopathic violent prisoners? Crim Behav Ment
     Health 20(2):100–111, 2010 20352647
Polaschek DLL, Skeem JL: Treatment of adults and juveniles with psychopathy, in Handbook
     of Psychopathy, 2nd Edition. Edited by Patrick CJ. New York, Guilford, 2018, pp 710–731
Power P: Doctors tortured patients at Ontario mental-health centre, judge rules. The Globe and
     Mail, June 7, 2017. Available at: www.theglobeandmail.com/news/national/doctors-at-
     ontario-mental-health-facility-tortured-patients-court-finds/article35246519. Accessed
     April 20, 2021.
Reidy DE, Kearns MC, DeGue S: Reducing psychopathic violence: a review of the treatment lit-
     erature. Aggress Violent Behav 18(5):527–538, 2013 29593447
Rice ME, Harris GT, Cormier CA: An evaluation of a maximum security therapeutic commu-
     nity for psychopaths and other mentally disordered offenders. Law Hum Behav 16(4):399–
     412, 1992
Ross EC, Polaschek DLL, Ward T: The therapeutic alliance: a theoretical revision for offender
     rehabilitation. Aggress Violent Behav 13(6):462–480, 2008
Ross J, Quayle E, Newman E, et al: The impact of psychological therapies on violent behaviour
     in clinical and forensic settings: a systematic review. Aggress Violent Behav 18(6):761–773,
     2013
Salekin RT: Psychopathy and therapeutic pessimism: clinical lore or clinical reality? Clin Psy-
     chol Rev 22(1):79–112, 2002 11793579
Salekin RT, Worley C, Grimes RD: Treatment of psychopathy: a review and brief introduction
     to the mental model approach for psychopathy. Behav Sci Law 28(2):235–266, 2010
     20422648
Skeem JL, Monahan J, Mulvey EP: Psychopathy, treatment involvement, and subsequent vio-
     lence among civil psychiatric patients. Law Hum Behav 26(6):577–603, 2002 12508696

Swogger MT, Conner KR, Caine ED, et al: A test of core psychopathic traits as a moderator of the efficacy of a brief motivational intervention for substance-using offenders. J Consult Clin Psychol 84(3):248–258, 2016 26727409

Tennet G, Tennent D, Prins H, et al: Is psychopathic disorder a treatable condition? Med Sci Law 33(1):63–66, 1993 8429770

Thylstrup B, Hesse M: Impulsive lifestyle counseling to prevent dropout from treatment for substance use disorders in people with antisocial personality disorder: a randomized study. Addict Behav 57:48–54, 2016 26882500

Thylstrup B, Schrøder S, Hesse M: Psycho-education for substance use and antisocial personality disorder: a randomized trial. BMC Psychiatry 15:283, 2015 26573140

Thylstrup B, Schrøder S, Fridell M, et al: Did you get any help? A post-hoc secondary analysis of a randomized controlled trial of psychoeducation for patients with antisocial personality disorder in outpatient substance abuse treatment programs. BMC Psychiatry 17(1):7, 2017 28068951

Trestman RL, Lazrove S: Commentary: On the coming of age of antisocial personality disorder: a commentary on the NICE treatment guidelines for antisocial personality disorder. Personal Ment Health 4:12–15, 2010

Tyrer P, Tom B, Byford S, et al: Differential effects of manual assisted cognitive behavior therapy in the treatment of recurrent deliberate self-harm and personality disturbance: the POPMACT study. J Pers Disord 18(1):102–116, 2004 15061347

Tyrer P, Duggan C, Cooper S, et al: The successes and failures of the DSPD experiment: the assessment and management of severe personality disorder. Med Sci Law 50(2):95–99, 2010 20593601

van den Bosch LMC, Rijckmans MJN, Decoene S, et al: Treatment of antisocial personality disorder: development of a practice focused framework. Int J Law Psychiatry 58:72–78, 2018 29853015

Walton A, Jeglic EL, Blasko BL: The role of psychopathic traits in the development of the therapeutic alliance among sexual offenders. Sex Abuse 30(3):211–229, 2018 27000265

Weisman R: Reflections on the Oak Ridge experiment with mentally disordered offenders, 1965–1968. Int J Law Psychiatry 18(3):265–290, 1995 7591397

Wilson HA: Can antisocial personality be treated? A meta-analysis examining the effectiveness of treatment in reducing recidivism for individuals diagnosed with ASPD. Int J Forensic Ment Health 13(1):36–46, 2014

Wilson NJ, Tamatea A: Challenging the "urban myth" of psychopathy untreatability: the High-Risk Personality Programme. Psychol Crime Law 19(5–6):493–510, 2013

Wong SCP: Treatment of violence-prone individuals with psychopathic personality traits, in Integrated Treatment for Personality Disorder: A Modular Approach. Edited by Livesley WJ, Dimaggio G, Clarkin JF. New York, Guilford, 2016, pp 345–376

Wong S, Gordon A, Gu D, et al: The effectiveness of violence reduction treatment for psychopathic offenders: empirical evidence and a treatment model. Int J Forensic Ment Health 11(4):336–349, 2012

Woodall WG, Delaney HD, Kunitz SJ, et al: A randomized trial of a DWI intervention program for first offenders: intervention outcomes and interactions with antisocial personality disorder among a primarily American-Indian sample. Alcohol Clin Exp Res 31(6):974–987, 2007 17403067

Woody GE, McLellan AT, Luborsky L, et al: Sociopathy and psychotherapy outcome. Arch Gen Psychiatry 42(11):1081–1086, 1985 4051686

Pharmacological Treatment of Antisocial Personality Disorder

Mario Moscovici, M.D.

Roland M. Jones, M.B.Ch.B., B.Sc., M.Sc., Ph.D., FRCPsych

People with antisocial personality disorder (ASPD) are disproportionately high users of both medical and mental health care services (Black 2015); however, few individuals ever seek help for the primary disorder. The functional impairment and increased rates of mortality and morbidity from accidents, suicide, traumatic injuries, hepatitis, and HIV (Black 2015), as well as the high societal impact, highlight the need for effective treatments for this disorder (National Collaborating Centre for Mental Health 2010).

The characteristic features of ASPD include a pervasive pattern of rule-breaking, deceitfulness, impulsivity, aggression, recklessness, irresponsibility, lack of remorse, and lack of empathy for which no licensed pharmacological treatments are available. People who have ASPD also may experience dysphoria, depressed mood, and anxiety (American Psychiatric Association 2013) or have comorbid diagnoses of substance use disorders, ADHD, major mood disorders, or psychosis. Pharmacological treatments are available for these conditions, but they are rarely researched specifically in people who have ASPD.

Current guidelines do not recommend routine use of pharmacological therapy for ASPD and often suggest nonpharmacological interventions first (National Institute for Health and Care Excellence 2009) because of the limited evidence base for pharmacotherapy in this population. The scarcity of evidence for pharmacological treatment in people with ASPD was borne out in a systematic review of the literature in 2010, which reported only eight randomized controlled studies carried out in patients who had ASPD. In fact, none of the studies identified in the review had selected participants primarily on the basis of a diagnosis of ASPD, but rather selected patients with substance use disorders who had a comorbid personality disorder (Khalifa et al. 2010). The review was updated in 2020 and identified three further papers (Khalifa et al. 2020). In total, only two studies reported outcomes that were directly relevant to ASPD, and only one of these found any improvement between treatment and control groups. That study found a reduction in impulsive aggression among prisoners with ASPD who took the anticonvulsant medication phenytoin compared with placebo (Barratt et al. 1997). The only other study identified in the systematic review as having outcomes relevant to ASPD reported no difference in illegal activities among patients prescribed either the tricyclic antidepressant desipramine or placebo (Arndt et al. 1994).

Although there has been little research into pharmacological treatments specifically for people with ASPD, research is accumulating on treatments for some of the manifestations of the disorder, particularly impulsivity and aggression; however, these manifestations are not specific to ASPD. There have been steady advances in the understanding of the neurobiology and psychopharmacology of aggression and impulsivity, and targeted treatments to modulate these biological networks are being investigated in animal and human studies (Rosell and Siever 2015). The neurobiological basis of other human characteristics relevant to ASPD, such as morality (Fede and Kiehl 2020) and deception (Karim et al. 2017), are also becoming better understood but have not yet reached the stage where pharmacological agents to target such deficits have been studied.

In this chapter, we review the evidence for the role of pharmacological treatments for ASPD and some of the manifestations of ASPD, particularly impulsive aggression. Medications that have been proposed as being of benefit in ASPD are mainly antidepressants, mood stabilizers, anticonvulsants, and antipsychotics, and we describe the evidence that currently exists for each class of medication.

Antidepressants

Antisocial Personality Disorder and Aggression

A correlation between aggressive behavior and low serotonin levels in the cerebrospinal fluid (CSF) (Brown et al. 1979; Gerard and Moeller 2007) in both animal (Kästner et al. 2019) and human (Duke et al. 2013) studies has led to the hypothesis that there is a causal relationship between the two, accompanied by interest in the investigation of pharmacological agents that may reduce aggression via action on the serotonergic system. Most antidepressants increase central serotonin availability by preventing neuronal reuptake of synaptic serotonin. It has been suggested that antidepressants, specifically selective serotonin reuptake inhibitors (SSRIs), most commonly prescribed for the treatment of depression and anxiety, can be used to increase central serotonin levels and possibly reduce aggression. A small number of trials have been carried out using antidepressants and other pharmacological agents that increase serotonin, although very few studies of these agents were done in people with ASPD.

One potentially relevant study, although not specifically carried out among participants with ASPD, investigated the SSRI paroxetine as a potential treatment for impulsive aggression in a small study of 12 patients with conduct disorder and antisocial behavior. In this study, impulsivity and impulsive aggression were measured using the Point Subtraction Aggression Paradigm (PSAP; Cherek et al. 1996). This is a laboratory measure in which participants play a game against a fictitious (i.e., computer-simulated) opponent. Aggression is measured as the degree to which participants steal points from their opponent in response to provocation. Participants were randomly assigned to receive either 20 mg of paroxetine or a placebo over a 21-day period, and those who received paroxetine showed a significant reduction in aggressive responses by the end of the study (Cherek et al. 2002b). In a more recent double-blind, placebo-controlled trial, the effect of paroxetine in reducing impulsive aggression compared with placebo was investigated in a sample of community volunteers with psychopathic traits, also during a simulated game (Fanning et al. 2014). In this study, 47 individuals were randomly assigned to receive a single 40-mg dose of paroxetine or placebo prior to the game. Results indicated that volunteers who had received paroxetine had significantly attenuated aggressive behavior in response to provocation.

Both of the previous studies investigated measures of aggression in laboratory conditions, and it could be argued that their observations might not generalize to real-world situations of physical violence. However, there have also been some studies of aggressive behavior in clinical settings involving treatment with the SSRIs citalopram (Armenteros and Lewis 2002), sertraline (Dunlop et al. 2011), and fluoxetine (Coccaro and Kavoussi 1997). None of these studies were specifically aimed at people who had ASPD, and the studies were generally small, providing weak evidence (Table 18–1). In the absence of larger studies, we present the evidence that exists for these medications, which might be relevant to ASPD.

Citalopram has been studied in relation to impulsive aggression in multiple conditions, including dementia (Porsteinsson et al. 2014), schizophrenia (Vartiainen et al. 1995), and, indeed, people with no DSM diagnosis (American Psychiatric Association 2013; Kamarck et al. 2009). In a small open-label study, 12 children and adolescents with antisocial behavior and impulsive aggression were studied for 6 weeks (Armenteros and Lewis 2002). The dose of citalopram was increased by 10 mg each week to a maximum daily dose of 40 mg. There was reportedly a significant reduction in aggression scores as well as aggressive outbursts at the end of the 6-week study period.

Fluoxetine is used mainly for the treatment of depression in both adult and adolescent populations as well as for generalized anxiety disorder, obsessive-compulsive disorder, and PTSD (Katzman et al. 2014; Kennedy et al. 2016). In relation to the treatment of aggression, an initial open-label study examined the efficacy of fluoxetine in three patients with a Cluster B personality disorder, one of whom met criteria for ASPD (Coccaro et al. 1990). Results indicated that during a 6-week trial with all individuals receiving 60 mg/day of fluoxetine, two of the patients had a significant reduction in aggression, as measured by the Modified Overt Aggression Scale (OAS-M; Yudofsky et al. 1986), and global self-reported aggression. Subsequently, Coccaro and Kavoussi (1997) conducted a double-blind, placebo-controlled trial to test the effect of fluoxetine on impulsive aggression. In their study of 40 patients with personality disorders treated with fluoxetine 40 mg/day or higher, in which only 4 met criteria for ASPD (none had depression, bipolar disorder, or schizophrenia), they reported a significant reduction in aggression at 2 months as measured by OAS-M, which was sustained for the remainder of the 3-month study. Coccaro et al. (2009) also studied the effect of fluoxetine on impulsive aggression in the treatment of intermittent explosive disorder. This double-blind, placebo-controlled study included 100 individuals with

TABLE 18–1. **Summary of pharmacological treatments for antisocial personality disorder (ASPD)**

Medication	Dose	Effects	References
Antidepressants			
Paroxetine	20 mg	Reduction in impulsive aggression in patients with conduct disorder and antisocial behavior	Cherek et al. 2002b
	40 mg	Reduction in aggressive behavior in response to provocation	Fanning et al. 2014
	40 mg	Reduction in suicidal behavior in patients with Cluster B personality disorders	Verkes et al. 1998
Fluoxetine	20–60 mg	Reduction in impulsive aggression in patients with Cluster B personality disorders	Coccaro and Kavoussi 1997; Coccaro et al. 1990
	20–60 mg	Reduction in impulsive aggression in patients with intermittent explosive disorder	Coccaro et al. 2009
Sertraline	50–200 mg	Reduction in psychopathy personality inventory scores	Dunlop et al. 2011
Citalopram	20–40 mg	Reduction in impulsive aggression in patients with conduct disorder and antisocial behavior	Armenteros and Lewis 2002
Amitriptyline	50–150 mg	Reduction in depressive symptoms in patients with comorbid personality disorder	Patience et al. 1995
Nortriptyline	25–75 mg	Reduction in multiple alcohol severity variables for patients with comorbid ASPD	Powell et al. 1995
Mood stabilizers			
Lithium	Serum 0.6–1.0 mEq/L	Reduction in impulsive aggression in patients with antisocial behavior; no exclusion for bipolar disorder	Sheard 1971; Sheard et al. 1976; Tupin et al. 1973
		Reduction in abusive behavior toward children	do Prado-Lima et al. 2001
Valproate	500–1,500 mg	Reduction in impulsive aggression in patients with conduct disorder	Donovan et al. 2000; Steiner et al. 2003

TABLE 18–1.   **Summary of pharmacological treatments for antisocial personality disorder (ASPD)** *(continued)*

Medication	Dose	Effects	References
Mood stabilizers *(continued)*			
Phenytoin	300 mg	Reduction in impulsive aggression but not premeditated aggression in patients with antisocial behavior in the prison population	Barratt et al. 1991, 1997; Stanford et al. 2005
Carbamazepine	~800 mg	Reduction in aggressive behavior in patients with Cluster B personality disorders but not in those with conduct disorder	Cueva et al. 1996; Mattes 1990; Stanford et al. 2005
Oxcarbazepine	1,200–2,400 mg	Reduction in impulsive aggression in patients with Cluster B personality disorders	Mattes 2005
Topiramate	200–300 mg	Increase in aggressive behavior in patients with ASPD and comorbid substance use	Lane et al. 2009
	>400 mg	Reduction in aggressive behavior in patients with ASPD and comorbid substance use	
Levetiracetam	<3,000 mg	No significant reduction in aggression	Mattes 2008
Gabapentin	200–800 mg	Reduction in aggression for 800-mg dose but no significant changes for lower doses	Cherek et al. 2004
Antipsychotics			
Risperidone	<6 mg	Reduction in aggressive behavior in patients with ASPD	Hirose 2001
	<4 mg	Reduction in self-reported aggression	Rocca et al. 2002
Olanzapine	5–10 mg	Reduction in aggressive behavior in patients with conduct disorder and antisocial behavior	Gerra et al. 2006; Masi et al. 2006
Quetiapine	600–800 mg	Reduction in impulsivity and aggression in patients with ASPD	Walker et al. 2003
Clozapine	100–325 mg	Reduction in violent incidents in patients with ASPD and high degree of psychopathy	Brown et al. 2014

TABLE 18–1.   **Summary of pharmacological treatments for antisocial personality disorder (ASPD)** *(continued)*

Medication	Dose	Effects	References
Other pharmacotherapies			
Propranolol	10–160 mg	Reduction in impulsive aggression in patients with ASPD	Mattes 1990
Nadolol	80–120 mg	No significant effect on aggression	Alpert et al. 1990
Oxazepam	<120 mg	Reduction in chronic aggression	Lion 1979
Baclofen	0.07–0.28 mg/kg	Reduction in aggressive behavior in laboratory measures	Cherek et al. 2002a
D-fenfluramine	0.1–0.4 mg/kg	Reduction in aggressive behavior in laboratory measures	Cherek and Lane 2001
Oxytocin	12–48 IU	Mixed effect on aggressive behavior in patients with ASPD	Alcorn et al. 2015; Timmermann et al. 2017
Tiagabine	4–12 mg	Reduction in aggressive behavior in laboratory measures	Gowin et al. 2012

Note.   Doses outlined are based on average doses used in the studies.

a diagnosis of intermittent explosive disorder and showed a significant reduction in OAS-M scores as early as 2 weeks regardless of the effect on anxiety or depressive symptoms. The study included 12 individuals with a diagnosis of ASPD, but no direct analysis was performed on these participants.

Although there is some evidence for the role of antidepressants in reducing impulsive aggression among patients with Cluster B personality disorders, more evidence exists for the role of antidepressants in the reduction of aggression in other populations. A systematic review of studies of pharmacological agents that increase serotonin found 16 studies in which the target outcome was a reduction in aggression, anger, or hostility (Duke et al. 2013). There were 395 participants in the combined studies. Seven of the studies were carried out in healthy adults; in three studies, the participants had a criminal history or conduct disorder; in the remaining studies, the study group had diagnoses of either schizophrenia or anxiety or alcohol use disorders. Various pharmacological agents were used in the 16 studies, the most common being D-fenfluramine (previously marketed but no longer licensed as an appetite suppressant), which is thought to increase serotonin release and inhibit reuptake (Pine et al. 1997). Other agents included *m*-chlorophenylpiperazine, ipsapirone, buspirone, citalopram, escitalopram, paroxetine, fluvoxamine, fluoxetine, zolmitriptan, and tryptophan. Although there were mixed findings in the primary studies, the meta-analysis found a small but significant overall effect in reducing aggression among these diverse drugs and samples.

Antisocial Personality Disorder and Depression

With regard to the treatment of depression among people with ASPD, most studies targeting depression specifically exclude comorbid conditions such as personality disorders to avoid potential confounding of the treatment effect, and therefore the evidence is very limited. The studies discussed in the previous subsection provide some indication as to the current evidence for SSRIs in reducing impulsive aggression, and SSRIs also have been studied in Cluster B personality disorders (although not specifically ASPD) in relation to depression and suicidal behavior. In one study, paroxetine at a dose of 40 mg was compared with placebo in a double-blind study of 91 patients, of whom 74 were classified as having Cluster B personality disorders (although the number with ASPD was not reported). Over a 1-year period, a reduction in suicide attempts was seen among participants taking paroxetine. However, paroxetine was found to be significantly more effective among those with a lower rather than a higher number of Cluster B symptoms (Verkes et al. 1998).

Another study examined the effect of the tricyclic antidepressant amitriptyline on depressive symptoms among 113 patients, of whom 38 had a diagnosis of a personality disorder, and the differences in response between the various personality disorders (Patience et al. 1995). The authors showed that a diagnosis of ASPD was not associated with more severe depression. However, compared with participants without a personality disorder, significantly poorer social functioning was reported at 12 months, with nonsignificant differences in work, money, and use of leisure time. Nonetheless, the study demonstrated that amitriptyline was equally effective in treating depressive symptoms among people with and without ASPD.

Finally, sertraline has been studied in patients with major depressive disorder to investigate changes in psychopathic traits (Dunlop et al. 2011). A total of 84 patients were recruited who met criteria for a nonpsychotic major depressive disorder. They completed a study in which sertraline was prescribed in combination with either thyroid hormone or placebo. Sertraline was prescribed as open label with weekly dose adjustments (between 50 mg and 200 mg daily), and participants were randomly assigned to receive either thyroid hormone or placebo in combination with sertraline. This study found reductions in both groups in self-reported impulsivity and increases in "fearless dominance," which comprises social skillfulness, general fearlessness, and stress immunity as measured by the Psychopathic Personality Inventory (Lilienfeld and Andrews 1996). The observed effects were independent of the effect on mood.

Antisocial Personality Disorder and Alcohol Use Disorders

Although ASPD is commonly associated with alcohol use disorders, the comorbid conditions have rarely been studied together in pharmacological trials. In one study, the tricyclic antidepressant nortriptyline was investigated among patients with ASPD for its effect on their alcohol use disorder (Powell et al. 1995). The study examined the effect of nortriptyline or bromocriptine, a dopamine D_2 receptor agonist, in 216 male patients with alcohol use disorder. The study presented data from a large trial conducted between 1988 and 1993, which commenced before the availability of SSRIs, hence the choice of nortriptyline. The patients were divided into three groups: alcohol use, alcohol use and a depressive or anxiety disorder, and alcohol use and ASPD. At the end of a 6-month follow-up period, the study showed that the only significant positive effect was in reducing alcohol use among individuals with ASPD treated with nortriptyline, and it was hypothesized that nortriptyline reduced impulsivity and, hence, reduced impulsive drinking in patients with ASPD.

In summary, the evidence base for the use of antidepressants in ASPD is weak. No evidence suggests that antidepressants are any more or less effective in treating depression among people with ASPD. Few studies specifically selected people with ASPD for treatment. However, some evidence indicates that antidepressants might be helpful in reducing reactive or impulsive aggression, which could be relevant to individuals with ASPD. The hypothesis linking impulsive aggression and the serotonergic system has received some traction, but pharmacological treatments that increase serotonin have not yet been sufficiently studied among persons with ASPD to make any recommendations in regard to therapy. Caution is required in interpreting the findings in relation to antidepressants and aggression because the effect sizes are quite small, many of the studies are small or open label, and whether the findings would generalize to individuals with ASPD is unclear.

Although there is increasing understanding of the role of serotonin in aggression, the relationship is likely to be far more complex than originally proposed. Seven different families of serotonin receptors have now been identified, with at least 14 receptor subtypes, some of which have opposing effects (Quadros et al. 2010). For example, serotonin type 1A and 1B (5-HT_{1A} and 5-HT_{1B}) receptors are thought to reduce aggressive behavior, whereas the 5-HT_{2A} and 5-HT_{2C} receptors are thought to increase it (Quadros et al. 2010).

In addition, some evidence has shown an increase in violence associated with treatment with SSRIs. A systematic review of 70 trials including more than 18,000 people who received either SSRI or placebo found a doubling of suicidality and aggression among children and adolescents taking SSRIs but no difference among adults (Sharma et al. 2016). A systematic review of adverse outcomes in randomized controlled trials of SSRIs given to healthy volunteers included 11 published trials and 2 unpublished clinical study reports (Bielefeldt et al. 2016). The authors reported a twofold increased rate of adverse events (typically, tremor, agitation, restlessness, or nightmares) among the treatment group compared with the placebo group, reported as symptomatic precursors to suicidality and violence. A better understanding of both risks and benefits is needed before recommendations for off-label prescribing can be made in this patient group.

Although the biological underpinnings of ASPD are still being elucidated, there will need to be a focus on research to unpack the effects of different pharmacological agents on specific receptor subtypes in order to understand their effect on aggression in people with ASPD. Of the antidepressants tested thus far, some SSRIs (citalopram, fluoxetine, and paroxetine) have shown some promise in reducing impulsive aggression and aggression in response to provocation. However, larger, higher-quality studies are needed to produce a more definitive answer as to whether antidepressants should be used as a treatment option for the ASPD patient population.

Mood Stabilizers and Anticonvulsants

For the purpose of this chapter, we define a *mood stabilizer* as a pharmacological treatment that is used to treat both mania and depression in bipolar disorder and an *anti-*

convulsant as a medication for the control of epileptic seizures. Many, but not all, mood stabilizers are also anticonvulsants. Antipsychotic medications also have been used for their mood-stabilizing properties; however, we review this class of medication in a later section. Although no studies have used mood stabilizers specifically for the treatment of ASPD, mood stabilizers have been used for a variety of indications, including for the treatment of impulsivity and aggression (Jones et al. 2011) and to reduce self-harm (Kessing et al. 2005).

Lithium was the first medication to be used as a mood stabilizer, having been serendipitously discovered in 1847, and it has been in widespread use since 1949 (Shorter 2009). Lithium is effective for treating mania and depression, and it prevents relapse of mood episodes in bipolar disorder (Won and Kim 2017). It has also been used for the treatment of aggression in Cluster B personality disorders (Ripoll et al. 2011). Despite the use of lithium for multiple indications, the exact mechanism by which the medication acts is unknown. Several hypotheses have been suggested, but none fully explains the efficacy of lithium across the variety of indications. One theory suggests that it reduces the excitatory effects of glutamate and dopamine neurons and increases the activity of inhibitory neurons mediated by GABA (Malhi et al. 2013). Furthermore, lithium is also found to modulate intracellular signaling by affecting adenyl cyclase and protein kinase C, which may dampen the effects of these excitatory neurons (Malhi et al. 2013).

The earliest study of lithium relevant to ASPD investigated its effects in 12 maximum-security prisoners who had frequent violent outbursts (Sheard 1971). The inmates were randomly assigned to either placebo or lithium in a weekly alternating sequence lasting 8 weeks. Lithium concentration was maintained between 0.6 mEq/L and 1.5 mEq/L with an average dose of 1,200 mg/day. A decrease in violent incidents and outbursts as measured by weekly checklists and clinical interviews was reported. Sheard et al. (1976) conducted a subsequent double-blind, placebo-controlled trial for subjects with chronic aggression that excluded any patients with acute illness, including psychosis. This study included 66 male participants from a medium-security facility who were followed up for a 3-month period. A significant reduction in the number of infractions related to violence was reported in the group taking lithium. Doses of lithium were maintained between 1,200 mg and 1,600 mg to achieve serum levels between 0.6 mEq/L and 1.0 mEq/L. Participants received five capsules containing varying amounts of lithium carbonate depending on the target dose used for that week or five identical capsules containing placebo.

Another study also found a significant benefit of lithium over an 18-month period among 27 individuals with a recurrent pattern of violent infractions (Tupin et al. 1973). Patients had heterogeneous diagnoses including personality disorders and schizophrenia; however, there was no mention of bipolar disorder. The average lithium dose was 1,800 mg daily, with serum levels averaging 0.8 mEq/L. In this study, there was a significant reduction in violent incidents reported, replicating the previous findings of Sheard and colleagues (1976). Of note, however, it is difficult to draw a firm conclusion as to whether lithium was an effective treatment for reducing aggression independent of bipolar disorder diagnosis because none of these previous studies using lithium explicitly excluded this diagnosis.

A more recent study that examined eight mothers with recurrent abusive behavior toward their children showed a significant decrease in abusive and aggressive behavior independent of a diagnosis of bipolar disorder or schizophrenia or substance mis-use after treatment with lithium (do Prado-Lima et al. 2001). The open-label study was small, and more studies are needed to definitively determine whether lithium is effective for impulsivity and aggression, independent of a bipolar disorder diagnosis.

With regard to anticonvulsant medications, most of the studies that have investigated efficacy in treating impulsivity or aggression so far have been carried out in patients with borderline personality disorder, but even here the evidence is quite scant and has been drawn from mainly small-scale studies (Crawford et al. 2014). The mechanism of action of anticonvulsants as mood stabilizers is not clear. Similar to lithium, anticonvulsants have an indirect effect on enhancing inhibitory neurons through GABA activity. Most anticonvulsants enact this effect through voltage-gated sodium and calcium channels; for example, valproate reduces high-frequency action potentials through enhancing the inhibitory effect of sodium-gated ion channels and indirectly enhancing GABA function. Lamotrigine, on the other hand, has an effect on both sodium- and calcium-gated channels, which has a substantial effect on several neurotransmitters (Schloesser et al. 2012). However, how this relates to a potential mechanism for the treatment of impulsivity and aggression is not yet known.

Two studies of youths with conduct disorder showed reduced aggressive outbursts among those who received divalproex sodium. The first study was a randomized, double-blind, placebo-controlled crossover design, which included 20 participants ages 10–18 years who had a diagnosis of conduct disorder. It was reported that 8 of 10 participants who were prescribed divalproex responded to treatment, whereas none of the 10 participants in the control group responded to placebo in terms of reduced numbers of aggressive outbursts during the 6-week trial (Donovan et al. 2000). The second study was a larger randomized controlled study of 71 male youths with a diagnosis of conduct disorder and at least one criminal conviction. Low-dose divalproex sodium (250 mg daily) was compared with high-dose (500–1,500 mg daily) divalproex sodium in the treatment of impulsivity. A significant reduction in impulsive behavior was found for the high-dose group on the basis of self-report as well as a significant reduction in the Clinical Global Impression—Severity (CGI-S) score (Steiner et al. 2003).

Phenytoin is an anticonvulsant and is the only drug that has been studied in a prison population for both premeditated and impulsive aggression. An early study examined the effect of phenytoin on aggressive behavior in 13 maximum-security prisoners (Barratt et al. 1991). This double-blind study used a crossover design with 4 weeks for each condition and a 1-week washout period, randomizing the sequence of each condition for each participant: placebo or 100 mg or 300 mg daily of phenytoin. A significant reduction in aggressive incidents was seen in patients who were taking 300 mg of phenytoin daily but not for the other conditions. The results were replicated in a larger study that included 60 inmates with both premeditated and impulsive acts of aggression (Barratt et al. 1997). Again, the study used a crossover design and was double-blinded with 6 weeks for each condition: phenytoin 300 mg/day or placebo. There was a significant reduction in impulsive aggression but not in premeditated aggression. Unlike premeditated aggression, impulsive aggression may be due to frontal lobe dysfunction—in particular, ventromedial frontal cortex and dorsomedial frontal cortical dysfunction (Blair 2016). Phenytoin acts on sodium-gated channels, preventing repetitive firing (Yaari et al. 1986), which may increase the threshold for an aggressive response. On the contrary, premeditated aggression, which requires planning and is not associated with frustration or an immediate response (Siever 2008), likely does not share this dysfunction and will not respond to phenytoin.

Carbamazepine is another mood stabilizer used mainly in the treatment of bipolar disorder (Yatham et al. 2018) that has been studied in the treatment of aggression. A nonblinded study compared carbamazepine with propranolol for the treatment of aggression (Mattes 1990). The study included a total of 51 patients randomly assigned to either carbamazepine or propranolol and showed that both propranolol and carbamazepine reduced aggression by clinician-rated assessments. Carbamazepine dosages averaged approximately 800 mg total daily and were titrated on the basis of serum concentrations. Carbamazepine was also studied in conduct disorder for children ages 5–12 years but showed no significant reduction in aggressive behaviors (Cueva et al. 1996).

Few head-to-head studies have been carried out to compare the efficacy of different pharmacological agents in the treatment of aggression. One study that stands out in this regard compared phenytoin, sodium valproate, and carbamazepine as well as placebo. In this small study, a total of 29 patients were selected on the basis of having impulsive aggression, with 17 of the participants having a diagnosis of ASPD (Stanford et al. 2005). Even though the study was quite small, with a total of 7 patients per treatment arm, it found that each of these agents was equally effective (and superior to placebo) for the treatment of impulsive aggression.

Oxcarbazepine is a newer anticonvulsant that is derived from carbamazepine and has similar anticonvulsant efficacy (Koch and Polman 2009). This medication is not generally classified as a mood stabilizer but has been investigated as a treatment for bipolar disorder with mixed results (Vasudev et al. 2011). It has also been studied as a potential agent in reducing impulsive aggression. Although not specific for ASPD, some evidence indicates that oxcarbazepine is effective in intermittent explosive disorder and Cluster B personality traits (Mattes 2005). The patients in the study by Mattes (2005) showed significant improvement in aggression for doses between 1,200 mg and 2,400 mg daily. The same author conducted a similar study with another anticonvulsant, levetiracetam, up to a maximum dosage of 3,000 mg daily; however, no significant reduction in impulsive aggression occurred in this study (Mattes 2008). Neither of these studies was specific for ASPD, but they did include patients with Cluster B personality traits. These studies raise the question as to whether anticonvulsants in general have an effect on impulsive aggression and whether the mechanism for seizure activity has any similarity to that of impulsive aggression.

Topiramate is an anticonvulsant that has been studied as a mood stabilizer and also as a treatment for alcohol use disorder. There is mixed evidence for topiramate as a mood stabilizer, and it is generally not used in the treatment of bipolar disorder (Pigott et al. 2016); however, topiramate has been shown to be effective for alcohol use disorder by reducing the number of drinking days and reducing craving for alcohol. Topiramate acts as an allosteric GABA modulator, which causes chloride ions to influx into the cell, thereby increasing overall GABA inhibition. The exact mechanism on alcohol use disorder has remained speculative, but it is thought to blunt the reinforcing properties of alcohol in the reward circuit (Manhapra et al. 2019). Outside these indications, topiramate has been studied primarily in patients with borderline personality disorder and has been shown to be effective in reducing aggression in male (Nickel et al. 2005) and female (Nickel et al. 2004) patients. Topiramate also has been examined in a small study of 12 patients with ASPD who also met criteria for concurrent substance use disorder (Lane et al. 2009). This study showed that for doses between 200 mg and 300 mg, aggressive behavior increased, and for doses of 400 mg and higher, patients had a modest decrease in aggression.

Another anticonvulsant medication, gabapentin, also has been used for treatment of chronic pain, anxiety, and alcohol use disorder. It is understood that gabapentin binds to calcium channels and affects the influx of calcium into the neuron. The abundance of calcium channels throughout the body likely gives rise to the diversity of effects of gabapentin (Berlin et al. 2015). There has been some interest in evaluating the effect of gabapentin on aggression. Cherek and colleagues (2004) have examined the effect of gabapentin on aggression for patients with a diagnosis of conduct disorder and antisocial behavior who were on parole. A total of 20 patients with and without conduct disorder were randomly assigned to placebo or a single dose of gabapentin (200 mg, 400 mg, or 800 mg). Aggression response was tested in a laboratory setting using the PSAP. One-time administration of gabapentin reduced overall aggression response for the 800-mg dose but increased aggression responses for the lower doses. Therefore, a dose-dependent effect for both topiramate and gabapentin may be present that is not seen with other mood stabilizers.

Finally, tiagabine is an anticonvulsant medication that is used for the treatment of epilepsy (Adkins and Noble 1998). It also has been used as an off-label medication for the treatment of anxiety symptoms (Schaller et al. 2004). Gowin and colleagues (2012) studied the effect of tiagabine on impulsive aggression in a laboratory setting among 12 patients, 6 of whom met criteria for ASPD. Tiagabine, administered at doses of up to 12 mg, was found to be associated with a significant reduction in aggressive behavior as measured by the PSAP.

In summary, there is some evidence for the efficacy of mood stabilizers and anticonvulsants in the treatment of aggression, although not specifically for ASPD. Most of the available evidence for the use of mood stabilizers is for borderline personality disorder, and even then, the evidence is quite limited. More high-quality studies are needed to draw conclusions as to whether mood stabilizers or anticonvulsants should be used to treat aggression. Therefore, the routine use of these medications for ASPD is not recommended currently and should be evaluated on a case-by-case basis. Nonetheless, on the basis of the limited evidence available, phenytoin, divalproate sodium, lithium, carbamazepine, and gabapentin have relatively more evidence than do other mood stabilizers or anticonvulsants for efficacy in reducing impulsive aggression, albeit low-quality evidence. For patients with alcohol abuse issues, topiramate has been shown to have some efficacy at doses of 400 mg, but it is important to be cautious because aggression may worsen with lower doses. Of note, mood stabilizers and anticonvulsants are associated with significant potential side effects, and particular caution is required in prescribing, especially for women because of the risk of teratogenic effects in pregnancy. These risks are likely to outweigh any benefits for all but the most severely affected and those for whom other approaches have failed.

Antipsychotics

Antipsychotic medications, also referred to as neuroleptics, are indicated primarily for the treatment of psychotic disorders such as schizophrenia (Carpenter and Davis

2012), but some have been applied to a variety of other indications, including bipolar disorder, major depression, vocal tics, and hiccups (Yatham et al. 2018). The mechanism of action of antipsychotics is perhaps better understood than that of mood stabilizers or antidepressants. Antipsychotic medications have an antagonistic effect on dopamine receptors in the mesolimbic pathway, which are thought to be hyperactive in schizophrenia and contribute to the positive symptoms (Liemburg et al. 2012). Antipsychotic medications also have a relatively weaker effect on other receptors in the brain (notably, histamine H_1, muscarinic M_1, and α_1 receptors), which gives rise to some of the side effects of this medication class. Newer-generation antipsychotics also have an effect on serotonin receptors, in particular the $5\text{-}HT_{2A}$ receptor (Schmidt et al. 1995), and it is thought that the effect on serotonin receptors could contribute to the mood-stabilizing effects of the newer generation of antipsychotic medications.

As with other classes of medications, minimal evidence is available specifically for treatment of ASPD; however, evidence shows that antipsychotics, specifically risperidone, are effective in the treatment of aggression in patients with major neurocognitive disorder (Seitz et al. 2013) and autism spectrum disorder (Jesner et al. 2007). Risperidone also has been studied in borderline personality disorder, specifically for symptoms of impulsivity and aggression. Rocca et al. (2002) found that an average dose of 3.27 mg daily can have a substantial effect on borderline personality disorder symptoms. The study was conducted over an 8-week period with a total of 15 patients who had a personality disorder, 4 of whom met criteria for ASPD. Participants that met criteria for severe and persistent mental illness were excluded from the study. Aggression was assessed with the self-rated Aggression Questionnaire (Rocca et al. 2002). Although no study has specifically examined the efficacy of risperidone in ASPD, there are anecdotal reports of a significant decrease in impulsive behavior and aggression in ASPD when treatment with risperidone is applied (Hirose 2001).

A small study of 23 adolescents ages 11–18 years examined the effect of olanzapine (an atypical antipsychotic) on impulsive aggression, with a mean dose of 8 mg daily (Masi et al. 2006). Olanzapine was shown to have a beneficial effect; however, an important detail in this study is that all the participants had tried nonpharmacological interventions, as well as lithium and sodium valproate, which failed to reduce their aggressive behavior. Therefore, this sample may have had illness that was more treatment refractory than in other studies. Olanzapine also has been investigated in an open-label observational study of 67 patients with aggressive behavior and comorbid heroin use disorder (Gerra et al. 2006). Most patients had a personality disorder, with 20% of the participants meeting criteria for ASPD. The patients in this study showed a reduction in aggressive behavior and an improved overall outcome in heroin dependency.

A small case series of four patients reported on the efficacy of quetiapine in patients with a diagnosis of ASPD who were referred to a maximum-security psychiatric facility because of aggressive behavior (Walker et al. 2003). Doses of 600–800 mg daily resulted in a reduction in aggression, irritability, and impulsive behavior for all four patients in the case series, although this study was neither controlled nor blinded.

Clozapine is unique among antipsychotic agents in that it has weak affinity for dopamine D_2 receptors and has affinity for D_4 as well as the serotonin, histamine, and α_1-adrenergic receptor systems. It is associated with virtually no extrapyramidal side effects (Warnez and Alessi-Severini 2014) and has superior efficacy in treatment-resistant schizophrenia (Leucht et al. 2013). Clozapine also has been studied in the treatment of aggression in people with ASPD in a small case series of seven patients who also endorsed a high degree of psychopathic traits in high-security psychiatric facilities (Brown et al. 2014). The patients were reported to have had a significant reduction in violent incidents and CGI scores (Guy 1976) with a minimum treatment time of 7 weeks. The patients were prescribed minimum doses of 100 mg daily (range of 100–325 mg daily).

Some evidence indicates that clozapine may have specific antiaggressive effects separate from its antipsychotic or sedative effects (Frogley et al. 2012); however, the side-effect profile and restrictions on prescribing outside the primary indication for treatment-resistant schizophrenia limit utility in ASPD as the primary indication. In addition, the requirement for regular bloodwork for all patients taking clozapine would further limit the practical utility of prescribing clozapine for this indication.

In summary, evidence is currently insufficient to recommend the routine use of any antipsychotic medication for ASPD. However, on the basis of the limited available evidence, quetiapine, risperidone, olanzapine, and clozapine may have some efficacy, notwithstanding the likely problems regarding tolerability and adherence.

Other Pharmacotherapies

Most of the evidence that is available for the pharmacological treatment of ASPD is focused on three major classes of medications: antidepressants, mood stabilizers and anticonvulsants, and antipsychotic medications. A small number of trials using a variety of other medication classes also have been investigated in the treatment of aggression, including β-blockers, benzodiazepines, anti-inflammatories, and hormones.

β-Blockers are used mainly to treat cardiovascular conditions (Steenen et al. 2016), PTSD (Giustino et al. 2016), and akathisia in the context of medication side effects (Pringsheim et al. 2018). β-Blockers compete with catecholamines, such as adrenaline, at the receptor level. Theoretically, they can block the physiological effects associated with catecholamines, thereby treating physical symptoms associated with anxiety and impulsivity. Moreover, β-blockers have been shown to have central effects on blocking fear response and even blocking reconsolidation of certain memories associated with fear response (Steenen et al. 2016). Two studies have investigated β-blockers for the treatment of ASPD or aggression, with contrasting findings. A study previously described in the section "Mood Stabilizers and Anticonvulsants" found that propranolol was effective in treating impulsive aggression (Mattes 1990). However, the study was small and relied on clinician assessment as the primary outcome measure. Another small study showed that nadolol, which was effective for akathisia, did not show a statistically significant response for treatment of impulsive aggression (Alpert et al. 1990).

Benzodiazepines are often used for the treatment of acute agitation and aggression, mainly for their sedating effects. Benzodiazepines have a direct effect on the GABA receptor and have been used primarily in short-term treatment of anxiety or agitation (Yildiz et al. 2003), but it is unclear what role benzodiazepines may have for more chronic or recurrent aggression. Only one study has examined this use of benzodiazepines: 65 outpatients with histories of chronic and impulsive aggressive outbursts were treated for antisocial behavior with either oxazepam, chlordiazepoxide, or placebo (Lion 1979). Results showed some reduction in hostility among those receiving oxazepam. Most guidelines do not support the long-term use of benzodiazepines because of their addictive potential and their cognitive and motor side effects (Airagnes et al. 2019; Markota et al. 2016). In addition, multiple studies have shown that chronic benzodiazepine use can paradoxically increase aggression (Albrecht et al. 2014). Given the long-term risks, addictive potential, and potential paradoxical increase in aggression, benzodiazepines are not recommended for the treatment of chronic aggression. However, this class of medication still has an important indication for treatment of acute aggression.

Several studies have evaluated the efficacy of medications that are not generally used in psychiatric practice. Cherek and colleagues have studied the effect of both baclofen and D-fenfluramine in separate studies for the treatment of aggression in patients with conduct disorder (Cherek and Lane 2001; Cherek et al. 2002a). Baclofen, which is used as an anti-inflammatory, has a $GABA_B$ receptor antagonism. Stimulation of $GABA_B$ receptors has been implicated in reducing aggression (Cherek et al. 2004). D-fenfluramine was used as an appetite-suppressing drug but was discontinued because of cardiovascular adverse events. Interestingly, D-fenfluramine exerts its effect through the $5\text{-}HT_{2B}$ receptor, which was also implicated in aggression, as discussed in the section on antidepressants (Schoonjans et al. 2017). The studies of baclofen and D-fenfluramine investigated the acute effects of the medications on patients with conduct disorder in a laboratory setting using the PSAP (Cherek and Lane 2001; Cherek et al. 2002a). Both medications showed a reduction in aggressive responding on the PSAP. Nonetheless, further studies are needed to justify the clinical use of these medications. This is especially true for D-fenfluramine given its safety concerns.

Oxytocin, a neuropeptide produced by the hypothalamus, has a broad range of functions in humans, including being implicated in empathy response and nurturing behavior (Geng et al. 2018). Because of oxytocin's involvement in empathic responding, nurturing behavior, and suppressing aggression or violence, there has been increased interest in using it as a treatment for ASPD. A systematic review of the overall evidence for the use of oxytocin found that most studies were carried out in healthy participants (Gedeon et al. 2019). Only two studies tested oxytocin in ASPD, with mixed results (Alcorn et al. 2015; Timmermann et al. 2017). Some patients experienced a reduction in aggression, whereas others had an increase in violent behavior. It is unclear why oxytocin results in such mixed outcomes, and further studies are needed to demonstrate its clinical utility.

In summary, there are several studies of benzodiazepines and other pharmacotherapies that are not generally used in psychiatry but that have been applied for the treatment of ASPD. However, none of the studies presented here provide sufficient evidence to recommend routine use of these medications in individuals with ASPD. Studies of benzodiazepines, D-fenfluramine, and oxytocin also have reported conflicting results or significant safety concerns.

Case Example

Mr. G, a 34-year-old male inmate in a correctional facility, was diagnosed with ASPD and is serving a 5-year sentence for a violent offense. He has had extensive involvement with the criminal justice system, including multiple previous periods of incarceration with charges of assault, uttering threats, and breach of probation. He has been struggling intermittently with impulsive aggression, which has led to further incidents of institutional misconduct. He tried group therapy, which he was not able to complete because of interpersonal difficulties in the group. He also tried individual cognitive-behavioral therapy focusing on anger and aggression, which was not helpful.

Following a discussion of the available evidence with the psychiatrist, Mr. G expressed a strong preference to try a pharmacological agent for management of impulsive aggression. He also had been struggling with labile mood, which led to multiple interpersonal conflicts. Mood stabilizers were tried, including lithium and valproate. Unfortunately, neither of the agents was effective for the management of his impulsive aggression.

During follow-up appointments, Mr. G voiced depressive symptoms as he continued to struggle with interpersonal problems. An SSRI, paroxetine, was offered as an option. The medication was effective in improving mood, with some reported reduction in aggressive incidents. Although paroxetine was helpful in treating depressive symptoms, the early apparent improvement in aggression was not sustained, and Mr. G elected to discontinue taking it because of reported sexual side effects.

Conclusion

Overall, the evidence base for pharmacological treatment of ASPD is quite poor. Very few studies have recruited patients with ASPD, and most either included these patients as part of a larger group sample or focused on Cluster B traits or conduct disorder. In addition, most of the findings were based on relatively small samples. Nonetheless, on the basis of the limited evidence, a few medications from each class have relatively more evidence than others. From the antidepressant category, citalopram and fluoxetine have some limited data showing efficacy for aggression in ASPD as well as other disorders. For patients with recurrent suicide attempts, there is some evidence for efficacy of paroxetine. For the treatment of alcohol use disorder in ASPD, some evidence was found for the efficacy of nortriptyline. Mood stabilizers have been used for different personality disorders, including ASPD. However, it is difficult to recommend the routine use of mood stabilizers in ASPD because of concerns about side effects. Nonetheless, phenytoin shows some promise in the treatment of impulsive aggression. Other agents that have shown some evidence of efficacy include carbamazepine, valproate sodium, and gabapentin or topiramate if the patient has a comorbid alcohol use disorder. Antipsychotics have been used extensively for different indications, including mood disorders, neurocognitive disorders, autism spectrum disorder, and borderline personality disorder. The evidence for their use in ASPD is again quite limited, and routine use of antipsychotics is not recommended. However, risperidone, quetiapine, olanzapine, and clozapine have shown some promise in treating impulsivity and aggression.

Other pharmacotherapies such as β-blockers, benzodiazepines, and hormones have been tried in the treatment of ASPD. The results are mixed, and there are some concerns regarding the safe use of these medications. Overall, no studies have adequately compared the efficacy of medications between classes. Given this paucity of data, it is difficult to recommend which class or medication to use; moreover, consideration of acceptability and tolerability in relation to side-effect profile will be paramount on a case-by-case basis.

Most of the studies carried out to date have reported on changes in aggression or hostility, and it is likely that with further advances in understanding the biological basis of aggression, more targeted pharmacological treatments could be developed, especially in relation to impulsive aggression. However, over the past decade there have been virtually no pharmacological studies of treatments for the manifestations of ASPD, and at present there is little to indicate that this situation will change in the near future. Investment by large pharmacological companies in medication development for mental health has declined by as much as 70% over recent years, with some pharmaceutical companies ceasing neuropharmacological research altogether (Wentworth 2019). The main reasons for this are the very high cost of new drug development, the high percentage of failures in this area, the complexity of the CNS, the complex etiologies of mental disorders, and the lack of adequate animal models for many psychiatric conditions (Ghani 2014). Given the decline in investment in the development of drugs that are very widely used globally for conditions such as schizophrenia, bipolar disorder, or depression, there would appear to be little appetite for large-scale investment in potentially controversial drug treatments to modify antisocial personality because the number of those who might objectively benefit is low. Any breakthrough in drug development will likely arise from academic research that is not driven by profit, building on the rapidly expanding knowledge of the integration of behavior and the brain at the cellular level.

Of the currently available pharmacotherapies, mood stabilizers suggest perhaps the most promise in reducing impulsive aggression, but for the medications currently available, the benefits likely do not outweigh the risks in most cases. Nonetheless, further understanding of the mechanism of action of mood stabilizers in reducing impulsivity could lead to more targeted action with fewer side effects. Furthermore, the combination of pharmacotherapies with specific psychological skills–based interventions might well prove more effective than either intervention alone. In the absence of pharmacological breakthroughs, this might prove a fruitful avenue for further research. In addition, as the broader neurobiology of ASPD becomes better understood, in the future there could be targeted treatments for some of the primary manifestations of ASPD, such as reckless decision-making, deficits in empathy, or lack of remorse, and there is already some promising research into the effects of oxytocin in this regard. Should such interventions ever become possible, however, they would raise significant legal, ethical, and moral considerations around the treatment of ASPD.

Key Points

- The evidence for pharmacological treatment of antisocial personality disorder (ASPD) is poor. Very few studies have specifically recruited patients with ASPD, but manifestations of ASPD, primarily aggression and impulsivity, have been studied.

- Routine pharmacological treatment of ASPD is not recommended on the basis of the current evidence. If pharmacological treatment is considered, mood stabilizers, selective serotonin reuptake inhibitors, and antipsychotics have been shown to reduce impulsive aggression, although the quality of evidence overall is weak.

• Advances in the understanding of the neurobiology of other deficits in ASPD such as lack of empathy or lack of remorse may allow for novel treatments to be designed, but such treatments would be accompanied by significant ethical and practical concerns.

References

Adkins JC, Noble S: Tiagabine: a review of its pharmacodynamic and pharmacokinetic properties and therapeutic potential in the management of epilepsy. Drugs 55(3):437–460, 1998 9530548

Airagnes G, Lemogne C, Renuy A, et al: Prevalence of prescribed benzodiazepine long-term use in the French general population according to sociodemographic and clinical factors: findings from the CONSTANCES cohort. BMC Public Health 19(1):566, 2019 31088561

Albrecht B, Staiger PK, Hall K, et al: Benzodiazepine use and aggressive behaviour: a systematic review. Aust N Z J Psychiatry 48(12):1096–1114, 2014 25183003

Alcorn JL 3rd, Green CE, Schmitz J, et al: Effects of oxytocin on aggressive responding in healthy adult men. Behav Pharmacol 26(8 spec no):798–804, 2015 26241153

Alpert M, Allan ER, Citrome L, et al: A double-blind, placebo-controlled study of adjunctive nadolol in the management of violent psychiatric patients. Psychopharmacol Bull 26(3):367–371, 1990 2274638

American Psychiatric Association: Diagnostic and Statistical Manual of Mental Disorders, 5th Edition. Arlington, VA, American Psychiatric Association, 2013

Armenteros JL, Lewis JE: Citalopram treatment for impulsive aggression in children and adolescents: an open pilot study. J Am Acad Child Adolesc Psychiatry 41(5):522–529, 2002 12014784

Arndt IO, McLellan AT, Dorozynsky L, et al: Desipramine treatment for cocaine dependence: role of antisocial personality disorder. J Nerv Ment Dis 182(3):151–156, 1994 8113775

Barratt ES, Kent TA, Bryant SG, et al: A controlled trial of phenytoin in impulsive aggression. J Clin Psychopharmacol 11(6):388–389, 1991 1770157

Barratt ES, Stanford MS, Felthous AR, et al: The effects of phenytoin on impulsive and premeditated aggression: a controlled study. J Clin Psychopharmacol 17(5):341–349, 1997 9315984

Berlin RK, Butler PM, Perloff MD: Gabapentin therapy in psychiatric disorders: a systematic review. Prim Care Companion CNS Disord 17(5):10.4088/PCC.15r01821, 2015 26835178

Bielefeldt AØ, Danborg PB, Gøtzsche PC: Precursors to suicidality and violence on antidepressants: systematic review of trials in adult healthy volunteers. J R Soc Med 109(10):381–392, 2016 27729596

Black DW: The natural history of antisocial personality disorder. Can J Psychiatry 60(7):309–314, 2015 26175389

Blair RJR: The neurobiology of impulsive aggression. J Child Adolesc Psychopharmacol 26(1):4–9, 2016 26465707

Brown D, Larkin F, Sengupta S, et al: Clozapine: an effective treatment for seriously violent and psychopathic men with antisocial personality disorder in a UK high-security hospital. CNS Spectr 19(5):391–402, 2014 24698103

Brown GL, Goodwin FK, Ballenger JC, et al: Aggression in humans correlates with cerebrospinal fluid amine metabolites. Psychiatry Res 1(2):131–139, 1979 95232

Carpenter WT Jr, Davis JM: Another view of the history of antipsychotic drug discovery and development. Mol Psychiatry 17(12):1168–1173, 2012 22889923

Cherek DR, Lane SD: Acute effects of D-fenfluramine on simultaneous measures of aggressive escape and impulsive responses of adult males with and without a history of conduct disorder. Psychopharmacology (Berl) 157(3):221–227, 2001 11605076

Cherek DR, Schnapp W, Moeller FG, et al: Laboratory measures of aggressive responding in male parolees with violent and nonviolent histories. Aggress Behav 22:27–36, 1996

Cherek DR, Lane SD, Pietras CJ, et al: Acute effects of baclofen, a γ-aminobutyric acid-B agonist, on laboratory measures of aggressive and escape responses of adult male parolees with and without a history of conduct disorder. Psychopharmacology (Berl) 164(2):160–167, 2002a 12404078

Cherek DR, Lane SD, Pietras CJ, et al: Effects of chronic paroxetine administration on measures of aggressive and impulsive responses of adult males with a history of conduct disorder. Psychopharmacology (Berl) 159(3):266–274, 2002b 11862359

Cherek DR, Tcheremissine OV, Lane SD, et al: Acute effects of gabapentin on laboratory measures of aggressive and escape responses of adult parolees with and without a history of conduct disorder. Psychopharmacology (Berl) 171(4):405–412, 2004 13680071

Coccaro EF, Kavoussi RJ: Fluoxetine and impulsive aggressive behavior in personality-disordered subjects. Arch Gen Psychiatry 54(12):1081–1088, 1997 9400343

Coccaro EF, Astill JL, Herbert JL, et al: Fluoxetine treatment of impulsive aggression in DSM-III-R personality disorder patients. J Clin Psychopharmacol 10(5):373–375, 1990 2258454

Coccaro EF, Lee RJ, Kavoussi RJ: A double-blind, randomized, placebo-controlled trial of fluoxetine in patients with intermittent explosive disorder. J Clin Psychiatry 70(5):653–662, 2009 19389333

Crawford MJ, MacLaren T, Reilly JG: Are mood stabilisers helpful in treatment of borderline personality disorder? BMJ 349:g5378, 2014 25228296

Cueva JE, Overall JE, Small AM, et al: Carbamazepine in aggressive children with conduct disorder: a double-blind and placebo-controlled study. J Am Acad Child Adolesc Psychiatry 35(4):480–490, 1996 8919710

Donovan SJ, Stewart JW, Nunes EV, et al: Divalproex treatment for youth with explosive temper and mood lability: a double-blind, placebo-controlled crossover design. Am J Psychiatry 157(5):818–820, 2000 10784478

do Prado-Lima P, Knijnik L, Juruena M, et al: Lithium reduces maternal child abuse behaviour: a preliminary report. J Clin Pharm Ther 26(4):279–282, 2001 11493370

Duke AA, Bègue L, Bell R, et al: Revisiting the serotonin-aggression relation in humans: a meta-analysis. Psychol Bull 139(5):1148–1172, 2013 23379963

Dunlop BW, DeFife JA, Marx L, et al: The effects of sertraline on psychopathic traits. Int Clin Psychopharmacol 26(6):329–337, 2011 21909028

Fanning JR, Berman ME, Guillot CR, et al: Serotonin (5-HT) augmentation reduces provoked aggression associated with primary psychopathy traits. J Pers Disord 28(3):449–461, 2014 22984854

Fede SJ, Kiehl KA: Meta-analysis of the moral brain: patterns of neural engagement assessed using multilevel kernel density analysis. Brain Imaging Behav 14(2):534–547, 2020 30706370

Frogley C, Taylor D, Dickens G, et al: A systematic review of the evidence of clozapine's anti-aggressive effects. Int J Neuropsychopharmacol 15(9):1351–1371, 2012 22339930

Gedeon T, Parry J, Völlm B: The role of oxytocin in antisocial personality disorders: a systematic review of the literature. Front Psychiatry 10:76, 2019 30873049

Geng Y, Zhao W, Zhou F, et al: Oxytocin enhancement of emotional empathy: generalization across cultures and effects on amygdala activity. Front Neurosci 12:512, 2018 30108475

Gerard F, Moeller ACS: Pharmacotherapy of clinical aggression in individuals with psychopathic disorders, in The International Handbook of Psychopathic Disorders and the Law, Volume 1: Diagnosis and Treatment. Edited by Felthous AR, Saß H. Hoboken, NJ, Wiley, 2007, pp 397–416

Gerra G, Di Petta G, D'Amore A, et al: Effects of olanzapine on aggressiveness in heroin dependent patients. Prog Neuropsychopharmacol Biol Psychiatry 30(7):1291–1298, 2006 16766110

Ghani S: Psychiatric drug development: a dry pipeline? Health Management 14(4):30–31, 2014

Giustino TF, Fitzgerald PJ, Maren S: Revisiting propranolol and PTSD: memory erasure or extinction enhancement? Neurobiol Learn Mem 130:26–33, 2016 26808441

Gowin JL, Green CE, Alcorn JL, et al: Chronic tiagabine administration and aggressive responding in individuals with a history of substance abuse and antisocial behavior. J Psychopharmacol 26(7):982–993, 2012 21730016

Guy W (ed): Clinical global impressions, in ECDEU Assessment Manual for Psychopharmacology, Revised (DHEW Publ No ADM 76-338). Rockville, MD, National Institute of Mental Health, 1976, pp 217–222

Hirose S: Effective treatment of aggression and impulsivity in antisocial personality disorder with risperidone. Psychiatry Clin Neurosci 55(2):161–162, 2001 11285097

Jesner OS, Aref-Adib M, Coren E: Risperidone for autism spectrum disorder. Cochrane Database Syst Rev (1):CD005040, 2007 17253538

Jones RM, Arlidge J, Gillham R, et al: Efficacy of mood stabilisers in the treatment of impulsive or repetitive aggression: systematic review and meta-analysis. Br J Psychiatry 198(2):93–98, 2011 21282779

Kamarck TW, Haskett RF, Muldoon M, et al: Citalopram intervention for hostility: results of a randomized clinical trial. J Consult Clin Psychol 77(1):174–188, 2009 19170463

Karim A, Khalil R, Schneider M, et al: P111 Neurobiology of deception and moral cognition. Clin Neurophysiol 128(3):e68, 2017

Kästner N, Richter SH, Urbanik S, et al: Brain serotonin deficiency affects female aggression. Sci Rep 9(1):1366, 2019 30718564

Katzman MA, Bleau P, Blier P, et al: Canadian clinical practice guidelines for the management of anxiety, posttraumatic stress and obsessive-compulsive disorders. BMC Psychiatry 14 (suppl 1):S1, 2014 25081580

Kennedy SH, Lam RW, McIntyre RS, et al: Canadian Network for Mood and Anxiety Treatments (CANMAT) 2016 clinical guidelines for the management of adults with major depressive disorder, Section 3: pharmacological treatments. Can J Psychiatry 61(9):540–560, 2016 27486148

Kessing LV, Søndergård L, Kvist K, et al: Suicide risk in patients treated with lithium. Arch Gen Psychiatry 62(8):860–866, 2005 16061763

Khalifa N, Duggan C, Stoffers J, et al: Pharmacological interventions for antisocial personality disorder. Cochrane Database Syst Rev (8):CD007667, 2010 20687091

Khalifa NR, Gibbon S, Völlm BA, et al: Pharmacological interventions for antisocial personality disorder. Cochrane Database Syst Rev 9:CD007667, 2020 32880105

Koch MW, Polman SK: Oxcarbazepine versus carbamazepine monotherapy for partial onset seizures. Cochrane Database Syst Rev (4):CD006453, 2009 19821367

Lane SD, Gowin JL, Green CE, et al: Acute topiramate differentially affects human aggressive responding at low vs. moderate doses in subjects with histories of substance abuse and antisocial behavior. Pharmacol Biochem Behav 92(2):357–362, 2009 19353809

Leucht S, Cipriani A, Spineli L, et al: Comparative efficacy and tolerability of 15 antipsychotic drugs in schizophrenia: a multiple-treatments meta-analysis. Lancet 382(9896):951–962, 2013 23810019

Liemburg EJ, Knegtering H, Klein HC, et al: Antipsychotic medication and prefrontal cortex activation: a review of neuroimaging findings. Eur Neuropsychopharmacol 22(6):387–400, 2012 22300864

Lilienfeld SO, Andrews BP: Development and preliminary validation of a self-report measure of psychopathic personality traits in noncriminal populations. J Pers Assess 66(3):488–524, 1996 8667144

Lion JR: Benzodiazepines in the treatment of aggressive patients. J Clin Psychiatry 40(2):70–71, 1979 762032

Malhi GS, Tanious M, Das P, et al: Potential mechanisms of action of lithium in bipolar disorder: current understanding. CNS Drugs 27(2):135–153, 2013 23371914

Manhapra A, Chakraborty A, Arias AJ: Topiramate pharmacotherapy for alcohol use disorder and other addictions: a narrative review. J Addict Med 13(1):7–22, 2019 30096077

Markota M, Rummans TA, Bostwick JM, et al: Benzodiazepine use in older adults: dangers, management, and alternative therapies. Mayo Clin Proc 91(11):1632–1639, 2016 27814838

Masi G, Milone A, Canepa G, et al: Olanzapine treatment in adolescents with severe conduct disorder. Eur Psychiatry 21(1):51–57, 2006 16487906

Mattes JA: Comparative effectiveness of carbamazepine and propranolol for rage outbursts. J Neuropsychiatry Clin Neurosci 2(2):159–164, 1990 2136070

Mattes JA: Oxcarbazepine in patients with impulsive aggression: a double-blind, placebo-controlled trial. J Clin Psychopharmacol 25(6):575–579, 2005 16282841

Mattes JA: Levetiracetam in patients with impulsive aggression: a double-blind, placebo-controlled trial. J Clin Psychiatry 69(2):310–315, 2008 18232724

National Collaborating Centre for Mental Health: Interventions for People With Antisocial Personality Disorder and Associated Symptoms and Behaviours. London, British Psychological Society and Royal College of Psychiatrists, 2010

National Institute for Health and Care Excellence: Antisocial Personality Disorder: Prevention and Management (No CG77). London, National Institute for Health and Care Excellence, 2009

Nickel MK, Nickel C, Mitterlehner FO, et al: Topiramate treatment of aggression in female borderline personality disorder patients: a double-blind, placebo-controlled study. J Clin Psychiatry 65(11):1515–1519, 2004 15554765

Nickel MK, Nickel C, Kaplan P, et al: Treatment of aggression with topiramate in male borderline patients: a double-blind, placebo-controlled study. Biol Psychiatry 57(3):495–499, 2005 15737664

Patience DA, McGuire RJ, Scott AI, et al: The Edinburgh Primary Care Depression Study: personality disorder and outcome. Br J Psychiatry 167(3):324–330, 1995 7496640

Pigott K, Galizia I, Vasudev K, et al: Topiramate for acute affective episodes in bipolar disorder in adults. Cochrane Database Syst Rev 9:CD003384, 2016 27591453

Pine DS, Coplan JD, Wasserman GA, et al: Neuroendocrine response to fenfluramine challenge in boys: associations with aggressive behavior and adverse rearing. Arch Gen Psychiatry 54(9):839–846, 1997 9294375

Porsteinsson AP, Drye LT, Pollock BG, et al: Effect of citalopram on agitation in Alzheimer disease: the CitAD randomized clinical trial. JAMA 311(7):682–691, 2014 24549548

Powell BJ, Campbell JL, Landon JF, et al: A double-blind, placebo-controlled study of nortriptyline and bromocriptine in male alcoholics subtyped by comorbid psychiatric disorders. Alcohol Clin Exp Res 19(2):462–468, 1995 7625583

Pringsheim T, Gardner D, Addington D, et al: The assessment and treatment of antipsychotic-induced akathisia. Can J Psychiatry 63(11):719–729, 2018 29685069

Quadros IM, Takahashi A, Miczek KA: Serotonin and aggression, in Handbook of the Behavioral Neurobiology of Serotonin. Edited by Müller CP, Jacobs BL. San Diego, CA, Elsevier Academic Press, 2010, pp 687–713

Ripoll LH, Triebwasser J, Siever LJ: Evidence-based pharmacotherapy for personality disorders. Int J Neuropsychopharmacol 14(9):1257–1288, 2011 21320390

Rocca P, Marchiaro L, Cocuzza E, et al: Treatment of borderline personality disorder with risperidone. J Clin Psychiatry 63(3):241–244, 2002 11926724

Rosell DR, Siever LJ: The neurobiology of aggression and violence. CNS Spectr 20(3):254–279, 2015 25936249

Schaller JL, Thomas J, Rawlings D: Low-dose tiagabine effectiveness in anxiety disorders. MedGenMed 6(3):8, 2004 15520630

Schloesser RJ, Martinowich K, Manji HK: Mood-stabilizing drugs: mechanisms of action. Trends Neurosci 35(1):36–46, 2012 22217451

Schmidt CJ, Sorensen SM, Kehne JH, et al: The role of 5-HT2A receptors in antipsychotic activity. Life Sci 56(25):2209–2222, 1995 7791509

Schoonjans A-S, Marchau F, Paelinck BP, et al: Cardiovascular safety of low-dose fenfluramine in Dravet syndrome: a review of its benefit-risk profile in a new patient population. Curr Med Res Opin 33(10):1773–1781, 2017 28704161

Seitz DP, Gill SS, Herrmann N, et al: Pharmacological treatments for neuropsychiatric symptoms of dementia in long-term care: a systematic review. Int Psychogeriatr 25(2):185–203, 2013 23083438

Sharma T, Guski LS, Freund N, et al: Suicidality and aggression during antidepressant treatment: systematic review and meta-analyses based on clinical study reports. BMJ 352:i65, 2016 26819231

Sheard M: Effect of lithium on human aggression. Nature 230(5289):113–114, 1971 4927008

Sheard MH, Marini JL, Bridges CI, et al: The effect of lithium on impulsive aggressive behavior in man. Am J Psychiatry 133(12):1409–1413, 1976 984241

Shorter E: The history of lithium therapy. Bipolar Disord 11 (suppl 2):4–9, 2009 19538681

Siever LJ: Neurobiology of aggression and violence. Am J Psychiatry 165(4):429–442, 2008 18346997

Stanford MS, Helfritz LE, Conklin SM, et al: A comparison of anticonvulsants in the treatment of impulsive aggression. Exp Clin Psychopharmacol 13(1):72–77, 2005 15727506

Steenen SA, van Wijk AJ, van der Heijden GJMG, et al: Propranolol for the treatment of anxiety disorders: systematic review and meta-analysis. J Psychopharmacol 30(2):128–139, 2016 26487439

Steiner H, Petersen ML, Saxena K, et al: Divalproex sodium for the treatment of conduct disorder: a randomized controlled clinical trial. J Clin Psychiatry 64(10):1183–1191, 2003 14658966

Timmermann M, Jeung H, Schmitt R, et al: Oxytocin improves facial emotion recognition in young adults with antisocial personality disorder. Psychoneuroendocrinology 85:158–164, 2017 28865940

Tupin JP, Smith DB, Clanon TL, et al: The long-term use of lithium in aggressive prisoners. Compr Psychiatry 14(4):311–317, 1973 4724658

Vartiainen H, Tiihonen J, Putkonen A, et al: Citalopram, a selective serotonin reuptake inhibitor, in the treatment of aggression in schizophrenia. Acta Psychiatr Scand 91(5):348–351, 1995 7639092

Vasudev A, Macritchie K, Vasudev K, et al: Oxcarbazepine for acute affective episodes in bipolar disorder. Cochrane Database Syst Rev (12):CD004857, 2011 22161387

Verkes RJ, Van der Mast RC, Hengeveld MW, et al: Reduction by paroxetine of suicidal behavior in patients with repeated suicide attempts but not major depression. Am J Psychiatry 155(4):543–547, 1998 9546002

Walker C, Thomas J, Allen TS: Treating impulsivity, irritability, and aggression of antisocial personality disorder with quetiapine. Int J Offender Ther Comp Criminol 47(5):556–567, 2003 14526596

Warnez S, Alessi-Severini S: Clozapine: a review of clinical practice guidelines and prescribing trends. BMC Psychiatry 14:102, 2014 24708834

Wentworth S: Is pharma underinvesting in mental health? Toronto, ON, Canada, Six Degrees Medical, 2019. Available at: https://sixdegreesmed.com/2020/01/31/is-pharma-underinvesting-in-mental-health. Accessed August 6, 2020.

Won E, Kim Y-K: An oldie but goodie: lithium in the treatment of bipolar disorder through neuroprotective and neurotrophic mechanisms. Int J Mol Sci 18(12):E2679, 2017 29232923

Yaari Y, Selzer ME, Pincus JH: Phenytoin: mechanisms of its anticonvulsant action. Ann Neurol 20(2):171–184, 1986 2428283

Yatham LN, Kennedy SH, Parikh SV, et al: Canadian Network for Mood and Anxiety Treatments (CANMAT) and International Society for Bipolar Disorders (ISBD) 2018 guidelines for the management of patients with bipolar disorder. Bipolar Disord 20(2):97–170, 2018 29536616

Yildiz A, Sachs GS, Turgay A: Pharmacological management of agitation in emergency settings. Emerg Med J 20(4):339–346, 2003 12835344

Yudofsky SC, Silver JM, Jackson W, et al: The Overt Aggression Scale for the objective rating of verbal and physical aggression. Am J Psychiatry 143(1):35–39, 1986 3942284

CHAPTER 19

Treatment Issues With Antisocial Personality Disorder

Donald W. Black, M.D.

Treating antisocial personality disorder (ASPD) can be difficult and challenging. In this chapter, I focus on issues that directly or indirectly interfere with either accessing or delivering treatment, and although this discussion pertains mainly to psychotherapy, clinicians prescribing medication face many of the same issues. I also briefly discuss treatment settings and risk mitigation.

Impediments to Accessing or Providing Care

Impediments to accessing or providing treatment for individuals with ASPD include infrequency of diagnosis, therapeutic gloom, treatment rejection, and difficult patient characteristics.

Infrequency of Diagnosis

One impediment is the infrequency with which ASPD is diagnosed. Many mental health professionals fail to make the diagnosis, or ignore the diagnosis, even when obvious. This could relate to the well-documented stigma surrounding personality disorder diagnoses (Lewis and Appleby 1988). As shown with borderline personality disorder, many mental health professionals avoid caring for these individuals because of their negative attitudes toward the diagnosis (Black et al. 2011). If they do treat these patients, rather than making an ASPD diagnosis, many mental health professionals instead focus on isolated manifestations of the disorder such as anger outbursts, impulsivity, or recklessness rather than seeing them as part of a larger pattern.

Therapeutic Gloom

The therapeutic gloom (or nihilism) many mental health professionals associate with ASPD might prevent some of them from making the diagnosis. Antisocial individuals are unfairly labeled as unable to profit from therapy, which Beck et al. (2004) call the *untreatability myth*. As reviewed in Chapter 17, "Psychosocial Treatment of Antisocial Personality Disorder," empirical data suggest otherwise. But because these myths have long circulated among mental health professionals, they have likely contributed to the general pessimism toward ASPD treatment and may contribute to the lack of treatment research.

Treatment Rejection

Individuals with ASPD have been described as *treatment rejecting* (Tyrer et al. 2003). They rarely seek help for problems that arise from their personality disorder, in contrast to people with borderline personality disorder, who have high rates of health care use. This could be related to the antisocial person's tendency to externalize his or her difficulties (National Institute for Health and Care Excellence 2009). When persons with ASPD do present, their interest in and commitment to treatment are often minimal, perhaps because they feel coerced to seek treatment by family, friends, or the law (Black and Braun 1998). Comorbid conditions such as depression, suicidal thoughts or behaviors, substance misuse, anger outbursts, or marital problems are what typically lead these individuals to seek help (Black and Braun 1998), not the ASPD itself.

Difficult Patient Characteristics

Antisocial individuals bring with them a set of attitudes and behaviors that interfere with or otherwise complicate treatment (e.g., anger, blaming others, impulsivity) (Strasburger 1986). Rather than accepting responsibility for their actions, they blame others. Rather than following through with treatment, they quit abruptly. Rather than showing a willingness to engage in treatment, they lash out at the therapist. It is little wonder that many mental health professionals prefer not to work with these patients. These and other patient characteristics that contribute to the clinician's negative attitude toward such patients are outlined later in the chapter in the section "Challenges to Treatment."

Making the Diagnosis

It is important that ASPD be fully explained to the patient once a diagnosis has been made (Black 2003). The diagnosis should be presented in a straightforward, nonjudgmental manner that does not minimize the potentially devastating nature of the disorder. The onus for improvement should be placed on the patient. ASPD can be explained to patients as a *lifestyle disorder* that has affected their important life domains, placing them in conflict with society. It might be helpful to show patients and their family members (if present) the DSM-5 diagnostic criteria (American Psychiatric Association 2013). Some models for treating borderline personality disorder, such as Systems Training for Emotional Predictability and Problem Solving (STEPPS; Blum et al. 2008), recommend reviewing the diagnostic criteria and encouraging the person to "own" the disorder.

Treating Antisocial Personality Disorder

Therapists should be familiar with community resources that can assist in recovery, including support groups, vocational guidance, and other social services. They also should be accustomed to working with spouses, partners, and families; family involvement is important because the antisocial person will likely have disrupted important relationships. Some antisocial patients should be referred for neuropsychological testing because of frequent comorbidity with learning disorders that could interfere with treatment. Personality testing can also be helpful in selected individuals. The evaluation of antisocial patients is further discussed in Chapter 5, "Clinical Symptoms and Assessment of Antisocial Personality Disorder."

Care Settings

Most treatment can be delivered in an outpatient setting where an array of services is available, including psychotherapy, medication management, and case management. Because antisocial persons can be disruptive on inpatient units, it is best to avoid hospitalizing antisocial patients unless there is a specific reason to do so (Black 2003; Carney 1978). Reasons to hospitalize antisocial patients could include the presence of suicidal thoughts or a recent attempt, the need to protect others if the patient has thoughts or plans to harm others, the need to treat a disabling depression, or the need to be withdrawn from a substance under medical supervision (e.g., opioids). Because of the antisocial patient's impulsivity, the clinician should be prepared for abrupt discharges. High rates of hospital discharges against medical advice are well documented in these patients (Brook et al. 2006).

The following vignette shows how an antisocial patient can be disruptive on a psychiatric inpatient unit.

> Mr. H, a 46-year-old man, was admitted from the emergency department for observation and treatment after expressing suicidal thoughts and urges. He was recently discharged from a state prison and gave a history of violent behavior and assaults. Past medical records documented a lengthy history of misconduct, including criminality, violence, lying, and irresponsibility.
>
> The interview was remarkable for Mr. H's disrespectful attitude toward the clinicians and disdain for the admitting process. He appeared interested mainly in describing his history of aggression and showing off his recent "battle" scar received in a knife fight. A physical examination was remarkable for a 5-cm linear scar on his cheek and gang-related tattoos on his torso and upper arms.
>
> Mr. H reported having been previously diagnosed with an anxiety disorder and demanded treatment with benzodiazepines. Because of a history of substance abuse, he was informed that potentially addicting medications would not be prescribed, but other medications, such as buspirone, might help. Clearly unhappy with this response, he said that without such drugs he would become very angry.
>
> Mr. H had no obvious symptoms of depression, ate well, and slept soundly. His menacing attitude worried the other patients, who avoided him. On the third day of hospitalization, he threatened the attending psychiatrist with physical harm if he did not immediately prescribe benzodiazepines. Because there was no objective evidence of depression or suicidality, the psychiatrist discharged Mr. H after seeking support from the hospital security team.

In retrospect, Mr. H should not have been admitted to the inpatient unit, but many psychiatrists feel obligated to offer hospitalization to those who express suicidal thoughts or plans. Because there was no objective evidence of depressed mood or suicidality during the brief stay, it was clear that the patient was malingering, which is often comorbid with ASPD.

Risk Mitigation

Providing outpatient care necessitates that clinicians consider ways to minimize risk to self and others because many patients with ASPD have a history of violence (Table 19–1). For that reason, clinicians should be mindful of the patient's personal history of aggression and learn to balance the patient's needs against the clinician's needs to ensure a safe treatment environment. The clinician should see the patient in an outpatient clinic setting during regular work hours to ensure that others are around if problems arise. No new patient should be assumed to be safe in the absence of informants or confirmatory records. If in doubt, the interview room door should remain open, with the clinician seated near the door.

Some patients will manipulate therapists into violating boundaries by agreeing to see them after hours, on weekends, or in places outside the clinic. All these situations should raise a red flag to the clinician. Patients should be informed that treatment will take place only in the outpatient clinic during regular work hours.

Clinicians should convey an attitude of *respectful neutrality*, a term that indicates that he or she seeks information without making value judgments about its content. Patients should be reassured that what is said will remain confidential, but they also should be told that if the clinician has reason to believe that the patient presents a direct threat to others (e.g., has threatened to harm a specific person), then the law may require that confidentiality be broken and the intended victim warned (Appelbaum and Zoltek-Jick 1996; Felthous 2006). This stance on patient privacy ensures that paranoid beliefs are not reinforced while also allowing the clinician to maintain his or her legal and professional responsibilities (Davidson et al. 2010).

Maintaining a safe environment necessitates monitoring aggressive impulses by asking patients about their history of criminality, arrests, or incarceration; their history of aggression and violence; their violent urges or thoughts; and their access to guns or other dangerous weapons. Many of these questions should be repeated on an ongoing basis, just as depressed patients are recurrently asked about thoughts of harming themselves. This is one area in which many naïve therapists err in their judgment. They might surmise that the patient is safe or might fail to ask questions that they believe might interfere with rapport. Davidson et al. (2010) discussed this problem in the context of conducting their randomized clinical trial of cognitive-behavioral therapy: "One risk we encountered was the potential that therapists risked 'forgetting' that their patients with ASPD had a history of violence toward others…and that his propensity for violence may initially remain undiminished" (p. 90).

Challenges to Treatment

Mental health professionals understand that many antisocial patients have difficult and challenging behaviors that are part and parcel of the disorder. People with ASPD are impulsive; they blame others while avoiding taking responsibility for their actions, they display low frustration tolerance, and they have difficulty forming trust-

TABLE 19–1.	Risk mitigation strategies when treating antisocial personality disorder

Provide care in an outpatient setting during regular work hours to ensure that others are available if help is needed.

With new patients, consider leaving the office door open, and sit near the door. Remember the adage "Never let the patient get between you and the door."

Be knowledgeable of the patient's history of aggression and violence on the basis of previous medical records, public documents, or history provided by the patient, relatives, or friends.

Maintain an attitude of respectful neutrality.

Monitor the patient's aggressive impulses and behaviors the same way that you might monitor a depressed patient's suicidal thoughts or plans.

ing relationships. These traits can all interfere with treatment or prevent the patient from making progress. Furthermore, many antisocial individuals lack motivation to improve. They are notoriously poor self-observers, often not seeing themselves as the source of their difficulties even when this is obvious to everyone else.

Antisocial persons rarely see themselves as others do and are hard to convince that their self-image is distorted. Cleckley (1976) pointed out the antisocial person's specific lack of insight in *The Mask of Sanity*: "He has absolutely no capacity to see himself as others see him…. This is almost astonishing in view of the psychopath's perfect orientation, his ability and willingness to reason…and his perfect freedom from delusions and other signs of an ordinary psychosis" (p. 383).

Treatment sessions can end abruptly if the patient is challenged or provoked and could lead the patient to end therapy altogether. Dropout rates for outpatient therapy are high (Dolan and Coid 1993; Huband et al. 2007). Characteristics associated with high dropout rates include a hostile attributional style, low educational attainment, and impulsivity (National Institute for Health and Care Excellence 2009). On the other hand, antisocial individuals expect therapists to accommodate their demands and to be as interested in them as they are in themselves. Unrealistic about the goals of treatment, they may expect a quick solution to lifelong problems even while ignoring their therapists' recommendations. Sociologists William and Joan McCord described the challenge of treating these patients: "The psychopath is like a chow dog who may turn and bite the hand that pets it. The psychopath's hard emotional shell, his disturbing aggression, and his complete irresponsibility make therapy a thankless task" (McCord and McCord 1956, p. 84). Written in 1956, these observations, unfortunately, remain true today.

Countertransference Issues

Although they are trained to approach mental health problems in an objective, non-judgmental, and goal-oriented way, most therapists experience emotions—just like anyone else—in response to the antisocial patient's malevolent cognitions or disturbing behaviors. The term used to describe these emotions is *countertransference*. Although psychoanalysts use the term narrowly to refer to neurotic conflicts of the therapist reactivated by the patient, a more widely accepted use of the term is to define countertransference as "any emotional reaction the clinician has toward his patient" (Strasburger 1986, p. 195).

TABLE 19–2.   **Strasburger's seven countertransference reactions**

1. *Fear of assault or harm*: An emotional reaction among therapists is a feeling of fear, which may be rational if it is based on the patient's history of violence or aggression or if the patient has made implied or direct threats. The clinician's priority should be safety, and he or she should not be lulled into the belief that he or she is physically invulnerable.

2. *Helplessness and guilt*: A therapist might feel "impotent in his quest for change in the patient" (p. 198). The therapist might feel that his or her efforts to help are rejected or that he or she is devalued. In response, the patient's lack of improvement can fuel a sense of rage directed toward the patient.

3. *Feelings of invalidity and loss of identity*: Feelings of helplessness and guilt can arise when therapy proves slow, difficult, or unproductive, and the therapist's idealized self-image as kind and caring is undermined. As the patient disowns his or her problems and attributes them to the therapist, the therapist may feel that *he or she* owns the problems. The therapist may begin to doubt his or her sense of professional identity.

4. *Denial*: Denial of the patient's potential for violence could lead to a failure to ask about weapons, past criminality, and violence, thereby placing the therapist in a vulnerable position.

5. *Rejection:* Therapists might experience feelings of rejection, anger, or even hatred in the face of the patient's seemingly immovable personality or record of misdeeds. A therapist might reject a patient in subtle ways, such as acting bored during therapy sessions or being late for appointments or even ignoring the patient altogether.

6. *Hatred*: Therapists can develop a sense of revulsion for the patient based on his or her malevolent attitudes or past crimes. Furthermore, the patient's assaults on the therapist's self-esteem can arouse hatred.

7. *Rage and the wish to destroy*: "Whether it be through reactive mirroring the emotion of the patient or through the more complex route of identification with the aggressor the therapist will find anger to be a constant companion in the treatment of antisocial syndromes" (pp. 201–202).

Source.   Adapted from Strasburger 1986.

Strasburger (1986) outlined seven specific countertransference reactions that clinicians might experience (Table 19–2).

To these reactions, Meloy and Yakeley (2014) add several others. They describe *assumption of psychological maturity* as a subtle reaction whereby the clinician comes to believe that the patient is as developmentally mature and complex as is the clinician, and the patient's actual maturity needs to be facilitated or discovered in treatment. This reaction can be common when the patient has an above-average IQ. *Fascination*, *excitement*, and *sexual attraction* are other potential reactions in which the clinician is strongly drawn to the patient. The clinician provides an "eager audience" for an antisocial patient to regale him or her with tales of various exploits and misdeeds. In some situations, this countertransference can be sexualized, particularly between a male patient and a female therapist. In addition to these responses, Meloy and Yakeley (2014) add *therapeutic nihilism*, a reaction discussed earlier in the chapter.

Strasburger (1986) advised that mental health professionals who choose to work with antisocial individuals should be well versed in the disorder, should be able to anticipate their own emotions, and should present an attitude of acceptance without moralizing. They should understand their limits and have a sound sense of their professional identity, should be firm in dealing with manipulation, and should be willing to set limits. They should abandon rescue fantasies (e.g., "Only I can save this patient") and recognize that the onus for treatment success rests with the patient, not themselves.

Conclusion

As outlined in Chapter 17 and Chapter 18, "Pharmacological Treatment of Antisocial Personality Disorder," no standard or consistently effective treatments are available for ASPD. Stigma and therapeutic nihilism often prevent patients from seeking help or clinicians from offering to provide care. Antisocial patients can be treated in outpatient clinics, where an array of services can be provided. Antisocial individuals have many characteristics that have the potential to interfere with treatment or end it abruptly. Clinicians should be mindful of risk mitigation and take care to ensure that the treatment setting is safe.

Key Points

- Infrequency of diagnosis, therapeutic gloom, treatment rejection, and difficult patient characteristics can impede access to or provision of care for individuals with antisocial personality disorder (ASPD).

- The outpatient clinic is the most appropriate setting for care delivery. Risk mitigation strategies should be used to ensure a safe care environment.

- Hospitalization is appropriate only if the patient with ASPD is considered a danger to self or others, needs to be withdrawn from substances under medical supervision, or needs treatment of a disabling depression.

- Countertransference issues, such as fear of assault or harm and feelings of helplessness or guilt, can impede provision of care.

References

American Psychiatric Association: Diagnostic and Statistical Manual of Mental Disorders, 5th Edition. Arlington, VA, American Psychiatric Association, 2013

Appelbaum PS, Zoltek-Jick R: Psychotherapists' duties to third parties: Ramona and beyond. Am J Psychiatry 153(4):457–465, 1996 8599392

Beck AT, Freeman A, Davis DD, et al: Antisocial personality disorder, in Cognitive Therapy of Personality Disorders, 2nd Edition. New York, Guilford, 2004, pp 162–186

Black DW: Bad Boys, Bad Men: Confronting Antisocial Personality Disorder (Sociopathy), Revised and Updated. New York, Oxford University Press, 2013

Black DW, Braun D: Antisocial patients: a comparison of persons with and persons without childhood conduct disorder. Ann Clin Psychiatry 10(2):53–57, 1998

Black DW, Pfohl B, Blum N, et al: Attitudes toward borderline personality disorder: a survey of 706 mental health clinicians. CNS Spectr 16(3):67–74, 2011 24725357

Blum N, St John D, Pfohl B, et al: Systems Training for Emotional Predictability and Problem Solving (STEPPS) for outpatients with borderline personality disorder: a randomized controlled trial and 1-year follow-up. Am J Psychiatry 165(4):468–478, 2008 18281407

Brook M, Hilty DM, Liu W, et al: Discharge against medical advice from inpatient psychiatric treatment: a literature review. Psychiatr Serv 57(8):1192–1198, 2006 16870972

Carney FL: Inpatient treatment programs, in The Psychopath: A Comprehensive Study of Antisocial Disorders and Behaviors. Edited by Reid WH. New York, Brunner/Mazel, 1978, pp 261–285

Cleckley H: The Mask of Sanity: An Attempt to Clarify Some Issues About the So-Called Psychopathic Personality, 5th Edition. St. Louis, MO, CV Mosby, 1976

Davidson K, Halford J, Kirkwood L, et al: CBT for violent men with antisocial personality disorder: reflections on the experience of carrying out therapy in MASCOT, a pilot randomized controlled trial. Pers Ment Health 4:86–95, 2010

Dolan B, Coid J: Psychopathic and Antisocial Personality Disorders: Treatment and Research Issues. Glasgow, UK, Bell & Bain, 1993

Felthous AR: Warning a potential victim of a person's dangerousness: clinician's duty or victim's right? J Am Acad Psychiatry Law 34(3):338–348, 2006 17032958

Huband N, McMurran M, Evans C, et al: Social problem-solving plus psychoeducation for adults with personality disorder: pragmatic randomised controlled trial. Br J Psychiatry 190:307–313, 2007 17401036

Lewis G, Appleby L: Personality disorder: the patients psychiatrists dislike. Br J Psychiatry 153(153):44–49, 1988 3224249

McCord W, McCord J: Psychopathy and Delinquency. New York, Grune & Stratton, 1956, p 84

Meloy JR, Yakeley J: Antisocial personality disorder, in Gabbard's Treatment of Psychiatric Disorders, Fifth Edition. Edited by Gabbard GO. Washington, DC, American Psychiatric Publishing, 2014, pp 1015–1034

National Institute for Health and Care Excellence: Antisocial Personality Disorder: Prevention and Management (No CG77). London, National Institute for Health and Care Excellence, 2009

Strasburger LH: The treatment of antisocial syndromes: the therapist's feelings, in Unmasking the Psychopath: Antisocial Personality and Related Syndromes. Edited by Reid WH, Dorr D, Walker WI, et al. New York, WW Norton, 1986, pp 191–207

Tyrer P, Mitchard S, Methuen C, Ranger M: Treatment rejecting and treatment seeking personality disorders: type R and type S. J Pers Disorder 17(3):263–268, 2003

PART V

Special Problems,
Populations, and Settings

CHAPTER 20

Criminal Justice System and Antisocial Personality Disorder

Robert L. Trestman, M.D., Ph.D.

Elham Rahmani, M.D., M.P.H.

Nayan Bhatia, M.D.

To fully understand the interface of the criminal justice system with the individual diagnosed with antisocial personality disorder (ASPD), it is important to understand the role of each element. In general, the criminal justice system is broadly composed of the police (arrests), courts (trials, presentencing, sentencing, and drug courts), jails (detention or misdemeanant incarceration) and prisons (felony incarceration), and community corrections (parole and probation). Each of these justice systems serves different roles, including law enforcement, public protection, determination of guilt and sentencing, and, finally, rehabilitation of offenders and prevention of recidivism, respectively. Individuals with ASPD become involved in the justice system at rates greater than those without the diagnosis. There are contributing factors at each stage, which we discuss in turn in this chapter.

The National Epidemiologic Survey on Alcohol and Related Conditions–III (NESARC-III) was funded by the National Institute on Alcohol Abuse and Alcoholism (NIAAA) with supplemental support from the National Institute on Drug Abuse, National Institutes of Health, Bethesda, Maryland. This work was supported in part by the Intramural Programs of the National Institutes of Health, NIAAA. Data from the NESARC-III were analyzed using a limited access data set obtained from NIAAA. The NIH had no further role in study design; in the collection, analysis, and interpretation of data; in the writing of the chapter; or in the decision to submit the chapter for publication.

Antisocial Personality Disorder and Arrests

Rates of Arrest in Persons With Antisocial Personality Disorder

Individuals diagnosed with major mental disorders experience a 10%–20% greater likelihood of arrest in comparison to those without such disorders (Lurigio 2012; Markowitz 2011; Skeem et al. 2011). Of all individuals incarcerated in either federal or state prisons, the prevalence of serious mental disorders is 10%–15% in male prisoners and 20%–35% in female prisoners (Markowitz 2011). These individuals are also, on average, incarcerated for longer periods than individuals without mental disorders (Ballard and Teasdale 2016). In past versions of the *Diagnostic and Statistical Manual of Mental Disorders*, a diagnosis of ASPD required a prior developmental diagnosis of conduct disorder. Although this is no longer the case, studies have shown that individuals who have both diagnoses are usually about 13 years old when first arrested. Those without an antecedent diagnosis of conduct disorder but who have ASPD have, on average, a first arrest age of 20 years; for individuals with neither disorder, the average arrest age is 27 years (Delisi et al. 2018). The causes of higher and earlier arrest rates of individuals with ASPD are often viewed from either a criminalization perspective or a criminality perspective.

Criminalization Perspective

Proponents of a criminalization perspective assert that strict hospital admission criteria, war on drugs and crime, deinstitutionalization, and increased control of the criminal justice system have inordinately affected individuals with a mental disorder. It has been suggested that police officers may be unlikely to seek emergency psychiatric hospitalization because of strict admission criteria, and therefore an arrest ensues. Unfortunately, individuals with a history of violence co-occurring with personality disorders or substance use (even though admission criteria might otherwise be met) are frequently denied hospitalization because of their history (Ballard and Teasdale 2016).

Criminality Perspective

Proponents of a criminality perspective suggest that individuals with mental disorders are inclined to violence and defiance during encounters with law enforcement, leading to higher arrest rates. Various risk factors have been implicated in the explanation of these behaviors, including personality characteristics, psychosocial factors such as homelessness and poor socioeconomic status, and criminogenic needs (Ballard and Teasdale 2016).

Prevalence of Antisocial Personality Disorder in Arrestees

The lifetime prevalence of ASPD in the general population ranges from 2% to 4% in men and 0.5% to 1.0% in women (Compton et al. 2005; Sher et al. 2015). Both environmental and genetic factors play roles in the development of ASPD. The risk of developing ASPD in biological relatives of females with the disorder is much greater than in biological relatives of males with the disorder (Fazel and Danesh 2002). The gender-specific ASPD prevalence estimate in correctional settings is about 50% in males and 20% in females.

Four risk factors have consistently been shown to predict criminal conduct and elevated risk of arrest: history of antisocial behaviors, antisocial personality patterns, antisocial cognition, and antisocial associates (Andrews and Bonta 2010). Juvenile delinquents who are more sociable are less likely to be convicted of crimes than their less sociable counterparts (Henn et al. 1980). Antisocial behaviors have frequently been associated with a history of childhood trauma. Multiple studies have found that experiencing significant maltreatment during childhood and adolescence increases the risk of violence, drug use, delinquency, and, most importantly, arrest in comparison to those without a history of maltreatment (Ireland et al. 2002; Smith et al. 2005). Besides childhood trauma, multiple other risk factors include maternal prenatal depression, male gender, and maternal antisocial features (Hay et al. 2014).

Males and younger adults of both genders tend to have higher rates of arrests and incarcerations than do females and older adults. Observations dating back 50 years suggest that adults older than 60 years are treated much differently in comparison to younger counterparts. Officers tended to be much more compassionate and less stringent in their carrying out of normal procedures (Epstein et al. 1970). A strong criminogenic factor correlated with a higher rate of arrest is a history of arrests. In contrast to previous studies, more recent work has suggested that there is no association between arrest and individuals with ASPD when adjustment is made for prior arrests. Furthermore, no specific association was found between anger or aggressive traits and arrest history (Prins et al. 2015).

Antisocial Personality Disorder and Substance Use Disorders

It is estimated that approximately 5 million violent crimes and 8 million property crimes involved substance use within the United States (Miller et al. 2006). Although there is wide variability in rates of substance use comorbid with ASPD, in some studies it has been estimated that up to 90% of individuals who have been diagnosed with ASPD also have a comorbid substance use disorder. Substance use disorders, as well as ASPD, are associated with violent behavior as well as offending. The combination of alcohol misuse with ASPD is also linked to increased arrest rates, notably for intimate partner violence (Brem et al. 2018; Dykstra et al. 2015).

Antisocial Personality Disorder and the Court

Criminal sentencing has at least four distinct purposes: 1) punishing offenders with sentences that are equivalent to the seriousness of the crime committed, 2) incapacitating offenders to maintain the safety and well-being of the general public, 3) discouraging recidivism, and 4) rehabilitating offenders to enhance prosocial behavior and avoid reoffending (Fitch and Ortega 2000). We examine whether ASPD affects criminal sentencing and how individuals with ASPD do with rehabilitative efforts such as drug court.

Presentencing

The court functions to ensure that individuals who are at high risk to the community be physically detained in jails until they are tried. The system is also responsible for releasing lower-risk individuals on assurance that they will safely and reliably participate in the court proceeding while still at large in the community. In the United States, it has been estimated that approximately 63% of individuals held in jail are pretrial detainees (Clipper et al. 2017). Many of these individuals are released on bond set by the courts as a guarantee that the individual perceived to be involved in criminal activity will be present at trial. It has long been held (e.g., Callahan and Silver 1998) that individuals with substance abuse history and arrest history are relatively likely to be denied bond. Although there are no formal studies regarding the pretrial justice system and ASPD, given that individuals with ASPD often have prior arrests and become justice system involved at an early age, it is likely they are often less frequently released on bond.

In Court

Personality disorder diagnoses, including ASPD, are not a useful defense in court, either during the first phase, when guilt or innocence is determined, or subsequently at sentencing as a potential mitigating factor (Young et al. 2018). Nevertheless, a construct often used in discussions at court of individuals with ASPD is that of *psychopathy*. It has been postulated that having a psychopathy label may result in unjust and punitive outcomes. Various studies suggest that individuals assessed as having psychopathy are often seen as intelligent, bold, responsible for their own actions, and capable of making decisions on right and wrong. They are therefore often perceived as dangerous and evil (Edens et al. 2013). Because of this perceived dangerousness, individuals with psychopathic traits often receive longer and more severe sentences. In this context, the Hare Psychopathy Checklist–Revised (PCL-R; Hare et al. 1991) is increasingly being used and considered by the courts (DeMatteo et al. 2014).

Multiple studies have compared sentences given to individuals assessed as having psychopathy versus no diagnosis at all or psychopathy versus another psychiatric disorder. Although there have been a wide variety of conclusions from multiple studies, a meta-analysis of these studies concluded that there was a significant difference in sentencing for those with a label versus no label, and this was not specific to psychopathy. An assessment of psychopathy or of any other mental health label was associated with harsher punishment (Berryessa and Wohlstetter 2019). This finding speaks to the stigma associated with mental illness in general and mitigates to some degree the concerns that a psychopathy assessment leads to a longer sentence.

Typically, psychopathic traits such as callousness, lack of empathy, and manipulative tendencies are viewed as socially undesirable. In recent years, there is increasing evidence that jurors are influenced by these traits. Although studies suggest that, in general, this may not lead to a significantly worse outcome for the defendant, there are clearly concerning exceptions. One such instance is *Adams v. Texas* (1980). Mr. Adams was tried for the murder of a Dallas, Texas, police officer. The doctors involved in this case concluded that Mr. Adams had ASPD. Under Texas law at that time, if the death sentence were to be issued, it was the prosecutor's burden to prove that the defendant would be dangerous in the future. On the basis of a diagnosis of ASPD, the prosecution was able to convince the jury that Mr. Adams would kill again if given the opportunity. The jury returned a death sentence for Mr. Adams. Three days prior to his execution, the Supreme Court stayed the execution in order to review the lower court's decision. Later, he was found to be innocent, and the previous decision was overturned. As seen here, a diagnosis of ASPD can sometimes mean the difference between life and death.

Court-Mandated Substance Abuse Treatment in Antisocial Personality Disorder

Studies repeatedly find that drug screens of up to 60% of criminal offenders reveal various illicit substances at the time of arrest. The prevalence of comorbid ASPD and substance use disorder in some estimates is as high as 90%. Specialized drug courts were introduced as an alternative to incarceration in response to the increasing number of illicit drug cases presenting to the legal system (Somers and Holtfreter 2018). Specialized drug courts allow offenders to avoid incarceration or criminal records contingent on completing the substance abuse treatment and reoffending (Festinger et al. 2002). These specialized courts not only treat participants for substance use but also provide resources and help individuals obtain education, housing, and even employment. The prevalence of ASPD in individuals who are enrolled in drug treatment courts is usually estimated to be between 40% and 50% (Daughters et al. 2008).

Mandatory treatment may also be a reasonable and successful approach in this population. Individuals with ASPD mandated by the court to treatment in one study were less likely to drop out as compared with those who voluntarily joined the treatment program (Daughters et al. 2008). This is an important finding, because multiple studies have shown that individuals with comorbid ASPD and substance use do much better with contingency management, and in the case of these court-mandated treatments, individuals can avoid incarcerations and even have their records expunged.

Antisocial Personality Disorder and Incarceration

ASPD is common among incarcerated individuals; as many as 80% of prisoners have been reported to have presentations that meet this diagnosis (Ogloff 2006). However, different editions of DSM have used different definitions for ASPD, limiting the body of evidence using each variation. In contrast, the PCL-R (Hare et al. 1991) has provided a more stable standardized measure for studying the condition of psychopathy. Psychopathy is more specific than ASPD, and not all patients who can be diagnosed with ASPD based on DSM criteria will test positive for psychopathy on the PCL-R. Approximately 50%–80% of prisoners can have presentations that meet criteria for ASPD, while only approximately 15% of prisoners would test positive for psychopathy on the PCL-R (Ogloff 2006). The PCL-R focuses on affective, cognitive, and behavioral components, whereas the DSM criteria focus mainly on behavior. Despite these differences, numerous studies have demonstrated that the PCL-R is a reliable and valid measure, and it has been consistently associated with legal outcomes such as recidivism (Shepherd et al. 2018; Tengström et al. 2000). In this chapter, data associated with both ASPD and psychopathy are included when relevant.

Rates of Incarceration in Persons With Antisocial Personality Disorder

Rates of incarceration for individuals with ASPD are high, as pointed out by Robins (1966) in her 30-year follow-up study of former child guidance patients. She found that nearly three-quarters had spent 1 or more years behind bars, while almost 40% had been incarcerated for 5 years or longer. Black reported that nearly 87% of formerly hospitalized antisocial men in his nearly 30-year follow-up study (Black et al. 1995) had a history of incarceration (D.W. Black, personal communication, March 2020). More recently, data from the National Epidemiologic Survey on Alcohol and Related Conditions–III confirm high incarceration rates for adults across the spectrum of antisocial behavior (R.B. Goldstein, S.P. Chou, personal communication, February 2020). More than 36,000 subjects were asked if they had ever been "in jail, prison, or a juvenile detention center" both before age 18 and since age 18, as well as the length of the jailing or detention. Table 20–1 shows rates and lengths of incarceration for those individuals with ASPD, adult antisocial behavior, and conduct disorder without adult antisocial behavior, as compared with individuals without any antisocial syndrome. More than 50% of the individuals with ASPD had been incarcerated, including 44% during adulthood, for a mean of nearly 18 months. Antisocial men were more likely to have been incarcerated than antisocial women (58% vs. 40%). Lower rates were found in those with adult antisocial behavior and those with a history of conduct disorder but no evidence of adult antisocial behavior. In the general population, those without an antisocial syndrome were unlikely to have been incarcerated.

Prevalence of Antisocial Personality Disorder in Incarcerated Persons

Estimated rates of ASPD among incarcerated persons vary from 11% to 78% for men and 12% to 65% in women depending on the sample size, prison population sampled, and assessment method (Black et al. 2010). Blackburn and Coid (1999) reported in a study from the United Kingdom that 62% of 164 violent male offenders had antisocial behavior that met criteria for ASPD. Jordan et al. (1996) assessed 805 women entering prison in North Carolina and reported that 12% were antisocial, while Zlotnick (1999) reported that 40% of 85 women offenders incarcerated in Rhode Island had antisocial behavior that met criteria for ASPD. In a large survey of incarcerated persons in the United Kingdom, Singleton et al. (1997) determined that 56% of 2,371 men and 31% of 771 women were antisocial. Finally, in a sample of 320 offenders newly committed to the Iowa prison system, Black et al. (2010) found that 35% had antisocial behavior that met criteria for ASPD. All these studies point to the frequency with which ASPD is seen in prison settings. These figures are substantially higher than what has been reported in the general population.

Antisocial Personality Disorder, Incarceration, and Gender

Compared with incarcerated men, incarcerated women are less likely to be diagnosed with ASPD and more likely to be diagnosed with borderline personality disorder

TABLE 20–1. Prevalence and duration of juvenile[a] and adult[b] incarceration by antisocial syndrome and sex, National Epidemiologic Survey on Alcohol and Related Conditions–III

	Ever incarcerated in lifetime, % (SE)[c]	Ever incarcerated as juvenile, % (SE)	Duration of juvenile incarceration, months, mean (SE, median)	Ever incarcerated as adult, % (SE)	Duration of adult incarceration, months, mean (SE, median)
Total sample (N=36,309)					
ASPD (n=1,600)	52.8 (1.51)	28.2 (1.61)	9.7 (0.89, 1.0)	44.1 (1.76)	17.6 (1.56, 1.9)
AABS (n=7,470)	31.3 (0.86)	8.9 (0.52)	3.0 (0.30, 0.1)	27.5 (0.82)	8.9 (0.56, 0.1)
Conduct disorder, no AABS (n=154)	13.4 (3.20)	8.2 (2.69)	6.8 (3.86, 0.4)	5.7 (2.39)	2.6 (1.36, 0.03)
No lifetime antisocial syndrome (n=27,085)	4.9 (0.19)	1.2 (0.08)	3.4 (0.61, 0.1)	4.1 (0.15)	3.9 (0.43, 0.04)
Men (n=15,862)					
ASPD (n=1,077)	58.1 (2.08)	30.7 (1.95)	10.7 (0.96, 1.0)	50.3 (1.99)	19.7 (1.90, 2.8)
AABS (n=4,084)	37.5 (1.19)	10.7 (0.68)	3.2 (0.36, 0.1)	33.5 (1.16)	10.5 (0.70, 0.2)
Conduct disorder, no AABS (n=87)	15.1 (4.64)	7.5 (3.28)	9.1 (6.77, 0.1)	8.4 (3.59)	1.9 (1.07, 0.03)
No lifetime antisocial syndrome (n=10,614)	8.3 (0.34)	1.9 (0.15)	4.1 (0.85, 0.1)	7.1 (0.29)	4.6 (0.57, 0.04)
Women (n=20,447)					
ASPD (n=523)	39.7 (2.79)	22.1 (2.58)	6.3 (1.84, 0.5)	28.9 (2.41)	9.0 (1.37, 0.9)
AABS (n=3,386)	21.9 (0.90)	6.4 (0.52)	2.6 (0.52, 0.1)	18.5 (0.84)	4.5 (0.94, 0.1)
Conduct disorder, no AABS (n=67)	10.1 (4.34)	9.6 (4.32)	3.5 (1.24, 2.1)	0.5 (0.52)	—[d]
No lifetime antisocial syndrome (n=16,471)	2.4 (0.15)	0.6 (0.07)	1.9 (0.52, 0.1)	1.8 (0.13)	1.8 (0.50, 0.03)

Note. AABS=adulthood antisocial behavioral syndrome; ASPD=antisocial personality disorder.
[a]Before age 18 years.
[b]Since age 18 years.
[c]Either before or since age 18 years.
[d]Only one female respondent reported a duration of incarceration since age 18 so measures of central tendency and dispersion not relevant.
Source. Data courtesy of R.B. Goldstein, S.P. Chou, personal communication, February 2020.

(BPD) (Trestman et al. 2007). A systematic review of 62 surveys indicated that approximately one in two male prisoners can be diagnosed with ASPD, whereas only approximately one in five female prisoners can be diagnosed with this disorder (Fazel and Danesh 2002). However, this gap narrows among incarcerated women convicted of felonies. A similar pattern is found in studies of gender differences in men and women diagnosed with psychopathy, with the gender gap narrowing among those testing positive for psychopathy (Lewis 2015).

These findings may be explained using several different hypotheses. First, it may be hypothesized that women have a lower genetic and/or biological predisposition to antisocial behavior. However, this cannot explain the diminishing differences among men and women convicted of felonies or those testing positive for psychopathy. The other explanation may be that societal gender roles provide a differential pathway for similar pathophysiology to manifest in men and women. It also may be the case that in instances of similar manifestation, women's behavior may be interpreted differently. These hypotheses are in line with the finding that when the pathology becomes significant enough (felonies and psychopathy), the gender gap fades away.

Antisocial Personality Disorder, Incarceration, and Race

Prevalence estimates of ASPD among different racial groups of inmates are inconsistent among available studies. For instance, a study of inmates in Connecticut's jails found a higher prevalence of ASPD among Hispanic men compared with African American or white men (Trestman et al. 2007). On the other hand, a study on convicted driving while intoxicated offenders in New Mexico found that Hispanic men were less likely to be diagnosed with ASPD compared with non-Hispanic white men (C'de Baca et al. 2004). Differences in racial self-identification, diagnostic bias, and social, cultural, and regional legal factors may contribute to these inconsistencies.

Antisocial Personality Disorder, Incarceration, and Psychiatric Comorbidity

Studies on ASPD often focus on protecting society from individuals with these conditions. Some of the early definitions of psychopathy went as far as assuming that individuals with psychopathy were immune to suicide (Cleckley 1976). This is in sharp contrast with later studies that suggested an increased suicide risk among individuals diagnosed with ASPD or psychopathy (Black et al. 2010; Verona et al. 2001). In addition to a higher risk for suicide, Black et al. found that these patients had a lower quality of life and a higher likelihood of having comorbid psychiatric conditions such as mood and anxiety disorders, substance abuse, psychotic disorders, somatoform disorders, BPD, and ADHD.

Approximately one in two incarcerated offenders with ASPD may also have comorbid BPD, with higher prevalence among women (Black et al. 2010; Blackburn and Coid 1999). Comorbid ASPD and BPD in forensic populations can be associated with severe violence (defined by severity of violent behavior, quantity, and age at onset) (Howard et al. 2014). Of note is the high prevalence of ADHD comorbidity with ASPD. Different studies reflect that 35%–65% of incarcerated individuals with a diagnosis of ASPD have comorbid ADHD (Black et al. 2010; Semiz et al. 2008). Comorbid

ADHD and ASPD are associated with a higher rate of childhood neglect, self-harm behaviors, and suicide attempts (Semiz et al. 2008) as well as earlier onset of addiction and criminality (Mannuzza et al. 2004; Rutter et al. 2006).

Another group of comorbid conditions associated with poor outcome in ASPD is the anxiety disorders. Hodgins et al. (2010) found that in a group of 495 inmates, those with comorbid ASPD and anxiety disorders had an earlier onset of criminal behavior, higher rates of comorbid alcohol and/or drug abuse, a history of interpersonal violence, and suicide attempts.

In general, incarcerated individuals with a diagnosis of ASPD have high rates of psychiatric comorbidity that may contribute to higher risk for suicide attempts, self-harm behaviors, and lower quality of life as well as increased risk of violence. In the absence of highly effective treatments for ASPD, focusing on the treatment of these comorbid conditions may improve the mental health and quality of life of incarcerated individuals with ASPD while also potentially reducing the risk of violent and criminal behavior.

Parole and Probation

Different standardized personality assessment methods have recently been used to predict the risk of reoffending during probation, with limited agreement among different assessment methods (Shaw et al. 2012). However, as with recidivism in general, PCL-R scores have been shown to be strong predictors of recidivism during parole. In one study, those identified as psychopaths by PCL-R were recommitted four times more frequently than nonpsychopaths (Serin et al. 1999). Among men with sex offenses, those with high psychopathy scores and good treatment behavior were at a higher risk for reoffending. A study with Canadian male sex offenders (Porter et al. 2011) observed that those with high psychopathy scores were 2.5 times more likely to be granted conditional release while more likely to recommit both violent and nonviolent offenses. In this study, child molesters with high psychopathy scores were also more likely to be released, despite a higher risk of recommitting sexual offenses. These data emphasize the capabilities of individuals with high psychopathy scores to convince parole boards to release them despite their criminal history and high recidivism rates. As a result, better preparation and training may be necessary in the criminal justice system for dealing with individuals with psychopathic personalities.

Antisocial Personality Disorder and Institutional Misbehavior

There is limited evidence for an association between a DSM diagnosis of ASPD and institutional misbehavior (Edens et al. 2015), but psychopathy measures such as PCL-R scores are modestly associated with the risk of institutional misconduct, including physical aggression, verbal aggression, and nonaggressive infractions (Buffington-Vollum et al. 2002; Guy et al. 2005). Interestingly, these correlations are weakest when it comes to physical aggression. This may be due to relatively lower numbers of such incidents or to cultural or regional factors. For instance, a meta-analysis on the predictive validity of PCL-R for institutional misconduct found this scale to have a higher effect size for physical aggression in non-U.S. prison samples compared with U.S. samples (Buffington-Vollum et al. 2002).

Antisocial Personality Disorder and Recidivism

A diagnosis of ASPD is associated with a higher risk of reconviction and incarceration (Shepherd et al. 2018), and PCL-R scores have been shown to be a strong predictor of recidivism in multiple studies (Hemphill et al. 2011; Tengström et al. 2000). PCL-R scores are associated with general, violent, and sexual recidivism. Those testing positive for psychopathy are three times more likely to recidivate and four times more likely to violently recidivate within a year after their release (Hemphill et al. 2011).

Antisocial Personality Disorder, Genetics, and the Criminal Justice System

Genetic predisposition plays a significant role in an individual's susceptibility to ASPD. A meta-analysis of the available evidence (Ferguson 2010) demonstrated that 56% of the variance in antisocial personality and behavior can be explained by genetic factors. There is also some evidence for a potential synergistic interaction between genetic and environmental factors that significantly increases the risk of aggressive behavior (Cadoret et al. 1995).

Genetics and the Insanity Defense

If an individual is at increased risk for criminal behavior as a result of genetic factors, should he or she be held responsible for his or her behavior? In U.S. courtrooms, ASPD is simply not an allowed defense. Although we will not provide detailed legal arguments on this issue, several points of view are worth mentioning. Probably the most important point to keep in mind is that genetic predisposition is not deterministic. In other words, individuals who have a genetic predisposition for ASPD are not destined to engage in criminal behavior (DeLisi and Vaughn 2015). As a result, environmental factors (including legal consequences) can mitigate their risk. On the other hand, the challenges of the individuals who have personality disorders may arguably be considered at some level during the legal processes and used to better inform treatment and posttrial management (Kinscherff 2010).

Genetics and Risk Reduction

Should we identify individuals who are at genetically increased risk for ASPD for early intervention? This issue is of course highly controversial. Although several susceptibility alleles are associated with ASPD (Morley and Hall 2003), no single gene has been identified as causal. As a result, any genetic screening would be at best expensive and time-consuming. Moreover, any such screening will bring up significant ethical and privacy concerns, and most importantly, genetic screening would be effective only in the presence of well-studied and highly effective interventions. In the absence of such interventions, ethical, practical, and privacy risks will likely outweigh any potential benefits.

Conclusion

Just as there is a natural history to most illness, there is a natural history to the ontogeny of ASPD in any given individual (Black 2015). In parallel, there is all too frequently a natural history of justice involvement for many individuals with ASPD. This pattern of justice involvement is neither absolute nor unidimensionally linked to the diagnosis of ASPD. Genetics, developmental context, educational and therapeutic opportunities, and a broad array of social determinants each contribute to the evolution of criminality in those with ASPD (DeLisi and Vaughn 2015).

Key Points

- Genetics, developmental context, educational and therapeutic opportunities, and a broad array of social determinants contribute to the evolution of criminality in those with antisocial personality disorder (ASPD).

- Gender-specific ASPD prevalence estimates in correctional settings average about 50% of men and 20% of women.

- Antisocial behaviors are associated with a history of childhood maltreatment.

- The diagnosis of ASPD or psychopathy, or another psychiatric diagnosis, is associated with harsher judicial punishment.

- Individuals with ASPD court ordered to substance use disorder treatment are less likely to drop out as compared with those who enter treatment voluntarily.

- Individuals with comorbid ASPD and substance use disorders do much better with contingency management.

References

Adams v Texas, 448 US 38—Supreme Court 1980

Andrews DA, Bonta J: Rehabilitating criminal justice policy and practice. Psychol Public Policy Law 16(1):39–55, 2010

Ballard E, Teasdale B: Reconsidering the criminalization debate: an examination of the predictors of arrest among people with major mental disorders. Criminal Justice Policy Review 27(1):22–45, 2016

Berryessa CM, Wohlstetter B: The psychopathic "label" and effects on punishment outcomes: a meta-analysis. Law Hum Behav 43(1):9–25, 2019 30570278

Black DW: The natural history of antisocial personality disorder. Can J Psychiatry 60(7):309–314, 2015 26175389

Black DW, Baumgard CH, Bell SE: A 16- to 45-year follow-up of 71 men with antisocial personality disorder. Compr Psychiatry 36(2):130–140, 1995 7758299

Black DW, Gunter T, Loveless P, et al: Antisocial personality disorder in incarcerated offenders: psychiatric comorbidity and quality of life. Ann Clin Psychiatry 22(2):113–120, 2010 20445838

Blackburn R, Coid JW: Empirical clusters of DSM-III personality disorders in violent offenders. J Pers Disord 13(1):18–34, 1999 10228924

Brem MJ, Florimbio AR, Elmquist J, et al: Antisocial traits, distress tolerance, and alcohol problems as predictors of intimate partner violence in men arrested for domestic violence. Psychol Violence 8(1):132–139, 2018 29552375

Buffington-Vollum J, Edens JF, Johnson DW, et al: Psychopathy as a predictor of institutional misbehavior among sex offenders: a prospective replication. Criminal Justice and Behavior 29(5):497–511, 2002

C'de Baca J, Lapham SC, Skipper BJ, et al: Psychiatric disorders of convicted DWI offenders: a comparison among Hispanics, American Indians and non-Hispanic whites. J Stud Alcohol 65(4):419–427, 2004 15376815

Cadoret RJ, Yates WR, Troughton E, et al: Genetic-environmental interaction in the genesis of aggressivity and conduct disorders. Arch Gen Psychiatry 52(11):916–924, 1995 7487340

Callahan LA, Silver E: Revocation of conditional release: a comparison of individual and program characteristics across four U.S. states. Int J Law Psychiatry 21(2):177–186, 1998 9612717

Cleckley H: The Mask of Sanity: An Attempt to Clarify Some Issues About the So-Called Psychopathic Personality, 5th Edition. St. Louis, MO, CV Mosby, 1976, pp 338–339

Clipper SJ, Morris RG, Russell-Kaplan A: The link between bond forfeiture and pretrial release mechanism: the case of Dallas County, Texas. PLoS One 12(8):e0182772, 2017 28817579

Compton WM, Conway KP, Stinson FS, et al: Prevalence, correlates, and comorbidity of DSM-IV antisocial personality syndromes and alcohol and specific drug use disorders in the United States: results from the National Epidemiologic Survey on Alcohol and Related Conditions. J Clin Psychiatry 66(6):677–685, 2005 15960559

Daughters SB, Stipelman BA, Sargeant MN, et al: The interactive effects of antisocial personality disorder and court-mandated status on substance abuse treatment dropout. J Subst Abuse Treat 34(2):157–164, 2008 17869050

DeLisi M, Vaughn MG: Ingredients for criminality require genes, temperament, and psychopathic personality. Journal of Criminal Justice 43(4):290–294, 2015

Delisi M, Drury AJ, Caropreso D, et al: Antisocial personality disorder with or without antecedent conduct disorder: the differences are psychiatric and paraphilic. Criminal Justice and Behavior 45(6):902–917, 2018

DeMatteo D, Edens JF, Galloway M, et al: Investigating the role of the Psychopathy Checklist–Revised in United States case law. Psychol Public Policy Law 20:96–107, 2014

Dykstra RE, Schumacher JA, Mota N, et al: Examining the role of antisocial personality disorder in intimate partner violence among substance use disorder treatment seekers with clinically significant trauma histories. Violence Against Women 21(8):958–974, 2015 26084544

Edens JF, Clark J, Smith ST, et al: Bold, smart, dangerous and evil: perceived correlates of core psychopathic traits among jury panel members. Pers Ment Health 7(2):143–153, 2013 24343940

Edens JF, Kelley SE, Lilienfeld SO, et al: DSM-5 antisocial personality disorder: predictive validity in a prison sample. Law Hum Behav 39(2):123–129, 2015 25180763

Epstein LJ, Mills C, Simon A: Antisocial behavior of the elderly. Compr Psychiatry 11(1):36–42, 1970 5411213

Fazel S, Danesh J: Serious mental disorder in 23000 prisoners: a systematic review of 62 surveys. Lancet 359(9306):545–550, 2002 11867106

Ferguson CJ: Genetic contributions to antisocial personality and behavior: a meta-analytic review from an evolutionary perspective. J Soc Psychol 150(2):160–180, 2010 20397592

Festinger DS, Marlowe DB, Lee PA, et al: Status hearings in drug court: when more is less and less is more. Drug Alcohol Depend 68(2):151–157, 2002 12234644

Fitch WL, Ortega RJ: Law and the confinement of psychopaths. Behav Sci Law 18(5):663–678, 2000 11113967

Guy LS, Edens JF, Anthony C, et al: Does psychopathy predict institutional misconduct among adults? A meta-analytic investigation. J Consult Clin Psychol 73(6):1056–1064, 2005 16392979

Hare RD, Hart SD, Harpur TJ: Psychopathy and the DSM-IV criteria for antisocial personality disorder. J Abnorm Psychol 100(3):391–398, 1991 1918618

Hay DF, Waters CS, Perra O, et al: Precursors to aggression are evident by 6 months of age. Dev Sci 17(3):471–480, 2014 24612281

Hemphill JF, Hare RD, Wong S: Psychopathy and recidivism: a review. Legal Criminol Psychol 3(1):139–170, 2011

Henn FA, Bardwell R, Jenkins RL: Juvenile delinquents revisited: adult criminal activity. Arch Gen Psychiatry 37(10):1160–1163, 1980 7425800

Hodgins S, De Brito SA, Chhabra P, et al: Anxiety disorders among offenders with antisocial personality disorders: a distinct subtype? Can J Psychiatry 55(12):784–791, 2010 21172099

Howard RC, Khalifa N, Duggan C: Antisocial personality disorder comorbid with borderline pathology and psychopathy is associated with severe violence in a forensic sample. J Forens Psychiatry Psychol 25(6):658–672, 2014

Ireland TO, Smith CA, Thornberry TP: Developmental issues in the impact of child maltreatment on later delinquency and drug use. Criminology 40(2):359–400, 2002

Jordan BK, Schlenger WE, Fairbank JA, et al: Prevalence of psychiatric disorders among incarcerated women, II: convicted felons entering prison. Arch Gen Psychiatry 53(6):513–519, 1996 8639034

Kinscherff R: Proposition: a personality disorder may nullify responsibility for a criminal act. J Law Med Ethics 38(4):745–759, 2010 21105938

Lewis CF: Gender-specific treatment, in Oxford Textbook of Correctional Psychiatry. Edited by Trestman R, Appelbaum K, Metzner J. New York, Oxford University Press, 2015, pp 293–295

Lurigio AJ: Responding to the needs of people with mental illness in the criminal justice system: an area ripe for research and community partnerships. Journal of Crime and Justice 35:1–12, 2012

Mannuzza S, Klein RG, Abikoff H, et al: Significance of childhood conduct problems to later development of conduct disorder among children with ADHD: a prospective follow-up study. J Abnorm Child Psychol 32(5):565–573, 2004 15500034

Markowitz FE: Mental illness, crime, and violence: risk, context, and social control. Aggress Violent Behav 16(1):36–44, 2011

Miller TR, Levy DT, Cohen MA, et al: Costs of alcohol and drug-involved crime. Prev Sci 7(4):333–342, 2006 16845591

Morley K, Hall W: Is there a genetic susceptibility to engage in criminal acts? Trends Issues Crime Criminal Justice 110:1–6, 2003

Ogloff JR: Psychopathy/antisocial personality disorder conundrum. Aust N Z J Psychiatry 40(6–7):519–528, 2006 16756576

Porter S, Brinke L, Wilson K: Crime profiles and conditional release performance of psychopathic and non-psychopathic sexual offenders. Legal Criminol Psychol 14(1):109–118, 2011

Prins SJ, Skeem JL, Mauro C, et al: Criminogenic factors, psychotic symptoms, and incident arrests among people with serious mental illnesses under intensive outpatient treatment. Law Hum Behav 39(2):177–188, 2015 25133918

Robins LN: Deviant Children Grown Up. Baltimore, MD, Williams & Wilkins, 1966

Rutter M, Kim-Cohen J, Maughan B: Continuities and discontinuities in psychopathology between childhood and adult life. J Child Psychol Psychiatry 47(3–4):276–295, 2006 16492260

Semiz UB, Basoglu C, Oner O, et al: Effects of diagnostic comorbidity and dimensional symptoms of attention-deficit-hyperactivity disorder in men with antisocial personality disorder. Aust N Z J Psychiatry 42(5):405–413, 2008 18473259

Serin R, Peters R, Barbaree H: Predictors of psychopathy and release outcome in a criminal population. Psychol Assessment 2(4):419–422, 1999

Shaw J, Minoudis P, Craissati J: A comparison of the standardised assessment of personality – abbreviated scale and the offender assessment system personality disorder screen in a probation community sample. J Forens Psychiatry Psychol 23(2):156–167, 2012

Shepherd SM, Campbell RE, Ogloff JRP: Psychopathy, antisocial personality disorder, and reconviction in an Australian sample of forensic patients. Int J Offender Ther Comp Criminol 62(3):609–628, 2018 27288398

Sher L, Siever LJ, Goodman M, et al: Gender differences in the clinical characteristics and psychiatric comorbidity in patients with antisocial personality disorder. Psychiatry Res 229(3):685–689, 2015 26296756

Singleton N, Meltzer H, Gatward R, et al: Psychiatric Morbidity Among Prisoners: Summary Report. London, Government Statistical Services, 1997

Skeem JL, Manchak S, Peterson JK: Correctional policy for offenders with mental illness: creating a new paradigm for recidivism reduction. Law Hum Behav 35(2):110–126, 2011 20390443

Smith CA, Ireland TO, Thornberry TP: Adolescent maltreatment and its impact on young adult antisocial behavior. Child Abuse Negl 29(10):1099–1119, 2005 16233913

Somers LJ, Holtfreter K: Gender and mental health: an examination of procedural justice in a specialized court context. Behav Sci Law 36(1):98–115, 2018 29205471

Tengström A, Grann M, Långström N, et al: Psychopathy (PCL-R) as a predictor of violent recidivism among criminal offenders with schizophrenia. Law Hum Behav 24(1):45–58, 2000 10693318

Trestman RL, Ford J, Zhang W, et al: Current and lifetime psychiatric illness among inmates not identified as acutely mentally ill at intake in Connecticut's jails. J Am Acad Psychiatry Law 35(4):490–500, 2007 18086741

Verona E, Patrick CJ, Joiner TE: Psychopathy, antisocial personality, and suicide risk. J Abnorm Psychol 110(3):462–470, 2001 11502089

Young C, Habarth J, Bongar B, et al: Disorder in the court: Cluster B personality disorders in United States case law. Psychiatry Psychol Law 25(5):706–723, 2018 31984047

Zlotnick C: Antisocial personality disorder, affect dysregulation and childhood abuse among incarcerated women. J Pers Disord 13(1):90–95, 1999 10228930

CHAPTER 21

The Antisocial Child

Allan M. Andersen, M.D.

Samuel Kuperman, M.D.

The essential feature of conduct disorder (CD) is a repetitive and persistent pattern of behavior in which the basic rights of others or major age-appropriate societal norms or rules are violated (American Psychiatric Association 2013). The behaviors may entail aggressive conduct that causes or threatens harm to others or animals, nonaggressive behavior resulting in property damage, deceitfulness or theft, or serious violations of rules.

For DSM-5 (American Psychiatric Association 2013) criteria to be met, at least 3 of 15 antisocial behaviors must have been present within the preceding 12 months, and at least 1 in the past 6 months (Box 21–1). The specific behaviors listed are grouped under the categories of aggression to people and animals, destruction of property, deceitfulness or theft, and serious violations of rules. The behaviors must cause clinically significant impairment in functioning. Last, if the individual is 18 years or older, the criteria for antisocial personality disorder (ASPD) cannot be met. While CD technically can be diagnosed at any age, the intention of the final criterion is to describe a childhood behavioral syndrome that is the precursor to ASPD.

Box 21–1.   DSM-5 Diagnostic Criteria for Conduct Disorder

A. A repetitive and persistent pattern of behavior in which the basic rights of others or major age-appropriate societal norms or rules are violated, as manifested by the presence of at least three of the following 15 criteria in the past 12 months from any of the categories below, with at least one criterion present in the past 6 months:

Aggression to People and Animals

1. Often bullies, threatens, or intimidates others.
2. Often initiates physical fights.
3. Has used a weapon that can cause serious physical harm to others (e.g., a bat, brick, broken bottle, knife, gun).

  4. Has been physically cruel to people.
  5. Has been physically cruel to animals.
  6. Has stolen while confronting a victim (e.g., mugging, purse snatching, extortion, armed robbery).
  7. Has forced someone into sexual activity.

Destruction of Property

  8. Has deliberately engaged in fire setting with the intention of causing serious damage.
  9. Has deliberately destroyed others' property (other than by fire setting).

Deceitfulness or Theft

  10. Has broken into someone else's house, building, or car.
  11. Often lies to obtain goods or favors or to avoid obligations (i.e., "cons" others).
  12. Has stolen items of nontrivial value without confronting a victim (e.g., shoplifting, but without breaking and entering; forgery).

Serious Violations of Rules

  13. Often stays out at night despite parental prohibitions, beginning before age 13 years.
  14. Has run away from home overnight at least twice while living in the parental or parental surrogate home, or once without returning for a lengthy period.
  15. Is often truant from school, beginning before age 13 years.

B. The disturbance in behavior causes clinically significant impairment in social, academic, or occupational functioning.

C. If the individual is age 18 years or older, criteria are not met for antisocial personality disorder.

Specify whether:

312.81 (F91.1) Childhood-onset type: Individuals show at least one symptom characteristic of conduct disorder prior to age 10 years.

312.82 (F91.2) Adolescent-onset type: Individuals show no symptom characteristic of conduct disorder prior to age 10 years.

312.89 (F91.9) Unspecified onset: Criteria for a diagnosis of conduct disorder are met, but there is not enough information available to determine whether the onset of the first symptom was before or after age 10 years.

Specify if:

With limited prosocial emotions: To qualify for this specifier, an individual must have displayed at least two of the following characteristics persistently over at least 12 months and in multiple relationships and settings. These characteristics reflect the individual's typical pattern of interpersonal and emotional functioning over this period and not just occasional occurrences in some situations. Thus, to assess the criteria for the specifier, multiple information sources are necessary. In addition to the individual's self-report, it is necessary to consider reports by others who have known the individual for extended periods of time (e.g., parents, teachers, co-workers, extended family members, peers).

Lack of remorse or guilt: Does not feel bad or guilty when he or she does something wrong (exclude remorse when expressed only when caught and/or facing punishment). The individual shows a general lack of concern about the negative consequences of his or her actions. For example, the individual is not remorseful after hurting someone or does not care about the consequences of breaking rules.

Callous—lack of empathy: Disregards and is unconcerned about the feelings of others. The individual is described as cold and uncaring. The person appears more concerned about the effects of his or her actions on himself or herself, rather than their effects on others, even when they result in substantial harm to others.

Unconcerned about performance: Does not show concern about poor/problem-atic performance at school, at work, or in other important activities. The individual does not put forth the effort necessary to perform well, even when expectations are clear, and typically blames others for his or her poor performance.

Shallow or deficient affect: Does not express feelings or show emotions to others, except in ways that seem shallow, insincere, or superficial (e.g., actions contradict the emotion displayed; can turn emotions "on" or "off" quickly) or when emotional expressions are used for gain (e.g., emotions displayed to manipulate or intimidate others).

Specify current severity:

Mild: Few if any conduct problems in excess of those required to make the diagnosis are present, and conduct problems cause relatively minor harm to others (e.g., lying, truancy, staying out after dark without permission, other rule breaking).

Moderate: The number of conduct problems and the effect on others are intermediate between those specified in "mild" and those in "severe" (e.g., stealing without confronting a victim, vandalism).

Severe: Many conduct problems in excess of those required to make the diagnosis are present, or conduct problems cause considerable harm to others (e.g., forced sex, physical cruelty, use of a weapon, stealing while confronting a victim, breaking and entering).

Within DSM-5's classification scheme, CD is placed with disruptive and impulse-control disorders, including oppositional defiant disorder (ODD), intermittent explosive disorder, pyromania, and kleptomania. This group of "externalizing" disorders also includes ASPD, whose criteria are placed with the personality disorders. ODD has often been viewed as a developmental antecedent to CD, although as discussed later in this chapter, there is considerable discontinuity and heterogeneity with respect to individual trajectories among the three disorders.

The CD criteria represent an evolution from earlier DSM classification schemes. DSM-I (American Psychiatric Association 1952) included "conduct disturbance" within the category "adjustment reaction of childhood." Symptoms included truancy, stealing, destructiveness, cruelty, sexual offenses, or alcohol use. In DSM-II (American Psychiatric Association 1968), the category "behavior disorders of childhood and adolescence" was created. Two disorders were included within that category that are similar to today's CD: "unsocialized aggressive reaction" and "group delinquent reaction." The former was characterized by hostile disobedience, quarrelsomeness, stealing, lying, and teasing of others. The latter was characterized by gang loyalty and delinquent behaviors such as stealing, skipping school, and staying out late at night.

DSM-III formally introduced the term "conduct disorder" and included four subtypes based on a 2×2 matrix on the axes of socialization and aggressivity (American Psychiatric Association 1980). These subtypes derived from subtypes described in DSM-II, and symptoms and diagnostic thresholds were specified for each. The criteria were simplified in DSM-III-R (American Psychiatric Association 1987) to include a single set of symptoms; a group type and a solitary aggressive type were described. Each symptom had to be present for at least 6 months to reach diagnostic threshold. DSM-IV field trials supported adding bullying, threatening, or intimidating others to the criteria set, as well as often staying out after dark without permission beginning before age 13 years. These subtypes were discontinued in DSM-IV (American Psychiatric Association 1994) and replaced by the "childhood-onset" and "adolescent-onset" specifiers in recognition of research showing that early onset is a robust predictor of poor outcome (Moffitt 1993).

The criteria in DSM-5 are essentially unchanged from those in DSM-IV (see Box 21–1). In addition to maintaining the age-at-onset subtypes (childhood onset, adolescent onset), the "with limited prosocial emotions" specifier was added. Finally, severity of CD can be specified on the basis of the number of symptoms present and the severity of harm caused to others (i.e., mild, moderate, or severe). The equivalent of *psychopathy* in adults, the specifier is used to recognize children or adolescents who lack remorse or guilt, who are callous, and who lack concern with one's performance (e.g., at school, work). Research shows that the presence of limited prosocial emotions delineates a subtype that is particularly severe and recalcitrant. In addition, limited prosocial emotions are relatively stable from childhood to early adolescence and early adulthood (Frick et al. 2014).

Diagnostic criteria for CD in ICD-10 include the 8 DSM-IV criteria for ODD as well as 16 criteria that are essentially identical to DSM-IV's CD criteria, with an additional criterion used to distinguish theft in the home versus outside of the home (World Health Organization 1993). ICD-10's classification requires that at least 3 of the 6 required symptoms be drawn from the items corresponding to DSM-IV's CD criteria (items 9–24), whereas for criteria for ODD to be met, the child must exhibit no more than two of those symptoms. Similar to DSM, ICD-10 distinguishes between socialized and unsocialized CD.

Other proposed classifications of CD based on factor analyses have emphasized distinctions between covert, nonconfrontational behaviors, such as theft or status violations, and overt, confrontational behaviors, and destructive versus nondestructive behaviors (Frick et al. 1993). With specific respect to aggression, some schemes have made further distinctions between "hot" (impulsive, reactive) and "cold" (predatory, premeditated) types of aggression (McEllistrem 2004), proposing that these different patterns of behavior may stem from different causes, reflect distinct patterns of brain functioning (Atkins and Stoff 1993), and respond to different treatments (Steiner et al. 2011).

Epidemiology

Prevalence estimates for CD vary across geographic location, population, age range, and method of study but generally range from 1% to 10% (Costello et al. 2005; Dulcan et al. 2017; Maughan et al. 2004; Nock et al. 2006), with rates of 2%–5% being the most common (Canino et al. 2004; Costello et al. 2003; Fleitlich-Bilyk and Goodman 2004; Ford et al. 2003; Kessler et al. 2012; Leung et al. 2008; Sawyer et al. 2001). Rates of CD rise from childhood to adolescence, and in adults the 12-month prevalence of CD was 1% in the National Comorbidity Survey Replication (Kessler et al. 2005). Studies show a consistent male preponderance, with ratios of males to females ranging from approximately 2:1 to 4:1 (Maughan et al. 2004; Meltzer et al. 2000), while among those who commit violent crimes, the ratio of boys to girls is even greater (8:1) (Dulcan et al. 2017).

It has been suggested that the current diagnostic criteria overemphasize aspects of CD more typical of males (e.g., physical aggression rather than relational aggression) (Card et al. 2008; Pardini et al. 2010; Robins 1999). By contrast, rates of criminal behavior between boys and girls are more similar (2:1) when self-report data of misconduct and delinquent behaviors are used (Dulcan et al. 2017). Childhood-onset CD is more typically seen in boys and is associated with more frequent physical aggression, comorbid ADHD, worse peer relationships, and increased likelihood of progression to ASPD (Langbehn et al. 1998). Other factors known to affect the likelihood of an individual receiving a diagnosis of CD include class (Green et al. 2005), race (Nock et al. 2006), and urbanicity (Nock et al. 2006; Rutter 1973). Rates are also elevated in psychiatric hospital and clinic settings (Dulcan et al. 2017).

The public health burden of CD is substantial. A multisite, multicohort longitudinal study of 664 children at risk for emotional and behavior problems found that over 7 years of follow-up, additional costs in public service provision related to CD averaged more than $70,000 per child (Foster and Jones 2005). A U.K.–based longitudinal study of 142 children found similarly that by age 28, public service spending on children with CD was 10 times that of those with no behavior problems (Scott et al. 2001).

Risk factors for conduct disorder are summarized in Table 21–1.

Comorbidity

High rates of comorbidity between CD and other externalizing disorders are well established and could contribute to the severity and negative outcomes associated with the disorder (Krueger et al. 2002). Barkley and colleagues (2004) reported elevated rates of conduct-disordered behavior, arrests, and substance misuse in a group of children with ADHD followed up over 13 years into young adulthood compared with community control subjects. Individuals with CD have been reported to have a nearly 10-fold increase in rates of comorbid ADHD (Angold et al. 1999). Clinical samples of youths with "pure" CD unaccompanied by comorbid ADHD are rare (Dulcan et al. 2017). Adolescents with CD are four times as likely to have a substance use disorder as those without CD (Armstrong and Costello 2002), particularly when CD is also comorbid with ADHD (Brinkman et al. 2015). In females, substance misuse is strongly linked with CD (Moffitt et al. 2008). Most youths with CD also have presentations that meet criteria for ODD when structured instruments are used (Maughan et al. 2004), although the developmental relationship between ODD and CD is weaker in boys than in girls and when adjustment is made for preexisting CD symptoms (Rowe et al. 2010a).

In contrast to earlier assertions that antisocial individuals are protected against internalizing disorders (Cleckley 1951), children and adolescents with CD also have elevated rates of depression (Kessler et al. 2005; Morcillo et al. 2012). Individuals with CD have about a sevenfold increase in the risk for major depressive disorder (MDD) (Angold et al. 1999) and also higher rates of suicidal ideation, suicide attempts, and completed suicides (Bridge et al. 2006). Elevated rates of PTSD are seen (Keane and Kaloupek 1997), particularly among incarcerated youths (Wasserman and McReynolds 2011). Lastly, specific learning disorders, especially in reading, are also more common in CD than in the general population (Fergusson and Lynskey 1997; Kessler et al. 2012; Rutter et al. 1970).

TABLE 21–1.   Risk factors for conduct disorder (CD)

Category	Risk factor
Prenatal	Maternal prenatal smoking
	Poor maternal diet
Perinatal	Birth complication
	Low birth weight
Postnatal	Poor childhood health
	Head injury
	Early puberty (females)
Individual	Male sex
	Low IQ (especially verbal)
	Hyperactivity, impulsivity, inattention
	Aggressiveness
	Language and reading problems
	Low educational achievement
Family, home, and parents	Single or teenage mother at birth
	Parental disruption (separation, divorce, frequent changes in caregivers)
	Adoption
	Parental conflict
	Exposure to domestic violence
	Harsh and erratic discipline
	Physical and sexual abuse
	Cold/uncaring parenting style
	Poor supervision
	Biological parental psychopathology (ADHD, oppositional defiant disorder, CD, antisocial personality disorder, substance use disorder, depression, learning disability)
	Parental criminal behavior and imprisonment
	Large family
	Poverty
	Low cognitive stimulation
	Not taken to visit other families with children
	Modeling of aggressive, impulsive, antisocial behavior
	No modeling use of language to solve problems
Community and school	Poor schools
	Peer rejection
	Delinquent peer group
	High-crime neighborhood
	Intense exposure to media violence

In adulthood, a history of CD is associated with greater risk for bipolar disorder, psychotic disorders, and somatic symptom disorders (Kim-Cohen et al. 2003; Nock et al. 2006). CD also confers a substantially increased risk for substance use disorders in general (48% in men, 46% in women), and in particular alcohol use disorder (78% in men, 65% in women) (Morcillo et al. 2012).

Clinical Findings

Children and adolescents with CD often have aggression, impulsivity, recklessness, temper outbursts, sullenness, argumentativeness, poor school performance, truancy, lying, theft, and rule violations. These behaviors typically cause more distress to those around them than to the individuals themselves, hence the designation of CD as an "externalizing" disorder, indicating that distress caused by the disorder is directed outwardly and experienced by others rather than by the individual.

Temperamentally, people with CD have greater levels of trait neuroticism, low conscientiousness, and low agreeableness, manifesting as irritability, poor self-control, poor frustration tolerance, high novelty seeking, resistance in conforming to expected social norms, and insensitivity to punishment (Frick and Viding 2009). Although they may present themselves as rebellious and unconcerned, they often have low self-esteem and harbor distorted cognitions (suspiciousness, misattribution of hostile intent), responding with aggression in neutral situations (Dodge and Pettit 2003). Although children with CD have lower IQs on average, most are not intellectually disabled (Lunden 1964).

Relationships with family members, authority figures, and nondeviant peers are often troubled. Children with CD may become known as a neighborhood nuisance, while their disruptive behavior in school may cause alienation from peers and teachers, and result in suspensions and even dropping out of school (Black 2013). Conflict with family members might arise from their frequent lying, fights with siblings or parents, or defiance when confronted; defiance could lead the youth to run away from home. These factors contribute to the child or adolescent gravitating toward deviant peers. Research has consistently shown that troubled youths tend to seek out like peers, in all eventuality reinforcing the youth's deviant behavior (Gifford-Smith et al. 2005).

The following is a vignette of a patient treated at our child psychiatry outpatient clinic. The case demonstrates the chronicity of CD symptoms and the frustration experienced by his mother and treating clinician.

> Ike, a 7-year-old mixed race boy, was brought for evaluation and treatment of aggression and defiance. His mother was exhausted by her powerlessness and inability to control him. His birth was described as full term but complicated by meconium aspiration; Ike was otherwise healthy and had experienced normal motor and cognitive development. His father was described as a violent person and had a history of incarceration and drug addiction. His parents separated when Ike was 3 months old after his father physically assaulted his mother.
>
> Ike's behavior included constant lying, frequent irritability, and explosive outbursts. He would break objects, including his own toys, but also his mother's cherished dishes. He once threatened to stab his mother in her sleep, making her fearful of what he might

do. His misbehaviors occurred at home, school, and even grocery and other stores, leaving his mother afraid to take him anywhere.

Prior to entering kindergarten, Ike had attended a home-based preschool, and his transition to public school was difficult. Ike was placed in a "behavioral" classroom, where his deportment modestly improved. In school, his teachers observed interrupting others, impatience, blurting out, and difficulty sitting still. His mood was reportedly good, and he denied being sad or having crying spells.

Ike had been prescribed with risperidone during the last year, but it was hard to tell if he had improved because his behavior was still problematic and frequently threatening. He also received in-school counseling.

On initial evaluation, Ike was friendly and cooperated well. He explored the office, picking up and examining objects on the desk. He finally sat on the floor near a box of toys, which he promptly emptied out. As he played with the toys, he said that he never "felt like crying" and that he had many friends at school. He emphatically shook his head "no" when asked if he ever got into trouble or wanted to "hit other children."

Ike was diagnosed with CD, and because of his many ADHD symptoms, he was given a trial of methylphenidate in the hope that treating his attentional problems would reduce his impulsive aggression. The risperidone was continued. He was also referred to a therapist for individual and family therapy.

Ike did poorly over the next 11 years. By age 18, he had been hospitalized three times for violent behavior and had spent 2 years at a residential treatment facility. After returning home, he refused to enroll in school, and he and his mother argued about this, leading him to physically assault her. On several occasions, police were called, resulting in a brief stay in jail. Because he was not in school, he spent this time playing violent video games or hanging out with his troubled—and truant—peers. His mother expressed fear for her personal safety yet stated that she was unwilling to expel him from her home out of her concern for his welfare.

Course and Outcome

Children and adolescents with CD show impulsivity, aggression, and defiance as early as age 4 years, and sometimes at even younger ages (Waller et al. 2012). The child often displays symptoms of ADHD or ODD, both of which are common comorbidities and frequent developmental precursors to CD (Burke et al. 2005; Pardini et al. 2010). While most cases of ADHD and ODD will not progress to CD (Loeber et al. 1995; Rowe et al. 2010a), those that do are distinguished by the severity, persistence, and pervasive nature of the individual's behavior problems. By contrast, in typically developing children and adolescents, aggression, defiance, rebelliousness, and isolated delinquent behaviors are common within specific developmental phases but desist over time (Rey et al. 2018).

ADHD symptoms are more common than not in children who progress to CD. Overall, ODD appears to be a stronger predictor of CD than ADHD. In a study of developmental trajectories of ADHD, ODD, and CD symptoms, the association of ADHD and CD was largely accounted for by the presence of ODD symptoms (van Lier et al. 2007). Similarly, a cohort study of 140 children with ADHD and 120 control children by Biederman et al. (1996) found that 22% of children with ADHD had CD, but all but one child with CD had preexisting ODD.

Some ODD symptoms may be more predictive of progression to CD than others (Burke and Loeber 2010). In a study from the United Kingdom, Stringaris and Goodman (2009) examined three dimensions of ODD symptoms (i.e., irritable, headstrong, hurtful) in a sample of 18,415 subjects ages 5–16 years. They found that irritability was predictive of emotional disorders, and headstrong behaviors were most associated with ADHD, whereas hurtful behaviors were predictive of traits of callousness, cold-bloodedness, and aggression. Similarly, Leadbeater and Homel (2015) found that while irritability was predictive of both internalizing and externalizing symptoms, defiance was more specifically predictive of externalizing symptoms. A study by Biederman and colleagues (1996) cited earlier showed that children with ADHD and ODD that progressed to CD had greater baseline ODD severity, more severe Clinical Global Impression scores and Child Behavior Checklist scores, and greater psychiatric comorbidity than did those with ADHD and ODD or ADHD alone.

Although course of CD is highly variable, in most individuals, clinically significant behavioral symptoms first appear between late childhood and early adolescence (Keenan et al. 2011; Moffitt et al. 2008). Few children have symptoms that meet the criteria for CD before age 10 years, whereas the onset of symptoms after age 16 is unusual. Aggression is more commonly seen among those with childhood-onset CD, whereas status violations and nonaggressive conduct problems are more common in adolescent-onset CD (Maughan et al. 2004). When present, the most severe CD symptoms, such as sexual assault and robbery, typically emerge with physical maturity.

By early adulthood, most individuals with CD show significant desistance of symptoms and do not progress to ASPD (Glueck and Glueck 1950; Robins 1966; Stouthamer-Loeber et al. 2004). Henn et al. (1980) showed in a 10-year follow-up study of juvenile delinquents that those who were able to form relationships within a peer group and internalize social norms were less likely to have been convicted or incarcerated. Moffitt (1993) similarly described this "adolescence-limited" form of CD as being largely influenced by peer pressure and noted that a degree of antisocial behavior, particularly in boys, is common, associated with less psychosocial adversity and comorbidity, and likely to improve without intervention.

Childhood-onset CD; CD associated with limited prosocial emotions; and a greater number, frequency, and severity of CD symptoms all predict persistence and progression to ASPD (McMahon et al. 2010; Moffitt et al. 2008; Rowe et al. 2010a, 2010b). Boys are more likely than girls to progress to ASPD (Black and Andreasen 2014), consistent with the finding that nearly all childhood-onset cases of CD involve males (10:1), whereas adolescent-onset CD shows only a modest male preponderance (1.5:1) (Moffitt and Caspi 2001). Additional factors predicting a more persistent course of CD and worse outcomes include comorbid ADHD, parental ASPD, lower IQ, poor academic performance, and lower socioeconomic status (Black and Andreasen 2014; Loeber et al. 1995; Moffitt et al. 2008). Among boys with childhood-onset CD, treatment and incarceration do not appear to be linked with improvement of symptoms in adolescence (Lahey et al. 2002).

Adult Outcomes

Some individuals with CD are able to achieve stability in adulthood, particularly those with better social skills and a more positive peer group (Henn et al. 1980). As a whole, individuals with CD remain at risk for several negative outcomes, including educational failure, unemployment, teenage pregnancy, incarceration, and mental health problems, even when they do not progress to ASPD (Caspi et al. 1998; Fergusson and Lynskey 1998; Kim-Cohen et al. 2003; Morcillo et al. 2012; Robins and Price 1991). CD also confers increased risk for other psychiatric comorbidities, including major depressive disorder, psychotic disorders, substance use disorders, and suicidality (Morcillo et al. 2012). Conversely, psychiatrically ill populations have an elevated rate of CD. One longitudinal study found that among adults whose symptoms met criteria for one or more DSM-IV diagnoses, rates of childhood CD and ODD were as high as 25%–60% (Kim-Cohen et al. 2003).

Individuals with greater levels of "psychopathic" traits show an increased likelihood of engaging in criminal behavior and a higher risk for violent reoffending behavior compared with their peers with criminal offenses (Piquero et al. 2012). The small group of individuals (5%) with the most severe and persistent antisocial behavior has been termed *life-course persistent* by Terrie Moffitt (1993) and are estimated to account for 50% of all crimes committed.

Assessment

Because request for the assessment of a child with suspected CD may come from the child's parents, school, service agencies, or the law, it is important to clarify the purpose of the evaluation at the outset and review the limits of confidentiality. Regardless of context, assessment is typically challenging because youths may be understandably reluctant to divulge sensitive information on their behaviors. Sensitive but persistent probing by the clinician is needed to overcome a tendency to underreport symptoms. Hostility to authority figures and difficulty distinguishing the roles of the treating clinician from other involved adults such as probation officers or social workers may be additional obstacles. Because youths with CD are at elevated risk for other psychiatric disorders as well as sexual abuse and exposure to substance use in the home, efforts to build rapport are important. Youths with CD are more likely to report covert behaviors such as stealing or vandalism than overt behaviors such as aggression, which are more likely to be reported by parents or guardians.

Evaluation depends substantially on gathering collateral information from multiple sources, including teachers, parents, other family members, agency workers, and possibly agents of the legal system. Information from informants who have known the child or adolescent for an extended period of time is particularly important in the assessment of the "limited prosocial emotions" specifier, because this diagnosis relies on detailed knowledge of the individual's pattern of interpersonal and emotional functioning (American Psychiatric Association 2013).

Psychiatric evaluation should include assessment of the common comorbid conditions, including ADHD, substance use disorders, intellectual disability, learning disabilities, and mood and anxiety disorders (Steiner and Dunne 1997). The mental status examination may be challenging in these patients because of oppositionality, suspiciousness, or alexithymia. These may make it difficult to assess more subjective aspects of the child or adolescent's mental state such as mood, suicidality, or level of insight. However, objective components of the child's mental state, including his or her general cognitive ability, language, activity level, impulsivity, and attentional capacity, may be informative, helping to narrow down the differential diagnosis and identify comorbid issues in need of treatment.

Additional assessments by allied professionals, including psychologists, social workers, speech and language pathologists, and educational experts, may be needed to fully understand the complex dynamics of a child's dysfunction, particularly in more severe cases. Psychometric testing should be considered to assess for comorbid intellectual disability and learning disorders, which may be important factors in treatment planning and could affect legal decision making.

While mainly used in research, a variety of validated scales and questionnaires have been developed and might be useful in assessing the child with problematic behaviors. The Child Behavior Checklist (Achenbach et al. 1991) might be useful as a screening tool, while a structured instrument like the Kiddie Schedule for Affective Disorders and Schizophrenia (Kaufman et al. 1997), the Diagnostic Interview Schedule for Children (Shaffer et al. 1996), or the Diagnostic Interview for Children and Adolescents (Reich 2000) could be of use in assessing the full spectrum of behavior problems in the child. More detailed rating scales (Collett et al. 2003) for CD include the New York Teacher Rating Scale for Disruptive and Antisocial Behavior (Miller et al. 1995), Vitiello Aggression Scale (Vitiello et al. 1990), and for callous-unemotional traits, the Inventory of Callous-Unemotional Traits (Kimonis et al. 2008).

A physical examination is recommended as part of a comprehensive evaluation. Particular attention should be directed at detecting possible signs of sexually transmitted diseases, physical abuse, head trauma, and seizures, which unfortunately are all too common in children with CD. Lastly, urine drug screening should be strongly considered given the high rate of comorbidity of CD and substance use, but other laboratory testing is not typically indicated unless there is clinical suspicion. Brain imaging is not recommended unless there is a strong suspicion of a tumor or space-occupying lesion.

Differential Diagnosis

The differential diagnosis of CD includes disorders that may be associated with behavioral disturbances, such as mood disorders, psychotic disorders, impulse-control disorders, substance use disorders, and PTSD and adjustment disorders. Given the high rate of comorbidity of CD with other disorders, the clinician should ascertain if the disturbance is primarily due to the other disorder or is reflective of a persistent and pervasive pattern of behavior consistent with CD. Impulsive outbursts associated with aggression could point toward a diagnosis of ADHD or intermittent explosive disorder rather than CD, whereas episodic symptoms might point to the presence of a major depressive disorder or bipolar disorder. An individual with prodromal schizophrenia could also present with violent behavior (Gosden et al. 2005).

The relationship of CD to the new DSM-5 diagnosis disruptive mood dysregulation disorder (DMDD) is unclear, but high rates of comorbidity are to be expected given DMDD's strong associations with ADHD, ODD, and depression (Axelson 2013), all of which are also associated with CD. Of note, consistent with emerging evidence that ODD and CD consist of partially nonoverlapping domains of psychopathology (Pardini et al. 2010), DSM-5 no longer stipulates that the two disorders are mutually exclusive, and thus both disorders should be diagnosed if criteria are met. In clinical practice, however, it is unclear whether an additional diagnosis of ODD offers increased utility in the way of prognosis or treatment recommendations in individuals with CD.

Special care is needed in diagnosing CD in the presence of intellectual disability to ensure that problem behaviors are not primarily a result of lack of adequate educational supports or exposure to maladaptive peer influences, to which children and adolescents with intellectual disability may be particularly susceptible. However, when CD behaviors persist over time and across settings, the diagnosis may be warranted.

Consideration should be given to the child or adolescent's age, gender, and sociocultural context when a diagnosis of CD is being contemplated (American Psychiatric Association 2013). Disruptive behavior is common and developmentally normal in very young children as they learn to navigate the social world and deal with frustrations (i.e., the "terrible twos"); this behavior usually decreases by age 5 years (Liu et al. 2013). Aggression that continues or worsens after this period is more concerning. Although physical aggression is more common in boys, verbal and relational aggression is more prominent in girls and also should be assessed (Crick and Grotpeter 1995; Loeber et al. 2000). Lastly, in areas where disruptive behavior may be more normative (e.g., high-crime areas, war zones), a diagnosis of CD might be inappropriate (American Psychiatric Association 2013).

Clinical Management

The goal of treatment is to improve the child or adolescent's functioning, reduce CD behaviors, and prevent progression to adult ASPD, as well as prevent negative outcomes such as the development of a substance use disorder and criminal conduct. Broadly speaking, treatment categories for CD include individual- and family-level psychosocial interventions, higher-intensity multimodal interventions, and evidence-based treatment of any comorbid conditions. No FDA-approved medications are available for CD, but off-label use may be considered in selected cases.

Psychosocial Interventions

Treatment guidelines from the American Academy of Child and Adolescent Psychiatry were last updated in 1997 (Steiner and Dunne 1997), although newer guidelines were published in the United Kingdom in 2013 (National Collaborating Centre for Mental Health 2013), in Canada in 2015 (Gorman et al. 2015), and in the United States by the U.S. Department of Health and Human Services (Substance Abuse and Mental Health Services Administration 2011). In general, all the guidelines recommend psychosocial interventions as first-line treatment for CD that does not respond to treatment of comorbid disorders.

Therapies reported to be effective include anger management, social skills training, and problem-solving skills training (Buitelaar et al. 2013). A meta-analysis of 82 controlled trials (Brestan and Eyberg 1998) showed that problem-solving skills training, in which children learn to solve interpersonal conflicts through techniques such as role-play, stories, and social modeling, produces clinically meaningful improvements. A meta-analysis of cognitive-behavioral therapy modified for CD showed relatively modest effect sizes in decreasing antisocial behaviors (Bennett and Gibbons 2000).

Emerging evidence indicates that dialectical behavioral therapy could be helpful for children and adolescents who have disruptive behaviors (Nelson-Gray et al. 2006; Perepletchikova et al. 2017), even among those in detention (Shelton et al. 2011). It should be noted that, as with other forms of group therapy, a risk of worsening behavior could be present if delinquency is normalized and reinforced in the group setting because of inadequate structure or limit-setting by the therapist.

Parents should be encouraged to show warmth and empathy with the child, while avoiding harsh and inconsistent discipline. They should modulate their own expressed emotion, learn to communicate effectively, and seek care for their own mental health problems (Blair et al. 2014; Obsuth et al. 2006). Families could get emotional support through organizations such as NAMI (National Alliance on Mental Illness). Engaging in positive family activities such as playing games, exercising together, or watching an appropriate television show together provide an important foundation on which parents may build more effective disciplinary systems. The child with CD should have a high level of structure and supervision. Unsupervised access to electronic devices and social media should be discouraged, although limited and supervised access might help to reinforce positive behavior. Children should be steered away from violent video games that might promote a more hostile world view.

A treatment mainstay is parent management training (PMT), which aims to provide parents with tools to discipline children effectively and avoid coercive punishment cycles (Kazdin 1997). Relying on the behavioral principles of operant conditioning and social learning theory, PMT programs such as The Incredible Years (Webster-Stratton and Reid 2003) have a strong evidence base (Presnall et al. 2014) and have been shown to have robust effects on CD symptoms in randomized controlled trials (Bakker et al. 2017; Jones et al. 2008). Completion of PMT is associated with improvements in sibling behaviors, maternal psychopathology, and marital and family functioning (Scott 2005). PMT is less effective in children older than 8 years and may be less effective in children with callous-unemotional traits compared with those with impulsive aggression (Buitelaar et al. 2013). Other drawbacks include limited effectiveness in the most psychosocially disadvantaged families, high dropout rates and low motivation, and poor generalization to the school setting (Buitelaar et al. 2013).

In the school setting, the addition of problem solving and teacher training components to PMT has been shown to boost its effectiveness (Webster-Stratton et al. 2004; Woolgar and Scott 2005). Families and Schools Together (FAST) is a school-based multifamily group intervention program designed for children between ages 4 and 12 targeted at building school success that has shown evidence of effectiveness in several trials (Conduct Problems Prevention Research Group 2011; McDonald et al. 1997). Attention to learning disabilities, speech and language problems, and low cognitive ability are important and may require the implementation of a formal Individualized Education Program, or IEP. Assessment of behavioral patterns leading to escalations in the school setting may be analyzed through a Functional Behavioral Assessment performed by a trained psychologist and leads to the implementation of a Behavior Intervention Plan to address the disruptive behavior. Youths with CD may benefit from alternative curricula including vocational training. Increased supervision and monitoring in the school settings is recommended for all children with CD. Participation in positive group activities such as sports (Samek et al. 2015) and extracurricular programs such as Big Brothers Big Sisters of America (www.bbbsa.com)

may serve as a means of facilitating relationships within a positive peer group, known to be a protective factor in CD (Deković 1999).

For older and more severely affected youths, intensive multimodal interventions may be needed. The best-known model of this type is multisystemic therapy (MST), a demanding and resource intensive program involving daily, home-based systemic family therapy, behavioral modification, and direct involvement by the treatment team with the youth's social system and local agencies (Henggeler et al. 2009). Although a meta-analysis showed moderate effectiveness (effect sizes=0.4–0.9) in reducing antisocial behavior, widespread adoption of MST has been limited, in part because of cost (Olsson 2010). A second evidence-based multimodal intervention for severe and refractory CD known as the "Oregon model" involves out-of-home placement with specially trained therapeutic foster families that are supported by a team of therapists (Chamberlain and Smith 2003).

Hospitalization may be necessary in some cases if a child or an adolescent with aggressive or dangerous behavior presents a risk to the safety of self or others. The focus of treatment should be assessment, stabilization, treatment of comorbid conditions, and referral to an evidence-based psychosocial program. During hospitalization, behavioral strategies designed to avoid escalation of conflicts and coercive cycles are recommended, in keeping with PMT principles. Hospitalization is generally ineffective in itself in addressing or treating CD behaviors; furthermore, these patients could pose risks to other patients and staff (Black 2013). In some cases, a child or adolescent might need placement in a detention facility to help control incorrigible behavior, although it is unlikely to affect the progression of CD. Similarly, "boot camps" or "scared straight" programs are not recommended because they have not been shown to reduce future offending in youths with CD (Henggeler and Schoenwald 1994).

Pharmacotherapy

Evidence-based treatment of the comorbid psychiatric disorders in CD is recommended and could lead to improvements in the child's behavior (Buitelaar et al. 2013). Stimulant medications are recommended (Gorman et al. 2015) for treating comorbid ADHD and appear to have medium to large effect sizes on aggression above and beyond their effect on ADHD symptoms. Because of the potential for stimulant abuse in this population, it is recommended that a parent or guardian dispense the medication. For patients with comorbid substance use disorders, routine drug screening is recommended and also may allow the clinician to confirm adherence to some prescribed medications such as stimulants. Treatment of comorbid mood, anxiety, and psychotic disorders is also recommended. In cases in which epileptic phenomena are suspected, particularly in the presence of an abnormal electroencephalogram result, a trial of valproate or carbamazepine may be considered.

Second-generation antipsychotics (SGAs), adrenergic agents, and a variety of other medications have shown effectiveness in treating aggression and irritability in meta-analyses (Lettinga et al. 2011). Risperidone is the best studied SGA in youth populations generally because of its FDA approval for treating irritability and aggression in autism spectrum disorder, followed by aripiprazole (Findling 2008), which has the same FDA indication. Randomized controlled trials of risperidone for the treatment of CD, aggression, or other disruptive behavior disorders, often in the setting of intellectual deficiency, show effectiveness at doses ranging from 1 to 3 mg (Aman et al.

2002, 2014; Armenteros et al. 2007; Buitelaar et al. 2001; Findling et al. 2000; Reyes et al. 2006; Snyder et al. 2002; Van Bellinghen and De Troch 2001). The Treatment of Severe Childhood Aggression study showed medium effect sizes with the addition of risperidone (mean dose=1.7 mg) versus placebo to combination treatment with osmotic-release oral delivery methylphenidate and parent training by 3 weeks, although behavioral outcomes were not significantly different at 52 weeks (Gadow et al. 2009, 2016). Several open-label studies of aripiprazole have shown promise in the treatment of aggressive CD (Ercan et al. 2012; Findling et al. 2009; Kuperman et al. 2011).

A few other agents have been shown effective in CD (Lettinga et al. 2011). A double-blind, placebo-controlled study of children with CD showed that lithium was equal or superior to haloperidol in reducing aggression and caused fewer side effects (Campbell et al. 1995). Divalproex, an anticonvulsant, demonstrated effectiveness in two randomized placebo-controlled trials. In the study of Donovan and colleagues (2000), youths with CD or ODD had decreased outbursts and mood lability (mean blood drug level=82 µg/mL), while Blader and colleagues (2009) reported a decrease in aggression in children with ADHD (mean blood drug level=68 µg/mL). Finally, the antiadrenergic agents guanfacine and propranolol have shown effectiveness in reducing impulsive aggression and might also be considered for use in CD (Kuperman and Stewart 1987; Lettinga et al. 2011).

Prevention

Given the high societal costs of CD (Foster and Jones 2005) and the limitations of current treatments, preventive efforts may offer the most hope. One example of such an intervention is the Good Behavior Game (Barrish et al. 1969), a group-oriented contingency management procedure for classrooms with more than 30 years of outcome data (Kellam et al. 2011) in high-risk, inner-city individuals that has been described as a "universal behavioral vaccine" for the prevention of substance use and violent crime (Embry 2002). However, it is likely that meaningful reduction in the prevalence of CD will require not only widespread adoption of similar behavioral programs but also many other public health and policy initiatives targeting the multiple sources of risk for CD outlined earlier in this chapter, particularly at the family and community level. These might include improved prenatal care and mental health care for mothers, universal preschool, increased access to PMT programs, drug treatment programs, and job programs. Currently, the feasibility of such a program is not clear.

Key Points

- The DSM-5 conduct disorder (CD) specifier "with limited prosocial emotions" is equivalent to the adult construct of "psychopathy."

- Adolescents with CD are not "protected" from depression or anxiety; rather, they have higher rates of major depressive disorder, suicide, and PTSD.

- Childhood-onset CD; CD associated with limited prosocial emotions; and a greater number, frequency, and severity of CD symptoms are associated with progression to antisocial personality disorder.

- Assessment of CD requires gathering substantial collateral information because youths are less likely to accurately report their behavior or cooperate with a mental status examination.

- Clinical management of CD requires a multidisciplinary approach, with pharmacotherapy targeted at comorbid psychiatric disorders, which are common in CD.

References

Achenbach T, Achenbach T, Achenbach T: Integrative Guide to the 1991 CBCL/4–18, YSR, and TRF Profiles. Burlington, Department of Psychiatry, University of Vermont, 1991

Aman MG, De Smedt G, Derivan A, et al: Double-blind, placebo-controlled study of risperidone for the treatment of disruptive behaviors in children with subaverage intelligence. Am J Psychiatry 159(8):1337–1346, 2002 12153826

Aman MG, Bukstein OG, Gadow KD, et al: What does risperidone add to parent training and stimulant for severe aggression in child attention-deficit/hyperactivity disorder? J Am Acad Child Psychiatry 53(1):47.e41–60.e41, 2014 24342385

American Psychiatric Association: Diagnostic and Statistical Manual: Mental Disorders. Washington, DC, American Psychiatric Association, 1952

American Psychiatric Association: Diagnostic and Statistical Manual of Mental Disorders, 2nd Edition. Washington, DC, American Psychiatric Association, 1968

American Psychiatric Association: Diagnostic and Statistical Manual of Mental Disorders, 3rd Edition. Washington, DC, American Psychiatric Association, 1980

American Psychiatric Association: Diagnostic and Statistical Manual of Mental Disorders, 3rd Edition, Revised. Washington, DC, American Psychiatric Association, 1987

American Psychiatric Association: Diagnostic and Statistical Manual of Mental Disorders, 4th Edition. Washington, DC, American Psychiatric Association, 1994

American Psychiatric Association: Diagnostic and Statistical Manual of Mental Disorders, 5th Edition. Arlington, VA, American Psychiatric Association, 2013

Angold A, Costello EJ, Erkanli A: Comorbidity. J Child Psychol Psychiatry 40(1):57–87, 1999 10102726

Armenteros JL, Lewis JE, Davalos M: Risperidone augmentation for treatment-resistant aggression in attention-deficit/hyperactivity disorder: a placebo-controlled pilot study. J Am Acad Child Adolesc Psychiatry 46(5):558–565, 2007 17450046

Armstrong TD, Costello EJ: Community studies on adolescent substance use, abuse, or dependence and psychiatric comorbidity. J Consult Clin Psychol 70(6):1224–1239, 2002 12472299

Atkins MS, Stoff DM: Instrumental and hostile aggression in childhood disruptive behavior disorders. J Abnorm Child Psychol 21(2):165–178, 1993 8491930

Axelson D: Taking disruptive mood dysregulation disorder out for a test drive. Am J Psychiatry 170(2):136–139, 2013 23377631

Bakker MJ, Greven CU, Buitelaar JK, et al: Practitioner review: psychological treatments for children and adolescents with conduct disorder problems—a systematic review and meta-analysis. J Child Psychol Psychiatry 58(1):4–18, 2017 27501434

Barkley RA, Fischer M, Smallish L, et al: Young adult follow-up of hyperactive children: antisocial activities and drug use. J Child Psychol Psychiatry 45(2):195–211, 2004 14982236

Barrish HH, Saunders M, Wolf MM: Good behavior game: effects of individual contingencies for group consequences on disruptive behavior in a classroom. J Appl Behav Anal 2(2):119–124, 1969 16795208

Bennett DS, Gibbons TA: Efficacy of child cognitive-behavioral interventions for antisocial behavior: a meta-analysis. Child Fam Behav Ther 22(1):1–15, 2000

Biederman J, Faraone SV, Milberger S, et al: Is childhood oppositional defiant disorder a precursor to adolescent conduct disorder? Findings from a four-year follow-up study of children with ADHD. J Am Acad Child Adolesc Psychiatry 35(9):1193–1204, 1996 8824063

Black DW: Bad Boys, Bad Men: Confronting Antisocial Personality Disorder (Sociopathy), Revised and Updated. New York, Oxford University Press, 2013

Black DW, Andreasen NC: Introductory Textbook of Psychiatry, 6th Edition. Washington, DC, American Psychiatric Publishing, 2014

Blader JC, Schooler NR, Jensen PS, et al: Adjunctive divalproex versus placebo for children with ADHD and aggression refractory to stimulant monotherapy. Am J Psychiatry 166(12):1392–1401, 2009 19884222

Blair RJ, Leibenluft E, Pine DS: Conduct disorder and callous-unemotional traits in youth. N Engl J Med 371(23):2207–2216, 2014 25470696

Brestan EV, Eyberg SM: Effective psychosocial treatments of conduct-disordered children and adolescents: 29 years, 82 studies, and 5,272 kids. J Clin Child Psychol 27(2):180–189, 1998 9648035

Bridge JA, Goldstein TR, Brent DA: Adolescent suicide and suicidal behavior. J Child Psychol Psychiatry 47(3–4):372–394, 2006 16492264

Brinkman WB, Epstein JN, Auinger P, et al: Association of attention-deficit/hyperactivity disorder and conduct disorder with early tobacco and alcohol use. Drug Alcohol Depend 147:183–189, 2015 25487225

Buitelaar JK, van der Gaag RJ, Cohen-Kettenis P, et al: A randomized controlled trial of risperidone in the treatment of aggression in hospitalized adolescents with subaverage cognitive abilities. J Clin Psychiatry 62(4):239–248, 2001 11379837

Buitelaar JK, Smeets KC, Herpers P, et al: Conduct disorders. Eur Child Adolesc Psychiatry 22 (suppl 1):S49–S54, 2013 23224151

Burke J, Loeber R: Oppositional defiant disorder and the explanation of the comorbidity between behavioral disorders and depression. Clin Psychol Sci Pract 17:319–326, 2010

Burke JD, Loeber R, Lahey BB, et al: Developmental transitions among affective and behavioral disorders in adolescent boys. J Child Psychol Psychiatry 46(11):1200–1210, 2005 16238667

Campbell M, Adams PB, Small AM, et al: Lithium in hospitalized aggressive children with conduct disorder: a double-blind and placebo-controlled study. J Am Acad Child Adolesc Psychiatry 34(4):445–453, 1995 7751258

Canino G, Shrout PE, Rubio-Stipec M, et al: The DSM-IV rates of child and adolescent disorders in Puerto Rico: prevalence, correlates, service use, and the effects of impairment. Arch Gen Psychiatry 61(1):85–93, 2004 14706947

Card NA, Stucky BD, Sawalani GM, et al: Direct and indirect aggression during childhood and adolescence: a meta-analytic review of gender differences, intercorrelations, and relations to maladjustment. Child Dev 79(5):1185–1229, 2008 18826521

Caspi A, Wright BRE, Moffitt TE, et al: Early failure in the labor market: childhood and adolescent predictors of unemployment in the transition to adulthood. Am Sociol Rev 63:424–451, 1998

Chamberlain P, Smith DK: Antisocial behavior in children and adolescents: the Oregon Multidimensional Treatment Foster Care model, in Evidence-Based Psychotherapies for Children and Adolescents. Edited by Weisz JR, Kazdin AE. New York, Guilford, 2003, pp 282–300

Cleckley HM: The mask of sanity. Postgrad Med 9(3):193–197, 1951 14807904

Collett BR, Ohan JL, Myers KM: Ten-year review of rating scales, VI: scales assessing externalizing behaviors. J Am Acad Child Adolesc Psychiatry 42(10):1143–1170, 2003 14560165

Conduct Problems Prevention Research Group: The effects of the fast track preventive intervention on the development of conduct disorder across childhood. Child Dev 82(1):331–345, 2011 21291445

Costello EJ, Mustillo S, Erkanli A, et al: Prevalence and development of psychiatric disorders in childhood and adolescence. Arch Gen Psychiatry 60(8):837–844, 2003 12912767

Costello EJ, Egger H, Angold A: 10-year research update review: the epidemiology of child and adolescent psychiatric disorders, I: methods and public health burden. J Am Acad Child Adolesc Psychiatry 44(10):972–986, 2005 16175102

Crick NR, Grotpeter JK: Relational aggression, gender, and social-psychological adjustment. Child Dev 66(3):710–722, 1995 7789197

Deković M: Risk and protective factors in the development of problem behavior during adolescence. J Youth Adolesc 28(6):667–685, 1999

Dodge KA, Pettit GS: A biopsychosocial model of the development of chronic conduct problems in adolescence. Dev Psychol 39(2):349–371, 2003 12661890

Donovan SJ, Stewart JW, Nunes EV, et al: Divalproex treatment for youth with explosive temper and mood lability: a double-blind, placebo-controlled crossover design. Am J Psychiatry 157(5):818–820, 2000 10784478

Dulcan MK, Ballard RR, Jha P, et al: Concise Guide to Child and Adolescent Psychiatry, 5th Edition. Arlington, VA, American Psychiatric Association Publishing, 2017

Embry DD: The Good Behavior Game: a best practice candidate as a universal behavioral vaccine. Clin Child Fam Psychol Rev 5(4):273–297, 2002 12495270

Ercan ES, Uysal T, Ercan E, et al: Aripiprazole in children and adolescents with conduct disorder: a single-center, open-label study. Pharmacopsychiatry 45(1):13–19, 2012 21993869

Fergusson DM, Lynskey MT: Early reading difficulties and later conduct problems. J Child Psychol Psychiatry 38(8):899–907, 1997 9413790

Fergusson DM, Lynskey MT: Conduct problems in childhood and psychosocial outcomes in young adulthood: a prospective study. J Emot Behav Disord 6:2–18, 1998

Findling RL: Atypical antipsychotic treatment of disruptive behavior disorders in children and adolescents. J Clin Psychiatry 69 (suppl 4):9–14, 2008 18533763

Findling RL, McNamara NK, Branicky LA, et al: A double-blind pilot study of risperidone in the treatment of conduct disorder. J Am Acad Child Adolesc Psychiatry 39(4):509–516, 2000 10761354

Findling RL, Kauffman R, Sallee FR, et al: An open-label study of aripiprazole: pharmacokinetics, tolerability, and effectiveness in children and adolescents with conduct disorder. J Child Adolesc Psychopharmacol 19(4):431–439, 2009 19702495

Fleitlich-Bilyk B, Goodman R: Prevalence of child and adolescent psychiatric disorders in southeast Brazil. J Am Acad Child Adolesc Psychiatry 43(6):727–734, 2004 15167089

Ford T, Goodman R, Meltzer H: The British Child and Adolescent Mental Health Survey 1999: the prevalence of DSM-IV disorders. J Am Acad Child Adolesc Psychiatry 42(10):1203–1211, 2003 14560170

Foster EM, Jones DE: The high costs of aggression: public expenditures resulting from conduct disorder. Am J Public Health 95(10):1767–1772, 2005 16131639

Frick PJ, Viding E: Antisocial behavior from a developmental psychopathology perspective. Dev Psychopathol 21(4):1111–1131, 2009 19825260

Frick PJ, Lahey BB, Loeber R, et al: Oppositional defiant disorder and conduct disorder—a meta-analytic review of factor-analyses and cross-validation in a clinic sample. Clin Psychol Rev 13:319–340, 1993

Frick PJ, Ray JV, Thornton LC, et al: Annual research review: a developmental psychopathology approach to understanding callous-unemotional traits in children and adolescents with serious conduct problems. J Child Psychol Psychiatry 55(6):532–548, 2014 24117854

Gadow KD, Arnold LE, Molina BS, et al: Risperidone added to parent training and stimulant medication: effects on attention-deficit/hyperactivity disorder, oppositional defiant disorder, conduct disorder, and peer aggression. J Am Acad Child Psychiatry 53(9):948.e1–959.e1, 2009 19825260

Gadow KD, Brown NV, Arnold LE, et al: Severely aggressive children receiving stimulant medication versus stimulant and risperidone: 12-month follow-up of the TOSCA trial. J Am Acad Child Adolesc Psychiatry 55(6):469–478, 2016 27238065

Gifford-Smith M, Dodge KA, Dishion TJ, et al: Peer influence in children and adolescents: crossing the bridge from developmental to intervention science. J Abnorm Child Psychol 33(3):255–265, 2005 15957555

Glueck S, Glueck E: Unraveling Juvenile Delinquency. New York, Commonwealth Fund, 1950

Gorman DA, Gardner DM, Murphy AL, et al: Canadian guidelines on pharmacotherapy for disruptive and aggressive behaviour in children and adolescents with attention-deficit hyperactivity disorder, oppositional defiant disorder, or conduct disorder. Can J Psychiatry 60(2):62–76, 2015 25886657

Gosden NP, Kramp P, Gabrielsen G, et al: Violence of young criminals predicts schizophrenia: a 9-year register-based followup of 15- to 19-year-old criminals. Schizophr Bull 31(3):759–768, 2005 16123529

Green H, McGinnity Á, Meltzer H, et al: Mental Health of Children and Young People in Great Britain, 2004. New York, Palgrave Macmillan, 2005

Henggeler SW, Schoenwald SK: Boot camps for juvenile offenders: just say no. J Child Fam Stud 3(3):243–248, 1994

Henggeler SW, Schoenwald SK, Borduin CM, et al: Multisystemic Therapy for Antisocial Behavior in Children and Adolescents. New York, Guilford, 2009

Henn FA, Bardwell R, Jenkins RL: Juvenile delinquents revisited: adult criminal activity. Arch Gen Psychiatry 37(10):1160–1163, 1980 7425800

Jones K, Daley D, Hutchings J, et al: Efficacy of the Incredible Years Programme as an early intervention for children with conduct problems and ADHD: long-term follow-up. Child Care Health Dev 34(3):380–390, 2008 18410644

Kaufman J, Birmaher B, Brent D, et al: Schedule for Affective Disorders and Schizophrenia for School-Age Children-Present and Lifetime Version (K-SADS-PL): initial reliability and validity data. J Am Acad Child Adolesc Psychiatry 36(7):980–988, 1997 9204677

Kazdin AE: Parent management training: evidence, outcomes, and issues. J Am Acad Child Adolesc Psychiatry 36(10):1349–1356, 1997 9334547

Keane TM, Kaloupek DG: Comorbid psychiatric disorders in PTSD: implications for research. Ann NY Acad Sci 821:24–34, 1997 9238191

Keenan K, Boeldt D, Chen D, et al: Predictive validity of DSM-IV oppositional defiant and conduct disorders in clinically referred preschoolers. J Child Psychol Psychiatry 52(1):47–55, 2011 20738448

Kellam SG, Mackenzie AC, Brown CH, et al: The good behavior game and the future of prevention and treatment. Addict Sci Clin Pract 6(1):73–84, 2011 22003425

Kessler RC, Chiu WT, Demler O, et al: Prevalence, severity, and comorbidity of 12-month DSM-IV disorders in the National Comorbidity Survey Replication. Arch Gen Psychiatry 62(6):617–627, 2005 15939839

Kessler RC, Avenevoli S, Costello EJ, et al: Prevalence, persistence, and sociodemographic correlates of DSM-IV disorders in the National Comorbidity Survey Replication Adolescent Supplement. Arch Gen Psychiatry 69(4):372–380, 2012 22147808

Kim-Cohen J, Caspi A, Moffitt TE, et al: Prior juvenile diagnoses in adults with mental disorder: developmental follow-back of a prospective-longitudinal cohort. Arch Gen Psychiatry 60(7):709–717, 2003 12860775

Kimonis ER, Frick PJ, Skeem JL, et al: Assessing callous-unemotional traits in adolescent offenders: validation of the Inventory of Callous-Unemotional Traits. Int J Law Psychiatry 31(3):241–252, 2008 18514315

Krueger RF, Hicks BM, Patrick CJ, et al: Etiologic connections among substance dependence, antisocial behavior, and personality: modeling the externalizing spectrum. J Abnorm Psychol 111(3):411–424, 2002 12150417

Kuperman S, Stewart MA: Use of propranolol to decrease aggressive outbursts in younger patients: open study reveals potentially favorable outcome. Psychosomatics 28(6):315–319, 1987 3432546

Kuperman S, Calarge C, Kolar A, et al: An open-label trial of aripiprazole in the treatment of aggression in male adolescents diagnosed with conduct disorder. Ann Clin Psychiatry 23(4):270–276, 2011 22073384

Lahey BB, Loeber R, Burke J, Rathouz PJ: Adolescent outcomes of childhood conduct disorder among clinic-referred boys: predictors of improvement. J Abnorm Child Psychol 30(4):333–348, 2002 12108765

Langbehn DR, Cadoret RJ, Yates WR, et al: Distinct contributions of conduct and oppositional defiant symptoms to adult antisocial behavior: evidence from an adoption study. Arch Gen Psychiatry 55(9):821–829, 1998 9736009

Leadbeater BJ, Homel J: Irritable and defiant sub-dimensions of ODD: their stability and prediction of internalizing symptoms and conduct problems from adolescence to young adulthood. J Abnorm Child Psychol 43(3):407–421, 2015 25028284

Lettinga JR, Drent C, Hoekstra PJ, et al: Clinical pharmacology of conduct disorder: a critical review. Child and Adolescent Pharmacology News 16(6):1–10, 2011

Leung PW, Hung SF, Ho TP, et al: Prevalence of DSM-IV disorders in Chinese adolescents and the effects of an impairment criterion: a pilot community study in Hong Kong. Eur Child Adolesc Psychiatry 17(7):452–461, 2008 18427862

Liu J, Lewis G, Evans L: Understanding aggressive behaviour across the lifespan. J Psychiatr Ment Health Nurs 20(2):156–168, 2013 22471771

Loeber R, Green SM, Keenan K, et al: Which boys will fare worse? Early predictors of the onset of conduct disorder in a six-year longitudinal study. J Am Acad Child Adolesc Psychiatry 34(4):499–509, 1995 7751264

Loeber R, Burke JD, Lahey BB, et al: Oppositional defiant and conduct disorder: a review of the past 10 years, part I. J Am Acad Child Adolesc Psychiatry 39(12):1468–1484, 2000 11128323

Lunden WA: Statistics on Delinquents and Delinquency. Springfield, IL, Charles C Thomas, 1964

Maughan B, Rowe R, Messer J, et al: Conduct disorder and oppositional defiant disorder in a national sample: developmental epidemiology. J Child Psychol Psychiatry 45(3):609–621, 2004 15055379

McDonald L, Billingham S, Conrad T, et al: Families and schools together (FAST): integrating community development with clinical strategies. Families in Society 78(2):140–155, 1997

McEllistrem JE: Affective and predatory violence: a bimodal classification system of human aggression and violence. Aggress Violent Behav 10(1):1–30, 2004

McMahon RJ, Witkiewitz K, Kotler JS: Predictive validity of callous-unemotional traits measured in early adolescence with respect to multiple antisocial outcomes. J Abnorm Psychol 119(4):752–763, 2010 20939651

Meltzer H, Gatward R, Goodman R, et al: The Mental Health of Children and Adolescents in Great Britain. London, HM Stationery Office, 2000

Miller LS, Klein RG, Piacentini J, et al: The New York Teacher Rating Scale for disruptive and antisocial behavior. J Am Acad Child Adolesc Psychiatry 34(3):359–370, 1995 7896678

Moffitt TE: Adolescence-limited and life-course-persistent antisocial behavior: a developmental taxonomy. Psychol Rev 100(4):674–701, 1993 8255953

Moffitt TE, Caspi A: Childhood predictors differentiate life-course persistent and adolescence-limited antisocial pathways among males and females. Dev Psychopathol 13(2):355–375, 2001 11393651

Moffitt TE, Arseneault L, Jaffee SR, et al: Research review: DSM-V conduct disorder: research needs for an evidence base. J Child Psychol Psychiatry 49(1):3–33, 2008 18181878

Morcillo C, Duarte CS, Sala R, et al: Conduct disorder and adult psychiatric diagnoses: associations and gender differences in the U.S. adult population. J Psychiatr Res 46(3):323–330, 2012 22172996

National Collaborating Centre for Mental Health: Antisocial Behaviour and Conduct Disorders in Children and Young People: Recognition, Intervention, and Management, Volume 158. London, RCPsych Publications, 2013

Nelson-Gray RO, Keane SP, Hurst RM, et al: A modified DBT skills training program for oppositional defiant adolescents: promising preliminary findings. Behav Res Ther 44(12):1811–1820, 2006 16579964

Nock MK, Kazdin AE, Hiripi E, et al: Prevalence, subtypes, and correlates of DSM-IV conduct disorder in the National Comorbidity Survey Replication. Psychol Med 36(5):699–710, 2006 16438742

Obsuth I, Moretti MM, Holland R, et al: Conduct disorder: new directions in promoting effective parenting and strengthening parent-adolescent relationships. J Can Acad Child Adolesc Psychiatry 15(1):6–15, 2006 18392190

Olsson TM: MST with conduct disordered youth in Sweden: costs and benefits after 2 years. Res Soc Work Pract 20(6):561–571, 2010

Pardini DA, Frick PJ, Moffitt TE: Building an evidence base for DSM-5 conceptualizations of oppositional defiant disorder and conduct disorder: introduction to the special section. J Abnorm Psychol 119(4):683–688, 2010 21090874

Perepletchikova F, Nathanson D, Axelrod SR, et al: Randomized clinical trial of dialectical behavior therapy for preadolescent children with disruptive mood dysregulation disorder: feasibility and outcomes. J Am Acad Child Adolesc Psychiatry 56(10):832–840, 2017 28942805

Piquero AR, Farrington DP, Fontaine NMG, et al: Childhood risk, offending trajectories, and psychopathy at age 48 years in the Cambridge Study in Delinquent Development. Psychol Public Policy Law 18:577–598, 2012

Presnall N, Webster-Stratton CH, Constantino JN: Parent training: equivalent improvement in externalizing behavior for children with and without familial risk. J Am Acad Child Adolesc Psychiatry 53(8):879–887, 887.e1–887.e2, 2014 25062595

Reich W: Diagnostic Interview for Children and Adolescents (DICA). J Am Acad Child Adolesc Psychiatry 39(1):59–66, 2000 10638068

Rey J, Walter G, Soutullo C: Oppositional Defiant and Conduct Disorders, 5th Edition. Philadelphia, PA, Lippincott Williams & Wilkins, 2018

Reyes M, Buitelaar J, Toren P, et al: A randomized, double-blind, placebo-controlled study of risperidone maintenance treatment in children and adolescents with disruptive behavior disorders. Am J Psychiatry 163(3):402–410, 2006 16513860

Robins LN: Deviant Children Grown Up: A Sociological and Psychiatric Study of Sociopathic Personality. Baltimore, MD, Williams & Wilkins, 1966

Robins LN: A 70-year history of conduct disorder: variations in definition, prevalence, and correlates, in Historical and Geographical Influences on Psychopathology. Edited by Cohen P, Slomkowski C, Robins LN. Mahwah, NJ, Erlbaum, 1999, pp 37–56

Robins LN, Price RK: Adult disorders predicted by childhood conduct problems: results from the NIMH Epidemiologic Catchment Area project. Psychiatry 54(2):116–132, 1991 1852846

Rowe R, Costello EJ, Angold A, et al: Developmental pathways in oppositional defiant disorder and conduct disorder. J Abnorm Psychol 119(4):726–738, 2010a 21090876

Rowe R, Maughan B, Moran P, et al: The role of callous and unemotional traits in the diagnosis of conduct disorder. J Child Psychol Psychiatry 51(6):688–695, 2010b 20039995

Rutter M: Why are London children so disturbed? Proc R Soc Med 66(12):1221–1225, 1973 4777054

Rutter M, Tizard J, Whitmore K: Education, Health, and Behavior. London, Longman, 1970

Samek DR, Elkins IJ, Keyes MA, et al: High school sports involvement diminishes the association between childhood conduct disorder and adult antisocial behavior. J Adolesc Health 57(1):107–112, 2015 25937472

Sawyer MG, Arney FM, Baghurst PA, et al: The mental health of young people in Australia: key findings from the child and adolescent component of the national survey of mental health and well-being. Aust N Z J Psychiatry 35(6):806–814, 2001 11990891

Scott S: Do parenting programmes for severe child antisocial behaviour work over the longer term, and for whom? One year follow-up of a multi-centre controlled trial. Behav Cogn Psychother 33(4):403–421, 2005

Scott S, Knapp M, Henderson J, et al: Financial cost of social exclusion: follow up study of antisocial children into adulthood. BMJ 323(7306):191–194, 2001 11473907

Shaffer D, Fisher P, Dulcan MK, et al: The NIMH Diagnostic Interview Schedule for Children Version 2.3 (DISC-2.3): description, acceptability, prevalence rates, and performance in the MECA Study. Methods for the Epidemiology of Child and Adolescent Mental Disorders Study. J Am Acad Child Adolesc Psychiatry 35(7):865–877, 1996 8768346

Shelton D, Kesten K, Zhang W, et al: Impact of a Dialectic Behavior Therapy-Corrections Modified (DBT-CM) upon behaviorally challenged incarcerated male adolescents. J Child Adolesc Psychiatr Nurs 24(2):105–113, 2011 21501287

Snyder R, Turgay A, Aman M, et al: Effects of risperidone on conduct and disruptive behavior disorders in children with subaverage IQs. J Am Acad Child Adolesc Psychiatry 41(9):1026–1036, 2002 12218423

Steiner H, Dunne JE: Summary of the practice parameters for the assessment and treatment of children and adolescents with conduct disorder. J Am Acad Child Adolesc Psychiatry 36(10):1482–1485, 1997 9334562

Steiner H, Silverman M, Karnik NS, et al: Psychopathology, trauma and delinquency: subtypes of aggression and their relevance for understanding young offenders. Child Adolesc Psychiatry Ment Health 5:21, 2011 21714905

Stouthamer-Loeber M, Wei E, Loeber R, Mastenb AS: Desistance from persistent serious delinquency in the transition to adulthood. Dev Psychopathol 16(4):897–918, 2004 15704820

Stringaris A, Goodman R: Three dimensions of oppositionality in youth. J Child Psychol Psychiatry 50(3):216–223, 2009 19166573

Substance Abuse and Mental Health Services Administration: Interventions for disruptive behavior disorders evidence-based practices (EBP) KIT. 2011. Available at: http://store.samhsa.gov/product/Interventions-for-Disruptive-Behavior-Disorders-Evidence-Based-Practices-EBP-KIT/SMA11-4634. Accessed April 22, 2021.

Van Bellinghen M, De Troch C: Risperidone in the treatment of behavioral disturbances in children and adolescents with borderline intellectual functioning: a double-blind, placebo-controlled pilot trial. J Child Adolesc Psychopharmacol 11(1):5–13, 2001 11322745

van Lier PA, van der Ende J, Koot HM, et al: Which better predicts conduct problems? The relationship of trajectories of conduct problems with ODD and ADHD symptoms from childhood into adolescence. J Child Psychol Psychiatry 48(6):601–608, 2007 17537076

Vitiello B, Behar D, Hunt J, et al: Subtyping aggression in children and adolescents. J Neuropsychiatry Clin Neurosci 2(2):189–192, 1990 2136074

Waller R, Gardner F, Hyde LW, et al: Do harsh and positive parenting predict parent reports of deceitful-callous behavior in early childhood? J Child Psychol Psychiatry 53(9):946–953, 2012 22490064

Wasserman GA, McReynolds LS: Contributors to traumatic exposure and posttraumatic stress disorder in juvenile justice youths. J Trauma Stress 24(4):422–429, 2011 21800364

Webster-Stratton C, Reid MJ: The incredible years parents, teachers and children training series: a multifaceted treatment approach for young children with conduct problems, in Evidence-Based Psychotherapies for Children and Adolescents. Edited by Weisz JR, Kazdin AE. New York, Guilford, 2003, pp 122–141

Webster-Stratton C, Reid MJ, Hammond M: Treating children with early onset conduct problems: intervention outcomes for parent, child, and teacher training. J Clin Child Adolesc Psychol 33(1):105–124, 2004 15028546

Woolgar M, Scott S: Evidence-based management of conduct disorders. Curr Opin Psychiatry 18(4):392–396, 2005 16639131

World Health Organization: The ICD-10 Classification of Mental and Behavioural Disorders: Diagnostic Criteria for Research. Geneva, World Health Organization, 1993

CHAPTER 22

The Antisocial Woman

Brittany Bishop, M.Sc.F.S.

Birgit Völlm, M.D., Ph.D.

Najat Khalifa, M.D.

On a worldwide scale, the cost of antisocial behavior is immense. In 2012, the economic cost of violence containment[1] alone was estimated to be $9.46 trillion, approximately 11% of the Gross World Product (Institute for Economics and Peace 2013). Therefore, developing a more thorough understanding of antisocial behavior is critical in order to effectively prevent such behavior. Although research on antisocial behavior dates back to the early 1900s, research on antisocial patterns of behavior in women is a relatively new area of study, dating back to only the 1990s. Many of the first studies attempting to identify the key features of antisocial personality disorder (ASPD) were conducted on male-only samples, with only a few case examples of women to demonstrate that the disorder could occur in both genders (Cleckley 1976; Martens 2000; Rogstad and Rogers 2008). One reason that the research has focused on men is because ASPD is a heavily male-dominated disorder, with ASPD presenting in a 3:1 ratio of males to females, regardless of age or ethnicity (Alegria et al. 2013).

The gender difference in prevalence of ASPD may reflect some underlying differences in the presentation of the disorder in men and women, but differences also have been observed in the antecedents of the disorder, genetics, symptoms, and etiology. Several theories exist as to why these differences exist, including biological factors, the presence of gender bias in diagnosis, and compliance with traditional gender norms, but the actual reasons remain largely unknown. The current editions of both the *Diagnostic and Statistical Manual of Mental Disorders* (DSM-5; American Psychiatric Association 2013) and the *International Classification of Diseases* (ICD-10; World Health

---

[1] The Institute for Economics and Peace (2013) defined violence containment spending as "economic activity that is related to the consequences or prevention of violence where the violence is directed against people or property" (p. 4).

Organization 1992) recognize ASPD as a nosological entity, although ICD-10 uses the term *dissocial personality disorder* to denote the condition. Regardless of how the condition is classified, we summarize the evidence in the field to further explore the key gender differences in ASPD and examine the main theories as to why these differences exist. Although we also briefly focus on psychopathy, a condition that overlaps significantly with ASPD, providing a detailed account of the gender differences in psychopathy is beyond the scope of this chapter.

Prevalence of Antisocial Personality Disorder

Regardless of how ASPD is operationalized, across all settings the disorder is more prevalent in males than in females (Fazel and Danesh 2002; Robins and Regier 1991; Singleton et al. 1998; Swanson et al. 1994). The Epidemiologic Catchment Area survey reported that 2%–4% of men and 0.5%–1% of women had presentations that fulfilled DSM-III-R (American Psychiatric Association 1987) criteria for ASPD (Robins and Regier 1991). Another North American study reported prevalence rates of 6.8% among men and 0.8% among women (Swanson et al. 1994). A prevalence ratio of 3:1 of males to females with ASPD is commonly observed (Alegria et al. 2013).

In contrast, European studies reported lower prevalence rates among men (1.0%– 1.3%) and among women (0%–0.2%) (Coid et al. 2006; Torgersen et al. 2001). Naturally, rates are higher in the prison population, where, in the United Kingdom, 49% of male sentenced offenders and 31% of female prisoners had presentations that met DSM-IV (American Psychiatric Association 1994) criteria for ASPD (Singleton et al. 1998). In the United States, a study found the frequency of ASPD to be 37.1% among male offenders and 26.8% among female offenders (Black et al. 2010).

Antecedents of Antisocial Personality Disorder

The diagnosis of ASPD cannot be made before age 18 years, although the first signs of antisocial behavior manifest early in life. These signs tend to manifest later in childhood for girls than for boys (Robins 1966). One study of 3,258 randomly selected individuals from Edmonton, Ontario, showed that the first signs of antisocial behavior appeared at age 7.6 years for boys and at age 9.2 years for girls. The first signs generally start as behavior problems observed at home or at school (Martens 2000).

One disorder that is associated with many of the first indications of antisocial behavior in children and teens is conduct disorder (CD). Like much of the research on ASPD, research on CD also has been male-dominated, likely because of the lower base rate of CD among females, such that differences between male and female presentations of the disorder are not well known. In the United States, the estimated prevalence rates of CD are 12% for males and 0%–7.1% for females, with a median age at onset of 11.6 years. (Nock et al. 2006). Berkout et al. (2011) conducted a literature review of gender differences in CD and reported gender differences in multiple areas. In general, compared with females, males were found to be overall more physically aggressive than females, to be more impulsive, and to have more externalizing behaviors. Like males, females tend to develop the disorder before adolescence, but the ways in which they develop the disorder are not well understood, because they do not tend to follow the developmental trajectories established for males. In addition, males and females differ in the comorbidities associated with CD. While comorbid ADHD, substance use disorders, and anxiety disorders are highly prevalent among both males and females with CD, violent female juvenile offenders are three to five times more likely to endorse anxiety disorders than are violent male and nonviolent male and female offenders (Berkout et al. 2011). In fact, this association between anxiety and violent offending in females suggests that internalizing tendencies may be more strongly related to severe expressions of externalizing behavior in females compared with males (Wasserman et al. 2005).

Not all individuals with CD will go on to develop ASPD. The factors that determine who may subsequently develop ASPD have also been shown to have gender differences. Studies of children with CD reported evidence of lower resting levels of autonomic activity (as measured by heart rate and skin conductance) and to some extent autonomic reactivity to threatening stimuli compared with control children (Patrick 2008). In males, decreased emotional response to punishment has been related to development of antisocial behavior (Fowles and Dindo 2006). Anxiety is the only positive predictor found for females with CD who subsequently develop ASPD (Berkout et al. 2011). None of the other associations have been found in females, making it difficult to predict which young females with CD will go on to develop ASPD (Berkout et al. 2011).

Finally, it has been suggested that the diagnostic criteria for CD may need to be adjusted to adequately capture the female presentation of the disorder (Zoccolillo 1993). Although the diagnostic criteria were found to be valid for both genders, males with symptoms meeting criteria for CD present along a spectrum from mild to severe pathology, whereas most females with symptoms that meet criteria for CD are considered to have "severe" pathology. This suggests that the diagnostic criteria are not appropriate for identifying females with less severe presentations of the disorder (Berkout et al. 2011).

In summary, significant gaps remain in our understanding of the biological, psychological, social, and epidemiological differences in CD among males and females, which future studies in the field should endeavor to address. However, because CD is a prerequisite for a diagnosis of ASPD in DSM-5, it is reasonable to assume that ASPD also may manifest differently in females and males (Berkout et al. 2011).

Psychosocial Factors Associated With Antisocial Traits in Females

Although the developmental antecedents of ASPD in females remain unclear, some factors may increase the risk for developing antisocial behavior in females. For instance, a study by Dadds and colleagues (2009) underscored the roles of affective empathy (a tendency to feel and care about what others feel), cognitive empathy (being able to describe what and why other people feel), and callous-unemotional traits (a disregard for others with deficient empathy and affect) as reported by parents of 2,760 children ages 3–13 years. Overall, females showed higher levels of cognitive and affective empathy and lower levels of callous-unemotional traits than boys. Although boys with high levels of callous-unemotional traits had low cognitive empathy in early childhood, cognitive empathy reached normative levels by early adolescence (ages 9–13 years); however, girls with high callous-unemotional traits in early childhood continued to show lower cognitive empathy in early adolescence. Low affective empathy levels also were associated with higher psychopathic traits in males but not in females. The authors proposed that females may have a differential path for the development of antisocial behavior later in life, which is underpinned by a greater vulnerability to stress and emotion dysregulation rather than callousness or lack of empathy. However, this study was limited by parent reports and lack of long-term follow-up (Dadds et al. 2009).

Furthermore, for both males and females, family adversity and childhood abuse or neglect have been found to act as risk factors for the development of ASPD (Murray and Farrington 2010). However, the effect these have on the individual's risk for developing ASPD may be stronger for females. Alegria et al. (2013) used information from the National Epidemiologic Survey on Alcohol and Related Conditions (a large, nationally representative sample of the U.S. general population) to examine sex differences in ASPD, particularly adverse life events. They found more reports of both childhood and adulthood adverse life events in women, which included neglect, emotional abuse, sexual abuse, and physical abuse. This is consistent with the threshold-of-risk hypothesis, which posits that women may require a higher loading of risk factors before they present with the disorder (Alegria et al. 2013).

Moreover, some risk factors that have been identified in males may not play an important role in the development of ASPD in females. For instance, Krabbendam et al. (2015) examined the predictive value of trauma and mental health problems on the development of ASPD and borderline personality disorder (BPD) in a prospective study of 229 female juvenile offenders. They reported that posttraumatic stress, depressive symptoms, and dissociation increased the risk for developing BPD in adulthood, but neither conduct problems nor substance dependence predicted the development of ASPD (Krabbendam et al. 2015).

Finally, worthy of note is the role of protective factors for antisocial behavior. For example, positive parent training, particularly for parents of girls, can lead to a decrease in callous-unemotional traits over time (for boys, parental involvement has been found to be more important than positive parenting interventions) (Viding and McCrory 2012). Therefore, it has been suggested that family-based therapies may be effective early interventions for females with antisocial traits. Multi-Systemic Family Therapy, for example, has shown some benefits in reducing youth incarceration and offending behavior among chronic female offenders (Chamberlain et al. 2007; Leve et al. 2005). However, further research is required to further clarify the effectiveness that these treatments may have (Viding and McCrory 2012).

Genetics

Behavioral Genetic Studies

Research on sex differences in the heritability of ASPD is limited. Estimates of sex differences in the magnitude of genetic and environmental influences on antisocial behavior vary according to the operationalization of antisocial behavior (Rhee and Waldman

2002). Previous studies that examined these differences had mixed findings, with some reporting that the magnitude of genetic and environmental influences on antisocial behavior is equal for males and females (Rhee and Waldman 2002; Widom and Ames 1988) and others reporting a slightly higher magnitude for males than for females (Miles and Carey 1997). Furthermore, research evidence shows some support for a higher heritability of callous-unemotional traits for males (Fontaine et al. 2010), but other studies found little evidence of sex differences (Bezdjian et al. 2011; Larsson et al. 2006; Viding et al. 2007).

The polygenic multiple threshold model (Mednick et al. 1983; Sigvardsson et al. 1982) may provide one possible explanation for the lower prevalence rates of ASPD in females. This model suggests that it is the degree of liability rather than the magnitude of genetic or environmental influences that affects the development of the disorder (Rhee and Waldman 2002). In support of this theory is the fact that even though females are less affected by the disorder, they generally have more affected relatives than do males (Bagchi et al. 2013; McGuffin and Thapar 1992).

Molecular Genetic Studies

Some studies have examined which genes may influence the development of ASPD in females, in comparison to males; the same genes seem to be implicated in the development of ASPD in both males and females, suggesting similar underlying genetic influences for the disorder (Bagchi et al. 2013).

The Monoamine Oxidase A Gene

The monoamine oxidase A (MAO-A) gene (*MAOA*) is of interest in understanding the potential genetic underpinnings of both ASPD and BPD. Given some of the overlapping traits between BPD and ASPD (i.e., impulsivity, risk taking, anger), the same genes are often associated with the development of both disorders. Generally, the evidence suggests that females with the longer variation of *MAOA* are more prone to internalizing behaviors, such as depression, whereas men are more prone to externalizing behaviors, such as aggression (Beauchaine et al. 2009). Furthermore, the effects of *MAOA* seem to have a greater influence on males than on females, and the relationship between *MAOA* and aggression is clearer in males than in females. For example, in males with a variation of the *MAOA* promoter gene that is associated with decreased transcriptional efficiency, childhood maltreatment predicts future antisocial behavior to a greater extent compared with those without that variant (Caspi et al. 2002). Some studies have shown this same association in females. For example, Ducci et al. (2008) examined 291 females and found that having the low-activity *MAOA* genotype increases the individual's vulnerability to antisocial tendencies in those with a history of childhood maltreatment, much as in males. However, a meta-analysis of 12 papers involving 7,588 female subjects that examined the same trend in females found no association between lesser *MAOA* transcriptional efficiency and childhood maltreatment or antisocial behavior (Byrd and Manuck 2014). In fact, there was a weak association between antisocial behavior and the *MAOA* promoter gene with increased transcriptional efficiency in some of the studies of females, in contrast to the effect found in males. Later studies have also supported this finding that higher levels of *MAOA* promoter gene transcriptional efficiency appear to be associated with aggression in females (Godar et al. 2016).

What is evident is that *MAOA* can affect females differently than males, likely because of a lower-activity *MAOA* genotype, especially if this genotype is recessive (Bagchi et al. 2013). What remains unclear is why. One possible confounder is that *MAOA* is located on the X-chromosome, which raises several challenges for studies on females because of the lack of reliable information on dosage effects, making it difficult to interpret the actual levels of isoenzymes A and B in different genotypic classes (Craig 2007).

The Catechol O-Methyltransferase Gene

The catechol O-methyltransferase (COMT) gene (*COMT*) has been implicated in the development of both antisocial behavior and depression, which may be linked in part to sex differences in gene expression. One variation of the gene results in increased COMT enzymatic activity. In females, higher COMT activity has been found to be associated with increased rates of early-onset depression and increased vulnerability to mood episodes following stressful life events (Hatzimanolis et al. 2013). However, low enzyme activity of COMT has been associated with ASPD in males, likely by influencing dopamine reward pathways and modulating serotonin levels (Cuartas Arias et al. 2011). Therefore, differences in *COMT* expression due to genetic variations may lead to different symptom profiles and vulnerabilities between genders (Beauchaine et al. 2009).

The Serotonin Transporter Gene

Studies have shown consistently that low activity associated with the short variant of the serotonin transporter gene (*5HTT*) is associated with an increased risk for depression and anxiety and with the development of externalizing psychopathology, including violence (Mendoza and Casados 2014). However, this violence presents differently in males and females. The short variant of *5HTT* can lead to vulnerabilities to externalizing psychopathology in males but is associated with increased vulnerabilities to internalizing psychopathology in females. This is in keeping with the dimensional internalizing-externalizing model, which posits that observed gender differences in the prevalence rates of various mental disorders reflect underlying differences in latent internalizing and externalizing liability dimensions (Eaton et al. 2012). Furthermore, the long variant of *5HTT* has been associated with antisocial behavior and greater expression of callous-unemotional and narcissistic traits (Sadeh et al. 2010). Evidence suggests that the presence of two long alleles increases the risk for reduced emotional responding and psychopathic traits in the context of additional genetic and environmental factors (Glenn 2011).

Diagnosis and Assessment

Some researchers have questioned the validity of the diagnostic criteria and assessment tools that are routinely used for ASPD for women, because many of these measures were developed with male-only samples. Dolan and Völlm (2009) conducted a review to examine the validity and reliability of measures for assessment and diagnosis of ASPD and psychopathy in women. They examined the International Personality Disorder Examination (Loranger et al. 1994), the Structured Clinical Interview for DSM-IV Axis II Disorders (First et al. 1996) for ASPD, the Psychopathy Checklist–

Revised (PCL-R; Hare 2003), and the screening version of the Psychopathy Checklist (Hart et al. 1995). Overall, they found that the measures were generally sound but may require some adjustments to ensure that they properly capture the variations of the disorder in women. One of the main issues was the requirement for a diagnosis of childhood CD in order to qualify for a diagnosis of ASPD, according to DSM. The authors argued that a diagnosis of CD relies heavily on demonstrating physical aggression toward others, a behavior found more commonly in boys than in girls. This low rate of CD diagnosis for females necessitates a lower rate of ASPD in adults, even if women show other symptoms of ASPD (Dolan and Völlm 2009).

Burnette and Newman (2005) examined the association between CD and ASPD in women more closely, using a sample of 261 incarcerated women who screened positive for personality disorders. In this high-risk sample, approximately one-third of the women had presentations that met the full criteria for ASPD. Fewer than half (39.5%) had presentations that met criteria for CD, and most of these also had presentations that met criteria for ASPD. However, nearly half of the sample (47.5%) had presentations that met criteria for what the authors deemed "adult-onset" ASPD (i.e., adult diagnostic criteria were met, but no CD diagnosis had previously been made). They concluded that the requirement of a CD diagnosis as part of the diagnostic criteria for ASPD may lead to underdiagnosis of ASPD in women, who appear to have a later onset of symptoms (Burnette and Newman 2005).

Burnette and Newman (2005) also attempted to determine what other childhood factors predicted the disorder in females, given that CD was not enough. They found that certain patterns of behavior were better able to predict ASPD in girls than CD, with "destructive type" behaviors (property destruction, fire setting) being the strongest predictor. They also reported a high correlation in females between a diagnosis of childhood CD and borderline, histrionic, narcissistic, and paranoid personality disorders, indicating that CD may predict a wide range of personality psychopathology in females.

Dolan and Völlm (2009) also identified potential issues of gender bias in the assessment measures examined. For example, although the PCL-R was shown to have good reliability and construct validity for females, women tended to score differently on certain items compared with men and showed differences in item loading onto the different factors of the PCL-R. Items such as "criminal versatility," "juvenile delinquency," "revocation on conditional release," and "failure to accept responsibility" seemed less applicable to women, whereas "promiscuity" appeared to be more strongly related to the concept of psychopathy in women (Dolan and Völlm 2009). Goldstein et al. (1996) demonstrated that women tended to score higher on the items that relate to "financial irresponsibility," "failure to plan ahead/impulsivity," and "lack of remorse," whereas men scored higher on items of "irritability/aggressiveness" and "recklessness." In a more recent review, Efferson and Glenn (2018) reported that even though both males and females scoring higher in psychopathy have decreased brain responses in post error processing, deficits in emotional processing, passive avoidance errors, and response perseveration are less prominent in females.

In summary, traits shared by men and women may be expressed differently (e.g., impulsivity leads to self-harming behavior in women but to violence against others in men). Therefore, it has been suggested that measures such as the PCL-R and the DSM criteria may need to be revised to better reflect the female presentation of the disorder (Dolan and Völlm 2009). Dolan and Völlm (2009) suggested the removal of

450 Textbook of Antisocial Personality Disorder

the requirement of a diagnosis of CD as part of the criteria for ASPD and a lower clinical "cutoff" threshold on PCL measures to best reflect the presentation of the disorder in women. Their research also highlights the need to better understand the symptom profile and development of CD, ASPD, and psychopathy before a more appropriate measure for the diagnosis and assessment of these disorders in females can be created (Dolan and Völlm 2009).

Symptoms and Behavior

Table 22–1 summarizes differences in CD and ASPD symptoms. In short, females and males with CD or ASPD may present with different symptoms and behaviors, and this can cause problems in the accurate diagnosis of these disorders.

Even as children, the behaviors that antisocial boys and antisocial girls tend to engage in differ. Antisocial boys are more likely to engage in fighting, use weapons, engage in cruelty to animals, and set fires than are antisocial girls. Antisocial girls, on the other hand, are more likely to take part in "victimless" behavior, such as running away from home (Black et al. 2010).

In their examination of gender differences in symptoms and behaviors associated with ASPD, Alegria et al. (2013) found that, after controlling for the effects of sociodemographic characteristics (i.e., race, nativity [U.S. born vs. non–U.S. born], age, education, individual income, family income, and marital status) and several additional psychiatric disorders, women were more likely than men to have run away from home overnight, missed work or school, or been in a physical altercation that resulted in swapping blows with an intimate partner. Additionally, women were less likely than men to have put themselves into a dangerous situation, received three or more traffic tickets for reckless driving, had a driver's license suspended or revoked, destroyed others' property, deliberately started a fire, done something illegal, hit someone and injured him or her, harmed an animal on purpose, defrauded someone, or used a weapon in an altercation. In terms of symptoms, men and women did not differ on the number of criteria met, but sex differences were seen in terms of which criteria were more likely to be met. Women were more likely to have symptoms of deceitfulness and impulsivity and less likely to show irritability/aggressiveness and reckless disregard for the safety of self or others. Women also had significantly lower scores than men on the SF-12 Health Survey (a 12-item short-form questionnaire that assesses generic health outcomes from the patient's perspective; Ware et al. 2002) mental component summary, mental health scale, role emotional functioning scale, and social functioning scale; reported greater perceived stress; and had a lower score on the social network index. Overall, Alegria et al. (2013) concluded that women tended to participate in less violent antisocial behavior, whereas men participate in more violent and illegal behaviors. They hypothesized that this could lead to an underdiagnosis or misdiagnosis of the disorder in women because violent and more aggressive behaviors are more often associated with an ASPD diagnosis (Alegria et al. 2013).

Some studies have also identified that women tend to have more severe socioeconomic deprivation than men. In particular, women were shown to be more likely to be chronically unemployed, have higher rates of marital separation, and be reliant on state financial programs than their male counterparts (Rogstad and Rogers 2008).

TABLE 22–1.   **Gender differences in conduct disorder and antisocial personality disorder symptoms**

Symptoms	Female	Male
Conduct disorder		
Mean age at onset	9.2 years	7.6 years
Externalizing behaviors	Less physically aggressive, less impulsive, and more likely to play truant and to run away from home	More impulsive; more likely to engage in fighting, use weapons, engage in cruelty to animals, and set fires
Anxiety symptoms	Highly prevalent	Less prevalent
Symptom severity	Often severe	Mild to severe
Empathy	Higher levels of cognitive and affective empathy	Lower levels of cognitive and affective empathy
Callous-unemotional traits	Lower levels	Higher levels
Antisocial personality disorder		
Predisposing factors	More predisposing factors present (e.g., lower IQ, history of abuse, from low-income families), suggesting more predisposing factors required for the disorder to develop	Fewer predisposing factors present than in females
Offending behavior	More likely to desert their spouse, hit their spouse, or fail to work steadily	More likely to participate in more violent and illegal behaviors, engage in reckless driving, have a driver's license suspended or revoked, destroy others' property, deliberately start a fire, hit someone and injure him or her, harm an animal, defraud someone, or use a weapon
Deceitfulness and impulsivity	More likely to have these symptoms	Less likely to have these symptoms
Aggression and recklessness	Less likely to show irritability/aggressiveness and reckless disregard for the safety of self or others	More likely to show irritability/aggressiveness and reckless behavior
Relationship problems	Higher rates of marital separation	Higher rates of promiscuity
Substance misuse	Common, but conflicting evidence regarding gender differences	Highly prevalent
Comorbidity	More likely to have comorbid mood disorder, major depressive disorder, dysthymia, anxiety disorders, or PTSD	As likely to have bipolar disorder, social anxiety disorder, pathological gambling, ADHD, and any personality disorder
		More likely to have narcissistic personality disorder

The following composite case example illustrates a typical presentation of ASPD in women.

> Janet, a 30-year-old woman, grew up in a disturbed family home and witnessed her parents arguing and fighting. Her parents both abused alcohol and other substances. Her father had an extensive criminal history, and he abused her both physically and emotionally. For that reason, she was removed from the home at age 10 years and placed in an orphanage. She ran away several times and was often truant, but eventually she was placed in a foster home at age 11. In foster care, she had behavior problems and was diagnosed with CD and ADHD.
>
> Janet moved out at age 18 and has lived on her own, surviving through petty crime and by prostituting herself. She has never held a regular job. She reports having multiple one-night stands but no long-term relationships. She has an extensive criminal history with multiple convictions for theft and crimes of dishonesty but no history of violence.
>
> Janet first developed problems with drugs and alcohol during her teenage years. Additionally, she has a history of self-harming behavior, by cutting and overdosing, which has led to many admissions to psychiatric inpatient units. She has poor coping skills and significant issues with emotional dysregulation. She is unable to cope with stressful situations, which can trigger episodes of cutting.
>
> In addition to ASPD, Janet has received diagnoses of BPD, cannabis use disorder, alcohol use disorder, and drug-induced psychosis. She is now receiving treatment in a long-term psychiatric rehabilitation unit. With encouragement, she resumed her schooling and now has a high school equivalency degree and hopes to eventually become a hair stylist. Through therapy, she has learned to better control her emotional instability. She has abstained from drugs and alcohol and has abandoned her criminal career.

Comorbidity

Males and females with ASPD also differ in terms of their comorbidities. In men, the most prominent comorbidity is substance use disorder. Women also have high rates of substance use disorder, and in fact they may have even higher rates than men do. One study found that men with ASPD were 3 times more likely to abuse alcohol and 5 times more likely to abuse drugs than those without ASPD. Women with ASPD were 10–13 times more likely to abuse alcohol and 12 times more likely to abuse drugs than those without ASPD (Martens 2000). Lewis (2011) examined the relationship between substance use and ASPD in women more closely in a sample of 136 female offenders identified as being at high risk for ASPD or substance use. Of the 136 women, 41 had presentations that met criteria for ASPD. Of those 41 participants, 56.1% had a presentation that met criteria for alcohol dependence, 70.7% were dependent on at least one drug, and 52.6% had used drugs intravenously. The age at onset of substance dependence was relatively early, between 17 and 23.8 years, and ASPD symptom count was high for those with substance dependence, with average counts of about 3.6 (on a scale of 0 to 7). Women with ASPD had an increased risk of violence while under the influence of drugs or alcohol. The most common substances of dependence were cocaine (61% were dependent), alcohol (56.1% were dependent), and opiates (48.8% were dependent). These prevalence rates are much higher than what would be observed in a community sample for both men and women, and even when compared with samples of incarcerated men (Lewis 2011). The National Comorbidity Survey found that lifetime prevalence rates for alcohol dependence were 20.1% for males and 8.2% for females, and prevalence rates for drug dependence were 9.2% for males and 5.9% for females in the general population (Kessler et al. 1994). A more recent survey found that lifetime prevalence rates for alcohol dependence among people with lifetime exposure to substances were 19.6% for males and 10.3% for females. Prevalence rates for other substances varied by type, with the highest rates reported for heroin: 29.1% for males and 25.6% for females (Lev-Ran et al. 2013).

Overall, Lewis (2011) found that women with ASPD who used substances were likely to quickly develop substance dependence of substantial severity. They also had high comorbidity with other DSM-IV Axis I diagnoses. Lewis (2011) reported that the high number of comorbidities in women with ASPD suggests that these women could potentially be more difficult to treat, might require more services, could have worse outcomes, and could be at increased risk for suicide.

However, contradictory results suggesting that the rates of substance abuse in women with ASPD may be lower than those of men also have been presented. Alegria et al. (2013) found, in their general population study of 819 men and 407 women meeting DSM-IV ASPD criteria, that women with ASPD were, in fact, less likely than men to have alcohol or drug use disorders or dependency.

Women with ASPD also tend to show differences from males in other comorbid psychiatric disorders. Alegria et al. (2013) found that women with ASPD were more likely than men to have a comorbid diagnosis of any mood disorder, major depressive disorder, dysthymia, any anxiety disorder, panic disorder, specific phobias, PTSD, and generalized anxiety disorder. However, women and men were equally as likely to have any psychiatric disorder, any Axis I disorder, bipolar disorder, social anxiety disorder, pathological gambling, ADHD, and any personality disorder (except for narcissistic personality disorder, which was more common in men). Lewis (2011) also reported high prevalence rates of a major depressive episode (63.4%), PTSD (46.3%), and ADHD (22.0%), all higher than previously reported rates for women in community samples in the United States. Martens (2000), in a literature review of antisocial and psychopathic personality disorders, concluded that women with ASPD, compared with men with these disorders, had higher overall rates of comorbid disorders, including depression, anxiety, and suicidal behavior.

Besides comorbidities, women with ASPD have increased stress levels, decreased well-being, decreased social and emotional functioning, and increased mental health needs (Alegria et al. 2013; Ruan et al. 2008). Alegria et al. (2013) attributed the increased social impairment in this population to a greater level of rejections because of failure to conform with stereotypical gender-specific behavioral norms; a greater risk of relational aggression (i.e., targeting people they know, such as friends and relatives); and higher expectations regarding social ties with family and friends. Again, this information is consistent with the threshold risk hypothesis, stating that women require a higher loading of risk factors to develop ASPD (Alegria et al. 2013).

Treatment

There is a dearth of research on potential treatment options for ASPD or research on treatment options specific to females with the disorder. Two Cochrane systematic reviews reported on the use of pharmacological (Khalifa et al. 2010) and psychological interventions (Gibbon et al. 2010) for ASPD. Of the 19 studies included in the reviews, most participants were men (79.9% and 96.6% for psychological and pharmacological interventions, respectively). The reviews did not have sufficient power to conduct analysis by gender.

However, some researchers have pointed toward potentially beneficial treatment options for women, although these remain to be tested. For example, Alegria et al. (2013) suggested that interventions aimed at improving impulse control may be more beneficial for women with ASPD, whereas anger management may be more appropriate for men with ASPD. Because of the high number of comorbidities observed in women with ASPD (Alegria et al. 2013; Lewis 2011), the treatment of these other disorders obviously needs to be attended to and may render better outcomes. However, because of the severity of symptoms and interaction of various disorders, this group may be more challenging to treat and thus may require a multifaceted approach (Lewis 2011).

For children and adolescents, early identification of symptoms and early interventions could help to prevent a worsening of symptoms, which if untreated could potentially lead to criminality and increased mental health problems in adulthood. In addition, because females with CD who experience both internalizing and externalizing behaviors have been found to be more violent and more greatly impaired, treatment of associated internalizing disorders may be important for these girls (Berkout et al. 2011).

Finally, some research has suggested that females may be more likely than males to receive any sort of treatment. Some evidence suggests that there are gender biases in sentencing and that men and women who have committed the same crime and have similar mental health conditions may be subject to different outcomes, with women being less likely to receive a custodial sentence and more likely to receive treatment and men more likely to be incarcerated (Dolan and Völlm 2009).

Course and Outcomes

The outcomes of adolescents who present with antisocial behavior as they develop into adulthood have been examined. Pajer (1998) reviewed 20 studies examining adult outcomes of girls ages 13–18 years with antisocial behavior (i.e., those with CD or delinquency) and reported that as adults these females had increased rates of mortality, of criminality, and of psychiatric morbidity, along with more dysfunctional or violent relationships. Adult crime rates were reported to be 25%–46%, higher than in control girls or in girls with other psychiatric disorders. Between 14% and 60% of the girls with CD developed adult psychiatric disorders, compared with 0%–40% of the control girls, and nearly half of the antisocial girls developed substance abuse problems as adults. Finally, girls with antisocial behaviors were more likely than control girls or those with other psychiatric disorders to be diagnosed with ASPD as adults, with approximately one-third of the girls in the review eventually receiving this diagnosis (Pajer 1998).

In a separate study, Robins and Regier (1991) examined youths who developed ASPD to determine what type of antisocial behavior was more likely to lead to an adult diagnosis of ASPD. Results showed that 27% of the boys and 21% of the girls with three or more CD symptoms developed ASPD in adulthood, but 49% of the boys and 33% of the girls with six or more CD symptoms went on to develop ASPD. Delinquency before age 15 predicted later ASPD in 29% of the males and 13% of the females. These findings suggest that early life interventions may be critical in preventing further criminality and psychiatric problems in children with CD.

In terms of lifetime outcomes for women with ASPD, studies have shown that they have a relatively positive prognosis and more satisfactory long-term outcomes than men. One study showed that only 18% of females with criminal behavior and a diagnosis of ASPD were still engaged in criminal activity in the fourth decade of life (Martens 2000). The study found that 10% of women and 27% of men younger than 30 had presentations that met criteria for ASPD, whereas 5% of women and 20% of men between ages 30 and 44 had presentations that met the diagnostic criteria (Martens 2000). Martens (2000) even reported that none of the women in their research population ($n=3{,}258$) had the disorder past age 35 years.

Psychopathy

Psychopathy and ASPD are considered separate, yet related, conditions. Psychopathy in females is rare and less common than in males. When the traditional cutoff score of 30 on the PCL-R was used, diagnostic criteria were met in 7.7% of U.K. male prisoners but in only 1.6% of U.K. female prisoners (Coid et al. 2009). In violent offenders, 11% of women versus 31% of men had presentations that met criteria for psychopathy (Grann 2000).

Warren and South (2006) examined the relationship between ASPD and psychopathy in a sample of 802 incarcerated women divided into four categories: women with ASPD only ($n=23$; 16.8%), those with no ASPD and with a PCL-R score higher than 25 ($n=21$; 15.3%), those with both ASPD and psychopathy ($n=44$; 32.1%), and a control sample of women who did not receive either diagnosis ($n=49$; 35.8%). Results showed that it is possible to meet criteria for one disorder and not the other, suggesting that ASPD and psychopathy are likely separate entities. The length of sentence and rates of violent crime were approximately equal across all groups, suggesting that those with ASPD or psychopathy or both were not more violent than those without a diagnosis, in contrast to findings in men, in whom psychopathy was associated with increased violence (Warren and South 2006). Women with an ASPD diagnosis showed only higher rates of impulsivity, aggression, recklessness, and irresponsible behavior compared with those with psychopathy only and those with no diagnosis. Those who had both ASPD and psychopathy demonstrated higher degrees of deceitfulness and chronic breaking of social norms than those whose presentation did not meet criteria for either disorder. Those whose presentation met criteria for psychopathy only showed higher levels of remorselessness when compared with the ASPD-only group and with those with no diagnosis. The ASPD-only group also had greater comorbidity with other personality disorders and higher rates of psychological distress, paranoia and somatic anxiety, and childhood physical assault than any of the other groups. Although further research is required to confirm these findings, it does appear that psychopathy and ASPD are different constructs in women (Warren and South 2006).

There may also be differences in the expression of psychopathy between men and women. Rogstad and Rogers (2008) identified four key differences in the manifestation of the disorder between men and women: 1) differential expressions of psychopathic behavior (i.e., men tend to engage in impulsive and violent behavior, whereas women participate in manipulation and property crimes); 2) differences in interpersonal behavior (men are more likely to "con," whereas women are more likely to act flirtatious); 3) different psychological motivations (women may participate in promiscuous sexual behavior because of a drive to exploit their partners, whereas men may be driven by sensation seeking or a desire for sexual activity); and 4) potential bias in the assessment of psychopathy according to social norms (e.g., financial dependence can be seen as socially acceptable for women but as parasitic behavior for men).

Conclusion

Many gender differences have been observed in ASPD with regard to prevalence, risk factors, etiology, genetic underpinnings, comorbid disorders, prognosis, key traits and symptoms, and overall presentation of the disorder. The evidence reviewed in this chapter suggests that these differences are true and not artifactual. However, there is still a dearth of research regarding this unique population, and very little is understood about why these differences occur.

Even though the disorder is three times as prevalent in men as in women, a significant proportion of female offenders with the disorder would benefit from specific interventions and treatment programs, as well as customized assessment tools. Further research is required to better understand how these tools should be created and for best practices to be developed regarding assessment and treatment approaches.

Key Points

- Men with antisocial personality disorder (ASPD) have been researched far more than women with ASPD.

- ASPD is less frequent in women than in men, with an estimated 1:3 ratio.

- Gender differences have been observed in the prevalence, risk factors, proposed etiological mechanisms, genetics, comorbidity, course, key traits, and overall presentation.

- Women may need a higher loading for risk factors (e.g., genetic predispositions, childhood maltreatment) than men do in order to develop ASPD.

- DSM criteria may need to be modified to better account for gender differences in presentation.

References

Alegria AA, Blanco C, Petry NM, et al: Sex differences in antisocial personality disorder: results from the National Epidemiological Survey on Alcohol and Related Conditions. Pers Disord 4(3):214–222, 2013 23544428

American Psychiatric Association: Diagnostic and Statistical Manual of Mental Disorders, 3rd Edition, Revised. Washington, DC, American Psychiatric Association, 1987

American Psychiatric Association: Diagnostic and Statistical Manual of Mental Disorders, 4th Edition. Washington, DC, American Psychiatric Association, 1994

American Psychiatric Association: Diagnostic and Statistical Manual of Mental Disorders, 5th Edition. Arlington, VA, American Psychiatric Association, 2013

Bagchi P, Sushma N, Mahesh M, et al: The genetics of anti-social behavior with reference to forensic psychology: a review. International Journal of Pharmaceutical Sciences Review and Research 23(2):362–367, 2013

Beauchaine TP, Klein DN, Crowell SE, et al: Multifinality in the development of personality disorders: a biology x sex x environment interaction model of antisocial and borderline traits. Dev Psychopathol 21(3):735–770, 2009 19583882

Berkout OV, Young JN, Gross AM: Mean girls and bad boys: recent research on gender differences in conduct disorder. Aggress Violent Behav 16(6):503–511, 2011

Bezdjian S, Raine A, Baker LA, Lynam DR: Psychopathic personality in children: genetic and environmental contributions. Psychol Med 41(3):589–600, 2011 20482945

Black DW, Gunter T, Loveless P, et al: Antisocial personality disorder in incarcerated offenders: psychiatric comorbidity and quality of life. Ann Clin Psychiatry 22(2):113–120, 2010 20445838

Burnette ML, Newman DL: The natural history of conduct disorder symptoms in female inmates: on the predictive utility of the syndrome in severely antisocial women. Am J Orthopsychiatry 75(3):421–430, 2005 16060737

Byrd AL, Manuck SB: MAOA, childhood maltreatment, and antisocial behavior: meta-analysis of a gene-environment interaction. Biol Psychiatry 75(1):9–17, 2014 23786983

Caspi A, McClay J, Moffitt TE, et al: Role of genotype in the cycle of violence in maltreated children. Science 297(5582):851–854, 2002 12161658

Chamberlain P, Leve LD, DeGarmo DS: Multidimensional treatment foster care for girls in the juvenile justice system: 2-year follow-up of a randomized clinical trial. J Consult Clin Psychol 75:187–193, 2007 17295579

Cleckley H: The Mask of Sanity: An Attempt to Clarify Some Issues About the So-Called Psychopathic Personality, 5th Edition. St. Louis, MO, CV Mosby, 1976

Coid J, Yang M, Tyrer P, et al: Prevalence and correlates of personality disorder in Great Britain. Br J Psychiatry 188:423–431, 2006 16648528

Coid J, Yang M, Ullrich S, et al: Psychopathy among prisoners in England and Wales. Int J Law Psychiatry 32(3):134–141, 2009 19345418

Craig IW: The importance of stress and genetic variation in human aggression. BioEssays 29(3):227–236, 2007 17295220

Cuartas Arias JM, Palacio Acosta CA, Valencia JG, et al: Exploring epistasis in candidate genes for antisocial personality disorder. Psychiatr Genet 21(3):115–124, 2011 21519306

Dadds MR, Hawes DJ, Frost AD, et al: Learning to 'talk the talk': the relationship of psychopathic traits to deficits in empathy across childhood. J Child Psychol Psychiatry 50(5):599–606, 2009 19445007

Dolan M, Völlm B: Antisocial personality disorder and psychopathy in women: a literature review on the reliability and validity of assessment instruments. Int J Law Psychiatry 32(1):2–9, 2009 19042020

Ducci F, Enoch MA, Hodgkinson C, et al: Interaction between a functional MAOA locus and childhood sexual abuse predicts alcoholism and antisocial personality disorder in adult women. Mol Psychiatry 13(3):334–347, 2008 17592478

Eaton NR, Keyes KM, Krueger RF, et al: An invariant dimensional liability model of gender differences in mental disorder prevalence: evidence from a national sample. J Abnorm Psychol 121(1):282–288, 2012 21842958

Efferson LM, Glenn L: Examining gender differences in the correlates of psychopathy: a systematic review of emotional, cognitive, and morality-related constructs. Aggress Violent Behav 41:48–61, 2018

Fazel S, Danesh J: Serious mental disorder in 23000 prisoners: a systematic review of 62 surveys. Lancet 359(9306):545–550, 2002 11867106

First MB, Spitzer RL, Gibbon M, et al: Structured Clinical Interview for DSM-IV Axis I Disorders, Clinician Version (SCID-CV). Washington, DC, American Psychiatric Press, 1996

Fontaine NM, Rijsdijk FV, McCrory EJ, Viding E: Etiology of different developmental trajectories of callous-unemotional traits. J Am Acad Child Adolesc Psychiatry 49(7):656–664, 2010 20610135

Fowles DC, Dindo L: A dual deficit model of psychopathy, in Handbook of Psychopathy. Edited by Patrick CJ. New York, Guilford, 2006, pp 14–34

Gibbon S, Duggan C, Stoffers J, et al: Psychological interventions for antisocial personality disorder. Cochrane Database Syst Rev (6):CD007668, 2010 20556783

Glenn AL: The other allele: exploring the long allele of the serotonin transporter gene as a potential risk factor for psychopathy: a review of the parallels in findings. Neurosci Biobehav Rev 35(3):612–620, 2011 20674598

Godar SC, Fite PJ, McFarlin KM, et al: The role of monoamine oxidase A in aggression: current translational developments and future challenges. Prog Neuropsychopharmacol Biol Psychiatry 69:90–100, 2016 26776902

Goldstein RB, Powers SI, McCusker J, et al: Gender differences in manifestations of antisocial personality disorder among residential drug abuse treatment clients. Drug Alcohol Depend 41(1):35–45, 1996 8793308

Grann M: The PCL-R and gender. European Journal of Psychological Assessment 16(3):147–149, 2000

Hare RD: Manual for the Revised Psychopathy Checklist, 2nd Edition. Toronto, ON, Canada, Multi-Health Systems, 2003

Hart SD, Cox DN, Hare RD: Manual for the Hare Psychopathy Checklist: Screening Version (PCL:SV). Toronto, ON, Canada, Multi-Health Systems, 1995

Hatzimanolis A, Vitoratou S, Mandelli L, et al: Potential role of membrane-bound COMT gene polymorphisms in female depression vulnerability. J Affect Disord 148(2–3):316–322, 2013 23351565

Institute for Economics and Peace: The economic costs of violence containment: a comprehensive assessment of global cost of violence. 2013. Available at: http://economicsandpeace.org/wp-content/uploads/2015/06/The-Economic-Cost-of-Violence-Containment.pdf. Accessed April 22, 2021.

Kessler RC, McGonagle KA, Zhao S, et al: Lifetime and 12-month prevalence of DSM-III-R psychiatric disorders in the United States: results from the National Comorbidity Survey. Arch Gen Psychiatry 51(1):8–19, 1994 8279933

Khalifa N, Duggan C, Stoffers J, et al: Pharmacological interventions for antisocial personality disorder. Cochrane Database Syst Rev (8):CD007667, 2010 20687091

Krabbendam AA, Colins OF, Doreleijers TAH, et al: Personality disorders in previously detained adolescent females: a prospective study. Am J Orthopsychiatry 85(1):63–71, 2015 25420142

Larsson H, Andershed H, Lichtenstein P: A genetic factor explains most of the variation in the psychopathic personality. J Abnorm Psychol 115(2):221–230, 2006 16737387

Lev-Ran S, Le Strat Y, Imtiaz S, et al: Gender differences in prevalence of substance use disorders among individuals with lifetime exposure to substances: results from a large representative sample. Am J Addict 22(1):7–13, 2013 23398220

Leve LD, Chamberlain P, Reid JB: Intervention outcomes for girls referred from juvenile justice: effects on delinquency. J Consult Clin Psychol 73:1181–1185, 2005 16392991

Lewis CF: Substance use and violent behavior in women with antisocial personality disorder. Behav Sci Law 29(5):667–676, 2011 21928399

Loranger AW, Sartorius N, Andreoli A, et al: The International Personality Disorder Examination. The World Health Organization/Alcohol, Drug Abuse, and Mental Health Administration international pilot study of personality disorders. Arch Gen Psychiatry 51(3):215–224, 1994 8122958

Martens WHJ: Antisocial and psychopathic personality disorders: causes, course, and remission-a review article. International Journal of Offender Therapy and Comparative Criminology 44(4):406–430, 2000

McGuffin P, Thapar A: The genetics of personality disorder. Br J Psychiatry 160:12–23, 1992 1543993

Mednick SA, Gabrielli WF, Hutchings B: Genetic influences in criminal behavior: evidence from an adoption cohort, in Prospective Studies of Crime and Delinquency. Edited by Van Dusen KT, Mednick SA. Boston, MA, Kluwer-Nijhoff, 1983, pp 39–56

Mendoza THE, Casados JJP: Genetics of antisocial personality disorder: literature review. Salud Mental 37:83–91, 2014

Miles DR, Carey G: Genetic and environmental architecture of human aggression. J Pers Soc Psychol 72(1):207–217, 1997 9008382

Murray J, Farrington DP: Risk factors for conduct disorder and delinquency: key findings from longitudinal studies. Can J Psychiatry 55(10):633–642, 2010 20964942

Nock MK, Kazdin AE, Hiripi E, et al: Prevalence, subtypes, and correlates of DSM-IV conduct disorder in the National Comorbidity Survey Replication. Psychol Med 36(5):699–710, 2006 16438742

Pajer KA: What happens to "bad" girls? A review of the adult outcomes of antisocial adolescent girls. Am J Psychiatry 155(7):862–870, 1998 9659848

Patrick CJ: Psychophysiological correlates of aggression and violence: an integrative review. Philos Trans R Soc Lond B Biol Sci 363(1503):2543–2555, 2008 18434285

Rhee SH, Waldman ID: Genetic and environmental influences on antisocial behavior: a meta-analysis of twin and adoption studies. Psychol Bull 128(3):490–529, 2002 12002699

Robins LN: Deviant Children Grown Up: A Sociological and Psychiatric Study of Sociopathic Personality. Baltimore, MD, Williams & Wilkins, 1966

Robins LN, Regier DA: Psychiatric Disorders in America. New York, Free Press, 1991

Rogstad JE, Rogers R: Gender differences in contributions of emotion to psychopathy and antisocial personality disorder. Clin Psychol Rev 28(8):1472–1484, 2008 18945529

Ruan WJ, Goldstein RB, Chou SP, et al: The Alcohol Use Disorder and Associated Disabilities Interview Schedule-IV (AUDADIS-IV): reliability of new psychiatric diagnostic modules and risk factors in a general population sample. Drug Alcohol Depend 92(1–3):27–36, 2008 17706375

Sadeh N, Javdani S, Jackson JJ, et al: Serotonin transporter gene associations with psychopathic traits in youth vary as a function of socioeconomic resources. J Abnorm Psychol 119(3):604–609, 2010 20677849

Sigvardsson S, Cloninger CR, Bohman M, et al: Predisposition to petty criminality in Swedish adoptees, III: sex differences and validation of the male typology. Arch Gen Psychiatry 39(11):1248–1253, 1982 7138225

Singleton N, Meltzer M, Gatward R, et al: Psychiatric Morbidity Among Prisoners in England and Wales. London, The Stationery Office, 1998

Swanson MC, Bland RC, Newman SC: Epidemiology of psychiatric disorders in Edmonton: antisocial personality disorders. Acta Psychiatr Scand Suppl 376(suppl):63–70, 1994 8178687

Torgersen S, Kringlen E, Cramer V: The prevalence of personality disorders in a community sample. Arch Gen Psychiatry 58(6):590–596, 2001 11386989

Viding E, McCrory EJ: Genetic and neurocognitive contributions to the development of psychopathy. Dev Psychopathol 24(3):969–983, 2012 22781866

Viding E, Frick PJ, Plomin R: Aetiology of the relationship between callous-unemotional traits and conduct problems in childhood. Br J Psychiatry Suppl 49:S33–38, 2007 17470941

Ware JE, Kosinski M, Turner-Bowker DM, et al: How to Score Version 2 of the SF-12v2® Health Survey. Lincoln, RI, Quality Metric Incorporated, 2002

Warren JI, South SC: Comparing the constructs of antisocial personality disorder and psychopathy in a sample of incarcerated women. Behav Sci Law 24(1):1–20, 2006 16491474

Wasserman GA, McReynolds LS, Ko SJ, et al: Gender differences in psychiatric disorders at juvenile probation intake. Am J Public Health 95(1):131–137, 2005 15623873

Widom CS, Ames A: Biology and female crime, in Biological Contributions to Crime Causation. Edited by Moffitt TE, Mednick SA. Dordrecht, The Netherlands, Martinus Nijhoff, 1988, pp 308–331

World Health Organization: The ICD-10 Classification of Mental and Behavioural Disorders: Clinical Descriptions and Diagnostic Guidelines. Geneva, World Health Organization, 1992

Zoccolillo M: Gender and the development of conduct disorder. Dev Psychopathol 5(1–2):65–78, 1993

CHAPTER 23

The Antisocial Sexual Offender

Liam E. Marshall, Ph.D.

Sexual assault is a serious social problem. No other crime, perhaps even murder, evokes as strong an emotional response. Many websites and groups on social networking websites are dedicated to the vilification of sexual offenders. Despite clear evidence showing an overall drop in crime rates, including sexual offenses (Friedman et al. 2017; Gannon 2006), and a reduction in recidivism with treatment (Gannon et al. 2019), the general public has the perception that sexual crime is increasing in frequency and that the vast majority of sexual offenders will reoffend (Pfeiffer and Windzio 2006).

Although recent examinations of sexual offender recidivism show significant reductions in reoffending among those who receive psychological therapy, some sexual offenders refuse treatment, and some of those who participate in treatment do reoffend (Gannon et al. 2019; Olver et al. 2020). Thus, it is important to increase our understanding of the issues that lead to and maintain sexual offending. The prevalence and features of mental illness in sexual offenders have received significant research attention. This is likely, at least in part, because of increases in the use of civil commitment in the United States; for a sexual offender to qualify for commitment, a mental illness must be present (Levenson 2004a, 2004b; Levenson and Morin 2006).

Mental Illness in Offenders

The rate of mental illness in sexual offenders has not been satisfactorily established (Moulden and Marshall 2017). However, evidence has shown that rates of mental illness are increasing among those in the criminal justice system; for example, the prevalence of mental illness in incarcerated offenders increased from 4.7% in 1998 to 18.5% in 2008 (Abracen et al. 2012). In North American correctional institutions, rates of diagnosable psychiatric disorders are estimated to be up to three times greater than in the general population (Abracen et al. 2014; Gunter et al. 2008; Steadman et al. 2009). In Canada, a study of federal offenders (i.e., those with a more than 2-year sentence) showed that 84% of inmates had a current DSM-IV (American Psychiatric Association 1994) diagnosis, with substance use disorders being the highest at 75% (Booth 2011). Excluding substance use disorders, 43% of these inmates had a diagnosable psychiatric disorder and a suicide rate almost four times that of the general population.

Sexual offenders often present with personality disorders, including antisocial personality disorder (ASPD), borderline personality disorder (BPD), and avoidant personality disorder (Acha et al. 2011). Understanding which personality disorders are associated with a risk of reoffending is essential to better tailor treatment interventions and improve community risk management. Currently, the relationship between personality disorders and risk for reoffending is not well understood (Sigler 2017).

Many sexual offenders appear to meet criteria for ASPD, which is unsurprising. Many features of ASPD likely contribute to this association, including the individual's impulsivity, inherent aggression, and lack of empathy. A goal of many persons with ASPD is to dominate and control others, and sexual offending might be an expression of that tendency. Some also might be at an increased risk for committing a sexual offense because of impaired executive function, along with other features of ASPD (Walsh 2017). However, several factors must be considered when examining this assertion, including how well the specific criteria guide diagnostic decisions and whether the diagnoses, so guided, are reliable.

Diagnostic Assessment

Many clinicians working with men who commit sexual offenses are required by their work circumstances to apply a diagnosis to these patients, whereas others deem it essential to case formulation to provide proper treatment. Researchers examining the characteristics of those who offend sexually also typically use diagnostic descriptors, although they are not always careful to follow diagnostic criteria. In many cases, researchers could easily use behavioral or legal descriptors (e.g., child molesters, rapists), but there are times in research (depending on the topic) when diagnoses should be applied. Diagnoses are based on the careful application of criteria specified in DSM-5 (American Psychiatric Association 2013) or the *International Classification of Diseases*, 11th Revision (ICD-11; World Health Organization 2018).

DSM-5 does not have a category directly relevant to rapists, and many child molesters fail to meet diagnostic criteria for pedophilic disorder (American Psychiatric Association 2013). The authors of DSM have resisted calls to include rape as a diagnostic category (Abel and Rouleau 1990). A recent attempt to include "coercive paraphilia" as an official diagnosis in DSM-5 was rejected (Moser 2019). In terms of clinical practice, this has led many clinicians to use DSM-IV's diagnosis "paraphilia not otherwise specified" for persistent rapists, particularly in civil commitment cases (Doren 2002; Levenson 2004a). (In DSM-5, the equivalent diagnosis is either "specified" or "unspecified" paraphilic disorder depending on whether the clinician wishes to further describe the behavior.) This solution is not satisfactory because DSM offers no criteria in these categories for diagnosing rapists, and it likely was not the intention of the authors to have rape included in this catchall category (Black and Grant 2014).

Other disorders are often comorbid with sexual offending. A review of the literature reported by Marshall (2007) indicated, for example, that personality disorders commonly co-occur with sexual offending behaviors. Whenever a sexual offending patient has a comorbid personality disorder, it is necessary to design a treatment program to at least reduce the intensity of the disorder because often that personality disorder is functionally related to the offending behavior. Chen et al. (2016) reported that 59% of the sexual offenders in their study were diagnosed with a personality disorder. Kingston et al. (2015) found that 74% of the sexual offenders in their sample were diagnosed with a personality disorder, and 47% had received a diagnosis of ASPD. ASPD is commonly associated with sexual offenses, perhaps because antisocial persons can be deceitful, manipulative, and hostile and are likely to be involved with the criminal justice system (Fazel and Danesh 2002). However, other personality disorders are actually more frequent among sexual offenders. Craissati and Blundell (2013) found that avoidant, dependent, and obsessive-compulsive personality disorders were more frequent among sexual offenders. In the study by Chen et al. (2016), the most common diagnoses apart from ASPD were BPD and obsessive-compulsive personality disorder.

These studies suggest that, on average, more than 50% of those convicted of a sexual offense have a diagnosis of a personality disorder, with ASPD and BPD the most frequent. This rate is significantly higher than the estimate of 0.2%–3.3% prevalence of ASPD in the general population reported in DSM-5. Although personality disorder diagnoses are common among those convicted of a sexual offense, the diagnoses often differ depending on the type of crime the offender has committed. For example, in a small sample of those convicted for sexually offending, Aromäki et al. (2002) found that 70% of rapists met criteria for ASPD, compared with 30% of child molesters. In a different study on personality disorder diagnosis in sexual offenders, Francia et al. (2010) found, as the previous authors did, that ASPD was more common in those who offend against adult women (12.4%) than in those who offend against children (6.4%).

Factors Related to Recidivism

Personality disorders have been shown to increase the risk of recidivism among offending populations. Walter et al. (2011) reported that 69% of offenders with a diagnosis of a personality disorder and substance use disorder reoffended within 8 years of release. The reoffending rate for those with a personality disorder alone was 33%. In comparison, 25% of offenders without a personality disorder committed another crime. Violent recidivism, however, was highest in the group of offenders with only a personality disorder. Howard et al. (2013) found that nonsexual offenders with BPD reoffended at a faster rate (18.8 weeks) than those without BPD (42.2 weeks).

As it does for offenders in general, ASPD might provide insight into a sexual offender's risk of recidivism. As noted, Kingston et al. (2015) found that ASPD was a significant predictor of violent and general recidivism in sexual offenders but was not predictive of sexual recidivism. In fact, sexual offenders with ASPD were 1.79 times more likely to reoffend violently and 2.37 times more likely to reoffend generally than were sexual offenders with no such diagnosis. In a meta-analysis of 82 sexual offender recidivism studies conducted by Hanson and Morton-Bourgon (2005), antisocial orientation—comprising ASPD, antisocial traits, and history of rules violation—

was predictive of sexual, violent, and general recidivism. Among released sexual offenders, antisocial symptoms were a stronger predictor of violent ($d=0.54$) and general ($d=0.52$) recidivism than sexual recidivism ($d=0.23$).

Research has failed to adequately explain the risk of recidivism associated with ASPD in sexual offender populations. As discussed, ASPD appears to increase the risk of recidivism for all types of offending, including sexual reoffending, but ASPD was a stronger predictor of other forms of recidivism than of sexual recidivism. However, as seen in the research of Hanson and Morton-Bourgon (2005), ASPD is often confounded by other antisocial characteristics such as psychopathy and rules violations.

Etiology of Antisocial Personality Disorder in Sexual Offenders

Our group has described a theory of the etiology of sexual offending. Marshall and Barbaree (1990) wrote what has become known as the "integrated theory" of the etiology of sexual offending, which attempts to integrate inherited predispositions of self-interest, childhood learning experiences, and sociocultural influences. Later, Marshall and Marshall (2000) narrowed the focus to the influence of attachment problems. Ward and his colleagues pointed to what they saw as several flaws in these theories (Ward 2002; Ward et al. 2006). Noting the diversity of behaviors encompassed by the term *sexual offending*, they suggested that we had been too ambitious in attempting to explain all such acts within one theory. We agreed and in our most recent reformulation have addressed only the etiology of those who sexually abuse children (Gannon and Cortoni 2010). Furthermore, we restricted our focus to male offenders. Although we realize that women also molest children, we leave consideration of their etiology to those who work specifically with those offenders.

Ward et al. (2006) noted that we focused primarily on early childhood experiences while neglecting later life struggles. Some child abusers begin their offending while still young themselves, whereas others start abusing at various later stages in life, including old age (Marshall 2010; Smallbone and Wortley 2004). In response, our more recent version (Marshall and Marshall 2017) covered all life-stage developments. However, restricting our theory to child abusers still does not eliminate heterogeneity. Numerous studies have shown differences between offenders who molest children related to them (i.e., incest or familial offenders) and those who molest unrelated children (i.e., nonfamilial or stranger offenders), whereas other studies have found few or, in some cases, no differences between these groups. There appear to be problems in these studies that are primarily definitional. Some studies restrict incest offenders to only biological fathers, whereas others use a broader definition of "familial" to include uncles, grandfathers, and step, adoptive, or foster fathers, as well as cousins. The definitions of nonfamilial child abusers in these reports include men who are well known to the child (e.g., teachers, clergy, sports coaches, and other professionals working with children) and complete strangers. Both broad categories (i.e., familial vs. nonfamilial) seem likely to generate heterogeneous data, and that essentially is what has been found (Marshall et al. 2015). These data appear to suggest that child abusers who are known to their victims have more in common than any of them have with true stranger offenders.

In our latest reformulation regarding the etiology of sexual offending (Marshall and Marshall 2017), we view attachment issues to be critical and have addressed problems with attachments across the life span. An extensive body of literature attends to people's strengths and difficulties when attempting to understand the factors that influence the emergence of various clinical phenomena, including offending behaviors. This literature, largely neglected in the field of sexual offending, focuses on the development of resilience (i.e., protective strengths) and attends to factors that generate vulnerability (Rutter 2000, 2007). One of the formative and crucial factors that enhances resilience is affectionate and loving early attachments with caregivers. When childhood caregivers fail to provide love and security, this early experience entrenches vulnerability, which, fortunately, can be overcome by later positive relationship experiences (Luecken and Gress 2010).

The notion of resilience (i.e., strengths in the face of adversity) has a history dating to the 1970s. Its essence has been captured by Lutha and Cicchetti (2000), who declared it to be "a dynamic process wherein individuals display positive adaptation despite experiences of significant adversity or trauma" (p. 858). Early studies found that children who display resilience come from families who are warm, sensitive, and loving (Garmezy 1985). These resilient children are also involved in broader kinship networks similarly characterized by nurturance. The positive features of their community resources include safe neighborhoods, good-quality educational experiences and attentive teacher–child relationships, and the presence of other positive adults. Hence, good-quality attachments appear to be the basis on which people develop resilient attributes, such as a sense of mastery, self-regulatory mechanisms, a positive view of self, and moral competency (Masten 2001). Not surprisingly, the absence of these features markedly increases vulnerability.

The development of resilience or vulnerability is seen as an active dynamic process in which the meanings assigned to experiences influence the consequent responses. In this view, vulnerability and resilience vary over time and place. This may explain why affiliative child abusers, who are necessarily almost continually alone with children, do not always take advantage of every opportunity to offend and explains why most men in these situations never contemplate molesting a child. Presumably, on many occasions when opportunities to offend occur, fluctuating resilience or vulnerability factors enable men who might otherwise offend to resist these tempting circumstances. A strong adult affectionate relationship provides resilience by satisfying a range of needs (e.g., attachment, caregiving, sex) and by averting negative moods.

Numerous studies have pointed to the critical role of early attachments, and Rutter and Sroufe (2000) saw this as the most important developmental factor influencing later resilience or vulnerability. Problematic attachments with early caregivers are related to later problems of low self-worth (Sroufe 1983) and rejection by peers and teachers (Sroufe and Fleeson 1988), each of which predisposes the child to later conduct problems and to a higher risk of psychopathology (Belsky and Nezworski 1988). Parental crime and parental mental illness also increase vulnerability to subsequent adverse experiences. These effects result from disturbances in expressions of parental affection and from the inconsistent and inappropriate disciplinary practices of these parents (Cicchetti and Toth 1995).

Rutter's early review revealed that even markedly adverse early experiences on their own do not strongly predict problematic dispositions unless the individual experiences later consequences that are also adverse (Rutter 1981). Only in these circumstances do difficulties emerge and endure. In fact, even after early distressing experiences (e.g., poor attachments to caregivers), positive later events in adolescence (e.g., a supportive teacher) and adulthood (e.g., a harmonious marriage) can substantially enhance the self-concept and generate a positive cognitive set toward experience, thus reducing the effect of subsequent negative events (Luecken and Gress 2010). This, of course, suggests that attachment status may be a property of relationships rather than a property of an individual. People who have integrated a secure attachment model may, owing to disruptions in adult relationships, display insecure attachment behaviors. Similarly, individuals with an insecure attachment model may, as a result of being in a satisfying adult relationship, enact secure attachment behaviors. Thus, internal attachment models may not always be reflected in attachment behaviors. This explains why some affiliative child abusers who are characterized by secure attachment models nevertheless offend against children in their care: their secure model does not reflect their temporary insecure behaviors and their desperate need to seek affection and sex in inappropriate ways.

As Rutter and Sroufe (2000) noted, the development of all behavioral patterns (both positive and negative habits) is influenced at different stages of life by different factors, although they viewed attachments as basic. For example, a man might contemplate sexually abusing a child as a result of problematic relationship experiences, but a resilience feature (e.g., a strongly entrenched moral code) may block him from ever doing so. A man who has abused once, at a time when his vulnerability was transitorily high, might subsequently return to a greater state of resilience and never offend again. Of course, some child abusers clearly become entrenched in their abusive behaviors, and this might be more likely when victims continue to be readily available (as is true for affiliative offenders) and when the offender's intimacy needs are not being appropriately met. In any case, a theory of the etiology of child molestation must account for not only the initial onset of offending but also the subsequent desistance or persistence of the behavior. Presumably, the continuing absence of opportunities to develop resilience (e.g., the lack of availability of a loving relationship) leads to the persistence of offending propensities, whereas reestablishment of an affectionate adult relationship should result in desistance.

Resilience and vulnerability arise from many and varied experiences, but as Rutter and Sroufe (2000) noted, the main factors appear to revolve around the quality of attachments and the consequences of such attachments (e.g., self-confidence or lack thereof, good or poor emotional self-regulation, and an empathic or unempathic style). Breakdowns in attachments can occur at any point across the life span. An issue related to attachment, and to vulnerability and resilience, that has received increasing attention recently is the effect of early adverse experiences. There has long been interest in the relationship between adverse childhood experiences (ACEs) and sexual abuse and later engagement in sexually offensive behavior. The idea that being a victim of crime (Foa et al. 1999; Roth et al. 1997) and experiencing trauma increases the propensity to commit crime is a well-known phenomenon (Ardino 2011; Foy et al. 2011; Weeks and Widom 1998). Victims of violence and other forms of trauma can experience a myriad of negative outcomes, including dissociation, substance abuse, depression, and PTSD (Foa et al. 1999; Roth et al. 1997). Chronic and prolonged exposure to violence can evolve into a dysfunctional routine perpetrated in both family and community contexts, creating a "cycle of violence" in which the victim becomes the perpetrator (Garbarino et al. 2002). A considerable body of literature has documented the relationship between trauma/child abuse and subsequent aggressive and criminal behaviors (Smith et al. 2005; Widom and Maxfield 2001). Child abuse and neglect, poverty, sexual molestation, and witnessing violence are, among others, the most common risk factors for posttraumatic reactions, aggression, and antisocial behavior (Dong et al. 2004; Finkelhor and Dziuba-Leatherman 1994; Hussey et al. 2006).

Some theories on the etiology of sexual offending hypothesize that adverse early developmental experiences lead to a propensity for engaging in sexually offensive behavior in later life. As described in the "integrated theory" of sexual offending (Marshall and Barbaree 1990) and later revisions (Marshall and Marshall 2000, 2017), early problematic developmental experiences create vulnerability in the child that can, among other consequences, result in problems with socialization and the use of sex as a coping strategy. This combination of social problems and using sex for coping, along with environmental and other influences and conditions, has been hypothesized to cause the individual to seek out, or take advantage of, opportunities for sexual offending as an inappropriate strategy to resolve unmet needs. These early negative experiences, then, can be precursors of a risk for future sexual offending.

There is an emerging body of evidence on the prevalence and effect of ACEs in samples drawn from the general population (Centers for Disease Control and Prevention 2013a, 2013b), incarcerated offenders (Messina et al. 2007), and those who have offended sexually (Levenson et al. 2015, 2016). In studies with community-based respondents conducted by a health maintenance organization, Kaiser-Permanente, and later taken over by the Centers for Disease Control and Prevention (CDC), strong relationships were observed between an increase in the number of ACEs and poorer physical and mental health in later life (Anda et al. 2010). For example, a greater number of ACEs was found to be associated with a greater lifetime risk for substance abuse, suicide attempts, depression, smoking, obesity, domestic violence, and sexual promiscuity.

Few studies have been done on the prevalence and consequences of ACEs in general offenders. However, the results of those few studies have been consistent, with individuals who offend reporting a greater number of ACEs in comparison with non-offending samples. In one study, offender groups reported nearly four times as many ACEs as an adult male normative sample, with 8 of the 10 ACEs examined occurring at a significantly higher frequency among the offenders than in the normative comparison group (Reavis et al. 2013). In another study, among females who engaged in juvenile offending, an increase in the number of ACEs reported was strongly related to increased scores on scales of aggression and depression and to lower self-esteem (Matsuura et al. 2013). Total number of ACEs, aggression, and depression were also strongly positively correlated ($r=0.027$ to 0.35), and self-esteem was strongly negatively correlated to all these other variables ($r=-0.24$ to -0.47; $P<0.01$). Although ACEs have not yet been demonstrated to cause offending, these findings do suggest that they are a significant risk factor for offenders and the possible early development of ASPD.

Studies have also examined ACEs in individuals who offend sexually. The study of Reavis et al. (2013) cited earlier included a group of 61 men who had offended sexually. These authors found significantly higher rates of ACEs in all the offender groups than in those reported by the CDC (Centers for Disease Control and Prevention 2013b), with nearly 40% of the individuals who offend sexually reporting having experienced sexual abuse as a child. This prevalence rate is consistent with previous research (Dhawan and Marshall 1996; Hanson and Slater 1988). In separate examinations of males and females who have offended sexually, Levenson et al. (2015, 2016) reported significantly higher rates of ACEs than were reported by the CDC for community-based nonoffending males and females, respectively (Centers for Disease Control and Prevention 2013b). Levenson and colleagues noted an inverse correlation between ACEs and age of victim: the greater the number of ACEs experienced by the sexual offender, the younger the age of the victims in their offending. An increased number of ACEs was also related to an increased number of nonsexual arrests, greater violence in the commission of the offense, and increased risk for sexual reoffending, suggesting a possible link with ASPD. Of note, studies examining various populations (Table 23–1) have found high rates of all types of abuse (emotional, physical, and sexual), with individuals who offend sexually having significantly more ACEs than other groups.

DeLisi et al. (2019) recently described the etiology of ASPD as unknown. Like Marshall and Barbaree's (1990) integrated theory of the etiology of sexual offending, DeLisi and colleagues suggested that etiology is multifactorial, with biological and environmental bases. They provided citations of research showing the heritability of ASPD to be between 38% and 69% but noted that environmental causes also play an important role in the development of the disorder. They then cited two possible sources of environmental influence, namely ACEs and childhood psychopathologies such as ADHD, oppositional defiant disorder, and conduct disorder. The findings of this research showed ACEs and conduct disorder to be associated with ASPD. Of the various ACEs examined, physical abuse and sexual abuse were found to be related to a diagnosis of ASPD. This research shows support for the importance of these early experiences and how they may influence the development of ASPD; however, these authors appear to have not used the same ACEs scale used in the reports by the CDC, and other adverse experiences related to the development of ASPD may not have been examined.

DeLisi et al. (2019) reported that physical abuse engenders feelings of hostility, contempt, and distrust of adult authority figures, characteristics that set the stage for a personality style dominated by irritability, aggression, and rationalized indifference to others. Unlike emotional and verbal abuse, physical abuse also produces visible injuries that can serve as the impetus for out-of-home placement, which, for many offenders with severe conduct problems, is the first step in a long procession of institutional placement.

Evidence has shown that experiencing sexual abuse as a child has a disproportionate causal effect on sexual offending (DeLisi et al. 2014; Drury et al. 2017; Reavis et al. 2013; Widom et al. 2015) and a globally antisocial disposition, such as that embodied by ASPD, but not necessarily on generalized criminal offending. Like the relationship between childhood sexual abuse and adult sexual offending, a significant association exists between a history of sexual abuse and a formal diagnosis of ASPD. Sexual abuse is a severe example of an ACE; thus, it makes intuitive sense that it would be associated with a significant diagnostic condition. Overall, the significant effects of physical and sexual abuse are consistent with recent meta-analytic research that found sexual abuse and physical abuse, among various forms of maltreatment, to be more strongly linked to aggressive forms of deviance (Braga et al. 2017).

This information suggests that the development of the sexual offender with ASPD is similar to the path of both non-sexual-offending individuals with ASPD and sexual offenders who do not have a diagnosis of ASPD. The overlap in these groups could

TABLE 23–1.   Percentage of adverse childhood experiences (ACEs) reported in males

ACEs category	General population (Centers for Disease Control and Prevention; N=7,970)	Offenders (Messina et al.; N=425)	Sexual offenders (Levenson et al.; N=679)
Abuse			
Emotional abuse	7.6	[a]	53.3
Physical abuse	29.9	20.2	42.2
Sexual abuse	16.0	8.5	38.0
Neglect			
Emotional neglect	12.4	20.0	37.6
Physical neglect	10.7	4.9	15.9
Household dysfunction			
Mother treated violently	11.5	49.4	24.0
Household substance abuse	23.8	53.6	46.7
Household mental illness	14.8	NR	25.9
Parental separation or divorce	21.8	44.6	54.3
Incarcerated household member	4.1	41.6	22.6

Note.   NR=not reported.
[a]Included in emotional neglect total.
Source.   Centers for Disease Control and Prevention 2013b; Levenson et al. 2016; Messina et al. 2007.

be artifactual and related to poor reliability in the application of the diagnosis or perhaps to attrition in the study sample. Between 2009 and 2014, sexual assault cases experienced attrition at all levels of the criminal justice system. A suspect was identified in three of five (59%) sexual assault incidents reported by police, and fewer than half (43%) of sexual assault incidents resulted in a charge. Of these, 49% proceeded to court and 55% led to a conviction; 56% of those convicted were sentenced to custody (Rotenberg 2017). As is well known, many sexual assaults are never reported to the police; thus, sexual offenders with ASPD may be more likely to be incarcerated because of their general criminal disposition. Clearly, more research is needed on both the etiology and the epidemiology of sexual offending by persons with ASPD to better understand this group of sexual offenders.

Rockwood Treatment Program Outcome

Given the rates of ASPD among incarcerated sexual offenders, we are encouraged that our program might help these men avoid future offending. In several studies conducted since 2005, we have consistently found reductions in both sexual reoffending and other forms of offending among our sexual offender treatment program participants. In our most recently completed outcome study (Olver et al. 2020), we compared the outcome for the Rockwood program (N=579; overall sexual recidivism rate=5.4%) with two groups matched for risk and time at risk: an untreated group (N=107; overall sexual recidivism rate=19.6%) and a group treated in the same prison system's (i.e., the Correctional Service of Canada) regular sexual offender program (N=625; overall sexual recidivism rate=12.6%). This comparison of groups was calculated to have a Collaborative Outcome Data Committee (2007) rating of "Good": "High confidence that the study has no more than a small amount of bias." In this study, the Rockwood program was found to have statistically significantly lower sexual recidivism rates than either of the two other groups: for the Rockwood program versus the Correctional Service of Canada sexual offender program, χ^2=14.1 and P<0.001; for the Rockwood program versus the untreated group, χ^2=27.3 and P<0.001. The Rockwood program demonstrated a medium effect size compared with the Correctional Service of Canada program (d=0.056) and a large effect size compared with the untreated group (d=0.088).

In this study (Olver et al. 2020), we also compared the fixed 8-year violent reconviction rate for the Rockwood program (N=381; overall violent recidivism rate=12.1%) with the two matched for risk and time at risk groups: the Correctional Service of Canada regular sexual offender program (N=616; overall violent recidivism rate=26.5%) and an untreated group (N=104; overall violent recidivism rate=44.2%) from the same prison service. The Rockwood program was found to have statistically significantly lower rates of violent recidivism than either of the two other groups: for the Rockwood program versus the Correctional Service of Canada program, OR=0.038 and P<0.001; for the Rockwood program versus the untreated group, OR=0.017 and P<0.001. This result can also be reported as the Rockwood program reducing violent reoffending by 62% compared with the prison system's regular treatment program and by 83% compared with the untreated group.

These results suggest that our approach to treatment may help sexual offenders with ASPD desist from offending. Based on these results, we adapted our treatment program for men who have been convicted of violent offenses and for men who were convicted of intimate partner violence. Both adapted programs' participants showed improvements in dynamic risk issues associated with violence (Robinson et al. 2011) and intimate partner violence (Gates et al. 2011). It is unclear whether our treatment program is effective in reducing the symptoms and problems associated with ASPD.

Anecdotal Clinical Description of Antisocial Sexual Offenders

Sexual offenders with ASPD tend to be qualitatively different from the other participants in our program. First, they are usually either unmotivated to participate or motivated only by external factors, most typically early release or pressure from their case managers. Second, they often actively work against the therapist(s) by making inappropriate statements about other group members and attempting to undermine the therapist(s)'s credibility. Finally, antisocial sexual offenders often have nonsexual convictions and will report that their sexual conviction resulted from a misinterpretation of their behavior by the police or other judicial or correctional staff. They often begin their time in treatment by claiming that they are not actually sexual offenders and are participating in the program only to be considered for an early release.

We have often seen antisocial sexual offenders in our unique "Categorical Denier Sexual Offender Treatment Program" (Marshall et al. 2001). This program was designed to provide treatment to offenders typically excluded from therapy because they deny having committed a sexual offense. Often these "deniers" will admit to other forms of criminality but will deny any sexual offending or sexual intent to their offending. Sexual offenders with ASPD present a significant challenge to therapists tasked with their care and strain limited resources.

In our experience, older sexual offenders with or without ASPD or a history of antisocial behavior are more likely to be both compliant and motivated to change. Several age-related factors are likely responsible for this improvement with age in compliance and motivation. An association between low self-control and criminal behavior has been sufficiently well-established for some to consider it to be the cause of crime (Gottfredson and Hirschi 1990). Self-control dramatically improves from adolescence to adulthood and continues to improve with age. This is supported by observed age-related decreases in sexual crimes (Barbaree et al. 2003; Hanson 2002) and reflected in actuarial risk assessment instruments (e.g., STATIC-99R; Helmus et al. 2012). Second, sex drive reduces with age (Kinsey et al. 1948; Panser et al. 1995); therefore, older treatment participants may be less resistant to the removal of deviant sexual interests.

We have developed strategies that are helpful in managing antisocial sexual offenders. Our treatment programs overall are strengths-based and focus on enhancing motivation for change (Marshall et al. 2011), which most sexual offenders find more inviting than other, more typical programs, as evidenced by our low refusal rate (<5%). However, we also have some specific strategies that are intended to assist with all participants with antisocial behaviors. First, we try to limit the number of these individuals in any one treatment group to no more than 10%–20% of group members. Second, we avoid exercises in the group that give them the opportunity to display their antisocial tendencies; this is particularly true of the empathy exercises. Lastly, we try to focus on here-and-now rewards because we find that these offenders are often more motivated by immediate rewards (e.g., getting parole, having better relationships, and being more sexually satisfied) than by long-term rewards, such as not reoffending in the future. These strategies are helpful, but sexual offenders with ASPD remain clinically challenging. However, it can be immensely rewarding for therapists when they succeed in helping these men make positive life changes and prevent future offending.

Conclusion

Sexual offending is a serious social issue. A better understanding of the features of sexual offenders could enable more effective programming to keep potential victims—usually women and children—safe from the harm this behavior can cause. Research on sexual offenders with ASPD is starting to emerge, and this can aid the treatment and management of this unique group of offenders. Theory from both the sexual offender field and those studying ASPD suggests great overlap in the etiology of these disorders, with early adverse developmental experiences playing a significant role. Although treatment programs have been shown to reduce future offending in antisocial sexual offenders, both fields would benefit from further examination of this problematic population.

Key Points

- More than 50% of those who commit sexual offenses meet criteria for a personality disorder, with antisocial personality disorder (ASPD) and borderline personality disorder being the most frequent.

- Rates of ASPD differ by the type of sexual offense, with those who offend against adults being more than twice as likely to be diagnosed with ASPD than those who offend against children.

- ASPD is associated with increased risk for all types of reoffending, including general, nonsexual violent, and sexual reoffending.

- Early childhood adversity and, in particular, being a victim of sexual abuse appear to play a role in the onset of ASPD and may be related to later sexual offending.

- Research suggests that treatment of these types of sexual offenders with ASPD can reduce recidivism of all types.

References

Abel GG, Rouleau JL: The nature and extent of sexual abuse, in Handbook of Sexual Assault: Issues, Theories, and Treatment of the Offender. Edited by Marshall DR, Barbaree HE. New York, Plenum, 1990, pp 9–21

Abracen J, Axford M, Gileno J: Changes in the Profile of Offender Populations Residing in Community Facilities: 1998 and 2008 (R-256). Ottawa, ON, Public Safety Canada, 2012

Abracen J, Langton CM, Looman J, et al: Mental health diagnoses and recidivism in paroled offenders. Int J Offender Ther Comp Criminol 58(7):765–779, 2014 23640808

Acha M, Rigonatti S, Saffi F, et al: Prevalence of mental disorders among sexual offenders and non-sexual offenders. Jornal Brasileiro de Psiquiatria 60(1):11–15, 2011

American Psychiatric Association: Diagnostic and Statistical Manual of Mental Disorders, 4th Edition. Washington, DC, American Psychiatric Association, 1994

American Psychiatric Association: Diagnostic and Statistical Manual of Mental Disorders, 5th Edition. Arlington, VA, American Psychiatric Association, 2013

Anda RF, Butchart A, Felitti VJ, et al: Building a framework for global surveillance of the public implications of adverse childhood experiences. Am J Prev Med 39(1):93–98, 2010 20547282

Ardino V: Post-traumatic stress in antisocial youth: a multifaceted reality, in Posttraumatic Syndromes in Childhood and Adolescence: A Handbook of Research and Practice. Edited by Ardino V. Chichester, UK, Wiley-Blackwell, 2011, pp 211–230

Aromäki AS, Lindman RE, Eriksson CJ: Testosterone, sexuality and antisocial personality in rapists and child molesters: a pilot study. Psychiatry Res 110(3):239–247, 2002 12127474

Barbaree HE, Blanchard R, Langton C: The development of sexual aggression throughout the lifespan: the effect of age on sexual arousal and recidivism among sex offenders, in Sexually Coercive Behavior: Understanding and Management. Edited by Prentky RA, Janus E, Seto M. New York, New York Academy of Sciences, 2003, pp 59–71

Belsky J, Nezworski T: Clinical Implications of Attachment. Hillsdale, NJ, Erlbaum, 1988

Black DW, Grant JE: DSM-5 Guidebook: The Essential Companion to the Diagnostic and Statistical Manual of Mental Disorders, 5th Edition. Washington, DC, American Psychiatric Publishing, 2014

Booth B: Secure units and mentally disordered offenders: a Canadian experience. Paper presented at the 32nd International Congress on Law and Mental Health Conference (IALMH), Humboldt University, Berlin, Germany, 2011

Braga T, Gonclaves LC, Basto-Pereira M, et al: Unraveling the link between maltreatment and juvenile antisocial behavior: a meta-analysis of prospective longitudinal studies. Aggress Violent Behav 33:37–50, 2017

Centers for Disease Control and Prevention: Adverse childhood experience study: major findings, 2013a. Available at: www.cdc.gov/ace/findings.htm. Accessed April 26, 2021.

Centers for Disease Control and Prevention: Adverse childhood experiences study: prevalence of individual adverse childhood experiences, 2013b. Available at: www.cdc.gov/ace/prevalence.htm. Accessed April 26, 2021.

Chen YY, Chen CY, Hung DL: Assessment of psychiatric disorders among sex offenders: prevalence and associations with criminal history. Crim Behav Ment Health 26(1):30–37, 2016 25125391

Cicchetti D, Toth SL: Developmental psychopathology and disorders of affect, in Developmental Psychopathology, Vol 2: Risk, Disorder, and Adaptation. Edited by Cicchetti D, Cohen DJ. New York, Wiley, 1995, pp 369–420

Collaborative Outcome Data Committee: Guidelines for the evaluation of sexual offender treatment outcome research, part 2: CODC guidelines (User Report 2007–03). Ottawa, ON, Public Safety and Emergency Preparedness Canada, 2007

Craissati J, Blundell R: A community service for high-risk mentally disordered sex offenders: a follow-up study. J Interpers Violence 28(6):1178–1200, 2013 23315709

DeLisi M, Kosloski AE, Vaughn MG, et al: Does childhood sexual abuse victimization translate into juvenile sexual offending? New evidence. Violence Vict 29(4):620–635, 2014 25199390

DeLisi M, Drury AJ, Elbert MJ: The etiology of antisocial personality disorder: the differential roles of adverse childhood experiences and childhood psychopathology. Compr Psychiatry 92:1–6, 2019 31079021

Dhawan S, Marshall WL: Sexual abuse histories of sexual offenders. Sex Abuse 8:7–15, 1996

Dong M, Anda RF, Felitti VJ, et al: The interrelatedness of multiple forms of childhood abuse, neglect, and household dysfunction. Child Abuse Negl 28(7):771–784, 2004 15261471

Doren DM: Evaluating Sex Offenders: A Manual for Civil Commitments and Beyond. Thousand Oaks, CA, Sage, 2002

Drury A, Heinrichs T, Elbert M, et al: Adverse childhood experiences, paraphilias, and serious criminal violence among federal sex offenders. J Crim Psychol 7(2):105–119, 2017

Fazel S, Danesh J: Serious mental disorder in 23000 prisoners: a systematic review of 62 surveys. Lancet 359(9306):545–550, 2002 11867106

Finkelhor D, Dziuba-Leatherman J: Victimization of children. Am Psychol 49(3):173–183, 1994 8192272

Foa EB, Ehlers A, Clark DM, et al: The Posttraumatic Cognitions Inventory (PTCI): development and validation. Psychol Assess 11(3):303–314, 1999

Foy DW, Furrow J, McManus S, et al: Exposure to violence, post-traumatic symptomatology, and criminal behaviors, in Post-Traumatic Syndromes in Children and Adolescents: A Handbook of Research and Practice. Edited by Ardino V. Chichester, UK, Wiley/Blackwell, 2011, pp 199–210

Francia C, Coolidge F, White L: Personality disorder profiles in incarcerated male rapists and child molesters. American Journal of Forensic Psychology 28(3):1–14, 2010

Friedman M, Grawert AC, Cullen J: Crime Trends: 1990–2016. New York, Brennan Center for Justice at New York University School of Law, 2017

Gannon M: Crime statistics in Canada, 2005. Statistics Canada (Catalogue 85-002-XIE, Vol 24, No 4), July 2006. Available at: www150.statcan.gc.ca/n1/en/pub/85-002-x/85-002-x2006004-eng.pdf?st=rhSiPHmA. Accessed April 26, 2021.

Gannon TA, Cortoni F: Female Sexual Offenders: Theory, Assessment, and Practice. Chichester, UK, Wiley, 2010

Gannon TA, Olver ME, Mallion JS, et al: Does specialized psychological treatment for offending reduce recidivism? A meta-analysis examining staff and program variables as predictors of treatment effectiveness. Clin Psychol Rev 73:101752, 2019 31476514

Garbarino J, Bradshaw CP, Vorrasi JA: Mitigating the effects of gun violence on children and youth. Future Child 12(2):72–85, 2002 12194614

Garmezy M: Stress-resistant children: the search for protective factors, in Recent Research in Developmental Psychopathology: Journal of Child Psychology and Psychiatry Book Supplement. Edited by Stevenson JE. Oxford, UK, Pergamon, 1985, pp 213–233

Gates M, Marshall LE, Alguire T: An examination of a treatment group for domestic violence in incarcerated mentally ill offenders. Paper presented to the Royal Ottawa Health Care Group, Brockville, Canada, 2011

Gottfredson MR, Hirschi T: A General Theory of Crime. Stanford, CA, Stanford University Press, 1990

Gunter TD, Arndt S, Wenman G, et al: Frequency of mental and addictive disorders among 320 men and women entering the Iowa prison system: use of the MINI-Plus. J Am Acad Psychiatry Law 36(1):27–34, 2008 18354120

Hanson RK: Recidivism and age: follow up data from 4,673 sexual offenders. J Interpers Violence 17(10):1046–1062, 2002

Hanson RK, Morton-Bourgon KE: The characteristics of persistent sexual offenders: a meta-analysis of recidivism studies. J Consult Clin Psychol 73(6):1154–1163, 2005 16392988

Hanson RK, Slater S: Sexual victimization in the history of child sexual abusers: a review. Ann Sex Res 1:485–499, 1988

Helmus L, Thornton D, Hanson RK, et al: Improving the predictive accuracy of Static-99 and Static-2002 with older sex offenders: revised age weights. Sex Abuse 24(1):64–101, 2012 21844404

Howard R, McCarthy L, Huband N, et al: Re-offending in forensic patients released from secure care: the role of antisocial/borderline personality disorder co-morbidity, substance dependence and severe childhood conduct disorder. Crim Behav Ment Health 23(3):191–202, 2013 23371302

Hussey JM, Chang JJ, Kotch JB: Child maltreatment in the United States: prevalence, risk factors, and adolescent health consequences. Pediatrics 118(3):933–942, 2006 16950983

Kingston D, Olver M, Harris M, et al: The relationship between mental disorder and recidivism in sexual offenders. Int J Ment Health 14(1):10–22, 2015

Kinsey AC, Pomeroy WB, Martin CE: Sexual Behavior in the Human Male. Philadelphia, PA, WB Saunders, 1948

Levenson JS: Reliability of sexually violent predator civil commitment criteria in Florida. Law Hum Behav 28(4):357–368, 2004a 15499820

Levenson JS: Sexual predator civil commitment: a comparison of selected and released offenders. Int J Offender Ther Comp Criminol 48(6):638–648, 2004b 15538023

Levenson JS, Morin JW: Factors predicting selection of sexually violent predators for civil commitment. Int J Offender Ther Comp Criminol 50(6):609–629, 2006 17068188

Levenson JS, Willis GM, Prescott DS: Adverse childhood experiences in the lives of female sex offenders. Sex Abuse 27(3):258–283, 2015 25210107

Levenson JS, Willis GM, Prescott DS: Adverse childhood experiences in the lives of male sex offenders: implications for trauma-informed care. Sex Abuse 28(4):340–359, 2016 24872347

Luecken LJ, Gress JL: Early adversity and resilience in emerging adulthood, in Handbook of Adult Resilience. Edited by Reich JW, Zautra AJ, Hall JS. New York, Guilford, 2010, pp 238–257

Luthar SS, Cicchetti D: The construct of resilience: implications for interventions and social policies. Dev Psychopathol 12(4):857–885, 2000 11202047

Marshall LE: Aging and sexual offending: an examination of older sexual offenders. Doctoral thesis, Queen's University, Kingston, ON, Canada, 2010

Marshall WL: Diagnostic issues, multiple paraphilias, and comorbid disorders in sexual offenders: their incidence and treatment. Aggress Violent Behav 12(1):16–35, 2007

Marshall WL, Barbaree HE: An integrated theory of sexual offending, in Handbook of Sexual Assault: Issues, Theories, and Treatment of the Offender. Edited by Marshall WL, Barbaree HE. New York, Plenum, 1990, pp 257–275

Marshall WL, Marshall LE: The origins of sexual offending. Trauma Violence Abuse 1(3):250–263, 2000

Marshall WL, Marshall LE: An attachment-based theory of the aetiology of affiliative child molestation: resilience/vulnerability factors across life-span development, in The Wiley-Blackwell Handbook on the Assessment, Treatment, and Theories of Sexual Offending. Edited by Ward T, Beech A. Chichester, UK, Wiley, 2017, pp 3–24

Marshall WL, Thornton D, Marshall LE, et al: Treatment of sexual offenders who are in categorical denial: a pilot project. Sex Abuse 13(3):205–215, 2001 11486714

Marshall WL, Marshall LE, Serran GA, et al: Rehabilitating Sexual Offenders: A Strength-Based Approach. Washington, DC, American Psychological Association, 2011

Marshall WL, Smallbone S, Marshall LE: A critique of current child molester subcategories: a proposal for an alternative approach. Psychol Crime Law 21:205–218, 2015

Masten AS: Ordinary magic: resilience processes in development. Am Psychol 56(3):227–238, 2001 11315249

Matsuura N, Hashimoto T, Toichi M: Associations among adverse childhood experiences, aggression, depression, and self-esteem in serious female juvenile offenders in Japan. J Forens Psychiatry Psychol 24(1):111–127, 2013

Messina N, Grella C, Burdon W, et al: Childhood adverse events and current traumatic distress: a comparison of men and women drug-dependent prisoners. Crim Justice Behav 34(11):1385–1401, 2007

Moser C: DSM-5, paraphilias, and the paraphilic disorders: confusion reigns. Arch Sex Behav 48(3):681–689, 2019 30790206

Moulden HM, Marshall LE: Major mental illness in those who sexually abuse. Curr Psychiatry Rep 19(12):105, 2017 29119325

Olver ME, Marshall LE, Marshall WL, et al: A long-term outcome assessment of the effects on subsequent reoffense rates of a prison-based CBT/RNR sex offender treatment program with strength-based elements. Sex Abuse 32(2):127–153, 2020 30362904

Panser LA, Rhodes T, Girman CJ, et al: Sexual function of men ages 40 to 79 years: the Olmsted County study of urinary symptoms and health status among men. J Am Geriatr Soc 43(10):1107–1111, 1995 7560700

Pfeiffer C, Windzio M: Crime statistics and public opinion: two pictures of one phenomenon. Paper presented at the 9th biannual conference of the International Association for the Treatment of Sexual Abusers, Hamburg, Germany, September 6–9, 2006

Reavis JA, Looman J, Franco KA, et al: Adverse childhood experiences and adult criminality: how long must we live before we possess our own lives? Perm J 17(2):44–48, 2013 23704843

Robinson J, Chagigiorgis H, Marshall LE: Treatment groups for anger management at a secure treatment unit for psychiatrically ill offenders. Paper presented at the Second North American Correctional and Criminal Justice Psychology Conference (NACCJPC). Toronto, ON, Canada, June 2–4, 2011

Rotenberg C: From arrest to conviction: court outcomes of police-reported sexual assaults in Canada, 2009 to 2014. Statistics Canada. 2017. Available at: www150.statcan.gc.ca/n1/pub/85-002-x/2017001/article/54870-eng.htm. Accessed April 26, 2021.

Roth S, Newman E, Pelcovitz D, et al: Complex PTSD in victims exposed to sexual and physical abuse: results from the DSM-IV Field Trial for Posttraumatic Stress Disorder. J Trauma Stress 10(4):539–555, 1997 9391940

Rutter M: Maternal Deprivation Reassessed, 2nd Edition. Harmondsworth, UK, Penguin, 1981

Rutter M: Resilience reconsidered: conceptual considerations, empirical findings, and policy implications, in Handbook of Early Childhood Intervention, 2nd Edition. Edited by Shonkoff JP, Meisels SJ. New York, Cambridge University Press, 2000, pp 651–682

Rutter M: Resilience, competence, and coping. Child Abuse Negl 31(3):205–209, 2007 17408738

Rutter M, Sroufe LA: Developmental psychopathology: concepts and challenges. Dev Psychopathol 12(3):265–296, 2000 11014739

Sigler A: Risk and prevalence of personality disorders in sexual offenders. CUNY Academic Works. 2017. Available at: https://academicworks.cuny.edu/jj_etds/23. Accessed April 26, 2021.

Smallbone SW, Wortley RK: Criminal diversity and paraphilic interests among adult males convicted of sexual offenses against children. Int J Offender Ther Comp Criminol 48(2):175–188, 2004 15070465

Smith CA, Ireland TO, Thornberry TP: Adolescent maltreatment and its impact on young adult antisocial behavior. Child Abuse Negl 29(10):1099–1119, 2005 16233913

Sroufe LA: Infant–caregiver attachment and patterns of adaptation in the preschool: the roots of maladaptation and competence, in Minnesota Symposia in Child Psychology, Volume 16: Development and Policy Concerning Children With Special Needs. Edited by Pearlmutter M. Hillsdale, NJ, Erlbaum, 1983, pp 41–83

Sroufe LA, Fleeson J: The coherence of family relationships, in Relationships Within Families: Mutual Influences. Edited by Hinde RA, Stevenson-Hinde J. Oxford, UK, Oxford University Press, 1988, pp 27–47

Steadman HJ, Osher FC, Robbins PC, et al: Prevalence of serious mental illness among jail inmates. Psychiatr Serv 60(6):761–765, 2009 19487344

Walsh K: Antisocial personality disorder and Donald DD: distinguishing the sex offender from the typical recidivist in the civil commitment of sex offenders. Fordham Urban Law Journal 44(3):867–917, 2017

Walter M, Wiesbeck GA, Dittmann V, et al: Criminal recidivism in offenders with personality disorders and substance use disorders over 8 years of time at risk. Psychiatry Res 186(2–3):443–445, 2011 20826002

Ward T: Marshall and Barbaree's integrated theory of child sexual abuse: a critique. Psychol Crime Law 8(3):209–229, 2002

Ward T, Polaschek DL, Beech AR: Theories of Sexual Offending. Chichester, UK, Wiley, 2006

Weeks R, Widom CS: Self-reports of early childhood victimization among incarcerated adult male felons. J Interpers Violence 13(3):346–361, 1998

Widom CS, Maxfield MG: An Update on the "Cycle of Violence." Washington, DC, US Department of Justice, Office of Justice Programs, National Institute of Justice, 2001

Widom CS, Czaja SJ, DuMont KA: Intergenerational transmission of child abuse and neglect: real or detection bias? Science 347(6229):1480–1485, 2015 25814584

World Health Organization: International Classification of Diseases, 11th Revision. 2018. Available at: http://icd.who.int. Accessed April 26, 2021.

CHAPTER 24

Prevention of Antisocial Personality Disorder

Eva R. Kimonis, Ph.D.
Georgette E. Fleming, Ph.D.

Antisociality in adulthood does not occur within a developmental vacuum. Antisocial personality disorder (ASPD) is widely considered the developmental culmination of externalizing disorders that onset during childhood and adolescence. From this perspective, prevention of ASPD necessitates timely and effective intervention for the symptoms of these early-onset disorders. In this chapter, we outline the typical developmental trajectory of ASPD, which often begins with externalizing problems emerging in the early childhood period. Accordingly, we argue that early-onset externalizing disorders represent a critical prevention target for ASPD and associated problems. Critically, we emphasize the existence of multiple, etiologically distinct developmental pathways leading to antisocial behavior and discuss the relative efficacy of traditional and novel interventions for childhood conduct problems along these pathways. Finally, we identify the next frontiers for the field to highlight critical future directions for research and practice with respect to preventing ASPD.

Externalizing Disorders of Childhood and Adolescence

The externalizing dimension of childhood and adolescent mental disorders is characterized by problems of conduct and aggression associated with oppositional defiant disorder (ODD) and conduct disorder (CD) (Boxes 24–1 and 24–2), as well as problems of inattention, impulsivity, and hyperactivity associated with ADHD.

Box 24–1.   DSM-5 Diagnostic Criteria for Oppositional Defiant Disorder

---

A. A pattern of angry/irritable mood, argumentative/defiant behavior, or vindictiveness lasting at least 6 months as evidenced by at least four symptoms from any of the following categories, and exhibited during interaction with at least one individual who is not a sibling.

Angry/Irritable Mood

1. Often loses temper.
2. Is often touchy or easily annoyed.
3. Is often angry and resentful.

Argumentative/Defiant Behavior

4. Often argues with authority figures or, for children and adolescents, with adults.
5. Often actively defies or refuses to comply with requests from authority figures or with rules.
6. Often deliberately annoys others.
7. Often blames others for his or her mistakes or misbehavior.

Vindictiveness

8. Has been spiteful or vindictive at least twice within the past 6 months.

Note: The persistence and frequency of these behaviors should be used to distinguish a behavior that is within normal limits from a behavior that is symptomatic. For children younger than 5 years, the behavior should occur on most days for a period of at least 6 months unless otherwise noted (Criterion A8). For individuals 5 years or older, the behavior should occur at least once per week for at least 6 months, unless otherwise noted (Criterion A8). While these frequency criteria provide guidance on a minimal level of frequency to define symptoms, other factors should also be considered, such as whether the frequency and intensity of the behaviors are outside a range that is normative for the individual's developmental level, gender, and culture.

B. The disturbance in behavior is associated with distress in the individual or others in his or her immediate social context (e.g., family, peer group, work colleagues), or it impacts negatively on social, educational, occupational, or other important areas of functioning.

C. The behaviors do not occur exclusively during the course of a psychotic, substance use, depressive, or bipolar disorder. Also, the criteria are not met for disruptive mood dysregulation disorder.

Specify current severity:
   Mild: Symptoms are confined to only one setting (e.g., at home, at school, at work, with peers).
   Moderate: Some symptoms are present in at least two settings.
   Severe: Some symptoms are present in three or more settings.

Source.   Reprinted from American Psychiatric Association: *Diagnostic and Statistical Manual of Mental Disorders,* 5th Edition. Arlington, VA, American Psychiatric Association, 2013. Copyright © 2013 American Psychiatric Association. Used with permission.

Box 24–2.   DSM-5 Diagnostic Criteria for Conduct Disorder

A. A repetitive and persistent pattern of behavior in which the basic rights of others or major age-appropriate societal norms or rules are violated, as manifested by the presence of at least three of the following 15 criteria in the past 12 months from any of the categories below, with at least one criterion present in the past 6 months:

Aggression to People and Animals

1. Often bullies, threatens, or intimidates others.
2. Often initiates physical fights.
3. Has used a weapon that can cause serious physical harm to others (e.g., a bat, brick, broken bottle, knife, gun).
4. Has been physically cruel to people.
5. Has been physically cruel to animals.
6. Has stolen while confronting a victim (e.g., mugging, purse snatching, extortion, armed robbery).
7. Has forced someone into sexual activity.

Destruction of Property

8. Has deliberately engaged in fire setting with the intention of causing serious damage.
9. Has deliberately destroyed others' property (other than by fire setting).

Deceitfulness or Theft

10. Has broken into someone else's house, building, or car.
11. Often lies to obtain goods or favors or to avoid obligations (i.e., "cons" others).
12. Has stolen items of nontrivial value without confronting a victim (e.g., shoplifting, but without breaking and entering; forgery).

Serious Violations of Rules

13. Often stays out at night despite parental prohibitions, beginning before age 13 years.
14. Has run away from home overnight at least twice while living in the parental or parental surrogate home, or once without returning for a lengthy period.
15. Is often truant from school, beginning before age 13 years.

B. The disturbance in behavior causes clinically significant impairment in social, academic, or occupational functioning.

C. If the individual is age 18 years or older, criteria are not met for antisocial personality disorder.

Specify whether:

312.81 (F91.1) Childhood-onset type: Individuals show at least one symptom characteristic of conduct disorder prior to age 10 years.

312.82 (F91.2) Adolescent-onset type: Individuals show no symptom characteristic of conduct disorder prior to age 10 years.

312.89 (F91.9) Unspecified onset: Criteria for a diagnosis of conduct disorder are met, but there is not enough information available to determine whether the onset of the first symptom was before or after age 10 years.

Specify if:

With limited prosocial emotions: To qualify for this specifier, an individual must have displayed at least two of the following characteristics persistently over at least 12 months and in multiple relationships and settings. These characteristics reflect the individual's typical pattern of interpersonal and emotional functioning over this period and not just occasional occurrences in some situations. Thus, to assess the criteria for the specifier, multiple information sources are necessary. In addition to the individual's self-report, it is necessary to consider reports by others who have known the individual for extended periods of time (e.g., parents, teachers, co-workers, extended family members, peers).

Lack of remorse or guilt: Does not feel bad or guilty when he or she does something wrong (exclude remorse when expressed only when caught and/or facing punishment). The individual shows a general lack of concern about the negative consequences of his or her actions. For example, the individual is not remorseful after hurting someone or does not care about the consequences of breaking rules.

Callous—lack of empathy: Disregards and is unconcerned about the feelings of others. The individual is described as cold and uncaring. The person appears more concerned about the effects of his or her actions on himself or herself, rather than their effects on others, even when they result in substantial harm to others.

Unconcerned about performance: Does not show concern about poor/problematic performance at school, at work, or in other important activities. The individual does not put forth the effort necessary to perform well, even when expectations are clear, and typically blames others for his or her poor performance.

Shallow or deficient affect: Does not express feelings or show emotions to others, except in ways that seem shallow, insincere, or superficial (e.g., actions contradict the emotion displayed; can turn emotions "on" or "off" quickly) or when emotional expressions are used for gain (e.g., emotions displayed to manipulate or intimidate others).

Specify current severity:

Mild: Few if any conduct problems in excess of those required to make the diagnosis are present, and conduct problems cause relatively minor harm to others (e.g., lying, truancy, staying out after dark without permission, other rule breaking).

Moderate: The number of conduct problems and the effect on others are intermediate between those specified in "mild" and those in "severe" (e.g., stealing without confronting a victim, vandalism).

Severe: Many conduct problems in excess of those required to make the diagnosis are present, or conduct problems cause considerable harm to others (e.g., forced sex, physical cruelty, use of a weapon, stealing while confronting a victim, breaking and entering).

Developmental Trajectory of Antisocial Personality Disorder

Of the 10 personality disorders described in DSM-5 (American Psychiatric Association 2013), ASPD is the only one that includes the presence of a childhood-onset disorder as part of its diagnostic criteria. This reflects the considerable evidence base indicating that childhood-onset CD commonly precedes the development of ASPD in adults (e.g., DeLisi et al. 2019). In a seminal study, Robins (1966) found that 31% of boys and 17% of girls referred to a mental health clinic for CD symptoms at an average age of 13 years were diagnosed with an antisocial disorder as adults. In addition, of the boys and girls with CD, 43% and 12%, respectively, were later imprisoned at least once as an adult. More recent longitudinal studies also support the predictive validity of CD for ASPD, finding that CD diagnosed between ages 7 and 17 years was highly predictive of an ASPD diagnosis during adulthood (Lahey et al. 2005; Loeber et al. 2002). Other studies have also demonstrated that ASPD in adulthood is more common among children with co-occurring CD and ADHD (Hofvander et al. 2009).

Consistent with this developmental perspective, research shows that CD is typically preceded by ODD, which tends to onset between ages 3 and 8 years (e.g., Burke et al. 2010). For many of these children, behaviors characteristic of ODD gradually escalate into more frequent and increasingly severe patterns of conduct problems (Shaw et al. 2003). Children who progress from ODD to CD do not change the types of behaviors they display but, rather, retain their ODD symptoms and add the more severe conduct problem behaviors to their existing behavioral repertoire (Kim-Cohen et al. 2009; Loeber et al. 1991). Although approximately 40% of children with ODD do not exhibit more severe conduct problems in later life (Shaw et al. 2003), research indicates a sharp increase in CD prevalence rates from age 4 years that continues to age 18 years (Erskine et al. 2013). The typical developmental course for chronic antisociality begins with severe hyperactive-impulsive behaviors in early childhood, followed by ODD at preschool age, childhood-onset CD at elementary school age, substance-related disorders in adolescence, and ASPD in adulthood (Beauchaine et al. 2010; Loeber et al. 2000).

Conduct problems characteristic of ODD and CD are considerably stable across development (Broidy et al. 2003; Shaw et al. 2003). In one study, 73% and 52% of preschoolers retained their ODD diagnosis when reassessed 1 and 3 years later, respectively (Keenan et al. 2011), whereas approximately half of the children diagnosed with CD retained this diagnosis at a follow-up assessment up to 5 years later (López-Romero et al. 2015; Raine et al. 2005; Robins 1966). On the other hand, a considerable proportion of children with ODD show a reduction in symptoms over the course of development, particularly those diagnosed during the preschool period (Kim-Cohen et al. 2009). However, longitudinal research indicates that even when conduct problems remit, these children remain at greater risk for adjustment problems in later development when compared with children who never had severe conduct problems (Bevilacqua et al. 2018; Kim-Cohen et al. 2009).

Childhood Conduct Problems as a Primary Prevention Target

Such longitudinal research findings underscore the importance of targeting conduct problems in childhood to prevent ASPD during adulthood. Furthermore, longitudinal research indicates that childhood conduct problems not only increase risk for later antisociality but also are frequently present early in the developmental trajectories of a host of other psychopathologies and adjustment problems. To illustrate, one follow-back study of a prospective longitudinal cohort found that children who had symptoms of ODD or CD were at increased risk for meeting diagnostic criteria for ASPD, anxiety disorders, depressive and manic episodes, substance dependence, eating disorders, and schizophreniform disorder in adulthood (Kim-Cohen et al. 2003). Relatedly, children whose conduct problems persisted across the lifetime were at significantly greater risk for not only later aggression but also poor educational and employment outcomes, economic problems, physical health problems, and greater use of health services (e.g., emergency department visits, prescription fills, injury insurance claims, and hospital bed nights) (Bevilacqua et al. 2018; Odgers et al. 2008; Rivenbark et al. 2018; Wertz et al. 2018) relative to those whose conduct problems were limited to childhood or onset during adolescence. Together, these data indicating the stability and multifinality associated with childhood conduct problems provide compelling support for prioritizing these problems in the prevention of ASPD and other serious psychosocial adversities.

Subtypes of Childhood Conduct Problems

Much of the stability in disorders related to childhood conduct problems is accounted for by a small group of children who show particularly severe and stable difficulties (Broidy et al. 2003; Moffitt 2003). There have been many attempts to uncover characteristics distinguishing more severe and chronic forms of conduct problems from more benign and transient forms. One of the more consistent predictors of poor outcome is the initial severity of the disorder—that is, the frequency and intensity of behavioral difficulties, the variety of symptoms, and the presence of symptoms in more than one setting are all linked to greater severity and persistence (Loeber et al. 2000). More distal factors also predict poorer outcomes for children with early-onset conduct problems, including family dysfunction and socioeconomic adversity (Moore et al. 2017; Pardini et al. 2015).

From a developmental perspective, one of the most consistent predictors of poor outcomes in adulthood is the age at which the child begins to show serious conduct problems. Robust longitudinal research indicates that conduct problems that onset prior to adolescence are associated with the greatest risk of psychosocial adversity. For example, a prospective study of adult outcomes of a birth cohort in New Zealand compared two groups of adults who had severe conduct problems as children, demonstrating that those whose conduct problems developed prior to puberty made up only 10% of the birth cohort but accounted for 43% of convictions for violent crimes (e.g., assault, robbery), 40% of drug convictions (e.g., using, trafficking), and 62% of convictions for violence against women during adulthood (Moffitt et al. 2002). In contrast, those adults whose conduct problems emerged during adolescence accounted for a larger proportion of the sample (26%) but were 50%–60% less likely to be convicted of an adulthood offense than the childhood-onset group (Moffitt et al. 2002). Moreover, the offenses of the adolescent-onset group tended to be less serious (e.g., minor theft, public drunkenness) and less violent (e.g., accounting for 50% of the convictions for property offenses) (Moffitt et al. 2002). The remainder of the cohort consisted of individuals who had conduct problems that were "childhood-limited" (8%), did not have conduct problems across childhood or adolescence (5%, called "abstainers"), or showed "normative" levels of antisocial behavior relative to the full cohort (51%) (Moffitt et al. 2002). These and related findings resulted in the distinction between childhood-onset and adolescent-onset subtypes of CD, first introduced in DSM-IV (American Psychiatric Association 1994) and retained in DSM-5 as a specifier denoting whether severe behavior problems began before or after age 10 years.

A problem with the approach to subtyping by age at onset is that important distinctions can also be made *within* the childhood-onset group. First, some children with childhood-onset CD do not continue to show problems into adulthood (Moore et al. 2017; Odgers et al. 2008). For example, in the aforementioned birth cohort of children in New Zealand, approximately one-quarter of the sample showed serious conduct problems that were limited to childhood, and these children experienced few physical or mental health problems as adults, with the possible exception of internalizing problems among men in middle adulthood (i.e., age 32 years) (Odgers et al. 2008). Second, although the childhood-onset group shows more dispositional risk factors than the adolescent-onset group, the type of dispositional risk factors may vary for subgroups of children and adolescents *within* the childhood-onset group, indicative of multiple and etiologically distinct developmental pathways leading to childhood conduct problems and later antisociality. This latter finding precipitated research exploring methods for distinguishing subgroups of children within the broader category of childhood-onset conduct problems.

The presence of a "callous" (e.g., lack of empathy, absence of guilt, uncaring attitudes) and "unemotional" (e.g., shallow or deficient emotional responses) interpersonal style has proven useful for designating a distinct subgroup of children with severe and chronic conduct problems and aggressive behaviors (for a review, see Frick et al. 2014). Subtyping children with conduct problems based on the presence of elevated callous-unemotional traits is based on a long history of clinical research showing that psychopathic traits characterize a distinct subgroup of adults with significant antisocial behavior (Cleckley 1941; Hare 1993; Lykken 1995). Psychopathy is a multidimensional personality disorder characterized by a narcissistic, deceitful, and manipulative interpersonal style; shallow and deficient affect; and impulsive, irresponsible, and antisocial behavior. Callous-unemotional traits are identified as the putative developmental precursor to adult psychopathy, capturing the deficient affect dimension of the construct (Frick and White 2008). An important aside relating to nomenclature is that although psychopathy and ASPD often overlap, these constructs are both conceptually and clinically distinct as operationalized using current diagnostic classification systems. The DSM-5 diagnostic criteria for ASPD capture the behavioral dimension of psychopathy (commonly referred to as "Factor 2" symptoms) but mostly neglect the interpersonal and affective dimensions (commonly referred to as "Factor 1" symptoms). In this way, although most individuals with psychopathy typically meet diagnostic criteria for ASPD, many individuals with ASPD do not evince psychopathy (Hare 1996).

Consideration of elevated childhood callous-unemotional traits is critical in the prevention of adult ASPD in light of evidence that these traits confer elevated risk for early starting, persistent, severe, and aggressive antisociality (Frick et al. 2014; McMahon et al. 2010). For example, relative to children with conduct problems and low callous-unemotional traits, those with elevated callous-unemotional traits show a greater number and variety of conduct problems, greater proactive aggression (i.e., planned, gainful), and higher self-reported general and violent delinquency (Frick et al. 2003, 2005). Although callous-unemotional traits are more common in CD with a childhood onset than an adolescent onset (Moffitt et al. 2002), evidence suggests that callous-unemotional traits retain their predictive utility for ASPD symptoms even when statistically controlling for childhood-onset CD (McMahon et al. 2010). Other longitudinal research also supports the utility of callous-unemotional traits for predicting severe conduct problems, delinquency, and criminality in later life. For example, children who have co-occurring conduct problems and callous-unemotional traits accounted for more than half of all police contacts across four yearly assessments in a longitudinal study of school-aged children (Frick et al. 2005). Childhood callous-unemotional traits also reliably predict psychopathic traits, externalizing and criminal behavior, and substance dependence in early adulthood (Hawes et al. 2017; Hyde et al. 2015; Pardini et al. 2018).

The utility of callous-unemotional traits for predicting a more severe course of antisociality has been found in samples of preschool children (Kimonis et al. 2006, 2016; Longman et al. 2016), elementary school–aged children (Fanti et al. 2017; Frick et al. 2005), and adolescents (Kruh et al. 2005; Muratori et al. 2016). It has also been found for both boys and girls (Pihet et al. 2015) and across countries, including the United States (Frick et al. 2005; Kimonis et al. 2008b), Australia (Dadds et al. 2005), the United Kingdom (Moran et al. 2008; Viding et al. 2009), Belgium (Roose et al. 2010), Germany (Essau et al. 2006), Cyprus (Kimonis et al. 2016), and Israel (Somech and Elizur 2009). Together, the strength of this evidence base precipitated incorporation of callous-unemotional traits into the diagnosis of CD in DSM-5 as a specifier of "with limited prosocial emotions." If a child meets diagnostic criteria for CD, the limited prosocial emotions specifier is assigned when two or more of the following characteristics are persistently displayed in multiple relationships and settings for 12 months or more: 1) lack of remorse or guilt, 2) callous—lack of empathy, 3) lack of concern about performance (at school, work, or in other important activities), and 4) shallow or deficient affect (American Psychiatric Association 2013).

Multiple Pathways to Severe Antisociality

More broadly, research pertaining to subtypes of childhood conduct problems highlights that many factors increase a child's risk for developing conduct problems and that these range from individual risk factors (e.g., poor impulse control, temperamental negative emotionality, punishment insensitivity, poor emotional regulation, insecure attachment, low intelligence, lack of social skills) to problems in the child's immediate psychosocial context (e.g., exposure to toxins, family poverty, parental psychopathology, inadequate parental discipline, association with deviant peers) and in the child's broader psychosocial context (e.g., living in a high-crime neighborhood, exposure to violence, lack of educational and vocational opportunities) (see Dadds and Frick 2019; Dodge and Pettit 2003 for reviews; Frick and Viding 2009). We are not likely able to weave this broad array of risk factors into a single, coherent, and comprehensive causal model for conduct problems because of the large number of factors and their variety. Moreover, risk factors are typically not independent of one another and likely operate in a transactional (i.e., one influencing another) or multiplicative (i.e., one interacting with another) manner (Dodge and Pettit 2003). The question of etiology is further complicated by evidence that the causal mechanisms leading to conduct problems may systematically differ across subgroups of children who have conduct problems. For example, childhood-onset CD is linked to many comorbid problems across multiple domains, including aggression, cognitive and neuropsychological disturbances (e.g., executive functioning deficits, autonomic nervous system irregularities), impulsivity, social alienation, and dysfunctional family backgrounds (Assink et al. 2015; Dandreaux and Frick 2009; Moffitt 2006), whereas adolescent-onset CD is associated with social causes, such as delinquent peer affiliations (Moffitt 2003, 2006, 2018). Furthermore, within the childhood-onset subgroup, research supports that callous-unemotional traits signify a unique constellation of causal risk factors relative to typical conduct problem presentations (Frick et al. 2014), with strong evidence that the genetic influence on childhood-onset CD is largely accounted for by children with significant levels of callous-unemotional traits (Larsson et al. 2006; Mann et al. 2018). Indeed, when heritability was examined in children with conduct problems, the genetic influence on these problems was more than twice as strong for those with co-occurring callous-unemotional traits relative to those with conduct problems alone, for whom these problems were more strongly related to environmental influences (Viding et al. 2005, 2008).

When taken together, research relating to subtype-specific risk factors indicates that children with conduct problems are a highly heterogeneous group for whom multiple developmental pathways lead to antisociality (Frick and White 2008). Importantly, the development of antisociality for any given child is likely the result of several different risk factors that accumulate and interact to increase that child's risk level, and these risk factors systematically differ among subgroups of children with conduct problems.

Treatment of Childhood Conduct Problems

The existence of multiple developmental pathways leading to antisociality has critical implications for treating childhood conduct problems and thus effectively preventing ASPD. That is, given the equifinality associated with childhood conduct problems, their treatment must be individualized to address the unique causal and maintaining factors among the various pathways. However, despite decades of compelling empirical support, traditional interventions for childhood conduct problems regularly fail to achieve this goal.

Traditional Interventions for Childhood Conduct Problems

Traditionally, evidence-based interventions for childhood conduct problems comprise both pharmacological and psychological approaches. Pharmacological interventions involve the use of psychotropic medications to reduce the disruptive behaviors and can include prescription of psychostimulants, α_2 agonists, antipsychotics, and mood stabilizers (Pringsheim et al. 2015a, 2015b). However, despite increasingly widespread prescription by medical professionals (Olfson et al. 2010; Zito et al. 2007), little evidence currently supports the efficacy and safety of most medications for reducing symptoms associated with ODD and CD (Gleason et al. 2007; Hambly et al. 2016).

In contrast, there is strong empirical support for the efficacy and acceptability of psychological treatments for childhood conduct problems (Comer et al. 2013; Eyberg et al. 2008). Evidence-based psychological interventions comprise direct child training programs, parent management training (PMT) programs, or a combination of the two (Eyberg et al. 2008; McCart et al. 2006). Direct child training programs incorporate cognitive-behavioral and contingency management approaches. The former targets deficits in social cognition, social problem-solving skills, and emotion regulation (McCart et al. 2006). This involves teaching the child or adolescent a series of problem-solving steps (e.g., how to recognize problems, consider alternative responses, and select the most adaptive solution) and overcoming deficits in how he or she processes social information, such as others' verbal and nonverbal cues (Larson and Lochman 2003). Contingency management approaches involve the use of individualized, structured behavior management systems across various contexts (e.g., home, school) to shape (e.g., gradually improve) and reinforce (e.g., reward) behavioral changes in an area of specific concern (e.g., noncompliance, aggression). Evidence supports the efficacy of contingency management approaches for improving conduct problems in a variety of settings, including the home (Henggeler 2015), school (Sanchez et al. 2018), and residential treatment centers (Lyman and Campbell 1996). The efficacy of direct child training programs is greater for older children and adolescents than for preschoolers and early elementary school–aged children, as the former are more able to reason, distinguish thoughts from feelings, and understand and use cognitive strategies and contingencies (Eyberg et al. 2008; McCart et al. 2006).

Conversely, PMT programs are the recommended first-line approach for treating conduct problems in preschoolers and early elementary school–aged children (Chorpita et al. 2011; Eyberg et al. 2008). Empirically supported PMT programs that have been widely disseminated include, but are not limited to, the Incredible Years Program (Webster-Stratton 2005), Parent-Child Interaction Therapy (PCIT; Brinkmeyer and Eyberg 2003); Parent Management Training–Oregon Model (PMTO; Forgatch and Patterson 2010), and the Triple P–Positive Parenting Program (Sanders 1999). Young children have particular potential to benefit from PMT given their reliance on caregiver fulfillment of basic needs and corresponding sensitivity to caregivers' use of behavioral contingency strategies. A robust evidence base supports the efficacy of PMT for improving conduct problems in young children (e.g., younger than 8 years), with meta-analytic findings favoring PMT over other treatment modalities, including nonbehavioral interventions (e.g., family systems approaches; within-subjects Hedges' g=0.88 vs. 0.42, respectively; Comer et al. 2013) and cognitive-behavioral therapy (within-subjects d=0.98 vs. 0.57, respectively; Chorpita et al. 2011), and evidence that PMT-related gains are maintained at follow-ups of various lengths (Lundahl et al. 2006; van Aar et al. 2017).

Broadly speaking, PMT derives from social learning theory, which integrates the operant learning principles of reinforcement and punishment (Skinner 1953) with the principle of vicarious learning (Bandura 1965, 1977). Practically, PMT teaches parents how to develop and implement structured contingency management programs in the home environment. Effective implementation of contingency management programs requires improvement in parents' ability to monitor and supervise child behavior; provide positive reinforcement for positive, prosocial behaviors; use differential attention approaches for socially maintained behaviors; and consistently use effective discipline strategies following disruptive behavior (McCart et al. 2006). Some PMT programs also emphasize improving the quality of the parent-child relationship as a means of shaping child behavior, driven by empirical findings indicating an association between insecure or disorganized attachment and childhood conduct problems (Fearon et al. 2010). Thus, effective prevention and intervention strategies for early-onset CDs focus heavily on family and parenting factors.

Limitations of Traditional Interventions for Childhood Conduct Problems

Despite compelling empirical support in some settings and for some patients, each of these interventions has substantial limitations (Bakker et al. 2017; Brestan and Eyberg

1998; Kazdin 1995). First, across interventions, a significant proportion of children with severe conduct problems do not show a positive response to treatment, called "nonresponders," and for those who do respond positively, their behavior problems are often not reduced to within normal limits. This is reflected in the percentage of children who do not show reliable and clinically significant change at posttreatment (Sheldrick et al. 2001). Second, a significant proportion of patients terminate treatment prematurely. For example, a recent systematic review reported that an average of 25% of eligible families chose not to enroll in a study of PMT, and a further 26% dropped out prior to or during the course of PMT (Chacko et al. 2016). This combined attrition rate of 51% indicated that more than half of families identified as suitable for PMT did not receive treatment or failed to experience its full benefit. Third, treatment is most effective with younger children (younger than 8 years) with less severe behavioral disturbances (Forehand et al. 2014), highlighting the importance of early identification and intervention. Fourth, the generalizability of treatment effects across settings and time tends to be poor. For example, treatments that are effective in changing a child's behavior in one setting (e.g., mental health clinics) often do not bring about changes in the child's behavior in other settings (e.g., home, school) (Naik-Polan and Budd 2008). Finally and more broadly, many evidence-based treatments for childhood conduct problems are not available or accessible in community settings, especially those that are rural or remote.

Altogether, these limitations mean that a significant proportion of children with antisocial behaviors fail to receive treatment, complete treatment, benefit from treatment, or benefit from treatment across settings and time. From a developmental perspective, these failures mean that this considerable proportion of children are at increased risk for developing ASPD during adulthood, relative to those who receive and comprehensively respond to treatment. The failure of traditional treatments to improve outcomes for all antisocial children is attributed in part to the "one-size-fits-all" approach that characterizes most interventions for childhood conduct problems. Although all of the traditional treatments described target basic processes that are theoretically important in the development and maintenance of conduct problems (e.g., dysfunctional parenting practices, cognitive biases), these treatments largely ignore the fact that severe conduct problems are generally caused by many different and interacting processes (Frick 2012). As a result, it is unlikely that any single intervention will be effective for all children with ODD or CD, resulting in systematically increased risk of later antisociality for some subgroups of children.

Failure of Traditional Interventions to Improve Outcomes Equally Across Levels of Callous-Unemotional Traits

In particular, research indicates that traditional treatments are less effective for improving the conduct problems of children with elevated callous-unemotional traits, relative to those with conduct problems but low callous-unemotional traits. Children with high callous-unemotional traits tend to enter treatment with more frequent and severe conduct problems, and although they can experience treatment-related improvement of considerable magnitude, they are systematically less likely to improve to within normal limits (Hawes et al. 2014; Waller et al. 2013). Moreover, accumulating evidence suggests that elevated callous-unemotional traits are associated with higher likelihood of premature attrition from treatment (Kimonis et al. 2014). This pattern of treatment nonresponse has been demonstrated in adolescent samples and using multimodal intervention delivery formats (Manders et al. 2013; Masi et al. 2013) and is consistent with findings in adult samples indicating the detrimental effect of psychopathic traits on treatment outcomes (Polaschek and Skeem 2018). Accumulating evidence indicates that callous-unemotional-related treatment nonresponse also occurs in studies of family-based PMT interventions involving younger samples (Hawes et al. 2014). For example, a seminal study investigated the effect of callous-unemotional traits on outcomes following the PMT program known as Integrated Family Intervention for Child Conduct Problems in a sample of boys ($n=56$; mean age=6.29 years; SD=1.55 years) with clinically significant conduct problems. This study found that boys with elevated callous-unemotional traits were more likely to receive a diagnosis of ODD at posttreatment than were boys with conduct problems and low callous-unemotional traits (Hawes and Dadds 2005). A similar pattern of impoverished treatment response was found in a sample of very young, developmentally delayed children ($n=28$; mean age=54.1 months; SD=10.0 months) receiving PCIT, such that elevated callous-unemotional traits were associated with significantly less treatment benefit and higher likelihood of attrition, relative to low callous-unemotional traits (Kimonis et al. 2014). A larger study of older children with clinically significant conduct problems ($n=323$; mean age=8.69 years; SD=2.14 years) found that higher ratings of observed child callousness predicted less parent- and teacher-rated treatment improvement following PMTO (Bjørnebekk and Kjøbli 2017). Altogether, these studies converge in finding that early intervention efforts may be less effective when callous-unemotional traits are elevated. This is a critical consideration for the prevention of ASPD given the importance of early intervention to reduce risk for later antisociality and other poor outcomes in adulthood (Dodge et al. 2015); children with conduct problems and elevated callous-unemotional traits may be at heightened risk for developing ASPD in adulthood *even with early intervention* compared with those with conduct problems only.

The failure of traditional interventions to improve outcomes equally across levels of callous-unemotional traits has been attributed to neglect of the unique emotional, cognitive, and psychobiological factors involved in the development and maintenance of conduct problems when callous-unemotional traits are elevated (Frick 2012; Kimonis et al. 2019). Accordingly, there has been increased focus on integrating knowledge about the causes of conduct problems with the development of innovative approaches to treatment aimed at improving treatment outcomes for those with elevated callous-unemotional traits (Frick 2012; Hyde et al. 2014). For example, interventions such as PMT rely heavily on improving the effectiveness and consistency of parental discipline to produce child behavior change, but elevated callous-unemotional traits are associated with a fearless temperamental style (Barker et al. 2011; Goffin et al. 2018) and reduced sensitivity to and learning following punishment (Byrd et al. 2014). On the contrary, using positive reinforcement within a parenting intervention was more effective than punishment-oriented behavioral modification methods for reducing disruptive behaviors among clinic-referred children with severe conduct problems and high callous-unemotional traits (Hawes and Dadds 2005). Similarly, an intensive treatment program administered to incarcerated adolescents with high psychopathic traits that used reward-oriented approaches, taught empathy skills, and targeted the youths' interests led to reductions in recidivism over a 2-year follow-up period (Caldwell et al. 2006). Together, these findings suggest that reward-focused intervention strategies are more beneficial for producing behavior change among children with elevated callous-unemotional traits than are punishment-based strategies.

Attempts to improve treatment outcomes for children with conduct problems and elevated callous-unemotional traits have also targeted low parental warmth and responsivity, a risk factor implicated in the development and maintenance of both callous-unemotional traits themselves and conduct problems when callous-unemotional traits are elevated (Frick et al. 2014; Waller et al. 2013, 2015). Although harsh, inconsistent, and coercive parenting is central to core developmental models of child conduct problems (Patterson 1982), this parenting style is less important for the development of conduct problems among children with high callous-unemotional traits (Pasalich et al. 2011; Wootton et al. 1997). Instead, warm and responsive parenting facilitates secure parent-child attachment that is the foundation for moral socialization and emotional learning, which are impaired in children with callous-unemotional traits (Emde et al. 1991; Kochanska 1993). Accordingly, reduced parental warmth is associated with increasing conduct problems when callous-unemotional traits are elevated (Pasalich et al. 2011). Thus, interventions that specifically target improvements in expressions of parental warmth and sensitivity may more effectively remediate conduct problems when callous-unemotional traits are elevated (e.g., Kimonis et al. 2019).

Finally, compelling evidence shows that children with conduct problems and elevated callous-unemotional traits uniquely demonstrate low emotional reactivity to aversive stimuli. For example, relative to children with conduct problems alone, those with elevated callous-unemotional traits are less accurate in recognizing emotional expressions and sadness and fear in particular (Marsh and Blair 2008), are less attentively engaged by others' distress cues (Kimonis et al. 2018) and less distressed by the negative effects of their behavior on others (Pardini et al. 2003), and are more impaired in their moral reasoning and empathic concern toward others (Pardini et al. 2003). Physiologically, relative to children with conduct problems alone, those with elevated callous-unemotional traits show less heart rate change to emotionally evocative films (de Wied et al. 2012) and less skin conductance reactivity when responding to peer provocation (Kimonis et al. 2008a). Neurologically, relative to children with conduct problems alone, those with callous-unemotional traits show deficits in brain areas associated with emotional, reward, and empathic processing (Viding and McCrory 2018; Viding et al. 2012). Despite this strong support for pervasive emotional deficits in children with conduct problems and elevated callous-unemotional traits, traditional interventions for childhood conduct problems rarely directly target children's emotional skills.

Accordingly, more recent approaches have incorporated strategies intended to remediate these emotional deficits. In one study, traditional PMT was augmented with a computerized emotion recognition training program, which was found to improve empathy and reduce conduct problems for those with elevated callous-unemotional traits in a sample of 6- to 16-year-old children ($n=195$; mean age=10.52 years; SD=2.6 years) (Dadds et al. 2012). Although other research has implicated eye gaze deficits in the emotional insensitivity of children with callous-unemotional traits (Dadds et al. 2006, 2008), a recent attempt to translate these findings into clinical intervention was not associated with sustained remediation of eye gaze deficits or with improvements in conduct problems and callous-unemotional traits above and beyond standard treatment (Dadds et al. 2019). This finding suggests that individualized interventions targeting single risk factors may be insufficient for improving treatment outcomes beyond the effect of traditional interventions. More encouraging outcomes have been found for comprehensive interventions targeting multiple risk factors involved in the development and maintenance of conduct problems when callous-unemotional traits are elevated (e.g., Kimonis et al. 2019; Kolko and Pardini 2010). For example, PCIT was adapted for children with elevated callous-unemotional traits to comprehensively target multiple putative causal and maintaining factors by increasing parental warmth, teaching reward-based strategies to manage problem behaviors, and improving children's emotional functioning (Fleming and Kimonis 2018). A small open trial of 3- to 6-year-old children ($n=23$; mean age=4.5 years; SD=0.92) with conduct problems and elevated callous-unemotional traits found that this PCIT–callous-unemotional intervention produced clinically significant decreases in child conduct problems and callous-unemotional traits (Kimonis et al. 2019).

Novel Approaches to Treating Childhood Conduct Problems

When taken together, the extant research clearly supports the use of comprehensive, individualized treatments for childhood conduct problems. It is important that this translational research has a specific focus on the treatment of conduct problems in young children for two primary reasons: 1) evidence supports the importance of early intervention for the prevention of antisociality during adulthood (Piquero et al. 2008); and 2) callous-unemotional traits, which uniquely increase risk for severe, stable, and persistent antisociality, are first detectable very early in life (Kimonis et al. 2016). Moreover, although the presence of callous-unemotional traits increases risk for treatment nonresponse, there is accumulating support that novel approaches to treating childhood conduct problems improve outcomes for this subgroup of children who have been traditionally earmarked as "treatment-resistant." In this way, dissemination and implementation of evidence-based interventions for childhood conduct problems—tailored to meet the unique needs of children with and without elevated callous-unemotional traits—in community settings are vital next steps in the process of preventing ASPD and its associated psychosocial adversities.

Case Example

At intake, Kyle was a 4-year, 10-month-old white boy referred to treatment by his parents because of severe behavior and emotional problems. Kyle lived with his mother, father, and 6-month-old brother, who was described as having significant health difficulties since birth. Kyle presented with significant conduct problems in both home and preschool contexts, including physical and verbal aggression toward family members, educators, and peers; chronic defiance and noncompliance with commands and rules; argumentativeness; emotion dysregulation characterized by frequent angry moods and temper tantrums; blaming others for his misbehavior; and lying and stealing. On one occasion, Kyle had intentionally thrown a hard block at an educator's head, causing her to sustain a concussion and leading to his expulsion from the daycare center. His parents and teachers described him as lacking in empathy and in remorse or guilt following misbehavior, noting that he often "taunted" peers, took joy in their distress, and rarely took responsibility or apologized for his actions. Many of these difficulties had been present since toddlerhood but had worsened significantly with the birth of Kyle's younger brother.

A comprehensive assessment of Kyle's behavioral and emotional symptoms was conducted by using a multi-informant and multimodal approach that assessed symptoms across settings. Kyle met diagnostic criteria for ODD (severe) and childhood-onset CD (mild) but not ADHD according to the National Institute of Mental Health's Diagnostic Interview Schedule for Children Version IV (DISC-IV; Shaffer et al. 2000) completed with his mother. Kyle's parents and teacher rated the intensity and problematic nature of his conduct problems as at or above the clinical cutoff *T*-score of 60 on the Eyberg Child Behavior Inventory (ECBI) and Sutter-Eyberg Student Behavior Inventory–Revised (SESBI-R; Eyberg and Pincus 1999), respectively (mother, father, and teacher Intensity *T*-scores: 62, 66, and 64, respectively; Problem *T*-scores: 61, 62, and 60, respectively). Two instruments were used to assess Kyle's level of callous-unemotional traits: the rater scale Inventory of Callous-Unemotional Traits (Kimonis et al. 2008b) and the Clinical Assessment of Prosocial Emotions: Version 1.1 (CAPE 1.1; Frick 2013), a clinician-administered interview and structured professional judgment tool. On the preschool version of the Inventory of Callous-Unemotional Traits that was completed by Kyle's mother, father, and teacher, Kyle demonstrated elevated levels of callous-unemotional traits, with scores of 27, 31, and 35, respectively. These scores correspond to an average informant response of *somewhat true* as rated by Kyle's parents and *very true* as rated by his teacher across Inventory of Callous-Unemotional Traits items. On the CAPE 1.1, administered to his mother, Kyle met diagnostic criteria for the "with limited prosocial emotions" specifier with three of the four diagnostic criteria endorsed: lack of remorse or guilt, callous—lack of empathy, and shallow or deficient affect. Thus, Kyle was assessed as meeting criteria for childhood-onset CD with limited prosocial emotions. Behavioral observation of Kyle with both parents using the *Dyadic Parent-Child Interaction Coding System,* 4th Edition (DPICS-IV; Eyberg et al. 2013), revealed coercive patterns of interaction when either parent gave Kyle an instruction and high levels of noncompliance, especially during a standardized clean-up task.

Kyle's family completed a PCIT version specifically adapted to address the unique risk and maintaining factors involved in the development of callous-unemotional–type conduct problems (Fleming and Kimonis 2018; Kimonis et al. 2019). Standard PCIT involves two treatment phases: 1) child-directed interaction, during which parents learn to apply differential attention strategies to reduce minor misbehavior, increase prosociality, and strengthen the parent–child relationship, and 2) parent-directed interaction, during which parents learn to apply effective, consistent discipline strategies (e.g., time-out) in response to noncompliance and aggression (Eyberg and Funderburk 2011). The adaptation of PCIT for children with callous-unemotional traits, called PCIT-CU, differs from standard PCIT in three key ways. First, PCIT-CU directly coaches parents to engage in warm, emotionally responsive parenting during the child-directed interaction phase, which is associated with reductions in conduct problems for children with callous-unemotional traits (Waller et al. 2013). Second, PCIT-CU systematically integrates an individualized reward-based system into the parent-directed interaction time-out sequence to address the punishment-insensitive and reward-dominant temperamental styles of children with callous-unemotional traits (Byrd et al. 2014). Finally, PCIT-CU delivers comprehensive emotional skill-building instruction in a supplemental module called Coaching and Rewarding Emotional Skills (CARES) to target the distinct core emotional deficits of these children (Datyner et al. 2016).

Kyle's family completed 21 PCIT-CU treatment sessions in total, including 7 sessions each of child-directed interaction, parent-directed interaction, and CARES, with assessments conducted at pretreatment, post–child-directed interaction, post–parent-directed interaction, post-CARES, and 3 months following treatment. Kyle's mother participated in all of the sessions, and his father attended 8 sessions because of work commitments.

At posttreatment, Kyle no longer met diagnostic criteria for ODD or CD according to the DISC-IV completed with his mother. Kyle's mother, father, and teacher rated the frequency of his disruptive behavior on the ECBI and SESBI-R Intensity scale as below the clinical cutoff (T-scores of 46, 44, and 50, respectively). They also reported greater tolerance for and less distress over his behaviors, as reflected by ECBI/SESBI-R Problem T-scores below the clinical cutoff (T-scores of 41, 42, and 46, respectively). Qualitatively, Kyle's mother reported that strategic ignoring was effective for reducing Kyle's temper tantrums when he did not get what he wanted when used in combination with descriptive praise and tangible rewards for calm behavior and asking nicely. Overall, Kyle's mother reported that he was extremely motivated by the token economy system, evidenced by reductions in his aggressive behavior and covert conduct problems (e.g., stealing, lying). On the CAPE 1.1, Kyle's mother reported significant improvement in his ability to accept responsibility for his misbehavior. She generated several examples of times when Kyle appeared to feel badly about hurting someone (e.g., younger brother); however, she reported that his refusal to apologize for his actions remained challenging. In contrast, she reported a marked improvement in his ability to empathize, especially with her own expressed emotions, and that she would no longer describe Kyle as being "mean" or "cruel." She reported several instances of spontaneous "nice" behavior; for example, wanting to take banana bread to a neighbor and expressing affection for an animal for the "first time ever." She also noted some improvement in his ability and willingness to express emotions, although he preferred to do so "in secret" to her.

Thus, although Kyle's emotional functioning still appeared to be below developmental expectations, he no longer met diagnostic criteria for the limited prosocial emotions specifier. Inventory of Callous-Unemotional Traits scores did not reflect as much positive change: parent ratings were stable and teacher ratings showed only a slight reduction, although it is possible that the restricted four-point response scale of the Inventory of Callous-Unemotional Traits was less effective at capturing treatment-related change. Finally, both parents demonstrated an improved ability to implement effective commands and to follow through calmly with the discipline procedure for noncompliance or with labeled praise and tangible reinforcer (i.e., token) for compliance, according to DPICS-IV observation at posttreatment. Treatment gains were maintained at 3-month follow-up.

Next Frontiers for the Prevention of Antisocial Personality Disorder

Finally, we outline some critical future research and practice directions in preventing ASPD. First, there is a clear need for continued translation of the robust research findings elucidating mechanisms in the development of conduct problem subtypes into targeted clinical interventions and for their iterative refinement and evaluation in large clinical research trials. It is essential that this research addresses whether targeted intervention (e.g., delivered according to presence or absence of co-occurring callous-unemotional traits) is superior to the predominating "one-size-fits-all" approach and identifies the active ingredients explaining behavior change in response to intervention. Second, targeted intervention for conduct problems will only be effective insofar as it reaches and adequately engages its intended population. Recent efforts to increase accessibility to general evidence-based interventions via online delivery offer a promising solution to the challenge of accessing care (e.g., Comer et al. 2017; Fleming et al. 2021; Sanders et al. 2012). However, even with increased accessibility, the problem of low treatment adherence and nonresponsiveness will remain if targeted interventions are not also adapted for online delivery (Fleming et al. 2017, 2020). Finally, long-term follow-up studies are needed to establish the longevity of intervention effects and to identify effective strategies for sustaining treatment benefits.

In regard to future practice, although PMT represents a first-line approach to treating early childhood conduct problems, it requires adaptation to better meet the needs of those with callous-unemotional traits. For older children and adolescents, this is likely to require supplementation with direct child training focused on the development of emotional skills, empathy, and prosocial behavior. Critically, the success of this approach rests on ensuring that the latest research developments in the assessment of conduct problem subtypes reach community practitioners. Assessment is vital for effective treatment planning, and it is critical that community practitioners know how and with what tools to evaluate the presence of clinically significant conduct problems and their diagnostic specifiers, including limited prosocial emotions. Parent and teacher rating measures are most common for screening childhood externalizing problems and can be used to identify those with subthreshold but impairing problems who are most amenable to preventive intervention. Ultimately, effectively bridging the research-to-practice gap is likely to yield the greatest effect on derailing children with severe, early-starting antisocial behavior from a developmental trajectory that is likely to culminate in adult ASPD.

Key Points

- Antisocial personality disorder (ASPD) is the developmental culmination of externalizing disorders that onset during childhood and adolescence.

- Prevention of ASPD necessitates timely and effective prevention of and intervention for symptoms of early-onset externalizing disorders.

- Traditional interventions for early-onset externalizing disorders (e.g., parent management training) are not equally effective among all children and adolescents, in part because traditional interventions fail to address the unique risk and maintaining factors involved in the development of externalizing symptoms for some children (i.e., those with co-occurring callous-unemotional traits).

- For effective prevention of ASPD, interventions for early-onset externalizing disorders require adaptation to more comprehensively address the factors involved in the development and maintenance of externalizing symptoms across the multiple etiological pathways leading to antisociality.

- Once determined to be efficacious for the population of interest, adapted interventions require dissemination to community practitioners to ensure that they are reaching individuals at greatest risk for ASPD.

References

American Psychiatric Association: Diagnostic and Statistical Manual of Mental Disorders, 4th Edition. Washington, DC, American Psychiatric Association, 1994

American Psychiatric Association: Diagnostic and Statistical Manual of Mental Disorders, 5th Edition. Arlington, VA, American Psychiatric Association, 2013

Assink M, van der Put CE, Hoeve M, et al: Risk factors for persistent delinquent behavior among juveniles: a meta-analytic review. Clin Psychol Rev 42:47–61, 2015 26301752

Bakker MJ, Greven CU, Buitelaar JK, et al: Practitioner review: psychological treatments for children and adolescents with conduct disorder problems—a systematic review and meta-analysis. J Child Psychol Psychiatry 58(1):4–18, 2017 27501434

Bandura A: Influence of models' reinforcement contingencies on the acquisition of imitative responses. J Pers Soc Psychol 1(6):589–595, 1965 14300234

Bandura A: Self-efficacy: toward a unifying theory of behavioral change. Psychol Rev 84(2):191–215, 1977 847061

Barker ED, Oliver BR, Viding E, et al: The impact of prenatal maternal risk, fearless temperament and early parenting on adolescent callous-unemotional traits: a 14-year longitudinal investigation. J Child Psychol Psychiatry 52(8):878–888, 2011 21410472

Beauchaine TP, Hinshaw SP, Pang KL: Comorbidity of attention-deficit/hyperactivity disorder and early-onset conduct disorder: biological, environmental, and developmental mechanisms. Clinical Psychology: Science and Practice 17(4):327–336, 2010

Bevilacqua L, Hale D, Barker ED, et al: Conduct problems trajectories and psychosocial outcomes: a systematic review and meta-analysis. Eur Child Adolesc Psychiatry 27(10):1239–1260, 2018 28983792

Bjørnebekk G, Kjøbli J: Observed callousness as a predictor of treatment outcomes in parent management training. Clin Child Psychol Psychiatry 22(1):59–73, 2017 26763014

Brestan EV, Eyberg SM: Effective psychosocial treatments of conduct-disordered children and adolescents: 29 years, 82 studies, and 5,272 kids. J Clin Child Psychol 27(2):180–189, 1998 9648035

Brinkmeyer MY, Eyberg SM: Parent-child interaction therapy for oppositional children, in Evidence-Based Psychotherapies for Children and Adolescents. Edited by Kazdin AE, Weisz JR. New York, Guilford, 2003, pp 204–223

Broidy LM, Nagin DS, Tremblay RE, et al: Developmental trajectories of childhood disruptive behaviors and adolescent delinquency: a six-site, cross-national study. Dev Psychol 39(2):222–245, 2003 12661883

Burke JD, Waldman I, Lahey BB: Predictive validity of childhood oppositional defiant disorder and conduct disorder: implications for the DSM-V. J Abnorm Psychol 119(4):739–751, 2010 20853919

Byrd AL, Loeber R, Pardini DA: Antisocial behavior, psychopathic features and abnormalities in reward and punishment processing in youth. Clin Child Fam Psychol Rev 17(2):125–156, 2014 24357109

Caldwell M, Skeem J, Salekin R, et al: Treatment response of adolescent offenders with psychopathy features: a 2-year follow-up. Criminal Justice and Behavior 33:571–596, 2006

Chacko A, Jensen SA, Lowry LS, et al: Engagement in behavioral parent training: review of the literature and implications for practice. Clin Child Fam Psychol Rev 19(3):204–215, 2016 27311693

Chorpita BF, Daleiden EL, Ebesutani C, et al: Evidence-based treatments for children and adolescents: an updated review of indicators of efficacy and effectiveness. Clinical Psychology: Science and Practice 18(2):154–172, 2011

Cleckley HM: The Mask of Sanity—An Attempt to Clarify Some Issues About the So-Called Psychopathic Personalities. St. Louis, MO, CV Mosby, 1941

Comer JS, Chow C, Chan PT, et al: Psychosocial treatment efficacy for disruptive behavior problems in very young children: a meta-analytic examination. J Am Acad Child Adolesc Psychiatry 52(1):26–36, 2013 23265631

Comer JS, Furr JM, Miguel EM, et al: Remotely delivering real-time parent training to the home: an initial randomized trial of Internet-delivered parent-child interaction therapy (I-PCIT). J Consult Clin Psychol 85(9):909–917, 2017 28650194

Dadds MR, Frick PJ: Toward a transdiagnostic model of common and unique processes leading to the major disorders of childhood: the REAL model of attention, responsiveness and learning. Behav Res Ther 119:103410, 2019 31176136

Dadds MR, Fraser J, Frost A, et al: Disentangling the underlying dimensions of psychopathy and conduct problems in childhood: a community study. J Consult Clin Psychol 73(3):400–410, 2005 15982138

Dadds MR, Perry Y, Hawes DJ, et al: Attention to the eyes and fear-recognition deficits in child psychopathy. Br J Psychiatry 189(3):280–281, 2006 16946366

Dadds MR, El Masry Y, Wimalaweera S, et al: Reduced eye gaze explains "fear blindness" in childhood psychopathic traits. J Am Acad Child Adolesc Psychiatry 47(4):455–463, 2008 18388767

Dadds MR, Cauchi AJ, Wimalaweera S, et al: Outcomes, moderators, and mediators of empathic-emotion recognition training for complex conduct problems in childhood. Psychiatry Res 199(3):201–207, 2012 22703720

Dadds MR, English T, Wimalaweera S, et al: Can reciprocated parent-child eye gaze and emotional engagement enhance treatment for children with conduct problems and callous-unemotional traits: a proof-of-concept trial. J Child Psychol Psychiatry 60(6):676–685, 2019 30697730

Dandreaux DM, Frick PJ: Developmental pathways to conduct problems: a further test of the childhood and adolescent-onset distinction. J Abnorm Child Psychol 37(3):375–385, 2009 18670873

Datyner AC, Kimonis ER, Hunt E, et al: Using a novel emotional skills module to enhance empathic responding for a child with conduct problems with limited prosocial emotions. Clinical Case Studies 15(1):35–52, 2016

de Wied M, van Boxtel A, Matthys W, et al: Verbal, facial and autonomic responses to empathy-eliciting film clips by disruptive male adolescents with high versus low callous-unemotional traits. J Abnorm Child Psychol 40(2):211–223, 2012 21870040

DeLisi M, Drury AJ, Elbert MJ: The etiology of antisocial personality disorder: the differential roles of adverse childhood experiences and childhood psychopathology. Compr Psychiatry 92:1–6, 2019 31079021

Dodge KA, Pettit GS: A biopsychosocial model of the development of chronic conduct problems in adolescence. Dev Psychol 39(2):349–371, 2003 12661890

Dodge KA, Bierman KL, Coie JD, et al: Impact of early intervention on psychopathology, crime, and well-being at age 25. Am J Psychiatry 172(1):59–70, 2015 25219348

Emde RN, Biringen Z, Clyman RB, et al: The moral self of infancy: affective core and procedural knowledge. Developmental Review 11(3):251–270, 1991

Erskine HE, Ferrari AJ, Nelson P, et al: Epidemiological modelling of attention-deficit/hyperactivity disorder and conduct disorder for the Global Burden of Disease Study 2010. J Child Psychol Psychiatry 54(12):1263–1274, 2013 24117530

Essau CA, Sasagawa S, Frick PJ: Callous-unemotional traits in a community sample of adolescents. Assessment 13(4):454–469, 2006 17050915

Eyberg SM, Funderburk B: Parent–Child Interaction Therapy Protocol. Gainesville, FL, PCIT International, 2011

Eyberg SM, Pincus D: Eyberg Child Behavior Inventory and Sutter-Eyberg Student Behavior Inventory—Revised: Professional Manual. Odessa, FL, Psychological Assessment Resources, 1999

Eyberg SM, Nelson MM, Boggs SR: Evidence-based psychosocial treatments for children and adolescents with disruptive behavior. J Clin Child Adolesc Psychol 37(1):215–237, 2008 18444059

Eyberg SM, Nelson MM, Ginn NC, et al: Dyadic Parent-Child Interaction Coding System (DPICS): Comprehensive Manual for Research and Training, 4th Edition. Gainesville, FL, PCIT International, 2013

Fanti KA, Colins OF, Andershed H, et al: Stability and change in callous-unemotional traits: longitudinal associations with potential individual and contextual risk and protective factors. Am J Orthopsychiatry 87(1):62–75, 2017 27046166

Fearon RP, Bakermans-Kranenburg MJ, van Ijzendoorn MH, et al: The significance of insecure attachment and disorganization in the development of children's externalizing behavior: a meta-analytic study. Child Dev 81(2):435–456, 2010 20438450

Fleming GE, Kimonis ER: PCIT for children with callous-unemotional traits, in Handbook of Parent-Child Interaction Therapy: Innovations and Applications for Research and Practice. Edited by Niec LN. Cham, Switzerland, Springer, 2018, pp 19–34

Fleming GE, Kimonis ER, Datyner A, et al: Adapting Internet-delivered parent-child interaction therapy to treat co-occurring disruptive behavior and callous-unemotional traits: a case study. Clinical Case Studies 16(5):370–387, 2017

Fleming GE, Kimonis ER, Furr JM, et al: Internet-delivered parent training for preschoolers with conduct problems: do callous-unemotional traits moderate efficacy and engagement? J Abnorm Child Psychol 48(9):1169–1182, 2020 32533295

Fleming GE, Kohlhoff J, Morgan S, et al: An effectiveness open trial of Internet-delivered parent training for young children with conduct problems living in regional and rural Australia. Behav Ther 52(1):110–123, 2021 33483109

Forehand R, Lafko N, Parent J, et al: Is parenting the mediator of change in behavioral parent training for externalizing problems of youth? Clin Psychol Rev 34(8):608–619, 2014 25455625

Forgatch MS, Patterson GR: Parent management training—Oregon model: an intervention for antisocial behavior in children and adolescents, in Evidence-Based Psychotherapies for Children and Adolescents, 2nd Edition. Edited by Kazdin AE, Weisz JR. New York, Guilford, 2010, pp 159–177

Frick PJ: Developmental pathways to conduct disorder: implications for future directions in research, assessment, and treatment. J Clin Child Adolesc Psychol 41(3):378–389, 2012 22475202

Frick PJ: Clinical Assessment of Prosocial Emotions: Version 1.1 (CAPE 1.1). New Orleans, LA, University of New Orleans, 2013

Frick PJ, Viding E: Antisocial behavior from a developmental psychopathology perspective. Dev Psychopathol 21(4):1111–1131, 2009 19825260

Frick PJ, White SF: Research review: the importance of callous-unemotional traits for developmental models of aggressive and antisocial behavior. J Child Psychol Psychiatry 49(4):359–375, 2008 18221345

Frick PJ, Cornell AH, Barry CT, et al: Callous-unemotional traits and conduct problems in the prediction of conduct problem severity, aggression, and self-report of delinquency. J Abnorm Child Psychol 31(4):457–470, 2003 12831233

Frick PJ, Stickle TR, Dandreaux DM, et al: Callous-unemotional traits in predicting the severity and stability of conduct problems and delinquency. J Abnorm Child Psychol 33(4):471–487, 2005 16118993

Frick PJ, Ray JV, Thornton LC, et al: Can callous-unemotional traits enhance the understanding, diagnosis, and treatment of serious conduct problems in children and adolescents? A comprehensive review. Psychol Bull 140(1):1–57, 2014 23796269

Gleason MM, Egger HL, Emslie GJ, et al: Psychopharmacological treatment for very young children: contexts and guidelines. J Am Acad Child Adolesc Psychiatry 46(12):1532–1572, 2007 18030077

Goffin KC, Boldt LJ, Kim S, et al: A unique path to callous-unemotional traits for children who are temperamentally fearless and unconcerned about transgressions: a longitudinal study of typically developing children from age 2 to 12. J Abnorm Child Psychol 46(4):769–780, 2018 28608168

Hambly JL, Khan S, McDermott B, et al: Pharmacotherapy of conduct disorder: challenges, options and future directions. J Psychopharmacol 30(10):967–975, 2016 27436231

Hare RD: Without Conscience: The Disturbing World of the Psychopaths Among Us. New York, Pocket Books, 1993

Hare RD: Psychopathy and antisocial personality disorder: a case of diagnostic confusion. Psychiatric Times, February 1, 1996. Available at: www.sakkyndig.com/psykologi/artvit/hare1996.pdf. Accessed April 26, 2021.

Hawes DJ, Dadds MR: The treatment of conduct problems in children with callous-unemotional traits. J Consult Clin Psychol 73(4):737–741, 2005 16173862

Hawes DJ, Price MJ, Dadds MR: Callous-unemotional traits and the treatment of conduct problems in childhood and adolescence: a comprehensive review. Clin Child Fam Psychol Rev 17(3):248–267, 2014 24748077

Hawes SW, Byrd AL, Waller R, et al: Late childhood interpersonal callousness and conduct problem trajectories interact to predict adult psychopathy. J Child Psychol Psychiatry 58(1):55–63, 2017 27516046

Henggeler SW: Effective family based treatments for adolescents with serious antisocial behavior, in The Development of Criminal and Antisocial Behavior. Edited by Morizot J, Kazemian L. Cham, Switzerland, Springer International, 2015, pp 461–475

Hofvander B, Ossowski D, Lundström S, et al: Continuity of aggressive antisocial behavior from childhood to adulthood: the question of phenotype definition. Int J Law Psychiatry 32(4):224–234, 2009 19428109

Hyde LW, Waller R, Burt SA: Commentary: improving treatment for youth with callous-unemotional traits through the intersection of basic and applied science—reflections on Dadds et al. (2014). J Child Psychol Psychiatry 55(7):781–783, 2014 24946897

Hyde LW, Burt SA, Shaw DS, et al: Early starting, aggressive, and/or callous-unemotional? Examining the overlap and predictive utility of antisocial behavior subtypes. J Abnorm Psychol 124(2):329–342, 2015 25603360

Kazdin AE: Conduct Disorders in Childhood and Adolescence, 2nd Edition. Thousand Oaks, CA, Sage, 1995

Keenan K, Boeldt D, Chen D, et al: Predictive validity of DSM-IV oppositional defiant and conduct disorders in clinically referred preschoolers. J Child Psychol Psychiatry 52(1):47–55, 2011 20738448

Kim-Cohen J, Caspi A, Moffitt TE, et al: Prior juvenile diagnoses in adults with mental disorder: developmental follow-back of a prospective-longitudinal cohort. Arch Gen Psychiatry 60(7):709–717, 2003 12860775

Kim-Cohen J, Arseneault L, Newcombe R, et al: Five-year predictive validity of DSM-IV conduct disorder research diagnosis in 4(1/2)-5-year-old children. Eur Child Adolesc Psychiatry 18(5):284–291, 2009 19165535

Kimonis ER, Frick PJ, Boris NW, et al: Callous-unemotional features, behavioral inhibition, and parenting: independent predictors of aggression in a high-risk preschool sample. Journal of Child and Family Studies 15(6):745–756, 2006

Kimonis ER, Frick PJ, Munoz LC, et al: Callous-unemotional traits and the emotional processing of distress cues in detained boys: testing the moderating role of aggression, exposure to community violence, and histories of abuse. Dev Psychopathol 20(2):569–589, 2008a 18423095

Kimonis ER, Frick PJ, Skeem JL, et al: Assessing callous-unemotional traits in adolescent offenders: validation of the Inventory of Callous-Unemotional Traits. Int J Law Psychiatry 31(3):241–252, 2008b 18514315

Kimonis ER, Bagner DM, Linares D, et al: Parent training outcomes among young children with callous–unemotional conduct problems with or at risk for developmental delay. J Child Fam Stud 23(2):437–448, 2014 24511217

Kimonis ER, Fanti KA, Anastassiou-Hadjicharalambous X, et al: Can callous-unemotional traits be reliably measured in preschoolers? J Abnorm Child Psychol 44(4):625–638, 2016 26344015

Kimonis ER, Graham N, Cauffman E: Aggressive male juvenile offenders with callous-unemotional traits show aberrant attentional orienting to distress cues. J Abnorm Child Psychol 46(3):519–527, 2018 28374219

Kimonis ER, Fleming GE, Briggs N, et al: Parent-child interaction therapy adapted for preschoolers with callous-unemotional traits: an open trial pilot study. J Clin Child Adolesc Psychol 48 (suppl 1):S347–S361, 2019 29979887

Kochanska G: Toward a synthesis of parental socialization and child temperament in early development of conscience. Child Development 64(2):325–347, 1993

Kolko DJ, Pardini DA: ODD dimensions, ADHD, and callous-unemotional traits as predictors of treatment response in children with disruptive behavior disorders. J Abnorm Psychol 119(4):713–725, 2010 21090875

Kruh IP, Frick PJ, Clements CB: Historical and personality correlates to the violence patterns of juveniles tried as adults. Criminal Justice and Behavior 32:69–96, 2005

Lahey BB, Loeber R, Burke JD, et al: Predicting future antisocial personality disorder in males from a clinical assessment in childhood. J Consult Clin Psychol 73(3):389–399, 2005 15982137

Larson J, Lochman JE: Helping Schoolchildren Cope With Anger. New York, Guilford, 2003

Larsson H, Andershed H, Lichtenstein P: A genetic factor explains most of the variation in the psychopathic personality. J Abnorm Psychol 115(2):221–230, 2006 16737387

Loeber R, Lahey BB, Thomas C: Diagnostic conundrum of oppositional defiant disorder and conduct disorder. J Abnorm Psychol 100(3):379–390, 1991 1918617

Loeber R, Burke JD, Lahey BB, et al: Oppositional defiant and conduct disorder: a review of the past 10 years, part I. J Am Acad Child Adolesc Psychiatry 39(12):1468–1484, 2000 11128323

Loeber R, Burke JD, Lahey BB: What are adolescent antecedents to antisocial personality disorder? Crim Behav Ment Health 12(1):24–36, 2002 12357255

Longman T, Hawes DJ, Kohlhoff J: Callous–unemotional traits as markers for conduct problem severity in early childhood: a meta-analysis. Child Psychiatry Hum Dev 47(2):326–334, 2016 26123709

López-Romero L, Romero E, Andershed H: Conduct problems in childhood and adolescence: developmental trajectories, predictors and outcomes in a six-year follow up. Child Psychiatry Hum Dev 46(5):762–773, 2015 25354563

Lundahl B, Risser HJ, Lovejoy MC: A meta-analysis of parent training: moderators and follow-up effects. Clin Psychol Rev 26(1):86–104, 2006 16280191

Lykken DT: The Antisocial Personalities. Hillsdale, NJ, Erlbaum, 1995

Lyman RD, Campbell NR: Treating Children and Adolescents in Residential and Inpatient Settings. Thousand Oaks, CA, Sage, 1996

Manders WA, Deković M, Asscher JJ, et al: Psychopathy as predictor and moderator of multisystemic therapy outcomes among adolescents treated for antisocial behavior. J Abnorm Child Psychol 41(7):1121–1132, 2013 23756854

Mann FD, Tackett JL, Tucker-Drob EM, et al: Callous-unemotional traits moderate genetic and environmental influences on rule-breaking and aggression: evidence for gene×trait interaction. Clin Psychol Sci 6(1):123–133, 2018 30701129

Marsh AA, Blair RJR: Deficits in facial affect recognition among antisocial populations: a meta-analysis. Neurosci Biobehav Rev 32(3):454–465, 2008 17915324

Masi G, Muratori P, Manfredi A, et al: Response to treatments in youth with disruptive behavior disorders. Compr Psychiatry 54(7):1009–1015, 2013 23683839

McCart MR, Priester PE, Davies WH, et al: Differential effectiveness of behavioral parent-training and cognitive-behavioral therapy for antisocial youth: a meta-analysis. J Abnorm Child Psychol 34(4):527–543, 2006 16838122

McMahon RJ, Witkiewitz K, Kotler JS, et al: Predictive validity of callous-unemotional traits measured in early adolescence with respect to multiple antisocial outcomes. J Abnorm Psychol 119(4):752–763, 2010 20939651

Moffitt TE: Life-course persistent and adolescence-limited antisocial behavior: a 10-year research review and research agenda, in Causes of Conduct Disorder and Juvenile Delinquency. Edited by Lahey BB, Moffitt TE, Caspi A. New York, Guilford, 2003, pp 49–75

Moffitt TE: Life-course-persistent versus adolescence-limited antisocial behavior, in Developmental Psychopathology, Volume 3: Risk, Disorder, and Adaptation, 2nd Edition. Edited by Cicchetti D, Cohen DJ. Hoboken, NJ, Wiley, 2006, pp 570–598

Moffitt TE: Male antisocial behaviour in adolescence and beyond. Nat Hum Behav 2(3):177–186, 2018 30271880

Moffitt TE, Caspi A, Harrington H, et al: Males on the life-course-persistent and adolescence-limited antisocial pathways: follow-up at age 26 years. Dev Psychopathol 14(1):179–207, 2002 11893092

Moore AA, Silberg JL, Roberson-Nay R, et al: Life course persistent and adolescence limited conduct disorder in a nationally representative US sample: prevalence, predictors, and outcomes. Soc Psychiatry Psychiatr Epidemiol 52(4):435–443, 2017 28180930

Moran P, Ford T, Butler G, et al: Callous and unemotional traits in children and adolescents living in Great Britain. Br J Psychiatry 192(1):65–66, 2008 18174513

Muratori P, Lochman JE, Manfredi A, et al: Callous unemotional traits in children with disruptive behavior disorder: predictors of developmental trajectories and adolescent outcomes. Psychiatry Res 236:35–41, 2016 26791396

Naik-Polan AT, Budd KS: Stimulus generalization of parenting skills during parent-child interaction therapy. Journal of Early and Intensive Behavior Intervention 5(3):71–92, 2008

Odgers CL, Moffitt TE, Broadbent JM, et al: Female and male antisocial trajectories: from childhood origins to adult outcomes. Dev Psychopathol 20(2):673–716, 2008 18423100

Olfson M, Crystal S, Huang C, et al: Trends in antipsychotic drug use by very young, privately insured children. J Am Acad Child Adolesc Psychiatry 49(1):13–23, 2010 20215922

Pardini DA, Lochman JE, Frick PJ: Callous/unemotional traits and social-cognitive processes in adjudicated youths. J Am Acad Child Adolesc Psychiatry 42(3):364–371, 2003 12595791

Pardini DA, Waller R, Hawes SW: Familial influences on the development of serious conduct problems and delinquency, in The Development of Criminal and Antisocial Behavior. Edited by Morizot J, Kazemian L. New York, Springer International, 2015, pp 201–220

Pardini DA, Byrd AL, Hawes SW, et al: Unique dispositional precursors to early onset conduct problems and criminal offending in adulthood. J Am Acad Child Adolesc Psychiatry 57(8):583.e3–592.e3, 2018 30071979

Pasalich DS, Dadds MR, Hawes DJ, et al: Do callous-unemotional traits moderate the relative importance of parental coercion versus warmth in child conduct problems? An observational study. J Child Psychol Psychiatry 52(12):1308–1315, 2011 21726225

Patterson GR: Coercive Family Process. Eugene, OR, Castalia Publishing, 1982

Pihet S, Etter S, Schmid M, et al: Assessing callous-unemotional traits in adolescents: validity of the Inventory of Callous-Unemotional Traits across gender, age, and community/institutionalized status. J Psychopathol Behav Assess 37(3):407–421, 2015

Piquero AR, Farrington DP, Welsh BC, et al: Effects of early family/parent training programs on antisocial behavior and delinquency. Campbell Syst Rev 4(1):1–122, 2008

Polaschek D, Skeem JL: Treatment of adults and juveniles with psychopathy, in Handbook of Psychopathy, 2nd Edition. Edited by Patrick C. New York, Guilford, 2018, pp 710–731

Pringsheim T, Hirsch L, Gardner D, et al: The pharmacological management of oppositional behaviour, conduct problems, and aggression in children and adolescents with attention-deficit hyperactivity disorder, oppositional defiant disorder, and conduct disorder: a systematic review and meta-analysis, part 1: psychostimulants, alpha-2 agonists, and atomoxetine. Can J Psychiatry 60(2):42–51, 2015a 25886655

Pringsheim T, Hirsch L, Gardner D, et al: The pharmacological management of oppositional behaviour, conduct problems, and aggression in children and adolescents with attention-deficit hyperactivity disorder, oppositional defiant disorder, and conduct disorder: a systematic review and meta-analysis, part 2: antipsychotics and traditional mood stabilizers. Can J Psychiatry 60(2):52–61, 2015b 25886656

Raine A, Moffitt TE, Caspi A, et al: Neurocognitive impairments in boys on the life-course persistent antisocial path. J Abnorm Psychol 114(1):38–49, 2005 15709810

Rivenbark JG, Odgers CL, Caspi A, et al: The high societal costs of childhood conduct problems: evidence from administrative records up to age 38 in a longitudinal birth cohort. J Child Psychol Psychiatry 59(6):703–710, 2018 29197100

Robins LN: Deviant Children Grown Up: A Sociological and Psychiatric Study of Sociopathic Personality. Baltimore, MD, Williams & Wilkins, 1966

Roose A, Bijttebier P, Decoene S, et al: Assessing the affective features of psychopathy in adolescence: a further validation of the inventory of callous and unemotional traits. Assessment 17(1):44–57, 2010 19797326

Sanchez AL, Cornacchio D, Poznanski B, et al: The effectiveness of school-based mental health services for elementary-aged children: a meta-analysis. J Am Acad Child Adolesc Psychiatry 57(3):153–165, 2018 29496124

Sanders MR: Triple P-Positive Parenting Program: towards an empirically validated multilevel parenting and family support strategy for the prevention of behavior and emotional problems in children. Clin Child Fam Psychol Rev 2(2):71–90, 1999 11225933

Sanders MR, Baker S, Turner KM: A randomized controlled trial evaluating the efficacy of Triple P Online with parents of children with early onset conduct problems. Behav Res Ther 50(11):675–684, 2012 22982082

Shaffer D, Fisher P, Lucas CP, et al: NIMH Diagnostic Interview Schedule for Children Version IV (NIMH DISC-IV): description, differences from previous versions, and reliability of some common diagnoses. J Am Acad Child Adolesc Psychiatry 39(1):28–38, 2000 10638065

Shaw DS, Gilliom M, Ingoldsby EM, et al: Trajectories leading to school-age conduct problems. Dev Psychol 39(2):189–200, 2003 12661881

Sheldrick RC, Kendall PC, Heimberg RG: The clinical significance of treatments: a comparison of three treatments for conduct disordered children. Clinical Psychology: Science and Practice 8(4):418–430, 2001

Skinner BF: Science and Human Behavior. New York, Free Press, 1953

Somech LY, Elizur Y: Adherence to honor code mediates the prediction of adolescent boys' conduct problems by callousness and socioeconomic status. J Clin Child Adolesc Psychol 38(5):606–618, 2009 20183646

van Aar J, Leijten P, Orobio de Castro B, et al: Sustained, fade-out or sleeper effects? A systematic review and meta-analysis of parenting interventions for disruptive child behavior. Clin Psychol Rev 51:153–163, 2017 27930935

Viding E, McCrory EJ: Understanding the development of psychopathy: progress and challenges. Psychol Med 48(4):566–577, 2018 29032773

Viding E, Blair RJR, Moffitt TE, et al: Evidence for substantial genetic risk for psychopathy in 7-year-olds. J Child Psychol Psychiatry 46(6):592–597, 2005 15877765

Viding E, Jones AP, Frick PJ, et al: Heritability of antisocial behaviour at 9: do callous-unemotional traits matter? Dev Sci 11(1):17–22, 2008 18171362

Viding E, Simmonds E, Petrides KV, et al: The contribution of callous-unemotional traits and conduct problems to bullying in early adolescence. J Child Psychol Psychiatry 50(4):471–481, 2009 19207635

Viding E, Sebastian CL, Dadds MR, et al: Amygdala response to preattentive masked fear in children with conduct problems: the role of callous-unemotional traits. Am J Psychiatry 169(10):1109–1116, 2012 23032389

Waller R, Gardner F, Hyde LW: What are the associations between parenting, callous-unemotional traits, and antisocial behavior in youth? A systematic review of evidence. Clin Psychol Rev 33(4):593–608, 2013 23583974

Waller R, Gardner F, Shaw DS, et al: Callous-unemotional behavior and early childhood onset of behavior problems: the role of parental harshness and warmth. J Clin Child Adolesc Psychol 44(4):655–667, 2015 24661288

Webster-Stratton C: The incredible years: a training series for the prevention and treatment of conduct problems in young children, in Psychosocial Treatments for Child and Adolescent Disorders: Empirically Based Strategies for Clinical Practice. Edited by Hibbs ED, Jensen PS. Washington, DC, American Psychological Association, 2005, pp 507–555

Wertz J, Agnew-Blais J, Caspi A, et al: From childhood conduct problems to poor functioning at age 18 years: examining explanations in a longitudinal cohort study. J Am Acad Child Adolesc Psychiatry 57(1):54.e4–60.e4, 2018 29301670

Wootton JM, Frick PJ, Shelton KK, et al: Ineffective parenting and childhood conduct problems: the moderating role of callous-unemotional traits. J Consult Clin Psychol 65(2):301–308, 1997 9086694

Zito JM, Safer DJ, Valluri S, et al: Psychotherapeutic medication prevalence in Medicaid-insured preschoolers. J Child Adolesc Psychopharmacol 17(2):195–203, 2007 17489714

Index

*Page numbers printed in **boldface** type refer to tables or figures.*

Marriage. *See also* Assortative mating;
Divorce
clinical symptoms of ASPD and, 88
as predictor of ASPD outcome, 106–107
as protective factor in ASPD, 129–130
*The Mask of Sanity: An Attempt to Clarify Some
Issues About the So-Called Psychopathic
Personality* (Cleckley 1976), xvi, 4, 22, 401
Maudsley, Henry, **17,** 18
Mauritius, study of childbirth complications
as risk factor for antisocial behavior in
children, 165
McCord, William and Joan, 22, 401
Measurement
of ASPD, 116
neurophysiology and, 186–187, **188**
Media, and exposure to violence, 156, 302
Medical conditions. *See* Accidental injuries;
Sexually transmitted diseases;
Traumatic brain injury
comorbidity of with ASPD, 72–74
differential diagnosis of ASPD and, 94
Medical history, and assessment, 90
MEDLINE electronic database, 362
Mental Health Act (United Kingdom 1959),
21
Mental status examination, 92–93, 430
Mentalization-based treatment (MBT), **356**
Meta-analyses, and neurophysiology, 189
Meta-chlorophenylpiperazine (*m*-CPP), 296
Methylphenidate, 435
Meyer, Adolf, 4
Michigan Alcoholism Screening Test, 92
Military, disciplinary problems of individu-
als with ASPD in, 88. *See also* War
veterans
Millon Clinical Multiaxial Inventory, 62
Minnesota Multiphasic Personality Inven-
tory (MMPI), 91
Minnesota Twin Family Study (MTFS), 124,
126, 130
Mismatch negativity (MMN), and electro-
encephalographic studies of ASPD,
197–199, **205**
Mixed personality disorder, in ICD-10, 10
Modified Overt Aggression Scale (OAS-M),
377
Modified therapeutic community (MTC),
359
Molecular genetics, of ASPD.
See also Genetics
antisocial traits in women and, 447–448
brain imaging studies and, 144–145
dopaminergic genes and, 138–140
epigenetics and, 145–146, 153

genome-wide association studies and,
144
serotonergic genes and, 141–143
Monoamine oxidase A gene (*MAOA*),
142–143, 145, 146, 163, 259, 301, 303,
447–448
Monoamine system, and biomarkers for
ASPD, 225–227
Mood stabilizers, **378–379,** 382–386
Moral insanity, xv–xvi, 16, 17–19
Morbid liar and swindler, Kraepelin's use of
term, 19
Morel, Bénédict Augustin, **17,** 18, **21**
Motivation, and neurophysiology of ASPD,
201–203, **206,** 207
Motivational interviewing, **357, 361**
Motor vehicle accidents, ASPD as predictor
of, 72, 90
MRI, and neural abnormalities in psychopa-
thy, 318–319. *See also* Functional MRI
studies; Neuroimaging; Structural MRI
studies
Multiaxial system, and DSM-III, 6
Multiple threshold model, and behavioral
genetic studies, 447
Multisystemic therapy (MST), 434, 446

N100 (N1) and P200 (P2) intensity/sensitiv-
ity function, and electroencephalographic studies of ASPD, 193, **194, 204**
N200 (N2), and electroencephalographic
studies of ASPD, 199–200, **205**
Nadolol, **380**
Naltrexone, 61
Narcissistic personality disorder (NPD),
59–60, 68, 70
NASA Twins Study, 128
National Alliance on Mental Illness (NAMI),
433
National Comorbidity Survey (NCS), 30, 40,
424, 452
National Epidemiologic Survey on Alcohol
and Related Conditions (NESARC), 29,
30, 36, 37, 39, 40, 84, 86, 99, 104, 106, 107,
446
National Epidemiologic Survey on Alcohol
and Related Conditions-III (NESARC-
III), 29, 30, 32, 34, 36, 39, 40, 44, 99, 105,
412
National Institute on Alcohol Abuse and
Alcoholism (NIAAA), 29, 30
National Institute on Drug Abuse, 29, 30, 99
National Institute for Health and Care Excel-
lence (NICE) website, 367
National Institute of Mental Health, xiii, 304

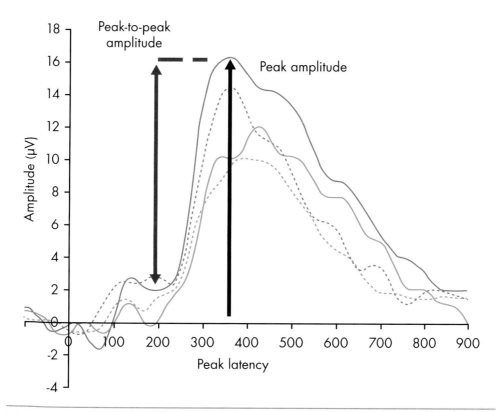

PLATE 1. *Figure 11–1* Example of a P300 (P3) event-related potential (ERP).

An ERP is a small part of electroencephalography (EEG) that is time-locked to an event (e.g., a stimulus or a response). The ERP reflects multiple stages of information processing before and after an event. The time before the event serves as baseline. The most frequently used measures of the ERP are the amplitude of an ERP component (wave) that is measured from either baseline or a prior peak and the time (latency) of the peak. The amplitude is measured in microvolt (μV), and the latency is measured in milliseconds (ms). This shows that neuronal activity measured by EEG sensors placed on the scalp is very small and that the dynamics of neuronal processes related to information processing are very fast.

Source. Adapted from Lijffijt M, Swann AC, Moeller FG: "Biological Substrate of Personality Traits Associated With Aggression," in *The SAGE Handbook of Personality Theory and Assessment: Volume 1—Personality Theories and Models.* Edited by Boyle GJ, Matthews G, Saklofske DH. Thousand Oaks, CA, Sage, 2008, pp. 334–356. Used with permission.

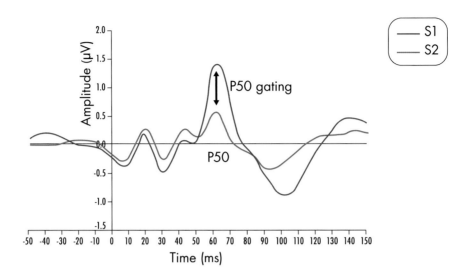

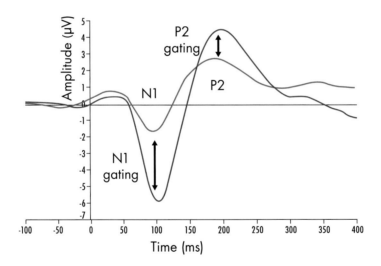

PLATE 2. *Figure 11–2* Sensory gating of the auditory P50 (*top graph*) and the N100 (N1) and P200 (P2) (*bottom graph*).

P50 rides on top of the beginning of N1 and is therefore more difficult to analyze. To better visualize and analyze the P50, researchers often filter the data between 10 and 50 Hz (band-pass filter with zero-phase shift). This significantly diminishes the influence of the N1 and P2 on the P50. To visualize and analyze the N1 and P2, the signal can be analyzed by applying a band-pass filter set between 1 and 30 Hz. The figure shows the P50-N1-P2 auditory evoked potential to S1 of the paired-click paradigm. A small P50-N1-P2 auditory event-related potential is evoked by S2. The difference between the amplitudes of S1 and S2 is interpreted as sensory gating.

Source. Adapted from Lijffijt M, Lane SD, Meier SL, et al.: "P50, N100, and P200 Sensory Gating: Relationships With Behavioral Inhibition, Attention, and Working Memory." *Psychophysiology* 46(5):1059–1068, 2009. Copyright © 2009 John Wiley and Sons. Used with permission.

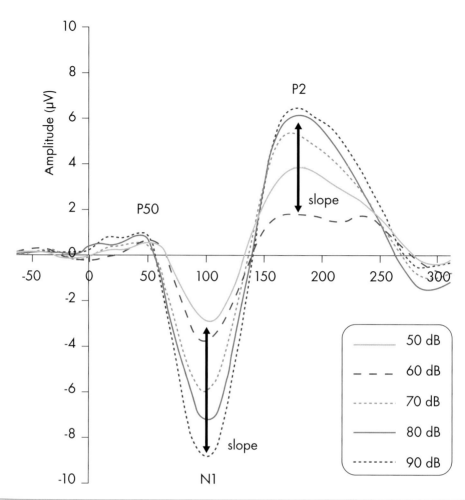

PLATE 3. *Figure 11–3* N100 (N1) and P200 (P2) intensity sensitivity function is expressed as the linear slope for N1 or P2 peak amplitude as a function of stimulus loudness or stimulus brightness.

In this example, N1 and P2 were evoked by auditory stimuli. The N1 and the P2 amplitude can be taken from baseline or from the P50 and N1, respectively.

Source. Adapted from Lijffijt M, Lane SD, Moeller FG, et al: "Trait Impulsivity and Increased Pre-Attentional Sensitivity to Intense Stimuli in Bipolar Disorder and Controls." *Journal of Psychiatric Research* 60:73–80, 2015. Copyright © 2015 Elsevier. Used with permission.

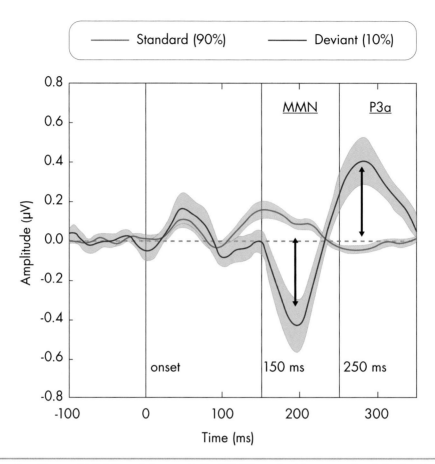

PLATE 4. *Figure 11–5* Mismatch negativity (MMN) evoked in a passive listening task by deviant stimuli presented randomly among standard stimuli.

The deviant stimulus can differ from the standard stimulus in pitch, duration, or any other property. The deviant stimulus elicits a negativity between 100 and 250 ms poststimulus compared with a standard stimulus. Following the MMN is a P3a, which is also enhanced for deviant compared with standard stimuli. The MMN and P3a are studied often as a difference wave by subtracting the event-related potential (ERP) of the standard from the ERP of the deviant stimulus.

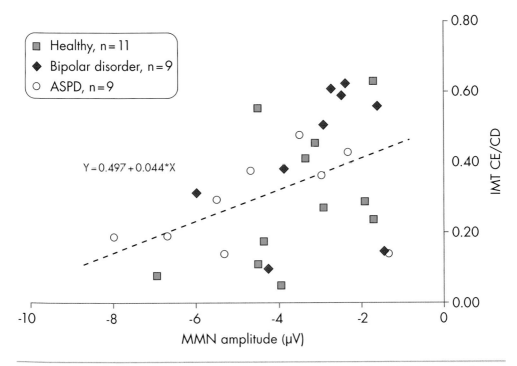

PLATE 5. *Figure 11–6* **Association between mismatch negativity (MMN) amplitude and impulsive action.**

Significant correlation between MMN amplitude and impulsive action measured as Immediate Memory Task (IMT) commission errors corrected for correct detections (CE/CD ratio) ($r=0.52$; $P=0.005$) across 11 healthy volunteers and 18 patients with impulsivity-related disorders (9 with bipolar disorder; 9 with antisocial personality disorder [ASPD]).

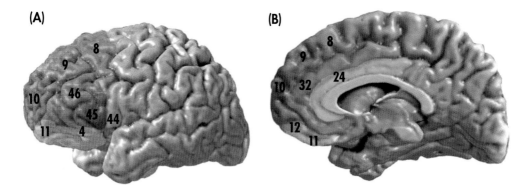

PLATE 6. *Figure 13–1* Lateral (A) and medial (B) illustration of the Brodmann areas (BA) in the orbitofrontal, dorsolateral prefrontal, ventrolateral prefrontal, medial prefrontal, and anterior cingulate cortices.

The orbitofrontal cortex included BA 11, 12, and 47. The dorsolateral prefrontal cortex included BA 8, 9, 10, and 46. The ventrolateral prefrontal cortex included BA 44 and 45. The medial prefrontal cortex included BA 8, 9, 10, 11, and 12. The anterior cingulate cortex included BA 24 and 32.

Source. Reprinted from Yang Y, Raine A: "Prefrontal Structural and Functional Brain Imaging Findings in Antisocial, Violent, and Psychopathic Individuals: A Meta-Analysis." *Psychiatry Research* 174(2):81–88, 2009. Copyright © 2009 Elsevier. Used with permission.

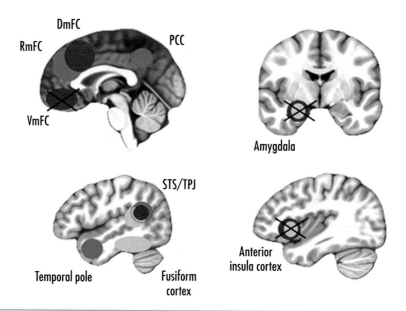

PLATE 7. *Figure 14–1* Core regions implicated in representing the beliefs and knowledge of others (*blue*), the emotional states of others (*red*), and the emotional expressions of others (*orange*).

Size of colored region is not indicative of strength of association. Crosses indicate regions that show significant deficient recruitment in patients with antisocial personality disorder/psychopathy/conduct disorder during relevant tasks.

DmFC=dorsomedial frontal cortex; PCC=posterior cingulate cortex; RmFC=rostromedial frontal cortex; STS/TPJ=superior temporal sulcus/temporal-parietal junction; VmFC=ventromedial frontal cortex.

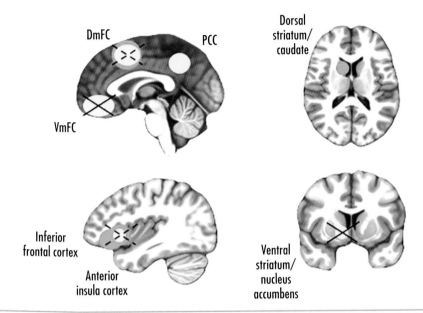

PLATE 8. *Figure 14–2* Core regions implicated in response control (*green*) and reinforcement-based decision-making (*yellow*).

Crosses indicate regions that show significant deficient recruitment in patients with antisocial personality disorder/psychopathy/conduct disorder during relevant tasks (hashed crosses indicate less consistent data).

DmFC=dorsomedial frontal cortex; PCC=posterior cingulate cortex; VmFC=ventromedial frontal cortex.